Hypoxia and the Circulation

Hypoxia and the Circulation

Editor: Stephan Blackwood

AMERICAN MEDICAL PUBLISHERS
www.americanmedicalpublishers.com

AMERICAN
MEDICAL PUBLISHERS
www.americanmedicalpublishers.com

Cataloging-in-Publication Data

Hypoxia and the circulation / edited by Stephan Blackwood.
p. cm.
Includes bibliographical references and index.
ISBN 979-8-88740-198-0
1. Anoxemia. 2. Blood--Circulation. 3. Exercise--Physiological aspects.
I. Blackwood, Stephan.
RC103.A4 H97 2023
616.989 3--dc23

American Medical Publishers,
41 Flatbush Avenue,
1st Floor, New York,
NY 11217, USA

ISBN 979-8-88740-198-0 (Hardback)

Contents

Preface

Hypoxia refers to a condition in which the body or some part of the body does not receive enough oxygen supply at the tissue level. It can be categorized as either generalized, where entire body is affected, or localized, where a part of the body is affected. It is a pathological condition including changes in the arterial oxygen concentrations. These types of changes can also occur during normal physiology, such as while doing vigorous physical activity and hypoventilation training. Hypoxia can be caused due to the failure in the delivery of oxygen to the cells. This condition results in increased heart rate and aortic blood flow, and it decreases the peripheral resistance. Oxygen supply and blood flow is increased towards the vital organs, which is an indicator that redistribution of blood flow is essential for the oxygen supply. This book unravels the recent studies on hypoxia and circulation. It consists of contributions made by international experts. This book will serve as a valuable source of reference for graduate and post graduate students.

Various studies have approached the subject by analyzing it with a single perspective, but the present book provides diverse methodologies and techniques to address this field. This book contains theories and applications needed for understanding the subject from different perspectives. The aim is to keep the readers informed about the progresses in the field; therefore, the contributions were carefully examined to compile novel researches by specialists from across the globe.

Indeed, the job of the editor is the most crucial and challenging in compiling all chapters into a single book. In the end, I would extend my sincere thanks to the chapter authors for their profound work. I am also thankful for the support provided by my family and colleagues during the compilation of this book.

Editor

1

MiR-29a Suppresses Spermatogenic Cell Apoptosis in Testicular Ischemia-Reperfusion Injury by Targeting TRPV4 Channels

Jin-zhuo Ning[1†], Wei Li[2†], Fan Cheng[1], Wei-min Yu[1], Ting Rao[1], Yuan Ruan[1], Run Yuan[1], Xiao-bin Zhang[1], Dong Zhuo[3], Yang Du[1] and Cheng-cheng Xiao[1]*

[1] Department of Urology, Renmin Hospital of Wuhan University, Wuhan, China, [2] Department of Anesthesiology, Renmin Hospital of Wuhan University, Wuhan, China, [3] Department of Urology, Wannan Medical College, Wuhu, China

***Correspondence:**
Fan Cheng
chenfan_93@126.com

† These authors have contributed equally to this work.

Background: MicroRNAs (miRNAs) have emerged as gene expression regulators in the progression of ischemia-reperfusion injury (IRI). Accumulating evidences have indicated miR-29a play roles in myocardial and cerebral IRI. However, the role of miR-29a in testicular IRI has not been elucidated.

Methods: Changes in expression of miR-29a and Transient Receptor Potential Vanilloid 4 (TRPV4) in animal samples and GC-1 spermatogenic cells were examined. The effects of miR-29a on spermatogenic cell apoptosis in testicular IRI were analyzed both *in vitro* and *in vivo*.

Results: The expression of MiR-29a was negatively correlated with the expression of TRPV4 and significantly downregulated in animal samples and GC-1 cells as testicular IRI progressed. Further studies revealed TRPV4 as a downstream target of miR-29a. Inhibition of miR-29a expression increased the expression of TRPV4 and promoted spermatogenic cell apoptosis, whereas overexpression of miR-29a downregulated TRPV4 expression and suppressed spermatogenic cell apoptosis caused by testicular IRI *in vitro* and *in vivo*.

Conclusion: Our results suggest that miR-29a suppresses apoptosis induced by testicular IRI by directly targeting TRPV4.

Keywords: miR-29a, TRPV4, testicular, IRI, apoptosis

INTRODUCTION

Testicular torsion is the most common cause of urological emergency in young and adolescent males (Tuglu et al., 2016). Once diagnosed, clinical treatment should be adopted to restore blood flow to the testis within an appropriate time frame (Kim et al., 2016). Testicular torsion/detorsion (T/D) is considered to be the primary pathophysiologic event that induces ischemia-reperfusion injury (IRI), which causes an enhancement of apoptosis and testicular spermatogenesis dysfunction (Meštrović et al., 2014). Therefore, elucidating the mechanism underlying cell apoptosis is critical to helping better understand the progression of testicular IRI and to identification of effective therapeutic targets.

Transient Receptor Potential Vanilloid 4 (TRPV4) is a primary member of the transient receptor potential (TRP) channels family (Fusi et al., 2014). TRPV4 is a non-selective cation channel activated by a wide range of stimuli, including heat, cell swelling, temperature changes, pH, anandamide, arachidonic acid metabolites, and other factors (Vergnolle, 2014). TRPV4 plays a key role in regulating various cellular activities and has been found to be expressed in the kidneys, brain, lungs, skin, heart, liver, and testes (Xu et al., 2009; Wei et al., 2015; Tsuno et al., 2016). Notably, it has been reported that excessive activation of this channel is related to renal, lung, and cerebral IRI (Townsley et al., 2010; Kassmann et al., 2013; Ding et al., 2015), suggesting that TRPV4 may be an important target for mediating reperfusion injury following ischemia in many organs.

MicroRNAs (miRNAs) are endogenous, single-stranded non-coding RNAs with a length of 18–25 nucleotides (Zhang et al., 2012). They are capable of downregulating gene expression by targeting specific mRNAs located mostly in 3′-untranslated-regions (Berezikov et al., 2005), thereby participating in a wide range of biological processes, including cell proliferation, development, differentiation and apoptosis (Zhang et al., 2010; Bao et al., 2012). Previous studies have reported that miRNAs are tightly associated with apoptosis during the progression of IRI. For example, miR-499 alleviates apoptosis by downregulating PDCD4 in myocardial IRI (Zhu et al., 2016), miR-200c regulates apoptosis of hepatic IRI by targeting ZEB1 (Wu et al., 2016), and miR-30 decreases apoptosis in renal IRI by repressing DRP1 (Gu et al., 2016). Although recent studies have shown that miR-29a plays a role in apoptosis during myocardial and cerebral IRI (Ye et al., 2010; Ouyang et al., 2013; Wang et al., 2015), the biological effect of miR-29a in testicular IRI and the interrelation between miR-29a and TRPV4 have not been described.

In the present study, we found that the expression of miR-29a was obviously reduced while TRPV4 expression was significantly enhanced in testicular IRI. Moreover, we identified miR-29a regulates TRPV4 expression by directly binding to it and demonstrated that miR-29a plays a key role in regulating IR-induced apoptosis by targeting TRPV4 in the testes. These results suggest that miR-29a may be used as a potential therapeutic option to inhibit apoptosis during the progression of testicular IRI.

MATERIALS AND METHODS

Animals and Surgical Protocols

All experimental procedures were adhered to the National Institutes of Health Guide for the Care and Use of Laboratory Animals and were approved by the Animal Care and Use Committee of Wuhan University. Male C57BL/6 mice (20–25 g) were obtained from the Hubei Center for Disease Control. Prior to experiments, all rats were caged in a standard temperature-controlled room (22 ± 2°C) and were subjected to alternating 12-h light/dark cycles. They also had free access to food and water. The rats were anesthetized by the intraperitoneal administration of 2% sodium phenobarbital (50 mg kg-1) and were then placed on a homeothermic table to maintain a rectal temperature of 37–38°C. The left testis was twisted 720° clockwise and fixed to the scrotal skin with 5/0 silk. After 1 h of torsion, the testis was allowed to recover to the natural position for 0, 4, 8, 16, or 24 h. In the sham group, the testis was localized via a left-sided scrotal incision. The incision was then sutured with 5/0 silk without additional intervention. Additionally, 1–2 µg of mouse miR-29a agomir and its negative control (RiboBio, Guangzhou, China) was injected into seminiferous tubules using an injection pipette (Liang et al., 2012).

Oxygen Glucose Deprivation/Reperfusion (OGD/R) in GC-1 Cells

Mouse GC-1 spermatogenic cells were purchased from ATCC (American Type Culture Collection, Manassas, VA, USA) and maintained in Dulbecco's modified Eagle's medium(DMEM; GIBCO, MA, USA) supplemented with 10% fetal bovine serum (FBS) at 37°C under normoxic conditions (5% CO_2, 95% O_2). Cells were transfected with pri-miR-29a, anti-miR-29a, siTRPV4, TRPV4-overexpression(GC-1/TRPV4) and their respective negative controls using Lipofectamine 2000 (Invitrogen, Carlsbad, CA, USA) according to the manufacturer's protocol. Then, 48 h after transfection, cells were maintained under hypoxic conditions with glucose-free DMEM for 3 h. After OGD treatment, GC-1 cells were placed in glucose-containing DMEM under normoxic conditions.

Plasmid Construction and Luciferase Reporter Assays

The putative and mutated miR-29a target binding sequence in TRPV4 were synthesized and cloned into luciferase reporter to generate the wild-type (TRPV4-Wt) or mutated-type (TRPV4-Mut) reporter plasmids. The mutant 3′UTR sequence of TRPV4 was generated using overlap extension PCR, and then both the wild-type and mutant sequences were cloned into a psiCHECK-2 vector (Promega, Madison, WI, USA).

For the luciferase reporter assay, GC-1 cells were seeded on a 24-well plate. The cells were then co-transfected with miR-29a mimics or miR-29a negative control using Lipofectamine 2000 (Invitrogen, USA). Luciferase assay was performed 48 h after transfection using a Dual-Luciferase Reporter Assay System (Promega, Madison, WI, USA).

Western Blot Analysis

Proteins from testicular tissues or cultured GC-1 cells were extracted using RIPA Lysis Buffer (P0013B, Beyotime Institute of Biotechnology), and protein concentration was qualified using a bicinchoninic acid assay kit (BCA; Beyotime, Shanghai, China). Briefly, Equivalent amounts of protein samples were separated by 10% sodium dodecyl sulfate-polyacrylamide (SDS-PAGE) gels electrophoresis, and transferred to (polyvinylidene fluoride) PVDF membranes subsequently. After that, the membrane was blocked with 5% non-fat milk in Tris-buffered saline and 0.1% Tween 20 (TBST) buffer and incubated with the following primary antibodies against TRPV4(ab94868; Abcam, Cambridge, UK), caspase-3 (sc7148; Santa Cruz, CA), Bax (sc493; Santa Cruz, CA) and Bcl-2 (sc7382; Santa Cruz, CA) at 4°C overnight. GAPDH was used as an internal control. After being rinsed three times with TBST buffer, the membranes were incubated with secondary antibodies at room temperature for 1 h. Target proteins were visualized using an ECL system kit (Pierce Biotechnology, Beijing, China). Optical densities were detected by enhanced chemiluminescent (ECL) and qualified using ImageJ software (NIH, Bethesda, MD, USA).

Quantitative Real-Time PCR

Total RNA was isolated from GC-1 cells and testis samples using TRIzol reagent (Invitrogen Life Technologies, Carlsbad, CA, USA), and the concentration of RNA was determined by a DU800 UV/Vis Spectrophotometer (Beckman Coulter, CA, USA). Total cellular RNAs were reversed transcribed into cDNA using reverse transcription reagent kit (Takara Biotechnology, Dalian China). Real-time quantitative PCR was performed via a Applied Biosystems SYBR Green mix kit and the ABI 7900 Real-Time PCR system (Applied Biosystems Life Technologies, Foster City, CA, USA). Relative miR-29a or TRPV4 mRNA expression were normalized to snRNA U6 (for miRNAs) or GAPDH (for mRNAs), respectively. The quantitative analysis was calculated by using $2^{-\Delta\Delta Ct}$ method (Rao et al., 2013). The primer sequences used are shown in **Table 1**.

Immunohistochemistry

The expression of TRPV4, Bax and Bcl-2 was detected by immunohistochemical staining. Tissues were fixed in 4% paraformaldehyde, embedded in paraffin and then cut in 4 μm thickness. Immunohistochemical staining was performed using rabbit polyclonal anti-TRPV4 (ab94868; Abcam, Cambridge, UK), rabbit polyclonal anti-Bax (sc493; Santa Cruz, CA) and mouse monoclonal anti-Bcl-2 (sc7382; Santa Cruz, CA). After being washed three times with PBS, all sections were incubated in diaminobenzidine (DAB) reagents and counterstained with haematoxylin.

TUNEL Assays

A TUNEL assay was performed to evaluate spermatogenic cell apoptosis in testicular tissues using a transferase-mediated dUTP nick-end labeling (TUNEL) method with a detection kit (Roche, Mannheim, Germany) following the manufacturer's protocol. The nuclei that stained brown were considered TUNEL-positive cells. Five visual fields were randomly selected in each slice, and the average number of apoptosis cells per 200 cells was counted. The apoptosis index (AI) was determined as follows: AI = (the number of positive cells/the total number of counted cells) × 100%.

TABLE 1 | RT-PCR primer sequences.

Gene	Primer sequences (5′-3′)
TRPV4	F: CGCTCCTTCCCCGTATTCCT R: TTGATGATGCCCAAGTTCTGGTT
miR-29a	F: UAGCACCAUCUGAAAUCGGUUA R: ACCGUGCUCGACUUUCCGG
U6 snRNA	F: CTCGCTTCGGCAGCACATATACT R: ACGCTTCACGAATTTGCGTGTC
GAPDH	F: ACAGCAACAGGGTGGTGGAC R: TTTGAGGGTGCAGCGAACTT

Cell Apoptosis Analysis

Cell apoptosis was performed using Annexin V-FITC/Propidium Iodide (PI) staining (BD PharMingen, San Jose, CA, USA). GC-1 cells were seeded in 6-well plates at a concentration of 10^6 cells mL-1. The cells were labeled with Annexin V-FITC for 5 min in the dark. Then, 5 mg ml-1 PI was added to each sample for 30 min so that flow cytometry could be performed (BD PharMingen, San Jose, CA, USA).

Statistical Analysis

All data are presented as the mean ± SD. Differences were assessed by one-way analysis of variance (ANOVA), followed by all pairwise multiple-comparison procedures using the Bonferroni test. A value of $P < 0.05$ was considered statistically significant. All experiments were performed at least 3 times. Statistical analysis was performed using SPSS 19.0 (SPSS Inc, Chicago, IL, USA).

RESULTS

Enhanced Expression of TRPV4 in Testicular IRI Correlates with Downregulation of miR-29a Expression

To investigate if TRPV4 and miR-29a are involved in testicular IRI, we examined their expression levels in animal samples by immunohistochemistry staining, qRT-PCR and western blot. The samples were collected and assayed for expresssion at 0, 4, 8, 16, or 24 h of reperfusion after 1 h ischemia (Aslan Koşar et al., 2015). The results showed that TRPV4 expression increased gradually and peaked at 16 h of reperfusion compared with the sham group (**Figures 1A–D**, $n = 5$ per group). On the other hand, miR-29a expression decreased significantly during the progression of IRI (**Figure 1E**, $n = 5$ per group). A two-tailed Pearson's correlation analysis was performed to further investigate the interrelation between miR-29a and TRPV4 expression (**Figure 1F**). Therefore, the expression of miR-29a is negatively correlated with the expression of TRPV4 *in vivo*.

miR-29a Is Negatively Correlated with the Expression of TRPV4 *in Vitro*

To further explore the possibility that miR-29a might negatively correlates with the expression of TRPV4 *in vitro*, we examined the expression of TRPV4 and miR-29a in GC-1 cells under different reoxygenation conditions (0, 6, 12, 24, and 48 h) after 3 h OGD exposure. Consistent with the *in vivo* studies, the qRT-PCR and western blot results showed that miR-29a expression was inversely correlated with the expression of TRPV4 at different reoxygenation time intervals (**Figures 2A–D**, $n = 6$ per group). We next transfected the GC-1 cells with pri-miR-29a and examined TRPV4 expression by western blot and qRT-PCR at 3 h of OGD followed by 24 h of reoxygenation. We found that overexpression of miR-29a led to a significant downregulation of TRPV4 expression. Further, GC-1 cells transfected with a miR-29a inhibitor, displayed a moderate upregulation of TRPV4 expression (**Figures 2E–G**, $n = 6$ per group).

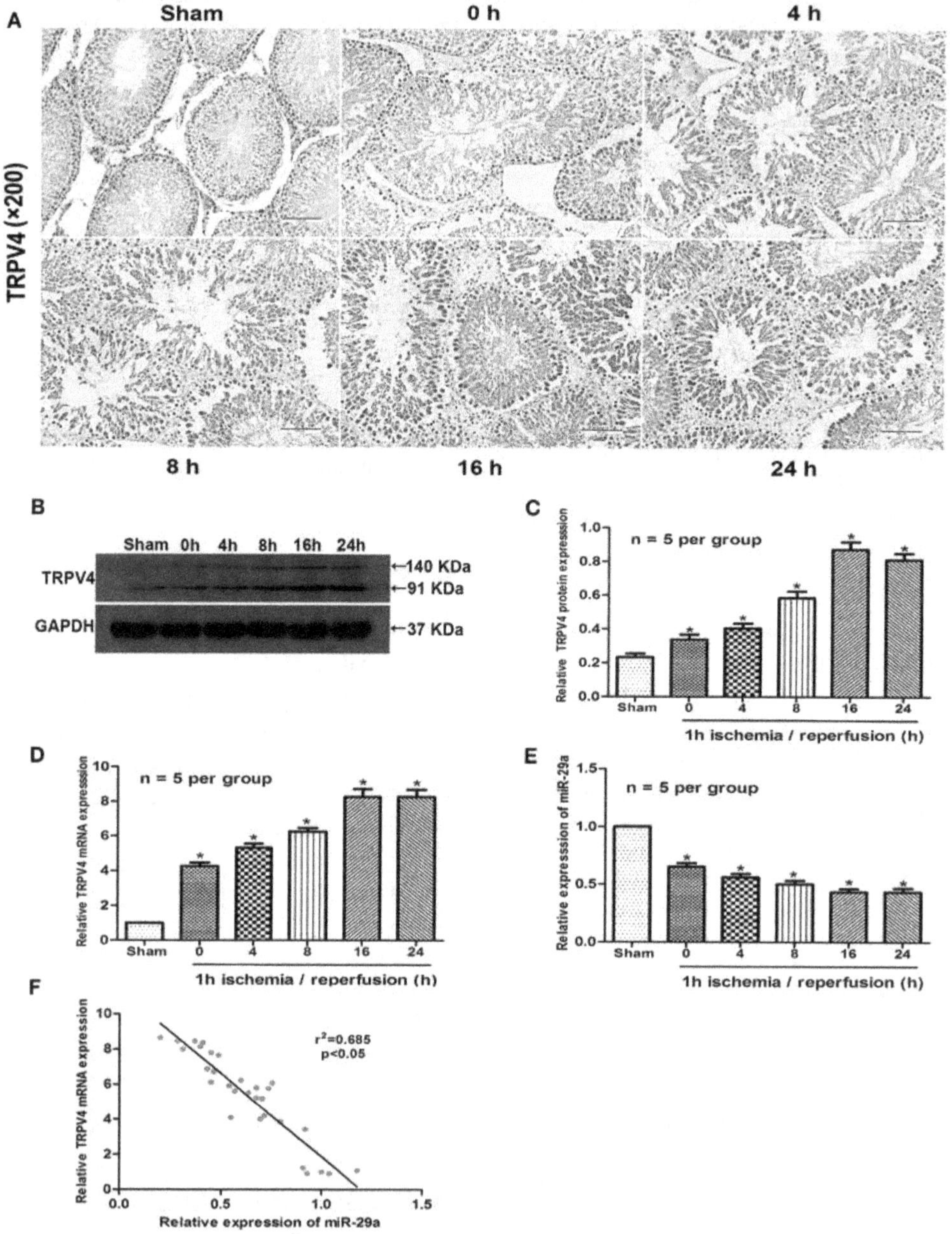

FIGURE 1 | High expression of TRPV4 in testicular IRI correlates with downregulation of miR-29a. **(A)** Immunohistochemistry staining of TRPV4 in the testis exposed to 1 h ischemia followed by reperfusion of different durations. $n = 5$ per group; **(B–E)** QRT-PCR and western blot analysis of miR-29a and TRPV4 expression at different reperfusion times after 1 h ischemia in animal samples. $^{*}p < 0.05$ vs. sham, $n = 5$ per group; **(F)** A two-tailed Pearson's correlation analysis reveals that the mRNA expression of miR-29a is inversely correlated with the expression of TRPV4 ($p < 0.05$).

Influence of miR-29a and TRPV4 on GC-1 Cell Apoptosis *in Vitro*

To investigate the effect of miR-29a on OGD/R cell injury, we used pri-miR-29a and anti-miR-29a to change miR-29a levels in GC-1 cells. Indeed, pri-miR-29a and anti-miR-29a markedly increased and decreased miR-29a levels at 3 h of OGD/24 h of reoxygenation, respectively when compared with their negative controls (**Figure 3A**, $n = 6$ per group). Flow cytometry data also showed that GC-1 cell apoptosis was induced by 3 h of OGD/24 h of reoxygenation. Transfection of pri-miR-29a inhibited cell apoptosis, while transfection of anti-miR-29a promoted GC-1 cell apoptosis induced by 3 h of OGD/24 h of reoxygenation (**Figures 3B,C**, $n = 6$ per group). In addition, western blot analysis showed that overexpression of miR-29a and knockdown of TRPV4 decreased the expression of Bax and caspase-3 and increased the expression of Bcl-2, respectively. Consistent with this result, inhibition of miR-29a and overexpression of TRPV4 in GC-1 cells resulted in an increase in Bax and

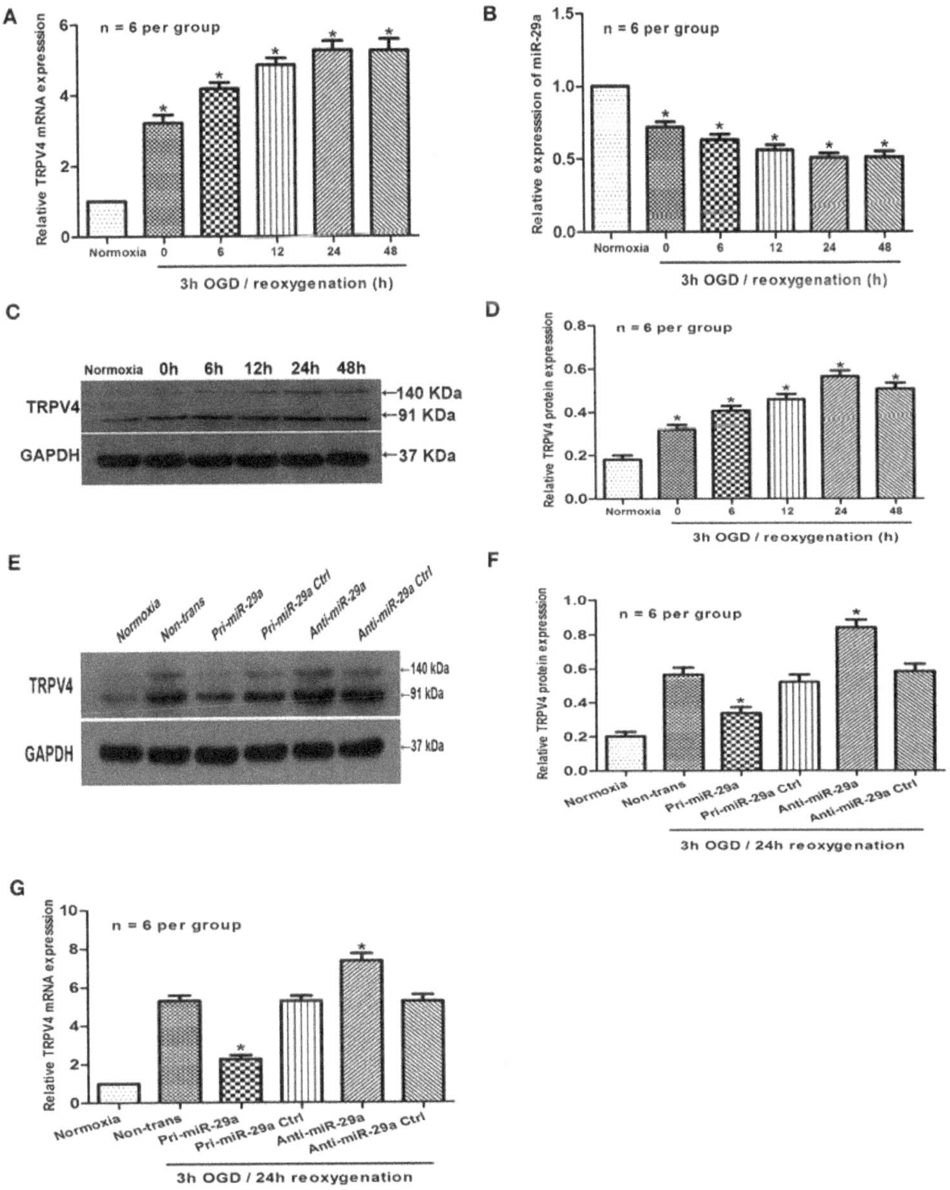

FIGURE 2 | MiR-29a is negatively correlated with the expression of TRPV4 in GC-1 cells. **(A–D)** QRT-PCR and western blot analysis of miR-29a and TRPV4 expression under different reoxygenation conditions after 3 h OGD exposure. $^*p < 0.05$ vs. normoxia, n =6 per group; **(E–G)** GC-1 cells were transfected with pri-miR-29a or anti-miR-29a. Western blot and qRT-PCR analysis were performed to examine TRPV4 mRNA expression in normoxia and 3 h OGD/24 h reoxygenation treatments. $^*p < 0.05$ vs. non-trans (3 h OGD/24 h reoxygenation treatment), $n = 6$ per group.

caspase-3 levels and a decrease in Bcl-2 expression, respectively (**Figures 3D–K**, $n = 6$ per group). These results suggest that miR-29a suppresses cell apoptosis and TRPV4 promotes cell apoptosis *in vitro*.

miR-29a Directly Targets TRPV4 and Alleviates Apoptosis *in Vitro*

To further explore the relationship between miR-29a and TRPV4, an *in silico* prediction was performed using open access software (TargetScan, PicTarget, and miRanda). A putative binding site for miR-29a was identified within the 3′UTR of TRPV4. To verify this prediction, we cloned a luciferase reporter sequence in the 3′UTR of TRPV4, which contains the putative miR-29a binding sites. A mutant reporter vector of the 3′UTR of TRPV4 containing luciferase reporter was used as negative control. Data from luciferase reporter assay showed that overexpression of miR-29a significantly decreased reporter vector activity of TRPV4 3′UTR in GC-1 cells but had no effect on the mutated reporter vector (**Figures 4A,B**, $n = 6$ per group). To further investigate whether

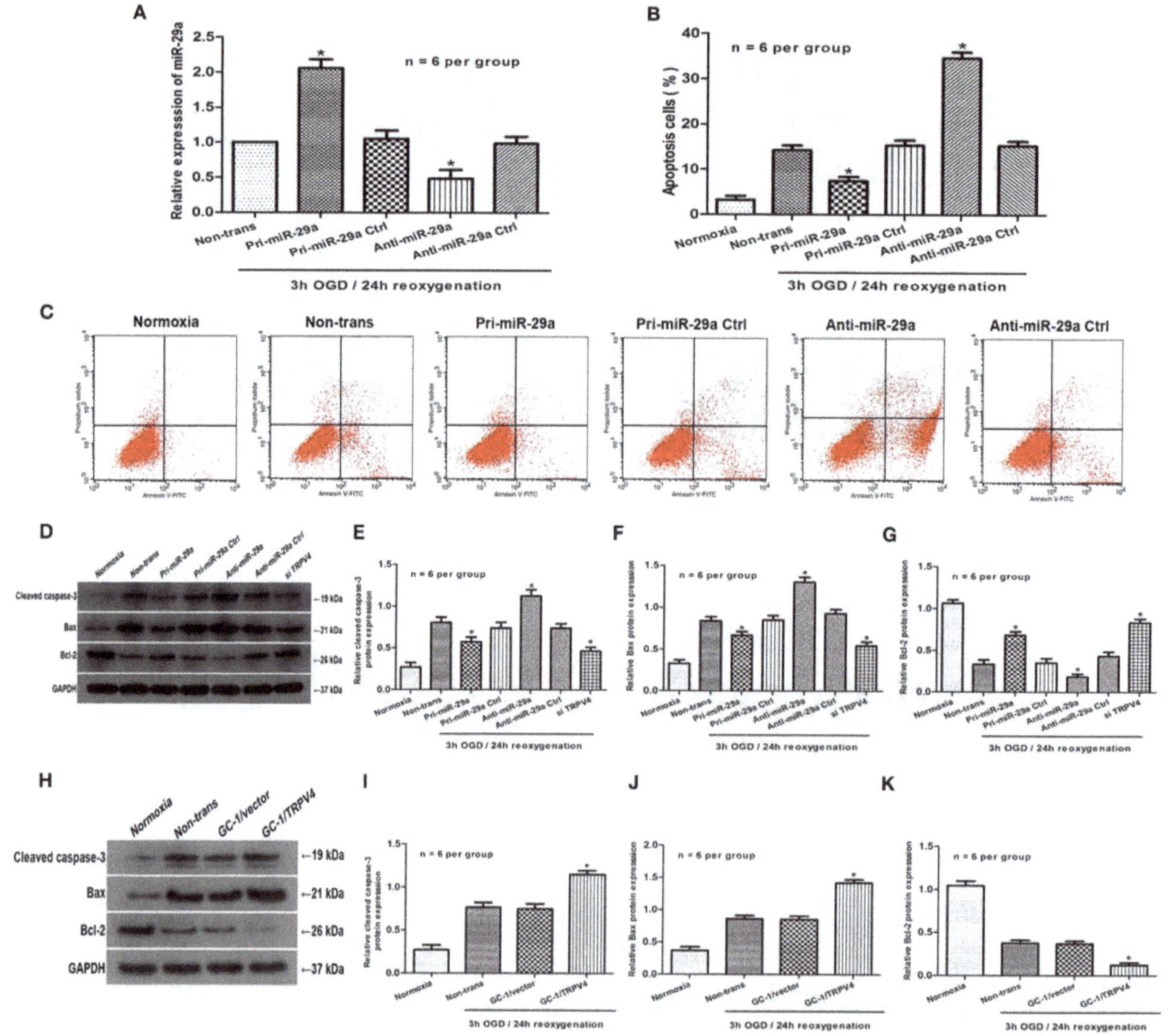

FIGURE 3 | Influence of MiR-29a and TRPV4 on GC-1 cell apoptosis *in vitro* **(A)** qRT-PCR assays were performed to analyze the expression level of miR-29a after transfection with pri-miR-29a or anti-miR-29a in 3 h OGD/24 h reoxygenation treatments. $^{*}p < 0.05$ vs. non-trans, $n = 6$ per group; **(B,C)** Flow cytometry assays were performed to show the cell apoptosis after transfection with pri-miR-29a or anti-miR-29a in normoxia and 3 h OGD/24 h reoxygenation treatments. $^{*}p < 0.05$ vs. non-trans, $n = 6$ per group; **(D–K)** Cleaved caspase-3, Bax and Bcl-2 protein levels transfected with pri-miR-29a, anti-miR-29a, TRPV4 siRNAs, or TRPV4-overexpression(GC-1/TRPV4) were examined in normoxia and 3 h OGD/24 h reoxygenation treatments by western blot analysis. $^{*}p < 0.05$ vs. non-trans, $n = 6$ per group.

miR-29a regulates apoptosis in testicular IRI via targeting TRPV4, we employed immunoblotting assays to determine apoptosis related proteins after cells were transfected with pri-miR-29a or anti-miR-29a and TRPV4 siRNAs or TRPV4 overexpression (GC-1/TRPV4). We found that overexpression of miR-29a markedly suppresses apoptosis, whereas TRPV4 overexpression abrogated such decrease in apoptosis induced by miR-29a (**Figures 4C–F**, $n = 6$ per group). On the other hand, knockdown of miR-29a led to an increase in apoptosis, while which could be rescued by TRPV4 inhibition (**Figures 4G–J**, $n = 6$ per group). Together, these results suggest that miR-29a directly targets TRPV4 and alleviates apoptosis *in vitro*.

miR-29a Inhibits Spermatogenic Cell Apoptosis via Downregulation of TRPV4 *in Vivo*

To further determine the effect of miR-29a expression on spermatogenic cell apoptosis *in vivo*, miR-29a agomir was injected into the seminiferous tubules to increase miR-29a expression. A TUNEL assay was used to determine whether

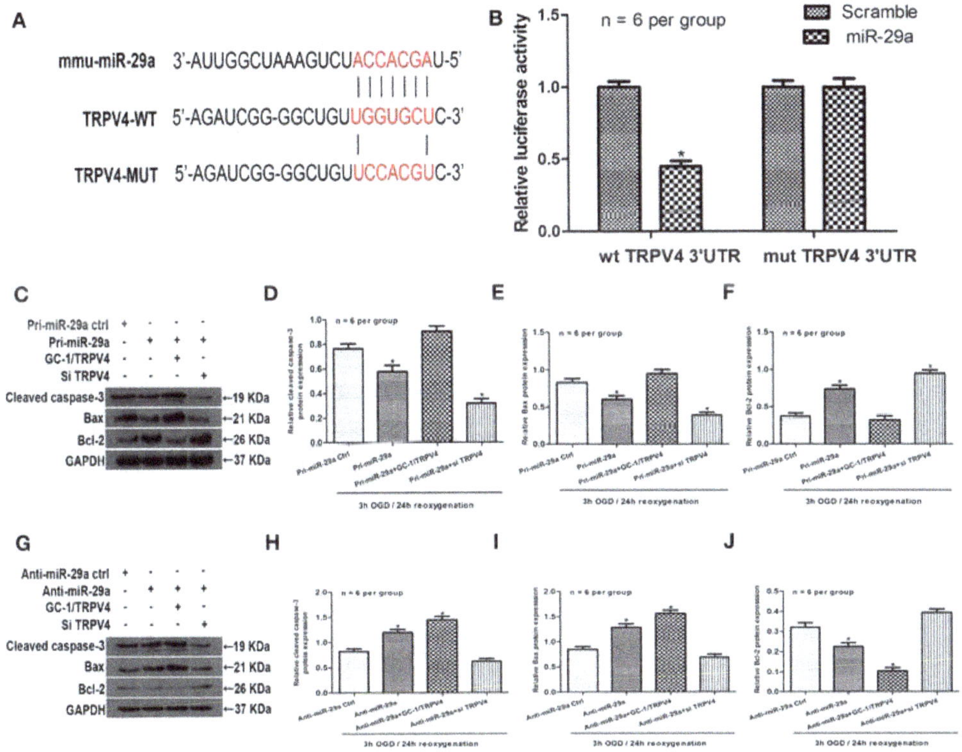

FIGURE 4 | MiR-29a directly targets TRPV4 and alleviates apoptosis *in vitro.* **(A)** Sequence alignment of predicted miR-29a binding sites within the TRPV4 3′UTR and its mutated sequence for luciferase reporter assay; **(B)** Luciferase reporter assay was performed in GC-1 cells that were co-transfected with pri-miR-29a and reporter vectors containing TRPV4 3′UTR or mutated TRPV4 3′UTR. Relative luciferase activities are presented. $^*p < 0.05$, $n = 6$ per group. **(C–F)** Cleaved caspase-3, Bax and Bcl-2 protein levels of GC-1 cells co-transfected with pri-miR-29a and TRPV4 siRNAs or TRPV4 overexpression (GC-1/TRPV4) in 3 h OGD/24 h reoxygenation treatments by western blot analysis. $^*p < 0.05$ vs. pri-miR-29a ctrl, $n = 6$ per group. **(G–J)** Cleaved caspase-3, Bax and Bcl-2 protein levels of GC-1 cells co-transfected with anti-miR-29a and TRPV4 siRNAs or TRPV4-overexpression(GC-1/TRPV4) in 3 h OGD/24 h reoxygenation treatments by western blot analysis.$^*p < 0.05$ vs. anti-miR-29a ctrl, $n = 6$ per group.

miR-29a could affect spermatogenic cell apoptosis in response to a 1 h of ischemia/16 h of reperfusion treatment. The TUNEL assay showed no obvious apoptotic cells in the sham group. Compared with negative control group, the effect of miR-29a overexpression dramatically reduced the number of apoptotic cells (**Figures 5A,B**, $n = 5$ per group). Immunohistochemistry staining revealed that overexpression of miR-29a resulted in lower expression levels of Bax and a higher expression level of Bcl-2 in comparison with negative control group (**Figure 5C**, $n = 5$ per group). Moreover, western blot data showed that overexpression of miR-29a decreased protein levels of TRPV4 and caspase-3 when compared to the negative control group (**Figures 5D–F**, $n = 5$ per group). Together, our results suggest that miR-29a suppresses apoptosis *in vivo*.

DISCUSSION

The pathophysiological mechanisms of testicular T/D result from direct damage induced by ischemia during torsion and a secondary effect attributed to enhanced blood flow with reperfusion during detorsion (Huang et al., 2012). Testicular IRI triggers apoptosis-related signaling pathways and further negatively affects spermatogenesis, eventually leading to male infertility (Hadziselimovic et al., 1998; Meštrović et al., 2014). The two major factors affecting testicular damage are the degree and duration of spermatic cord torsion (Cvetkovic et al., 2015). Timely treatment of testis torsion is a crucial issue, and currently both manipulative reduction and orchiectomy treatment are known to cause injury to the bilateral testis (Dursun et al., 2015). Thus, understanding the mechanisms underlying apoptosis in testicular IRI and exploring new molecular interactive targets will help to develop effective therapeutics. Previous studies have demonstrated that miRNA can regulate apoptosis process in organ IRI by targeting mRNAs of specific genes (Berezikov et al., 2005). Based on this information, we tried to identify miRNAs that bind the TRPV4 gene and to determine the regulatory relationship in the progression of testicular IRI.

MicroRNA expression is highly related to apoptosis in the progression of organs IRI. It has been shown that abnormally expressed miRNAs can regulate RNA networks during IRI progression, and a single miRNA may function in pro-apoptosis or anti-apoptosis roles under different contexts (Andreeva et al., 2015). Previous studies have demonstrated that overexpression of miR-29a promotes myocardial apoptosis by directly targeting

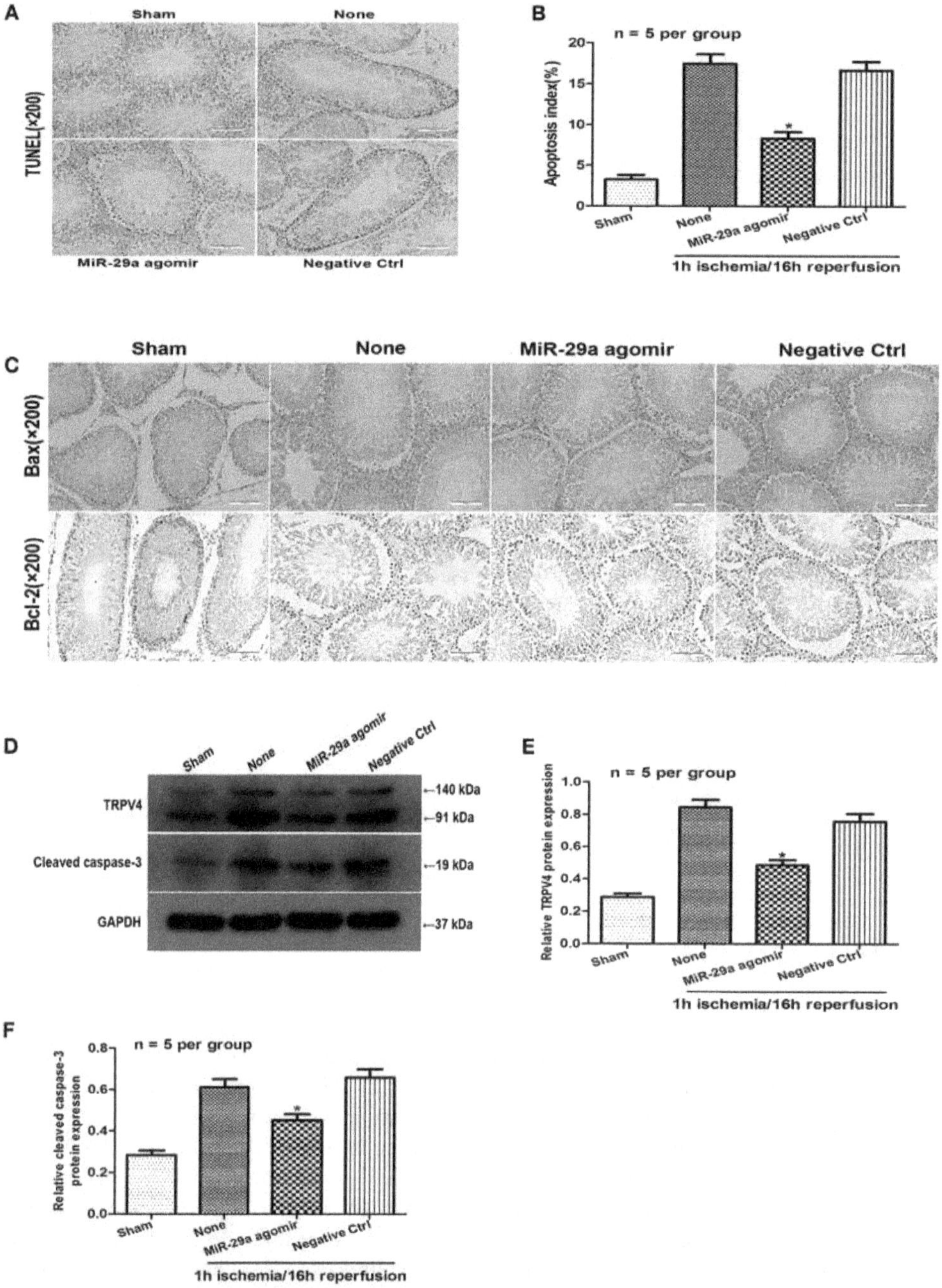

FIGURE 5 | MiR-29a inhibits apoptosis of testicular IRI via downregulation of TRPV4 *in vivo.* **(A,B)** TUNEL assays were performed to investigate the cell apoptosis after injection with miR-29a agomir and its negative ctrl at 16 h of reperfusion after 1 h ischemia. $^*p < 0.05$ vs. none(1 h ischemia/16 h reperfusion treatment), $n = 5$ per group; **(C)** Immunohistochemistry staining of Bax and Bcl-2 after injection with miR-29a agomir and its negative ctrl at 1 h of ischemia/16 h of reperfusion. $n = 5$ per group; **(D–F)** TRPV4 and Cleaved caspase-3 protein level expression after injection with miR-29a agomir and its negative ctrl were detected at 1 h of ischemia followed by 16 h of reperfusion by western blot analysis. $^*p < 0.05$ vs. none, $n = 5$ per group.

IGF-1 and Mcl-1 depending on activation of P13K/Akt signaling pathways (Ye et al., 2010; Wang et al., 2015). Furthermore, a recent study suggested that miR-29a suppresses apoptosis by negatively regulating PUMA in cerebral IRI (Ouyang et al., 2013). In our studies, we analysed animal samples at different time points of reperfusion. Our data demonstrated that miR-29a expression is significantly downregulated in the progression of testicular IRI and that lower expression of miR-29a is negatively correlated with expression of TRPV4 channels.

TRPV4 has been reported to be upregulated during the progression of IRI and to be involved in apoptosis via multiple signaling pathways (Ye et al., 2012; Hong et al.,

2016). For example, TRPV4 expression is upregulated during the progression of IRI and involved in apoptosis via multiple signaling pathways (Jie et al., 2015). Inhibition of TRPV4 reduces neurological injury after cerebral infarction, and leads to apoptosis of mouse retinal ganglion cells, which may contribute to the activation of $Ca2^{+}$-dependent signaling pathways (Ryskamp et al., 2011). In our *in vitro* studies, we further confirmed the opposite relationship between TRPV4 and miR-29a expression in the GC-1 cells. We found that overexpression of miR-29a suppressed TRPV4 expression and that inhibition of miR-29a promoted TRPV4 expression. More important, we have identified TRPV4 as a direct downstream target of miR-29a using a luciferase reporter assay. These data provide evidence that miR-29a negatively regulates the expression of TRPV4 in the GC-1 cells, which is consistent with findings from *in vivo* studies.

Apoptosis is a form of cell death based on genetic mechanisms and plays an important role by inducing a series of pathophysiologic changes (Vaux and Korsmeyer, 1999), and it has been generally accepted that the mitochondrial signaling pathway is the major channel for apoptosis, which is regulated by precise gene expression (Desagher and Martinou, 2000). The Bcl-2 family is composed of pro-apoptotic factors (e.g., Bax) and anti-apoptotic factors (e.g., Bcl-2). The ratio of Bcl-2/Bax is a regulator of spermatogenic cell apoptosis and determines the extent of apoptosis in spermatogenic cells exposed to damage (Liang et al., 2013). Moreover, caspase-3 is an inactive zymogen located in the cytoplasm and serves as the convergence point of multiple apoptotic stimuli signals. Its activation signals irreversible commitment to cell apoptosis, leading to changes in cell shrinkage, chromatin condensation and DNA fragmentation (Zheng et al., 2008). In our *in vitro* studies, we have demonstrated that overexpression of miR-29a and knockdown of TRPV4 reduce cell apoptosis, while inhibition of miR-29a and overexpression of TRPV4 have an opposite effect. Moreover, data from *in vivo* studies also support that increased expression of miR-29a produces a decrease in apoptosis by downregulating the TRPV4 gene expression. Together, these data suggest that miR-29a-mediated inhibition of TRPV4 is associated with cell apoptosis in testicular IRI.

CONCLUSIONS

In conclusion, our study revealed a negative correlation between the expression of miR-29a and TRPV4 during the progression of IRI. In addition, we showed that miR-29a alleviated apoptosis by directly targeting TRPV4 both *in vitro* and *in vivo*. These findings suggest that miR-29a might serve as an effective therapeutic target to suppress spermatogenic cell apoptosis in testicular IRI.

AUTHOR CONTRIBUTIONS

JN and WL, Conception and design of the study, data collection and analysis, manuscript writing. FC, WY, TR, and DZ, Design of the study, critical revision, supervised all phases of the study. RY, YR, XZ, YD, and CX, Data collection.

REFERENCES

Andreeva, K., Soliman, M. M., and Cooper, N. G. (2015). Regulatory networks in retinal ischemia-reperfusion injury. *BMC Genet.* 16, 43. doi: 10.1186/s12863-015-0201-4

Aslan Koşar, K. P., Tuncer, H., Cihangir, U. A., Espino, P. J., Darici, H., Onaran, I., et al. (2015). The efficiency of Poly(ADP-Ribose) Polymerase (PARP) cleavage on detection of apoptosis in an experimental model of testicular torsion. *Int. J. Exp. Pathol.* 96, 294–300. doi: 10.1111/iep.12137

Bao, J., Li, D., Wang, L., Wu, J., Hu, Y., Wang, Z., et al. (2012). MicroRNA-449 and microRNA-34b/c function redundantly in murine testes by targeting E2F transcription factor-retinoblastoma protein (E2F-pRb) pathway. *J. Biol. Chem.* 287, 21686–21698. doi: 10.1074/jbc.M111.328054

Berezikov, E., Guryev, V., van de Belt, J., Wienholds, E., Plasterk, R. H., and Cuppen, E. (2005). Phylogenetic shadowing and computational identification of human microRNA genes. *Cell* 120, 21–24. doi: 10.1016/j.cell.2004.12.031

Cvetkovic, T., Stankovic, J., Najman, S., Pavlovic, D., Stokanovic, D., Vlajkovic, S., et al. (2015). Oxidant and antioxidant status in experimental rat testis after testicular torsion/detorsion. *Int. J. Fertil. Steril.* 9, 121–128. doi: 10.22074/ijfs.2015.4216

Desagher, S., and Martinou, J. C. (2000). Mitochondria as the central control point of apoptosis. *Trends Cell Biol.* 10, 369–377. doi: 10.1016/S0962-8924(00)01803-1

Ding, H., Lin, Y. X., Shen, Q. W., Pan, Z., Wang, Z. C., and Chen, L. (2015). Research progress of TRPV4 and cerebral ischemic reperfusion injury. *Sheng Li Xue Bao* 67, 527–532. doi: 10.13294/j.aps.2015.0065

Dursun, R., Zengin, Y., Gündüz, E., Içer, M., Durgun, H. M., Daggulli, M., et al. (2015). The protective effect of goji berry extract in ischemic reperfusion in testis torsion. *Int. J. Clin. Exp. Med.* 8, 2727–2733.

Fusi, C., Materazzi, S., Minocci, D., Maio, V., Oranges, T., Massi, D., et al. (2014). Transient receptor potential vanilloid 4 (TRPV4) is downregulated in keratinocytes in human non-melanoma skin cancer. *J. Invest. Dermatol.* 134, 2408–2417. doi: 10.1038/jid.2014.145

Gu, D., Zou, X., Ju, G., Zhang, G., Bao, E., and Zhu, Y. (2016). Mesenchymal stromal cells derived extracellular vesicles ameliorate acute renal ischemia reperfusion injury by inhibition of mitochondrial fission through miR-30. *Stem Cells Int.* 2016:2093940. doi: 10.1155/2016/2093940

Hadziselimovic, F., Geneto, R., and Emmons, L. R. (1998). Increased apoptosis in the contralateral testes of patients with testicular torsion as a factor for infertility. *J. Urol.* 160, 1158–1160. doi: 10.1016/S0022-5347(01)62725-3

Hong, Z., Tian, Y., Yuan, Y., Qi, M., Li, Y., Du, Y., et al. (2016). Enhanced oxidative stress is responsible for TRPV4-induced neurotoxicity. *Front. Cell. Neurosci.* 10:232. doi: 10.3389/fncel.2016.00232

Huang, K. H., Weng, T. I., Huang, H. Y., Huang, K. D., Lin, W. C., Chen, S. C., et al. (2012). Honokiol attenuates torsion/detorsion-induced testicular injury in rat testis by way of suppressing endoplasmic reticulum stress-related apoptosis. *Urology* 79, 967.e5–11. doi: 10.1016/j.urology.2011.11.027

Jie, P., Hong, Z., Tian, Y., Li, Y., Lin, L., Zhou, L., et al. (2015). Activation of transient receptor potential vanilloid 4 induces apoptosis in hippocampus through downregulating PI3K/Akt and upregulating p38 MAPK signaling pathways. *Cell Death Dis.* 6:e1775. doi: 10.1038/cddis.2015.146

Kassmann, M., Harteneck, C., Zhu, Z., Nürnberg, B., Tepel, M., and Gollasch, M. (2013). Transient receptor potential vanilloid 1 (TRPV1), TRPV4, and the kidney. *Acta Physiol. (Oxf)* 207, 546–564. doi: 10.1111/apha.12051

Kim, H. J., Lee, J. W., Hwang, B. R., Lee, Y. A., Kim, J. I., Cho, Y. J., et al. (2016). Protective effect of pterostilbene on testicular ischemia/reperfusion injury in rats. *J. Pediatr. Surg.* 51, 1192–1196. doi: 10.1016/j.jpedsurg.2016.01.009

Liang, H., Yu, F., Tong, Z., Yuan, B., and Wang, C. (2013). Effect of ischemia post-conditioning on skeletal muscle oxidative injury, mTOR, Bax, Bcl-2 proteins expression, and HIF-1α/β-actin mRNA, IL-6/β-actin mRNA and caveolin-3/β-actin mRNA expression in ischemia-reperfusion rabbits. *Mol. Biol. Rep.* 40, 507–514. doi: 10.1007/s11033-012-2087-9

Liang, X., Zhou, D., Wei, C., Luo, H., Liu, J., Fu, R., et al. (2012). MicroRNA-34c enhances murine male germ cell apoptosis through targeting ATF1. *PLoS ONE* 7:e33861. doi: 10.1371/journal.pone.0033861

Meštrović, J., Drmić-Hofman, I., Pogorelić, Z., Vilović, K., Šupe-Domić, D., Šešelja-Perišin, A., et al. (2014). Beneficial effect of nifedipine on testicular torsion-detorsion injury in rats. *Urology* 84, 1194–1198. doi: 10.1016/j.urology.2014.07.022

Ouyang, Y. B., Xu, L., Lu, Y., Sun, X., Yue, S., Xiong, X. X., et al. (2013). Astrocyte-enriched miR-29a targets PUMA and reduces neuronal vulnerability to forebrain ischemia. *Glia* 61, 1784–1794. doi: 10.1002/glia.22556

Rao, X., Huang, X., Zhou, Z., and Lin, X. (2013). An improvement of the $2^{(}-\delta\delta CT)$ method for quantitative real-time polymerase chain reaction data analysis. *Biostat. Bioinforma. Biomath.* 3, 71–85.

Ryskamp, D. A., Witkovsky, P., Barabas, P., Huang, W., Koehler, C., Akimov, N. P., et al. (2011). The polymodal ion channel transient receptor potential vanilloid 4 modulates calcium flux, spiking rate, and apoptosis of mouse retinal ganglion cells. *J. Neurosci.* 31, 7089–7101. doi: 10.1523/JNEUROSCI.0359-11.2011

Townsley, M. I., Morisseau, C., Hammock, B., and King, J. A. (2010). Impact of epoxyeicosatrienoic acids in lung ischemia-reperfusion injury. *Microcirculation* 17, 137–146. doi: 10.1111/j.1549-8719.2009.00013.x

Tsuno, N., Yukimasa, A., Yoshida, O., Ichihashi, Y., Inoue, T., Ueno, T., et al. (2016). Discovery of novel 2′,4′-dimethyl-[4,5′-bithiazol]-2-yl amino derivatives as orally bioavailable TRPV4 antagonists for the treatment of pain: part 1. *Bioorg. Med. Chem. Lett.* 26, 4930–4935. doi: 10.1016/j.bmcl.2016.09.013

Tuglu, D., Yuvanc, E., Ozan, T., Bal, F., Yilmaz, E., Atasoy, P., et al. (2016). Protective effects of udenafil citrate, piracetam and dexmedetomidine treatment on testicular torsion/detorsion-induced ischaemia/reperfusion injury in rats. *Andrologia* 48, 676–682. doi: 10.1111/and.12499

Vaux, D. L., and Korsmeyer, S. J. (1999). Cell death in development. *Cell* 96, 245–254. doi: 10.1016/S0092-8674(00)80564-4

Vergnolle, N. (2014). TRPV4: new therapeutic target for inflammatory bowel diseases. *Biochem. Pharmacol.* 89, 157–161. doi: 10.1016/j.bcp.2014.01.005

Wang, L., Niu, X., Hu, J., Xing, H., Sun, M., Wang, J., et al. (2015). After myocardial ischemia-reperfusion, miR-29a, and Let7 could affect apoptosis through regulating IGF-1. *Biomed Res. Int.* 2015:245412. doi: 10.1155/2015/245412

Wei, Z. L., Nguyen, M. T., O'Mahony, D. J., Acevedo, A., Zipfel, S., Zhang, Q., et al. (2015). Identification of orally-bioavailable antagonists of the TRPV4 ion-channel. *Bioorg. Med. Chem. Lett.* 25, 4011–4015. doi: 10.1016/j.bmcl.2015.06.098

Wu, Y., Gu, C., and Huang, X. (2016). Sevoflurane protects against hepatic ischemia/reperfusion injury by modulating microRNA-200c regulation in mice. *Biomed. Pharmacother.* 84, 1126–1136. doi: 10.1016/j.biopha.2016.10.024

Xu, Z. P., Gao, W. C., Wang, H. P., and Wang, X. H. (2009). [Expression of transient receptor potential subfamily mRNAs in rat testes]. *Nan Fang Yi Ke Da Xue Xue Bao* 29, 519–520.

Ye, L., Kleiner, S., Wu, J., Sah, R., Gupta, R. K., Banks, A. S., et al. (2012). TRPV4 is a regulator of adipose oxidative metabolism, inflammation, and energy homeostasis. *Cell* 151, 96–110. doi: 10.1016/j.cell.2012.08.034

Ye, Y., Hu, Z., Lin, Y., Zhang, C., and Perez-Polo, J. R. (2010). Downregulation of microRNA-29 by antisense inhibitors and a PPAR-gamma agonist protects against myocardial ischaemia-reperfusion injury. *Cardiovasc. Res.* 87, 535–544. doi: 10.1093/cvr/cvq053

Zhang, H., Wu, J., Keller, J. M., Yeung, K., Keller, E. T., and Fu, Z. (2012). Transcriptional regulation of RKIP expression by androgen in prostate cells. *Cell. Physiol. Biochem.* 30, 1340–1350. doi: 10.1159/000343323

Zhang, S., Chen, L., Jung, E. J., and Calin, G. A. (2010). Targeting microRNAs with small molecules: from dream to reality. *Clin. Pharmacol. Ther.* 87, 754–758. doi: 10.1038/clpt.2010.46

Zheng, Y., Zhang, X., Zhou, J., Cheng, F., and Zhou, B. (2008). Effects on the ipsilateral testis during progression of experimental varicocele in rat. *Med. Sci. Monit.* 14, BR122-126.

Zhu, J., Yao, K., Wang, Q., Guo, J., Shi, H., Ma, L., et al. (2016). Ischemic postconditioning-regulated mir-499 protects the rat heart against ischemia/reperfusion injury by inhibiting apoptosis through PDCD4. *Cell. Physiol. Biochem.* 39, 2364–2380. doi: 10.1159/000452506

2

Arachidonic Acid Metabolism Pathway is not Only Dominant in Metabolic Modulation but Associated with Phenotypic Variation After Acute Hypoxia Exposure

Chang Liu[1,2,3], Bao Liu[1,2,3,4], Lu Liu[1,2,3], Er-Long Zhang[1,2,3], Bind-da Sun[1,2,3], Gang Xu[1,2,3], Jian Chen[1,2,3] and Yu-qi Gao[1,2,3]**

[1] Institute of Medicine and Hygienic Equipment for High Altitude Region, College of High Altitude Military Medicine, Army Medical University, Third Military Medical University, Chongqing, China, [2] Key Laboratory of High Altitude Environmental Medicine, Army Medical University, Third Military Medical University, Ministry of Education, Chongqing, China, [3] Key Laboratory of High Altitude Medicine, People's Liberation Army, Chongqing, China, [4] The 12th Hospital of Chinese People's Liberation Army, Kashi, China

***Correspondence:**
Jian Chen
jchenone@163.com
Yu-qi Gao
gaoy66@yahoo.com

Background: The modulation of arachidonic acid (AA) metabolism pathway is identified in metabolic alterations after hypoxia exposure, but its biological function is controversial. We aimed at integrating plasma metabolomic and transcriptomic approaches to systematically explore the roles of the AA metabolism pathway in response to acute hypoxia using an acute mountain sickness (AMS) model.

Methods: Blood samples were obtained from 53 enrolled subjects before and after exposure to high altitude. Ultra-performance liquid chromatography-quadrupole time-of-flight mass spectrometry and RNA sequencing were separately performed for metabolomic and transcriptomic profiling, respectively. Influential modules comprising essential metabolites and genes were identified by weighted gene co-expression network analysis (WGCNA) after integrating metabolic information with phenotypic and transcriptomic datasets, respectively.

Results: Enrolled subjects exhibited diverse response manners to hypoxia. Combined with obviously altered heart rate, oxygen saturation, hemoglobin, and Lake Louise Score (LLS), metabolomic profiling detected that 36 metabolites were highly related to clinical features in hypoxia responses, out of which 27 were upregulated and nine were downregulated, and could be mapped to AA metabolism pathway significantly. Integrated analysis of metabolomic and transcriptomic data revealed that these dominant molecules showed remarkable association with genes in gas transport incapacitation and disorders of hemoglobin metabolism pathways, such as ALAS2, HEMGN. After detailed description of AA metabolism pathway, we found that the molecules of 15-d-PGJ2, PGA2, PGE2, 12-O-3-OH-LTB4, LTD4, LTE4 were significantly up-regulated after hypoxia stimuli, and increased in those with poor response manner to hypoxia particularly. Further analysis in another cohort showed that genes in AA metabolism pathway such as PTGES, PTGS1, GGT1, TBAS1 et al. were excessively elevated in subjects in maladaptation to hypoxia.

Conclusion: This is the first study to construct the map of AA metabolism pathway in response to hypoxia and reveal the crosstalk between phenotypic variation under hypoxia and the AA metabolism pathway. These findings may improve our understanding of the advanced pathophysiological mechanisms in acute hypoxic diseases and provide new insights into critical roles of the AA metabolism pathway in the development and prevention of these diseases.

Keywords: metabolomics, transcriptomics, WGCNA, hypoxia, arachidonic acid

INTRODUCTION

Hypoxia is a common phenomenon associated with multiple pathophysiological processes, including inflammation, necrosis, and apoptosis, and observed in various clinic conditions such as myocardial ischemia and reperfusion as well as stroke (Michiels, 2004). The arachidonic acid (AA) metabolism pathway was shown to exhibit remarkable metabolic alterations after hypoxia exposure, but its role is controversial (Liao et al., 2016). As a part of the innate immune response, AA and its metabolites are known to induce or suppress inflammation (Bennett and Gilroy, 2016). In addition, the products of the AA cascade are shown to display multidirectional and often conflicting roles in endothelial and nerve cells, such as inhibition or promotion of cell proliferation and aggravation or alleviation of oxidative stress, in response to stimuli (Bogatcheva et al., 2005; Rink and Khanna, 2011). Although the partial function of this pathway was identified, the mechanism underlying the expression of the AA metabolism pathway and its role under acute hypoxic conditions are questionable.

Acute hypobaric hypoxia, one of the most common hypoxia types, occurs in response to the exposure to high altitude and initiates systematic pathophysiological alterations. Acute hypobaric hypoxia may serve as a principal etiological factor for acute mountain sickness (AMS) (Sun et al., 2017). Therefore, AMS is considered as a potent channel and an *in vivo* model to improve our understanding of the various acute hypoxic diseases with high-quality samples from self-controlled studies (Subudhi et al., 2010). In addition, mal-adaptation to hypoxia is characterized by symptoms such as headache, nausea, and vomiting that may progress into high altitude pulmonary edema or high altitude cerebral edema-the leading lethal diseases for mountaineers (Johnson and Luks, 2016). With $\sim$15 million people traveling to areas of high altitude (>2,500 m) annually in China alone (Gonggalanzi et al., 2016), it is important to unravel the mechanisms underlying AMS.

The technical platforms of system biology allow researchers to explore systematic alterations under hypoxia exposure. Metabolomic studies have demonstrated that metabolic reprogramming with dramatic turbulence in various metabolic pathways, including linoleic acid metabolism, purinergic signaling, and glycolysis, was implied in response to acute hypoxia (D'Alessandro et al., 2016; Liao et al., 2016). In addition, a recent study on acute hypoxia stimuli based on RNA-seq approach indicated that the disturbance in the inflammation response presented by the reduction in interleukin (IL)-10 was highly related to AMS incidences (Liu et al., 2017a). However, studies based on a single set of omics technology failed to extensively explain the alterations occurring at different levels during physiologic or pathophysiological responses, such as disabilities in interpreting metabolic regulatory processes in metabolomics (Kan et al., 2017). The development of efficient analysis methods and algorithms allows better insights, beyond those available from individual strategies through the integration of diverse omics (Li et al., 2016; Sun and Hu, 2016). In particular, the method of weighted gene co-expression network analysis (WGCNA), which could exhibit multiple network-level interactions, is effective for the identification of gene-to-metabolite relations and construction of the underlying complex regulatory networks (Acharjee et al., 2016; Liu et al., 2017b).

Here, we aimed to integrate clinical features, metabolomic datasets, and transcriptome profiling for the construction of the co-expression network to provide a better understanding of the AA metabolism pathway after acute hypoxia exposure. Our results identified that the AA metabolism pathway, a highly regulated metabolic pathway, was essential in response to acute hypoxia. Furthermore, the AA metabolism pathway may account for variations in response patterns after acute hypoxia stimuli. Our results may improve the understanding of AMS and provide new clues to counteract the effects of hypoxic diseases.

MATERIALS AND METHODS

Enrolled Subjects and Experimental Procedures

We enrolled 53 male subjects with intact clinical phenotype data of heart rate (HR), oxygen saturation (SpO_2), Lake Louise score (LLS), systolic blood pressure (SBP), diastolic blood pressure (DBP), and hemoglobin (HB) before and after high altitude exposure (5,300 m). These subjects were covered in our previous study (Liao et al., 2016). Physical and physiological characteristics [mean $\pm$ standard deviation (SD)] for enrolled subjects were as follows: age, 21.6 $\pm$ 2.0 years; height, 172 $\pm$ 1 cm; and body weight, 64.9 $\pm$ 2.3 kg. Exclusion criteria included prior exposure to high altitude, presence of cardiovascular pathologies or other diseases, and history of drug prescribed for high altitude. These volunteers traveled to an area of 5,300 m from the starting point of 1,400 m within 4 days, as illustrated in our previous article (Liao et al., 2016). Their clinical symptoms of HR, SpO_2, LLS, SBP, DBP, HB were monitored before and after hypoxia stimuli. The local ethics committee of the Third Military Medical University approved the experimental design, methods of clinical data collection, and strategies of data evaluation. These procedures were performed in accordance with the approved guidelines. Written informed consents were obtained from all participants.

Metabolomics Analysis

Metabolic profiling was performed, and metabolic data were obtained as previously described (Liao et al., 2016). Briefly, blood was drawn from a peripheral vein in the morning soon after waking before ascending to high altitudes and after 3 days high-altitude exposures. Blood samples were centrifuged to separate serum at 14,000 × g for 15 min at 4°C. Then, these plasma samples were delivered to Chongqing for further metabolomics analysis in the courier filed with dry ice.

Metabolomics analysis was conducted on an Agilent 1290 Infinity LC system (Agilent, Santa Clara, CA, USA). Chromatographic separations were performed on an ACQUITY UHPLC HSS T3 C18 column (2.1 × 100 mm, 1.8 μm; Waters, Milford, Ireland) at 45°C. The metabolomics detection was performed totally in accordance to the manufacturers' protocols of all devices. Raw LC-MS data were converted to mzData formats via Agilent MassHunter Qualitative software (Agilent, Santa Clara, CA, USA). The program XCMS (version 1.40.0) (https://xcmsonline.scripps.edu/) was used to preprocess the raw data, including peak detection, peak matching, matched filtration, and nonlinear alignment of data, with the default parameters (and snthresh, 5; bw, 10; fwhm, 10).

The resulting matrix from 53 subjects comprising retention time, mass-to-charge ratio (m/z), and normalized ion intensities was introduced into the subsequent analysis based on R platform (https://www.r-project.org). The model of partial squares discriminant analysis (OPLS-DA) was carried out to separate pre- and post-hypoxia in metabolic profiling. Variable importance project (VIP) was used to reveal discriminatory metabolites which were enrolled in the classification effects of hypoxia was calculated. In addition, adjusted p-value from the paired t-test and fold-change value (FC) were executed to discovery dominant metabolites. Pathway analysis was established by MetaboAnalyst platform (http://www.metaboanalyst.ca).

Transcriptomic Profiling Detection

To improve the reliability of the integrated analysis to uncover interactions at metabolic and transcriptional level, 11 individuals were randomly selected and subjected to metabolomic and RNA-seq detection (Li et al., 2016). RNA sequencing was performed as previously described (Liu et al., 2017a) with minor modifications. Briefly, after extraction, total RNA was quantified by spectrophotometer (NanoDrop 200, Thermo Scientific, Delaware, USA). mRNA-seq libraries were constructed according to the TruSeq RNA Sample Prep Kit v2 (Illumina) and sequenced on an Illumina HiSeq 2000 sequencer, following the manufacturer's instructions. after filtered, the clean reads were aligned to human genome hg19 based on HISAT and assembled by Stringtie (Li et al., 2014). The expression value of each transcript was subsequently calculated based on methods of Fragments Per Kilobase of exon model per Million mapped fragments (FPKM). In addition, GSE52209 datasets of blood samples from individuals suffering from adaptation or mal-adaptation to high altitude exposure were downloaded from Gene Expression Omnibus (GEO) datasets. After annotation, limma package was employed to normalize and detect the significantly differential genes involved in diverse response manner to hypoxia (Ritchie et al., 2015). ClusterProfiler package was used to determine enriched Gene Ontology (GO) terms in differentially expressed gene sets (Yu et al., 2012).

Weighted Gene Co-expression Network Analysis (WGCNA)

WGCNA, a robust tool for the integrative network analysis, is widely used in complex network construction (Liu et al., 2017b). According to the WGCNA protocol, we constructed clusters of genes firstly based on the matrix of pairwise correlations calculated across the selected samples. Then, we performed the network construction and module detection based on an appropriate soft-thresholding power. The default minimum cluster merge height of 0.25 was retained. These clusters identified by WGCNA are called modules, which represented a group of highly interconnected genes with similar expression profiles across the enrolled subjects. Further, we determined correlations among expression modules and clinical traits for all subjects. Hub genes were identified based on the connectivity among all nodes. Network was illustrated by Cytoscape software (Smoot et al., 2011).

Statistical Analysis

Differences before and after hypoxia exposure were determined by paired t-test. The unpaired Student's t-test was used to compare the expression between subjects with diverse response patterns to hypoxia. Statistical analysis was performed by GraphPad software (GraphPad Prism, USA). The data in this study were presented as the mean ± SD. A two-tailed p value <0.05 was considered as significant, unless specifically indicated.

RESULTS

Baseline Clinical Characteristics of Enrolled Subjects

The response of subjects to acute hypobaric hypoxia was assessed by various physiological parameters. As shown in **Figure 1A**, SpO_2, reflective of the oxygen concentration in the blood, significantly declined under hypoxia environment ($p < 0.05$; Netzer et al., 2017). Among the essential compensatory

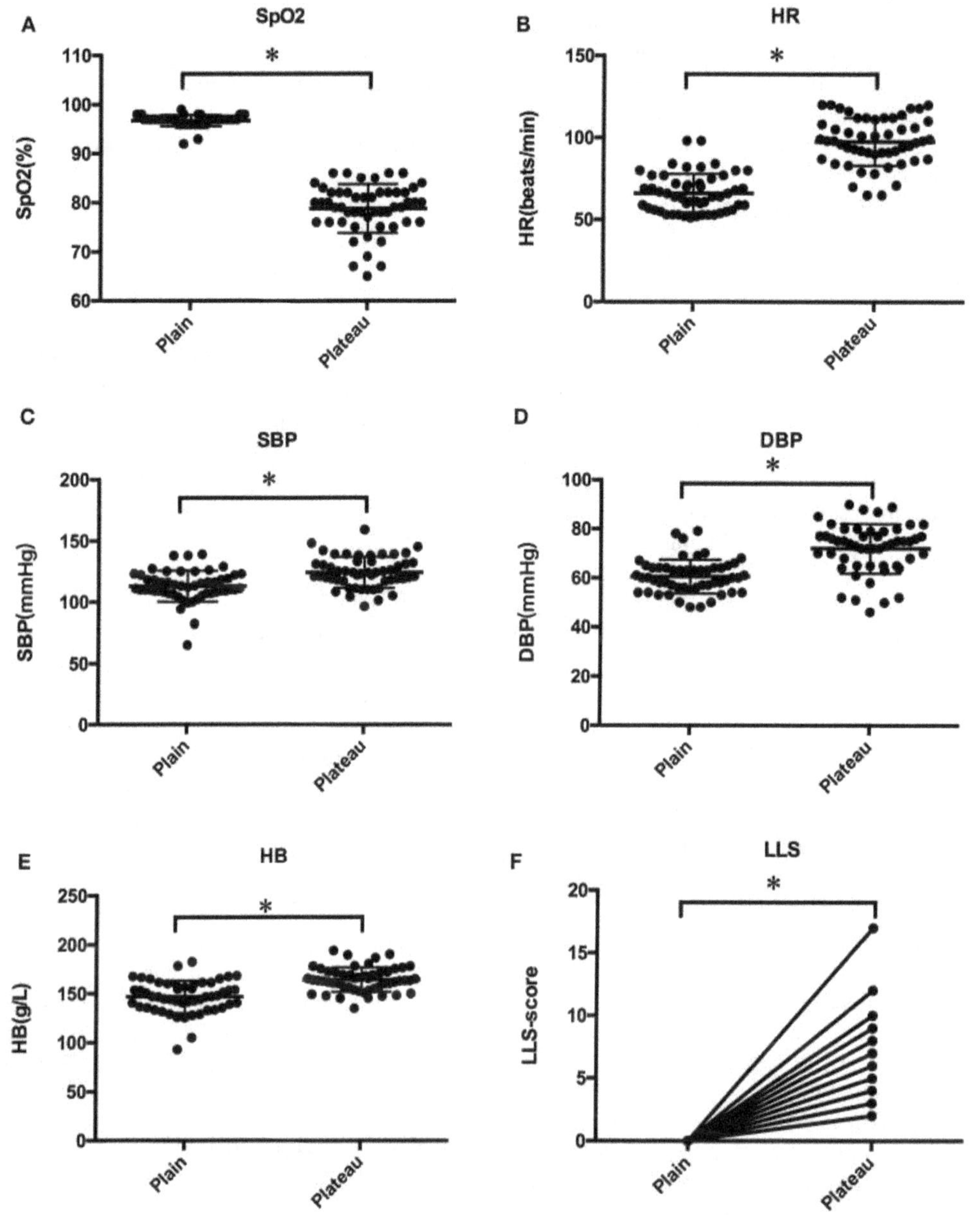

FIGURE 1 | Baseline clinical characteristics of SpO_2 **(A)**, HR **(B)**, SBP **(C)**, DBP **(D)**, HB **(E)**, and LLS **(F)** for enrolled subjects before and after high altitude exposure. Statistical significance is indicated as $^*p < 0.05$.

measurements, HR (**Figure 1B**), SBP (**Figure 1C**), DBP (**Figure 1D**), and HB (**Figure 1E**) increased along with hypoxia ($p < 0.05$), indicative of the comprehensive response manner to acute hypoxia stimuli. A significant increase in LLS was observed for all individuals (**Figure 1F**; $p < 0.05$).

Arachidonic Acid Metabolism Pathway Shows a Remarkable Correlation With Phenotypic Alterations After Hypoxia Exposure

Metabolomic analysis of blood samples from individuals before and after high altitude exposure revealed a total of 1,720 compounds. As indicated in **Figure 2A**, the method of WGCNA identified that four modules (MEgreen, MEred, MEmagenta, and MEblack) showed significant correlations with all clinical features of SBP, LBP, HR, SpO_2, LLS, and HB. To further explore influential metabolites in these modules, a volcano plot for these molecules was obtained (**Figure 2B**). At a cutoff point of $p < 0.05$, FC $\geq$ 1.5, and VIP > 1.5, a total of 36 metabolites showed significant alteration and comprised nine downregulated molecules and 27 elevated metabolites (**Table 1**). Moreover, the enrichment analysis demonstrated that AA metabolism pathway was particularly significant in the metabolic alterations in response to acute hypoxia (**Figure 2C**).

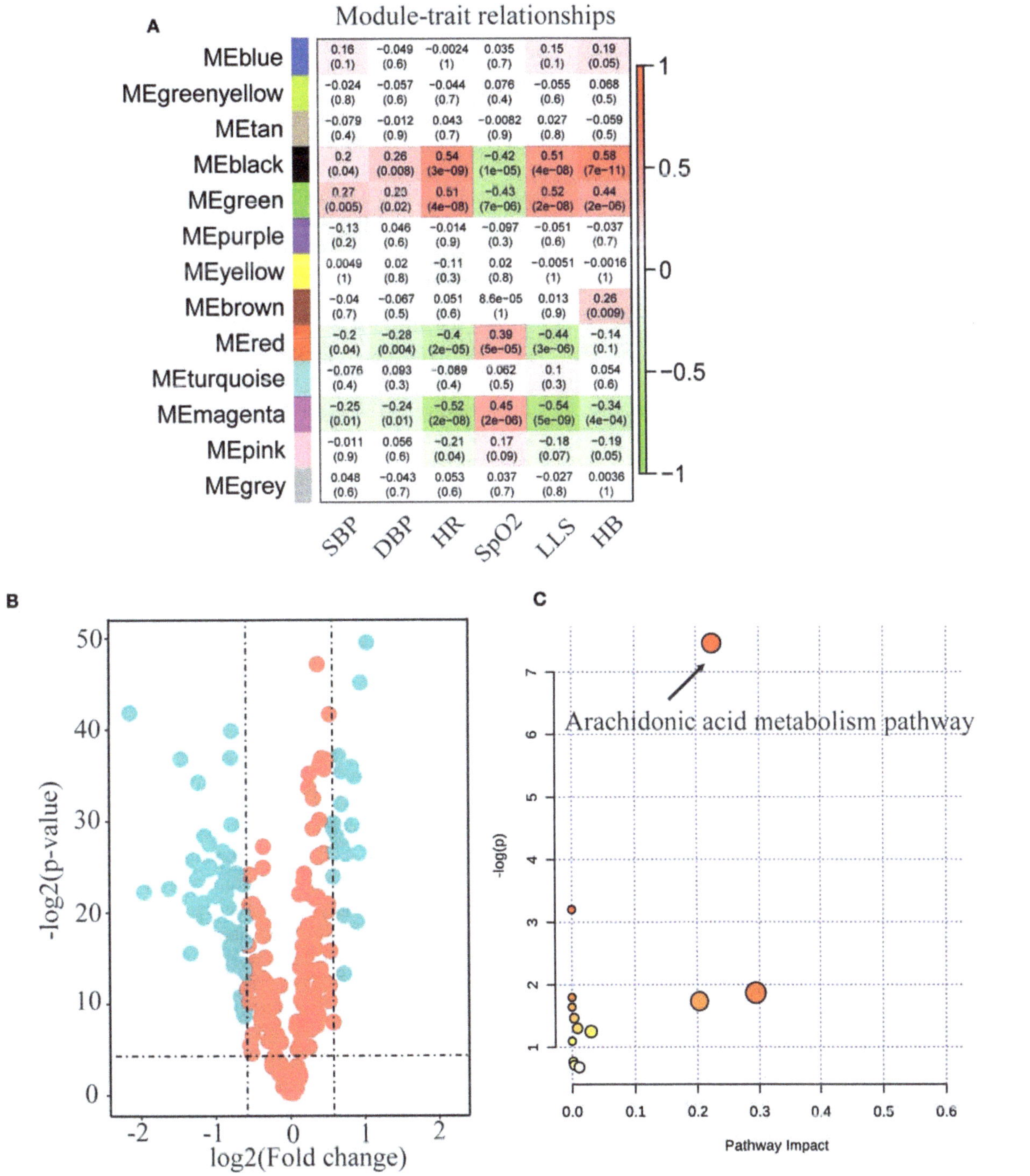

FIGURE 2 | Metabolic profiling analysis in response to acute hypoxia exposure. **(A)** WGCNA analysis identified four connectivity-based modules with high correlation to clinic features of heart rate (HR), oxygen saturation (SpO_2), Lake Louise score (LLS), systolic blood pressure (SBP), diastolic blood pressure (DBP), and hemoglobin (HB). High correlation values are indicated by red and negative correlations, in green color. **(B)** Comparison of all metabolites from plasma of subjects before and after hypoxia exposure. The volcano plot displays the relationship between fold change and significance using a scatter plot view. The green points in the plot represent the differential metabolites with statistical significance. **(C)** Enrichment pathway analysis for the dominant metabolites identified in the volcano plot before and after hypoxia exposure.

TABLE 1 | Summary of the influential metabolites in 53 subjects at high altitude relative to plain.

Metabolites	*P*-value	Fold change	VIP
12-Oxo-trihydroxy-leukotriene B4	2.04E-07	0.26	2.29
Bilirubin	1.57E-07	0.33	3.26
Undecanoylcarnitine	8.49E-12	0.37	1.75
15(S)-HETE	2.06E-05	0.40	1.85
Oleic acid	1.85E-08	0.41	4.47
L-Hexanoylcarnitine	8.01E-08	0.42	1.84
Ceramide (d18:1/16:0)	4.99E-11	0.43	2.20
15-Deoxy-d-12,14-PGJ2	4.84E-08	0.44	1.60
3, 5-Tetradecadiencarnitine	1.38E-06	0.45	2.33
20-Hydroxy-leukotriene E4	2.89E-09	0.45	1.57
Pimelylcarnitine	3.49E-08	0.48	2.23
3-hydroxydecanoyl carnitine	4.50E-09	0.48	2.25
9-Hexadecenoylcarnitine	5.37E-09	0.48	2.07
Dodecanoylcarnitine	2.75E-07	0.50	2.15
Decanoylcarnitine	2.35E-06	0.53	2.60
Tetradecanoylcarnitine	1.23E-07	0.54	1.73
trans-2-Dodecenoylcarnitine	2.80E-07	0.54	2.28
Linoleic acid	4.28E-08	0.55	4.33
DG(15:0/18:0/0:0)	2.29E-07	0.55	1.90
LysoPE(14:0/0:0)	1.35E-08	0.57	2.98
Palmitic acid	1.23E-05	0.57	2.87
N-methylphenylalanine	7.75E-12	0.58	1.55
Tiglylglycine	1.02E-12	0.58	2.93
21-Hydroxypregnenolone	8.95E-08	0.59	1.54
L-Octanoylcarnitine	5.25E-05	0.59	2.00
Arachidonic acid	1.17E-07	0.65	2.61
Alpha-Linolenic acid	8.90E-05	0.66	1.55
LysoPC(20:2)	6.82E-12	1.59	3.08
LysoPC(P-18:0)	2.57E-10	1.62	2.14
LysoPC(20:0)	6.09E-09	1.63	1.79
LysoPE(0:0/22:0)	2.17E-11	1.63	2.26
Stearoylcarnitine	1.22E-06	1.66	2.26
Glycocholic acid	1.14E-08	1.69	2.62
Deoxyinosine	3.28E-11	1.83	1.74
Deoxyribose 1-phosphate	1.92E-06	1.87	1.69
LysoPC(18:2(9Z,12Z))	1.23E-15	2.07	2.346

Integrative Network-Based Analysis Revealed Mechanisms of AA Metabolism Pathway

The physiological characteristics corresponding to SpO_2, HR, HB, LLS, SBP, and LBP for subjects evaluated by metabolomics and transcriptomics are listed in Supplemental Figure 1. These subjects chose for both omics detection, posed clinical features similar to those of the whole population after hypoxia stimuli. To provide a comprehensive interaction network between metabolomic and transcriptomic data sets, WGCNA was performed to identify connectivity-based modules comprising genes closely related to the aforementioned impact metabolites. As illustrated in **Figure 3A**, gene modules labeled by a violet frame were significantly correlated with these molecules, especially to metabolites of the AA metabolism pathway. As shown in **Figure 3B**, heme catabolism, gas transport, and porphyrin-related metabolism pathways were dominant in these gene modules after GO analysis ($p < 0.05$). To further clarify the mechanisms underlying the AA metabolism pathway after hypoxia exposure, genes with the highest connectivity from the co-expression network and a correlation coefficient >0.65 to at least one molecule among 13 metabolites in the AA metabolism pathway are circled in red in **Figure 3C**. These marked genes promoted proliferation and regulation of red blood cell metabolism. The detailed information is listed in **Figure 4**.

Detailed AA Metabolism Pathway Along With Hypoxia Stimuli

A map of metabolites in AA metabolism pathway was constructed in **Figure 4**. Alterations in these molecules before and after hypoxia exposure are listed in the blue box next to each metabolite. To elucidate the differences in subjects exhibiting diverse response patterns to hypoxia, these individuals were divided into two groups based on their LLS scores. Individuals with an LLS score lower than 4 were enrolled in the control group, while those with an LLS score higher than 9 were included in the group of mal-adaptation to hypoxia. Clinical characteristics of each group are listed in Supplemental Table 1. The metabolites exhibiting significant differences between control and mal-adjustment group are shown in the red box in **Figure 4**. As observed, the AA metabolism pathway was upregulated after hypoxia exposure and further elevated in those with poor response to hypoxia.

Validation of AA Metabolism Pathway in Another Dataset

We validated our findings in another population of GSE52209 from GEO database that comprised 14 subjects as the control group and 17 individuals suffering from mal-adaptation to high altitude. In comparison to individuals that adapted to hypoxia, those with poor response to acute hypoxia showed a significant upregulation ($p <$ 0.05, **Figure 5**) in the expression of genes such as *GGT1*, *PTGES*, *PTGS1*, *CBR1*, and *ALOX12* encoding key enzymes of the AA metabolism pathway. The effects of these genes on AA metabolism pathways are labeled with a yellow triangle in **Figure 4**.

DISCUSSION

Here, we performed an integrated analysis of metabolomic and transcriptomic expression profiling with the whole blood of individuals that experienced acute hypoxia. These approaches revealed pivotal roles of the AA metabolism pathway in the phenomenon of metabolic reprogramming during acute hypoxia exposure. Co-expression network analysis further identified that the AA metabolism pathway showed a significant positive correlation with transcriptional alterations, particularly with genes involved in porphyrin metabolism and gas transport pathways. Taken together, this is the first study to provide

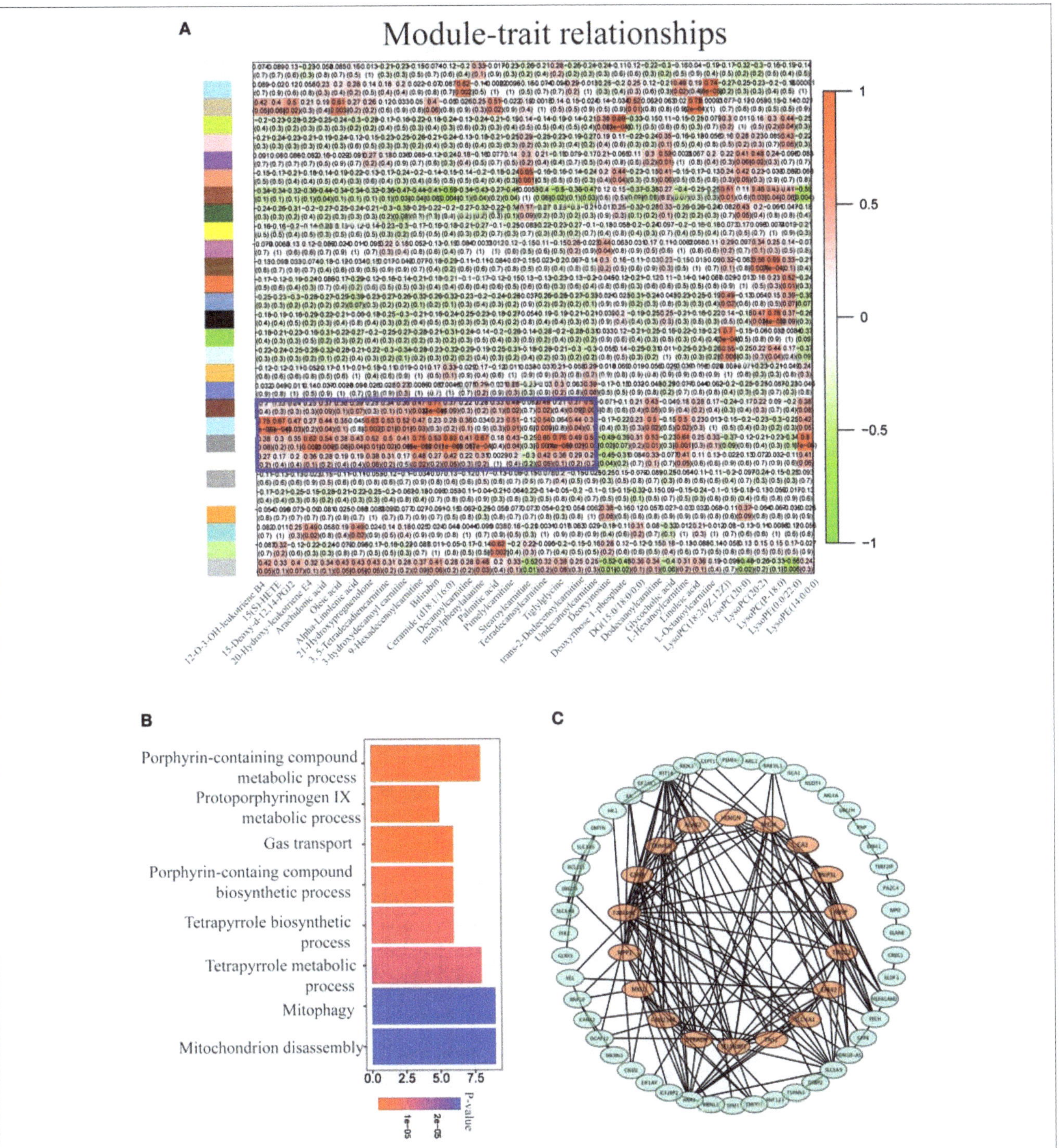

FIGURE 3 | Integrated analysis of metabolomic and transcriptomic profiling. **(A)** Unsupervised hierarchical cluster of correlation coefficients (kME and normalized metabolite values). High correlations are colored in red and low correlations, in green. **(B)** GO analysis for the modules inside the violet frame. **(C)** Network visualization of genes with high correlations to the AA metabolism pathway.

systematic changes in the AA metabolism pathway and reveal its potential mechanisms in response to hypoxia exposure.

We found an increase in the expression of molecules such as AA, prostaglandin A2 (PGA2), and cysteinyl leukotrienes (Cys-LTs) in AA metabolism pathway after hypoxia exposure. These molecules were important sources of pro-inflammatory mediators. The elevation in the inflammatory response and oxidative stress may be important in AMS pathogenesis (Boos et al., 2016; Liu et al., 2017a). AA has been demonstrated to activate p38 mitogen-activated protein kinase (MAPK) and

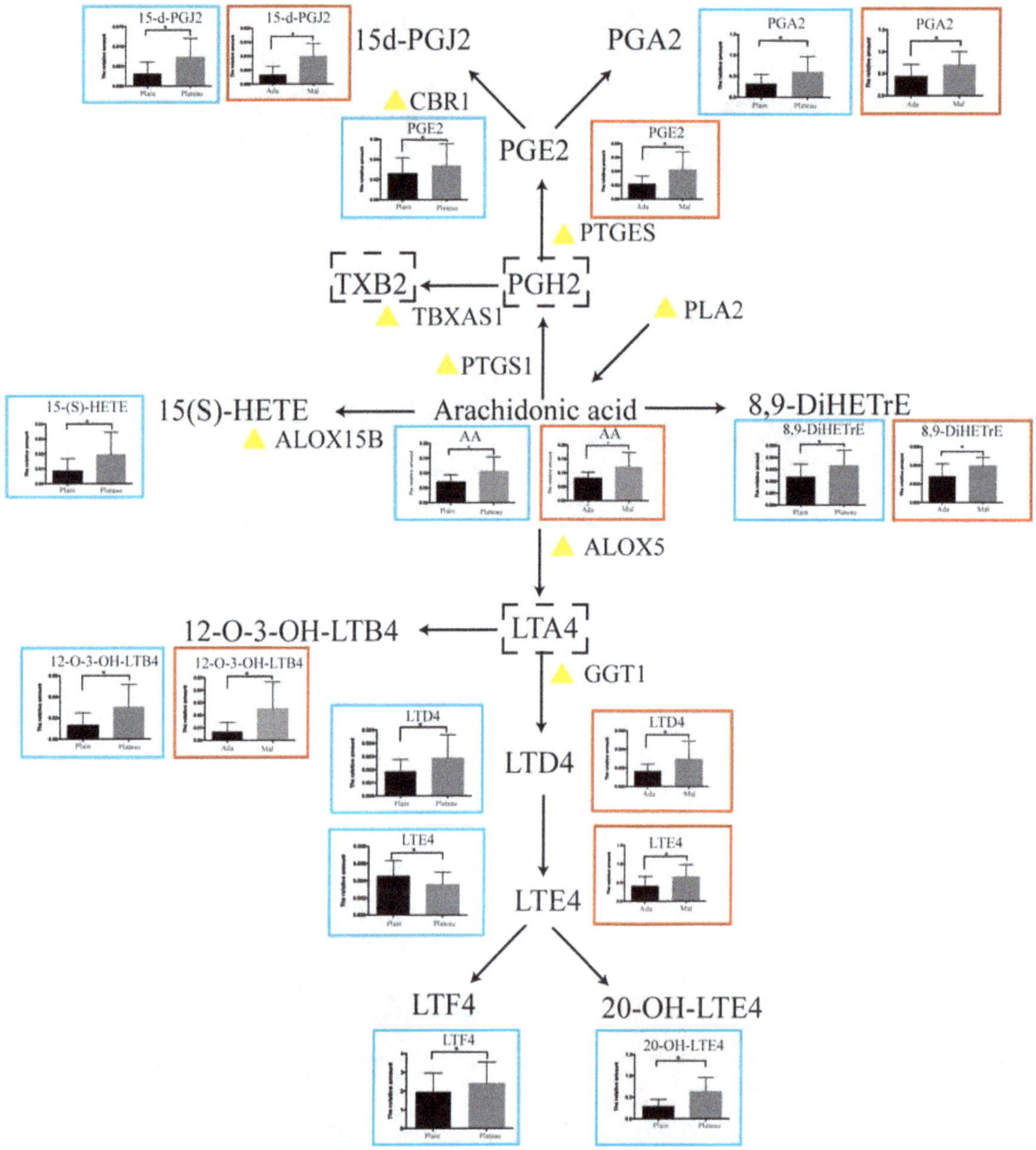

FIGURE 4 | Schematic overview of the AA metabolism pathway. The alterations in metabolites are shown in a blue frame (plain VS plateau), while the changes between adaptation(Ada) subjects and maladaptation(Mal) individuals to hypoxia are presented in a red box. The yellow triangle indicates the key enzymes validated in another cohort. The metabolites labeled by a dotted box represent no detection. Statistical significance is indicated as $^{*}p < 0.05$.

c-Jun N-terminal kinase (JNK), thereby directly promoting inflammation by increasing levels of tumor necrosis factor (TNF)-α (Saito et al., 2012). AA-derived metabolites such as leukotriene B4 (LTB4) and Cys–LTs from upregulated enzymes, including ALOX5 and GGT1, may operate as potent activators of and chemoattractants for leukocytes, eosinophils, and monocytes to propagate inflammation and oxidative stress (Rink and Khanna, 2011). Elevated PTGES may contribute to increased levels of PGE2 and PGA2, which activate IL-6 and nuclear factor kappa B (NF-κB) to promote vascular inflammation (Gomez et al., 2013). In addition to the biological effects of these metabolites, key enzymes in the AA metabolism pathway may directly trigger inflammation reactions and oxidative stress. Cyclooxygenase-2 (COX-2) contributes to the upregulation of TNF-α after hypoxia stimuli (Xing et al., 2015). The peroxidase activity of PTGS1 may serve as a source of oxygen radicals through the conversion of PGG2 to PGH2 by the removal of oxygen (Rink and Khanna, 2011). Moreover, phospholipase A2 may produce free radicals during the activation of arachidonic acid cascade under hypoxia environment (Tanaka et al., 2003).

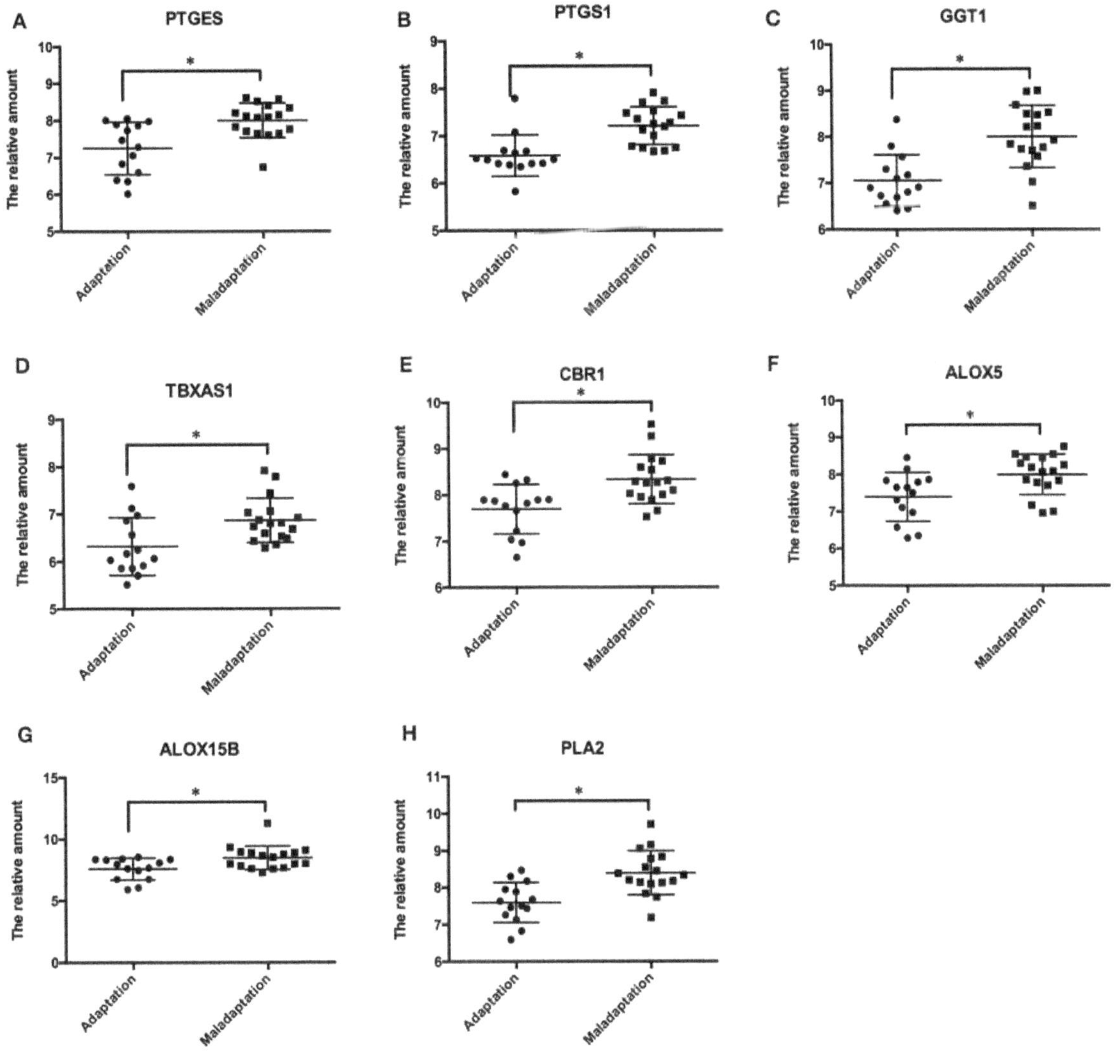

FIGURE 5 | Validation of the AA metabolism pathway in another cohort. The genes of PTGES **(A)**, PTGS1 **(B)**, GGT1 **(C)**, TBXAS1 **(D)**, CBR1 **(E)**, ALOX5 **(F)**, ALOX15B **(G)**, PLA2 **(H)** were significantly up-regulated in those who exhibited mal-adaptation to high altitude exposure. Statistical significance is indicated as $^{*}p < 0.05$.

With limited evidence focusing on the role of the AA metabolism pathway in the development of hypoxic diseases, our results systematically reveal the expression level of the AA metabolism pathway as well as its possible roles based on the AMS model and provide the basis for further research.

The increase in metabolites indicates the upregulation in sub-pathways activated by COX, lipoxygenase, and PLA2—the key enzymes of the AA metabolism pathway (Wong et al., 2003; Jantan et al., 2014). In line with previous studies, these proteins showed a hypoxia-regulated pattern. A recent study demonstrated that hypoxia-mediated extracellular signal-regulated kinase (ERK) activation may induce the activity of PLA2 in the erythrocyte membrane (Wu et al., 2016). In addition, as an essential oxygen-sensing molecule, heme oxygenase-1 was reported to act as an important mediator of transcription and translation of 15-lipoxygenase to promote lipoxins (Nie et al., 2013). Hypoxia-inducible factor-1 alpha (HIF-1a) was reported to directly stimulate COX enzymes after hypoxia exposure (Huang et al., 2016). However, we failed to detect the quantitative expression of the key enzymes in the AA metabolism pathway, owing to the limited blood sample during validation. An intervention experiment with drugs targeting the AA metabolism pathway in larger population samples is now being conducted by our group to verify these findings and search for effective prevention measures.

In our study, we demonstrated a crosstalk between response manners to acute hypoxia and expression level of the AA metabolism pathway. The excessive increase in the AA metabolism pathway after hypoxia stimuli may reflect mal-adaptation to hypoxia stimuli, as evident from the elevated levels of HR, HB, and LLS as well as the decreased level of SpO_2. These observations suggest impaired cardiopulmonary and hemoglobin function (Fuehrer and Huecker, 2017). For cardiopulmonary performance, the addition of AA was shown to aggravate respiration inhibition and decrease oxygen consumption at the mitochondrial level (Egorova et al., 2015), while targeting COX-2 improved hemodynamic parameters of cardiac output, left ventricular pressure, and LV*dp*/*dt* (Oshima et al., 2006). AA metabolism was also reported to influence heart rates by alerting histaminergic system (Altinbas et al., 2014). In addition, the elevated level of reactive oxygen species during AA metabolism was involved in the regulation of erythroid differentiation, and the activation of phospholipase A2 was shown to induce protein kinase C to increase erythrogenin level (Luo et al., 2017) (Mason-Garcia and Beckman, 1991). Furthermore, the process of reticulocyte maturation was dependent on phospholipase A2 during the remodeling of the plasma membrane by the removal of specific proteins (Blanc et al., 2007). As an irreversible pathological process with poor clinical outcomes caused by sustained hypoxia, elevated AA metabolism pathway may decrease the apoptosis of endothelial cells, induce the proliferation of pulmonary artery smooth muscle cells, activate angiogenesis, and influence the arterial vascular tonicity via K+ channels (Park et al., 2011; Zhang et al., 2011; Liu et al., 2012; Zhu and Ran, 2012; Pang et al., 2016). An excessive elevation in AA metabolism may result in poor response to acute hypoxia and even worse symptoms under chronic hypoxia environment.

The protective effects of anti-inflammatory molecules are increasingly recognized for the prevention of AMS. Apigenin targeting IL-1β, IL-6, and TNF-α was demonstrated to be effective in reducing the damage caused by acute hypoxia (Du et al., 2015). Recent pilot studies reported that ibuprofen, aspirin, and dexamethasone may be effective for the prevention and treatment of AMS, especially the syndrome of headache, although the underlying mechanisms remain largely unknown (Burtscher et al., 2001; Gertsch et al., 2012; Xiong et al., 2017). In this study, our results theoretically support anti-inflammatory drugs such as non-steroidal anti-inflammatory drugs (NSAIDS) and dexamethasone targeting the AA metabolism pathway for improving clinical symptoms of AMS. In addition, targeted therapies against specific enzymes or metabolites of the AA metabolism pathway may be beneficial in AMS prevention and demand further studies (Atluri et al., 2011). Given its close relationship with hemoglobin metabolism genes, the AA metabolism pathway may be an effective target for the prevention of hypoxia-induced erythrocytosis (Foley et al., 1978; Parise et al., 1991).

In summary, our integrated analysis of metabolomic and transcriptomic profiling revealed that the AA metabolism pathway was one of the most pivotal alterations after acute hypoxia exposure and may account for variations in response patterns to hypoxia stimuli. The detailed description of the AA metabolism pathway may offer the basis for follow-up mechanisms and drug screening.

AUTHOR CONTRIBUTIONS

YG and JC: Conceived and designed the study; CL and BL: Oversaw laboratory analyses and contributed the statistical analysis; LL, E-LZ, and BS: Contributed to sample and physical data collections; CL: Drafted the report. All authors reviewed and approved the manuscript.

ACKNOWLEDGMENTS

This work was supported by the Key Projects in the Military Science & Technology Pillar Program during the Thirteen 5-year Plan Period (AWS14C007&AWS16J023), by National Natural Science Foundation of China (J1310001).

REFERENCES

Acharjee, A., Kloosterman, B., Visser, R. G., and Maliepaard, C. (2016). Integration of multi-omics data for prediction of phenotypic traits using random forest. *BMC Bioinformatics* 17(Suppl. 5):180. doi: 10.1186/s12859-016-1043-4

Altinbas, B., Topuz, B. B., Ilhan, T., Yilmaz, M. S., Erdost, H., and Yalcin, M. (2014). Activation of the central histaminergic system mediates arachidonic-acid-induced cardiovascular effects. *Can. J. Physiol. Pharmacol.* 92, 645–654. doi: 10.1139/cjpp-2014-0043

Atluri, D. K., Prakash, R., and Mullen, K. D. (2011). Pathogenesis, diagnosis, and treatment of hepatic encephalopathy. *J. Clin. Exp. Hepatol.* 1, 77–86. doi: 10.1016/S0973-6883(11)60126-6

Bennett, M., and Gilroy, D. W. (2016). Lipid mediators in inflammation. *Microbiol. Spectr.* 4. doi: 10.1128/microbiolspec.MCHD-0035-2016

Blanc, L., Barres, C., Bette-Bobillo, P., and Vidal, M. (2007). Reticulocyte-secreted exosomes bind natural IgM antibodies: involvement of a ROS-activatable endosomal phospholipase iPLA2. *Blood* 110, 3407–3416. doi: 10.1182/blood-2007-04-085845

Bogatcheva, N. V., Sergeeva, M. G., Dudek, S. M., and Verin, A. D. (2005). Arachidonic acid cascade in endothelial pathobiology. *Microvasc. Res.* 69, 107–127. doi: 10.1016/j.mvr.2005.01.007

Boos, C. J., Woods, D. R., Varias, A., Biscocho, S., Heseltine, P., and Mellor, A. J. (2016). high altitude and acute mountain sickness and changes in circulating Endothelin-1, Interleukin-6, and Interleukin-17a. *High Alt. Med. Biol.* 17, 25–31. doi: 10.1089/ham.2015.0098

Burtscher, M., Likar, R., Nachbauer, W., Philadelphy, M., Pühringer, R., and Lämmle, T. (2001). Effects of aspirin during exercise on the incidence of high-altitude headache: a randomized, double-blind, placebo-controlled trial. *Headache* 41, 542–545. doi: 10.1046/j.1526-4610.2001.041006542.x

D'Alessandro, A., Nemkov, T., Sun, K., Liu, H., Song, A., Monte, A. A., et al. (2016). AltitudeOmics: red blood cell metabolic adaptation to high altitude hypoxia. *J. Proteome Res.* 15, 3883–3895. doi: 10.1021/acs.jproteome.6b00733

Du, H., Hao, J., Liu, F., Lu, J., and Yang, X. (2015). Apigenin attenuates acute myocardial infarction of rats via the inhibitions of matrix metalloprotease-9 and inflammatory reactions. *Int. J. Clin. Exp. Med.* 8, 8854–8859.

Egorova, M. V., Kutsykova, T. V., Afanas'ev, S. A., and Popov, S. V. (2015). Effect of arachidonic acid on the rate of oxygen consumption in isolated cardiomyocytes from intact rats and animals with ischemic or diabetic injury to the heart. *Bull. Exp. Biol. Med.* 160, 190–192. doi: 10.1007/s10517-015-3124-1

Foley, J. E., Gross, D. M., Nelson, P. K., and Fisher, J. W. (1978). The effects of arachidonic acid on erythropoietin production in exhypoxic polycythemic mice and the isolated perfused canine kidney. *J. Pharmacol. Exp. Ther.* 207, 402–409.

Fuehrer, J., and Huecker, M. R. (2017). *Altitude Illness, High Altitude Cardiopulmonary Diseases.* Treasure Island: FL: StatPearls.

Gertsch, J. H., Corbett, B., Holck, P. S., Mulcahy, A., Watts, M., Stillwagon, N. T., et al. (2012). Altitude sickness in climbers and efficacy of NSAIDs trial (ASCENT): randomized, controlled trial of ibuprofen versus placebo for prevention of altitude illness. *Wilderness Environ. Med.* 23, 307–315. doi: 10.1016/j.wem.2012.08.001

Gomez, I., Foudi, N., Longrois, D., and Norel, X. (2013). The role of prostaglandin E2 in human vascular inflammation. *Prostaglandins Leukot. Essent. Fatty Acids* 89, 55–63. doi: 10.1016/j.plefa.2013.04.004

Gonggalanzi, Labasangzhu, Nafstad, P., Stigum, H., Wu, T., Haldorsen, Ø. D., et al. (2016). Acute mountain sickness among tourists visiting the high-altitude city of Lhasa at 3658 m above sea level: a cross-sectional study. *Arch. Public Health* 74:23. doi: 10.1186/s13690-016-0134-z

Huang, M., Wang, L., Chen, J., Bai, M., Zhou, C., Liu, S., et al. (2016). Regulation of COX-2 expression and epithelial-to-mesenchymal transition by hypoxia-inducible factor-1α is associated with poor prognosis in hepatocellular carcinoma patients post TACE surgery. *Int. J. Oncol.* 48, 2144–2154. doi: 10.3892/ijo.2016.3421

Jantan, I., Bukhari, S. N., Adekoya, O. A., and Sylte, I. (2014). Studies of synthetic chalcone derivatives as potential inhibitors of secretory phospholipase A2, cyclooxygenases, lipoxygenase and pro-inflammatory cytokines. *Drug Des. Devel. Ther.* 8, 1405–1418. doi: 10.2147/DDDT.S67370

Johnson, N. J., and Luks, A. M. (2016). High-altitude medicine. *Med. Clin. North Am.* 100, 357–369. doi: 10.1016/j.mcna.2015.09.002

Kan, M., Shumyatcher, M., and Himes, B. E. (2017). Using omics approaches to understand pulmonary diseases. *Respir. Res.* 18:149. doi: 10.1186/s12931-017-0631-9

Li, B., Bi, C. L., Lang, N., Li, Y. Z., Xu, C., Zhang, Y. Q., et al. (2014). RNA-seq methods for identifying differentially expressed gene in human pancreatic islet cells treated with pro-inflammatory cytokines. *Mol. Biol. Rep.* 41, 1917–1925. doi: 10.1007/s11033-013-3016-2

Li, S., Todor, A., and Luo, R. (2016). Blood transcriptomics and metabolomics for personalized medicine. *Comput. Struct. Biotechnol. J.* 14, 1–7. doi: 10.1016/j.csbj.2015.10.005

Liao, W. T., Liu, B., Chen, J., Cui, J. H., Gao, Y. X., Liu, F. Y., et al. (2016). Metabolite modulation in human plasma in the early phase of acclimatization to hypobaric hypoxia. *Sci. Rep.* 6:22589. doi: 10.1038/srep22589

Liu, B., Chen, J., Zhang, L., Gao, Y., Cui, J., Zhang, E., et al. (2017a). IL-10 dysregulation in acute mountain sickness revealed by transcriptome analysis. *Front. Immunol.* 8:628. doi: 10.3389/fimmu.2017.00628

Liu, X., Hu, A. X., Zhao, J. L., and Chen, F. L. (2017b). Identification of key gene modules in human osteosarcoma by co-expression analysis weighted gene co-expression network analysis (WGCNA). *J. Cell. Biochem.* 118, 3953–3959. doi: 10.1002/jcb.26050

Liu, Y., Ma, C., Zhang, Q., Yu, L., Ma, J., Zhang, L., et al. (2012). The key role of transforming growth factor-beta receptor I and 15-lipoxygenase in hypoxia-induced proliferation of pulmonary artery smooth muscle cells. *Int. J. Biochem. Cell Biol.* 44, 1184–1202. doi: 10.1016/j.biocel.2012.04.009

Luo, S. T., Zhang, D. M., Qin, Q., Lu, L., Luo, M., Guo, F. C., et al. (2017). The promotion of erythropoiesis via the regulation of reactive oxygen species by lactic acid. *Sci. Rep.* 7:38105. doi: 10.1038/srep38105

Mason-Garcia, M., and Beckman, B. S. (1991). Signal transduction in erythropoiesis. *FASEB J.* 5, 2958–2964. doi: 10.1096/fasebj.5.14.1752362

Michiels, C. (2004). Physiological and pathological responses to hypoxia. *Am. J. Pathol.* 164, 1875–1882. doi: 10.1016/S0002-9440(10)63747-9

Netzer, N. C., Rausch, L., Eliasson, A. H., Gatterer, H., Friess, M., Burtscher, M., et al. (2017). SpO2 and heart rate during a real hike at altitude are significantly different than at its simulation in normobaric hypoxia. *Front. Physiol.* 8:81. doi: 10.3389/fphys.2017.00081

Nie, X., Hui, Y., Shi, S., Ma, J., Wang, S., Qiu, Z., et al. (2013). Heme oxygenase-1 induces 15-lipoxygenase expression during hypoxia-induced pulmonary hypertension. *Int. J. Biochem. Cell Biol.* 45, 964–972. doi: 10.1016/j.biocel.2013.01.017

Oshima, K., Takeyoshi, I., Tsutsumi, H., Mohara, J., Ohki, S., Koike, N., et al. (2006). Inhibition of cyclooxygenase-2 improves cardiac function following long-term preservation. *J. Surg. Res.* 135, 380–384 doi. 10.1016/j.jss.2006.03.044

Pang, L., Cai, Y., Tang, E. H., Yan, D., Kosuru, R., Li, H., et al. (2016). Cox-2 inhibition protects against hypoxia/reoxygenation-induced cardiomyocyte apoptosis via Akt-dependent enhancement of iNOS expression. *Oxid. Med. Cell. Longev.* 2016:3453059. doi: 10.1155/2016/3453059

Parise, P., Huybrechts, E., Grasselli, S., Falcinelli, F., Nenci, G. G., Gresele, P., et al. (1991). Generation of arachidonic acid metabolites from stimulated whole blood in patients with chronic myeloproliferative disorders. *Acta Haematol.* 85, 88–92. doi: 10.1159/000204863

Park, S. J., Yoo, H. Y., Earm, Y. E., Kim, S. J., Kim, J. K., and Kim, S. D. (2011). Role of arachidonic acid-derived metabolites in the control of pulmonary arterial pressure and hypoxic pulmonary vasoconstriction in rats. *Br. J. Anaesth.* 106, 31–37. doi: 10.1093/bja/aeq268

Rink, C., and Khanna, S. (2011). Significance of brain tissue oxygenation and the arachidonic acid cascade in stroke. *Antioxid. Redox Signal.* 14, 1889–1903. doi: 10.1089/ars.2010.3474

Ritchie, M. E., Phipson, B., Wu, D., Hu, Y., Law, C. W., Shi, W., et al. (2015). Limma powers differential expression analyses for RNA-sequencing and microarray studies. *Nucleic Acids Res.* 43:e47. doi: 10.1093/nar/gkv007

Saito, Y., Watanabe, K., Fujioka, D., Nakamura, T., Obata, J. E., Kawabata, K., et al. (2012). Disruption of group IVA cytosolic phospholipase A(2) attenuates myocardial ischemia-reperfusion injury partly through inhibition of TNF-α-mediated pathway. *Am. J. Physiol. Heart Circ. Physiol.* 302, H2018–H2030. doi: 10.1152/ajpheart.00955.2011

Smoot, M. E., Ono, K., Ruscheinski, J., Wang, P. L., and Ideker, T. (2011). Cytoscape 2.8: new features for data integration and network visualization. *Bioinformatics* 27, 431–432. doi: 10.1093/bioinformatics/btq675

Subudhi, A. W., Panerai, R. B., and Roach, R. C. (2010). Effects of hypobaric hypoxia on cerebral autoregulation. *Stroke* 41, 641–646. doi: 10.1161/STROKEAHA.109.574749

Sun, K., Liu, H., Song, A., Manalo, J. M., D'Alessandro, A., Hansen, K. C., et al. (2017). Erythrocyte purinergic signaling components underlie hypoxia adaptation. *J. Appl. Physiol* 123, 951–956. doi: 10.1152/japplphysiol.00155.2017

Sun, Y. V., and Hu, Y. J. (2016). Integrative analysis of multi-omics data for discovery and functional studies of complex human diseases. *Adv. Genet.* 93, 147–190. doi: 10.1016/bs.adgen.2015.11.004

Tanaka, E., Niiyama, S., Sato, S., Yamada, A., and Higashi, H. (2003). Arachidonic acid metabolites contribute to the irreversible depolarization induced by *in vitro* ischemia. *J. Neurophysiol.* 90, 3213–3223. doi: 10.1152/jn.00542.2003

Wong, R. K., Pettit, A. I., Quinn, P. A., Jennings, S. C., Davies, J. E., and Ng, L. L. (2003). Advanced glycation end products stimulate an enhanced neutrophil respiratory burst mediated through the activation of cytosolic phospholipase A2 and generation of Arachidonic acid. *Circulation* 108, 1858–1864. doi: 10.1161/01.CIR.0000089372.64585.3B

Wu, H., Bogdanov, M., Zhang, Y., Sun, K., Zhao, S., Song, A., et al. (2016). Hypoxia-mediated impaired erythrocyte lands' cycle is pathogenic for sickle cell disease. *Sci. Rep.* 6:29637. doi: 10.1038/srep29637

Xing, Y., Wang, R., Chen, D., Mao, J., Shi, R., Wu, Z., et al. (2015). COX2 is involved in hypoxia-induced TNF-α expression in osteoblast. *Sci. Rep.* 5:10020. doi: 10.1038/srep10020

Xiong, J., Lu, H., Wang, R., and Jia, Z. (2017). Efficacy of ibuprofen on prevention of high altitude headache: a systematic review and meta-analysis. *PLoS ONE* 12:e0179788. doi: 10.1371/journal.pone.0179788

Yu, G., Wang, L. G., Han, Y., and He, Q. Y. (2012). clusterProfiler: an R package for comparing biological themes among gene clusters. *OMICS* 16, 284–287. doi: 10.1089/omi.2011.0118

Zhang, Q., Wang, D., Singh, N. K., Kundumani-Sridharan, V., Gadiparthi, L., Rao Ch, M., et al. (2011). Activation of cytosolic phospholipase A2 downstream of the Src-phospholipase D1 (PLD1)-protein kinase C gamma (PKCgamma) signaling axis is required for hypoxia-induced pathological retinal angiogenesis. *J. Biol. Chem.* 286, 22489–22498. doi: 10.1074/jbc.M110.217786

Zhu, D., and Ran, Y. (2012). Role of 15-lipoxygenase/15-hydroxyeicosatetraenoic acid in hypoxia-induced pulmonary hypertension. *J. Physiol. Sci.* 62, 163–172. doi: 10.1007/s12576-012-0196-9

3

Skeletal Muscle Pyruvate Dehydrogenase Phosphorylation and Lactate Accumulation during Sprint Exercise in Normoxia and Severe Acute Hypoxia: Effects of Antioxidants

*David Morales-Alamo[1,2], Borja Guerra[1,2], Alfredo Santana[2,3], Marcos Martin-Rincon[1,2], Miriam Gelabert-Rebato[1,2], Cecilia Dorado[1,2] and José A. L. Calbet[1,2]**

[1] Department of Physical Education, University of Las Palmas de Gran Canaria, Las Palmas de Gran Canaria, Spain,
[2] Research Institute of Biomedical and Health Sciences, Las Palmas de Gran Canaria, Spain, [3] Clinical Genetics Unit, Complejo Hospitalario Universitario Insular-Materno Infantil de Las Palmas de Gran Canaria, Las Palmas de Gran Canaria, Spain

***Correspondence:**
José A. L. Calbet
lopezcalbet@gmail.com

Compared to normoxia, during sprint exercise in severe acute hypoxia the glycolytic rate is increased leading to greater lactate accumulation, acidification, and oxidative stress. To determine the role played by pyruvate dehydrogenase (PDH) activation and reactive nitrogen and oxygen species (RNOS) in muscle lactate accumulation, nine volunteers performed a single 30-s sprint (Wingate test) on four occasions: two after the ingestion of placebo and another two following the intake of antioxidants, while breathing either hypoxic gas (P_IO_2 = 75 mmHg) or room air (P_IO_2 = 143 mmHg). *Vastus lateralis* muscle biopsies were obtained before, immediately after, 30 and 120 min post-sprint. Antioxidants reduced the glycolytic rate without altering performance or VO_2. Immediately after the sprints, Ser^{293}- and Ser^{300}-PDH-E1α phosphorylations were reduced to similar levels in all conditions (~66 and 91%, respectively). However, 30 min into recovery Ser^{293}-PDH-E1α phosphorylation reached pre-exercise values while Ser^{300}-PDH-E1α was still reduced by 44%. Thirty minutes after the sprint Ser^{293}-PDH-E1α phosphorylation was greater with antioxidants, resulting in 74% higher muscle lactate concentration. Changes in Ser^{293} and Ser^{300}-PDH-E1α phosphorylation from pre to immediately after the sprints were linearly related after placebo ($r = 0.74$, $P < 0.001$; $n = 18$), but not after antioxidants ingestion ($r = 0.35$, $P = 0.15$). In summary, lactate accumulation during sprint exercise in severe acute hypoxia is not caused by a reduced activation of the PDH. The ingestion of antioxidants is associated with increased PDH re-phosphorylation and slower elimination of muscle lactate during the recovery period. Ser^{293} re-phosphorylates at a faster rate than Ser^{300}-PDH-E1α during the recovery period, suggesting slightly different regulatory mechanisms.

Keywords: sprint exercise, skeletal muscle, hypoxia, human, oxidative stress, pyruvate dehydrogenase, PDH

INTRODUCTION

During sprint exercise in normoxia lactate accumulates in the recruited skeletal muscles (Jones et al., 1985; Cheetham et al., 1986; Parolin et al., 1999; Morales-Alamo et al., 2012), indicating that the flux through the pyruvate dehydrogenase (PDH) is not sufficient to avoid pyruvate accumulation and its corresponding reduction to lactate (Howlett et al., 1999). Compared to sprint exercise in normoxia, sprint exercise in severe acute hypoxia is accompanied by increased lactate accumulation (McLellan et al., 1990; Morales-Alamo et al., 2012) and greater reactive nitrogen and oxygen species (RNOS) production and more oxidative stress (Cuevas et al., 2005; Morales-Alamo et al., 2012; Morales-Alamo and Calbet, 2014). Animal experiments have shown that excessive RNOS production may reduce PDH activity (Churchill et al., 2005). It remains unknown whether the increased lactate production during sprint exercise in severe acute hypoxia is due, at least in part, to reduced activation of PDH.

Putman et al. (1995) showed that during repeated 30-s isokinetic sprints in normoxia lactate production was not dependent on O_2 delivery. However, we have recently shown that during the last 15 s of a 30-s isokinetic sprint in severe acute hypoxia skeletal muscle VO_2 is indeed limited by O_2 delivery (Calbet et al., 2015). Moreover, during submaximal exercise at 55% of the VO_2max in acute hypoxia (F_iO_2: = 0.11), the level of PDH activation after 1 min cycling was lower than in normoxia (Parolin et al., 2000).

Increased acidification during exercise in hypoxia may reduce nicotinamide adenine dinucleotide phosphate-oxidase 2 (NOX2) activity, which is considered the main source of ion superoxide production during exercise (Simchowitz, 1985; Morgan et al., 2005; Brennan-Minnella et al., 2015), particularly during brief periods (10–15 min) of contractile activity (Jackson, 2015). Superoxide stimulates Ca^{2+} efflux through the ryanodine receptors of the sarcoendoplasmic reticulum (Jackson et al., 2007; Dulhunty et al., 2017). The increased (Ca^{2+}) in the sarcoplasm is necessary for the activation of PDH phosphatases, which dephosphorylate and activate PDH (Hucho et al., 1972; Wieland, 1983; Behal et al., 1993) (**Figure 1**). Thus, the increased muscle acidification during sprint exercise in hypoxia may reduce PDH activation by at least four mechanisms: (1) by decreasing Ca^{2+} efflux from the sarcoplasmic reticulum (Bailey et al., 2007; Dulhunty et al., 2017), (2) by inducing the activation of pyruvate dehydrogenase kinase (PDK) (Churchill et al., 2005; Wu et al., 2013), (3) by causing oxidative damage to the enzyme (Tabatabaie et al., 1996), and (4) by reducing PDH phosphatase activity (Radak et al., 2013). In the case of an inhibitory influence of exercise-induced RNOS on PDH activation, the ingestion of antioxidants before sprint exercise should enhance PDH dephosphorylation and activation, leading to lower accumulation of lactate.

Pyruvate dehydrogenase is activated by dephosphorylation of serine residues (Ser^{232}, Ser^{293}, Ser^{300}) located in the E1α subunit of PDH (Yeaman et al., 1978) (**Figure 1**). The balance between the activities of pyruvate dehydrogenase kinases (PDKs) and PDH phosphatases (PDP) determines the degree of PDH activation (Hucho et al., 1972; Wieland, 1983; Behal et al., 1993).

Therefore, the main aim of this study was to determine whether PDH activation, as determined by the assessment of its phosphorylation level, is reduced during sprint exercise in hypoxia compared to the same exercise performed in normoxia. Another aim was to ascertain whether antioxidants administration immediately before a sprint exercise in normoxia or hypoxia influences PDH activity during the subsequent recovery period.

MATERIALS AND METHODS

Subjects

Initially, 10 healthy male physical education students agreed to participate in this investigation, but completed data for all conditions were obtained in nine of them (age = 25 ± 5 year, height = 176.0 ± 5.1 cm, body mass = 79.4 ± 10.1 kg, body fat = 18.3 ± 6.7%, **Table 1**). The study was performed in accordance with the Declaration of Helsinki and was approved by the Ethical Committee of the University of Las Palmas de Gran Canaria (CEIH-2010-01). All subjects signed a written informed consent before entering the study.

General Procedures

Body composition was determined by dual-energy x-ray absorptiometry (Hologic QDR-1500, Hologic Corp., software version 7.10, Waltham, MA) as described elsewhere (Calbet et al., 1998). After familiarization, subjects reported to the laboratory to complete different tests on separate days. First their peak VO_2 (VO_2peak), maximal heart rate (HRmax) and maximal power output (Wmax) were determined in normoxia (F_IO_2: 0.21, P_IO_2: 143 mmHg) and severe acute hypoxia (F_IO_2: 0.105, P_IO_2: 75 mmHg) with an incremental exercise test to exhaustion (50 W/min), as previously described (Morales-Alamo et al., 2012, 2013, 2017). Hemoglobin oxygen saturation (SpO_2) was determined with a finger pulse oximeter (OEMIII module, 4549-000, Plymouth, MN). The main experiments consisted on a single 30-s isokinetic sprint at 100 revolutions per minute (Wingate Test) repeated on 4 different days, at least 1 week apart. The Wingate tests were carried out in normoxia (F_IO_2: 0.21, P_IO_2: 143 mmHg) and acute hypoxia (F_IO_2: 0.105, P_IO_2: 75 mmHg), both preceded by the ingestion of either placebo (200 mg of starch from corn, Sigma-Aldrich, ref. 14302) or antioxidants, with a double-blind design. Both the placebo and the antioxidants were introduced in microcrystalline cellulose capsules of identical characteristics.

Antioxidant supplements were administered in two doses separated by 30 min, with the first dose ingested 2 h before the sprint exercise, as previously reported (Morales-Alamo et al., 2017). The first dose contained 300 mg of α-lipoic acid, 500 mg vitamin C, and 200 IU vitamin E, whereas the second included 300 mg α-lipoic acid, 500 mg vitamin C, and 400 IU vitamin E (water dispersible). This antioxidant cocktail effectively decreases free radicals levels in blood as demonstrated by paramagnetic spin spectroscopy in humans (Richardson et al., 2007). We assume that similar effects were achieved in skeletal muscle as reflected by two facts. Firstly, these antioxidants blunted the RNOS-mediated signaling response elicited by sprint exercise

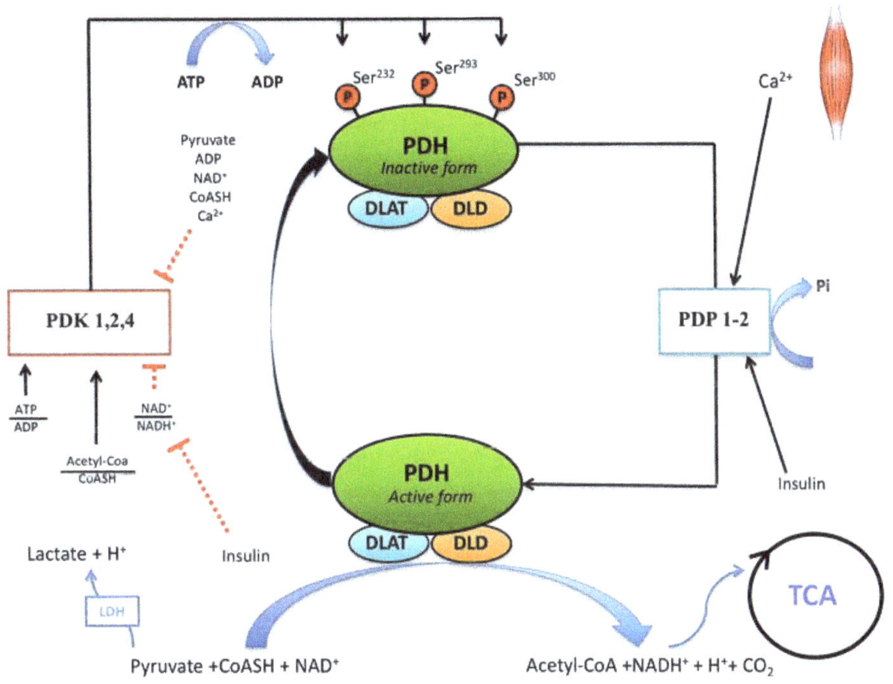

FIGURE 1 | Regulation of pyruvate dehydrogenase (PDH) activity in skeletal muscle. Pyruvate dehydrogenase complex (PDC) is regulated by phosphorylation and dephosphorylation by pyruvate dehydrogenase kinase (PDK) and pyruvate dehydrogenase phosphatase (PDP), respectively. PDC catalyzes the irreversible decarboxylation of pyruvate to Acetyl-CoA, which can be oxidized through the tricarboxylic acid cycle (TCA). DLAT, dihydrolipoamide S-acetyltransferase; DLD, dihydrolipoamide dehydrogenase; ATP, adenosine triphosphate; ADP, adenosine diphosphate; NAD, nicotinamide adenine dinucleotide; NADH, nicotinamide adenine dinucleotide reduced; CoASH, coenzyme A.

and, secondly, attenuated the formation of protein carbonyls in this study, as previously reported (Morales-Alamo et al., 2013, 2017).

The experimental days subjects reported to the laboratory early in the morning after a 12 h overnight fast. Then, an antecubital vein was catheterized and after 10 min of rest in the supine position a 20 ml blood sample was withdrawn and used to measure serum glucose and insulin. Right after, a muscle biopsy was obtained from the middle portion of the *Vastus lateralis* muscle using the Bergstrom's technique with suction (Guerra et al., 2011). After the resting muscle biopsy, the subjects sat on the cycle ergometer for 4 min while breathing either room air or a hypoxic gas mixture from a gas cylinder.

Within 10 s following the sprint, a second muscle biopsy was taken, and then another blood sample was obtained. During the following 2 h, the subjects had free access to water and sat quietly in the laboratory while two additional muscle biopsies and blood samples were obtained at 30 and 120 min post-Wingate. For the last two biopsies, a new incision was performed in the contralateral leg. To avoid injury-triggered activation of signaling cascades, the muscle biopsies were obtained at least 3 cm apart, using the procedures described by Guerra et al. (2011). The muscle specimens were fast cleaned to remove any visible blood, fat, or connective tissue. Then the muscle tissue was immediately frozen in liquid nitrogen and stored at −80°C for later analysis.

Oxygen Uptake

Oxygen uptake was measured with a metabolic cart (Vmax N29; Sensormedics, Yorba Linda, California, USA), as previously reported (Morales-Alamo et al., 2012, 2013, 2017). Respiratory variables were analyzed breath-by-breath and averaged every 5 s during the Wingate test and every 20 s during the incremental exercise tests (Calbet et al., 1997). The highest 20-s averaged VO_2 recorded in normoxia and hypoxia was taken as the normoxic and hypoxic VO_2peak values, respectively.

Muscle Metabolites

From each muscle biopsy, 30 mg of wet tissue were treated with 0.5 M $HClO_4$ and centrifuged at 15,000 g at 4°C for 15 min. The supernatant was neutralized with $KHCO_3$ 2.1M. Phosphocreatine (PCr), creatine (Cr), muscle glucose (GLU), glucose-6-phosphate (G6P), glucose-1-phosphate (G1P), fructose-6-phosphate (F6P), pyruvate (Pyr), and lactate (Lac) were enzymatically determined in neutralized extracts by fluorometric analysis (Lowry and Passonneau, 1972; Gorostiaga et al., 2010). Alanine (Ala) muscle accumulation was assumed to be equivalent to 1.43-fold that of pyruvate accumulation (Katz et al., 1986). Muscle metabolite concentrations were adjusted to the individual mean total creatine (PCr + Cr) because this mean should remain constant during the exercise (Harris et al., 1976). The adjustment to total creatine content accounts for variability in solid non-muscle constituents, which may be present in the biopsies (Parra et al., 2000). This correction was applied to all

TABLE 1 | Physical characteristics and ergoespirometric variables during incremental and sprint exercise in normoxia and severe acute hypoxia (mean ± SD).

	Normoxia	Hypoxia
Age (years)	25.2 ± 4.7	
Height (cm)	176.0 ± 5.1	
Weight (Kg)	80.2 ± 9.9	
% body fat	18.3 ± 6.7	
Two-Legs lean mass (Kg)	19.5 ± 2.4	
SHRpeak (Beats/min)	175.2 ± 8.0	173.5 ± 9.2*
VO_2max (L/min)	3.850 ± 0.308	2.586 ± 0.208*
Wmax (W)	356.3 ± 38.62	285.3 ± 32.1*
Wpeak (W)	999.11 ± 129.0	944.3 ± 131.3
Wpeak/Kg LLM (W/kg)	16.6 ± 2.0	15.6 ± 1.4
Wmean (W)	575.3 ± 60.7	539.8 ± 69.0*
Wmean/Kg LLM (W/kg)	9.56 ± 0.85	8.95 ± 0.78*
O_2 Demand (L/min)	8.390 ± 0.798	7.830 ± 0.765*
Accumulated VO_2 (L)	1.192 ± 0.406	0.847 ± 0.123*
O_2 deficit (L)	3.003 ± 0.498	3.068 ± 0.399
O_2 deficit/Wmean	5.24 ± 0.83	5.70 ± 0.45*
Wingate SpO_2	98.7 ± 0.6	80.6 ± 4.4*
Wingate $P_{ET}O_2$	114.1 ± 6.9	48.8 ± 3.3*

*SHRpeak, peak heart rate during the sprints; Wmax, maximal intensity during the incremental exercise test to exhaustion; Wpeak, peak power output during the Wingate test; LLM, lean mass of the lower extremities; Wmean, mean power output during the Wingate test; Accumulated VO_2, amount of O_2 consumed during the 30 s Wingate test; SpO_2, Hemoglobin saturation (pulse oximetry); $P_{ET}O_2$, end tidal O_2 pressure. *$P < 0.05$ compared to normoxia.*

metabolites including lactate. This assumes that the increase in interstitial lactate and intracellular water was similar in the four trials and that the majority of the lactate produced during the sprints was retained inside the muscle fibers (Calbet et al., 2003). The glycolytic rate (GR) was calculated as GR $= 0.5 \times (\Delta$ Lac $+ \Delta$ Pyr $+ \Delta$ Ala), and glycogenolytic rate (GGR) as GGR $= \Delta$ G1P $+ \Delta$ G6P $+ \Delta$ F6P $+ 0.5 \times (\Delta$ Lac $+ \Delta$ Pyr $+ \Delta$ Ala) (Chasiotis et al., 1982). The $NAD^+/NADH^+$ and ATP/ADP ratios were calculated as previously reported (Morales-Alamo et al., 2017).

Total Protein Extraction, Electrophoresis, and Western Blot Analysis

Muscle protein extracts were prepared as described previously (Guerra et al., 2007) with Complete protease inhibitor cocktail and PhosSTOP phosphatase inhibitor cocktail tablets (Roche Diagnostics, Mannheim, Germany). Total protein content was quantified using the bicinchoninic acid assay (Smith et al., 1985). Fifty microgram of each sample were subjected to immunobloting (Guerra et al., 2010) using Immun-BlotTM PVDF membranes from Bio-Rad Laboratories (Hemel Hempstead Hertfordshire, UK). Ser^{293}-PDH-E1α and Ser^{300}-PDH-E1α phosphorylation and total PDH were determined by western blot (50 μg in each lane) using specific antibodies (AP1062 and AP1064 from Calbiochem, Darmstadt, Germany; and sc-133898, Santa Cruz Biotechnology, CA, USA). Antibodies were diluted in 4% bovine serum albumin in Tris-buffered saline with 0.1% Tween 20 (TBS-T) (BSA-blocking buffer). To control for differences in loading and transfer efficiency, membranes were incubated with a monoclonal mouse anti-α-tubulin antibody (T-5168-ML, Sigma, St. Louis, MO, USA) diluted in TBS-T with 5% blotting grade blocker non-fat dry milk (blotto-blocking buffer). No significant changes were observed in α-tubulin protein levels during the experiments. Antibody-specific labeling was revealed by incubation with a HRP-conjugated goat anti-rabbit antibody (1:20,000; 111-035-144, Jackson ImmunoResearch, Baltimore, USA) antibody, both diluted in 5% blotto blocking buffer and specific bands were visualized with the Inmmun-Star™ WesternC™ kit, using the ChemiDoc XRS system (Bio-Rad Laboratories, Hercules, CA, USA) and analyzed with the image analysis program Quantity one© (Bio-Rad laboratories, Hercules, CA, USA). The densitometry analysis was carried out immediately before saturation of the immunosignal. Muscle-signaling data were represented as a percentage of immunostaining values obtained for the phosphorylated form of each kinase relative to the respective total form. Samples from each subject trial were run on the same gel. In addition, in all gels a human muscle sample obtained from a healthy young man was used as an internal control, to reduce inter-gel variability (Bass et al., 2017).

Statistics

Variables were checked for normal distribution by using the Shapiro-Wilks test. A three-way repeated-measures ANOVA was used with three within subject factors: F_IO_2 (with two levels: normoxia and hypoxia), antioxidants (with two levels: antioxidants and placebo), and time (with four levels: pre-exercise, end-exercise, 30 and 120 min recovery). The Mauchly's test of sphericity was run before the ANOVA, and in the case of violation of the sphericity assumption, the degrees of freedom were adjusted according to the Huynh and Feldt test. When a significant main effect or interaction was observed, specific pairwise comparisons were carried out with the least significant difference *post-hoc* test. The relationship between variables was determined using linear regression analysis. The areas under the curve (AUC) were determined using the trapezoidal rule and compared between conditions with paired Student *t*-tests. Values are reported as the mean ± standard deviation of the mean (unless otherwise stated). $P \leq 0.05$ was considered significant. Statistical analysis was performed using SPSS v.15.0 for Windows (SPSS Inc., Chicago, IL).

RESULTS

Performance and Metabolism

Part of the effects on performance (**Table 1**) and muscle metabolites (**Table 2**) have been published previously (Morales-Alamo et al., 2012, 2013, 2017) and are only summarized here. Peak power output was similar between conditions. Mean power output was reduced by 5.3% in hypoxia ($P = 0.03$) and was not affected by the ingestion of antioxidants (558 ± 62 and 559 ± 61 W, placebo and antioxidants, respectively $P = 0.81$). The

TABLE 2 | Muscle metabolites before, immediately after, and 30 min following a 30-s all-out sprint (Wingate test) in normoxia ($P_IO_2 = 143$ mmHg) and hypoxia ($P_IO_2 = 74$ mmHg), after the ingestion of antioxidants or placebo.

	Placebo		Antioxidants		Time	Antiox	Antiox × Time	F_IO_2	F_IO_2 × Time	Antiox × F_IO_2 × Time
	Hypoxia	Normoxia	Hypoxia	Normoxia						
Pre PCr	16.5 ± 1.5	16.0 ± 2.8	18.2 ± 2.3	17.8 ± 2.3	<0.001	0.12	0.78	0.49	0.75	0.97
Post PCr	6.0 ± 3.3[a]	5.0 ± 2.2[a]	6.8 ± 3.1[a]	6.0 ± 2.9[a]						
Post 30 min PCr	18.8 ± 4.0	18.4 ± 1.9	19.3 ± 2.0	19.6 ± 2.3						
Pre Cr	11.9 ± 1.5	12.4 ± 2.8	10.2 ± 2.3	10.6 ± 2.3	<0.001	0.12	0.78	0.49	0.75	0.97
Post Cr	22.4 ± 3.3[a]	23.5 ± 2.2[a]	21.6 ± 3.1[a]	22.4 ± 2.9[a]						
Post 30 min Cr	9.6 ± 4.0	10.1 ± 1.9	9.1 ± 2.0	8.8 ± 2.3						
Pre ATP	4.8 ± 1.0	5.1 ± 1.9	5.2 ± 1.2	5.0 ± 1.6	<0.001	0.41	0.009	0.9	0.016	0.37
Post ATP	3.2 ± 1.6[a]	2.4 ± 0.8[a]	3.1 ± 0.8[a]	3.5 ± 1.4[a]						
Post 30 min ATP	4.6 ± 2.0	3.5 ± 1.4	3.5 ± 1.1	4.8 ± 1.1						
Pre ADP	0.4 ± 0.2	0.5 ± 0.3	0.3 ± 0.2	0.3 ± 0.2	<0.001	0.4	0.85	0.074	0.76	0.047
Post ADP	0.9 ± 0.8	0.7 ± 0.5	0.4 ± 0.2	0.9 ± 0.8[a]						
Post 30 min ADP	0.3 ± 0.2	0.2 ± 0.1	0.2 ± 0.1	0.2 ± 0.2						
Pre ATP/ADP	13.6 ± 3.2	13.3 ± 5.6	18.3 ± 6.3	17.3 ± 6.8	<0.001	0.28	0.52	0.33	0.64	0.49
Post ATP/ADP	5.9 ± 3.8[a]	4.5 ± 2.5[a]	7.9 ± 2.9[ab]	6.0 ± 4.3[a]						
Post 30 min ATP/ADP	27.2 ± 25.2	18.3 ± 5.3	21.8 ± 7.9	22.8 ± 8.0						
Pre G1P	0.04 ± 0.05	0.02 ± 0.02	0.05 ± 0.04	0.06 ± 0.07	0.001	0.18	0.14	0.901	0.17	0.07
Post G1P	0.25 ± 0.30[a]	0.11 ± 0.10[a]	0.34 ± 0.21[a]	0.38 ± 0.32[a]						
Post 30 min G1P	0.05 ± 0.03	0.15 ± 0.16	0.10 ± 0.13	0.11 ± 0.12						
Pre G6P	0.50 ± 0.33	0.47 ± 0.38	0.46 ± 0.31	0.32 ± 0.37	<0.001	0.21	0.22	0.787	0.01	0.08
Post G6P	4.40 ± 3.21[a]	5.38 ± 1.97[a]	10.34 ± 6.98[a]	5.88 ± 4.77[a]						
Post 30 min G6P	1.21 ± 1.60	2.96 ± 6.37	1.44 ± 1.92	4.39 ± 5.29						
Pre F6P	0.08 ± 0.06	0.05 ± 0.06	0.06 ± 0.07	0.06 ± 0.06	0.005	0.06	0.2	0.098	0.34	0.96
Post F6P	0.24 ± 0.30	0.36 ± 0.32[a]	0.50 ± 0.41[a]	0.59 ± 0.42[a]						
Post 30min F6P	0.09 ± 0.11	0.22 ± 0.55	0.24 ± 0.32	0.59 ± 0.40						
Pre Pyr	0.14 ± 0.05	0.08 ± 0.04	0.09 ± 0.04	0.10 ± 0.07	0.02	0.16	0.08	0.09	0.11	0.11
Post Pyr	0.23 ± 0.07[a]	0.26 ± 0.13[a]	0.17 ± 0.07	0.27 ± 0.09[a]						
Post 30 min Pyr	0.07 ± 0.06	0.16 ± 0.10[a]	0.10 ± 0.09	0.13 ± 0.10						
Pre Lac	2.1 ± 1.3	2.6 ± 2.0	3.1 ± 2.0	2.4 ± 2.2	<0.001	0.06	0.002	0.009	0.002	0.26
Post Lac	55.4 ± 20.1[a,b,c]	38.2 ± 12.3[a]	38.3 ± 10.6[a,c]	34.1 ± 14.9[a]						
Post 30 min Lac	3.7 ± 2.9	5.0 ± 3.2	7.3 ± 8.8	8.9 ± 4.9[a]						
Pre $NAD^+/NADH^+ \times 10^{-7}$	897 ± 667	405 ± 250	339 ± 262	501 ± 363	<0.001	0.03	0.23	0.21	0.3	0.018
Post $NAD^+/NADH^+ \times 10^{-7}$	43 ± 21[a]	60 ± 22[a]	42 ± 16[a,b,c]	85 ± 51[a,d]						
Post 30 min $NAD^+/NADH^+ \times 10^{-7}$	256 ± 232[a]	350 ± 313	348 ± 421	153 ± 120[a]						

Values are means ± SD. Concentrations are reported in mmol.kg^{-1} muscle wet weight.
[a]*$P < 0.05$ Compared with Pre sprint.*
[b]*$P < 0.05$ compared with normoxia placebo at the same time point.*
[c]*$P < 0.05$ compared with normoxia antioxidants at the same time point.*
[d]*$P < 0.05$ compared with hypoxia placebo at the same time point. Pre, Pre sprint; Post, Post sprint; Post 30 min, 30 min into the recovery period; Antiox, antioxidants; Lac, lactate; Pyr, Pyruvate. n = 9.*

accumulated VO_2 during the Wingate test was reduced by 30% in hypoxia ($P = 0.006$) and was not altered by the ingestion of antioxidants (1.095 ± 0.242 and 1.098 ± 0.267 L, placebo and antioxidants, respectively $P = 0.99$). The mean muscle lactate concentration at the end of the sprint was 23% lower after the ingestion of antioxidants (46.8 ± 13.4 and 36.2 ± 12.1 mmol.kg wet^{-1}, mean of the two placebo and mean of the two antioxidants conditions, respectively, $P = 0.004$) and 30% higher in hypoxia than normoxia (46.9 ± 13.9 and 36.1 ± 12.2 mmol.kg wet^{-1}, mean of the two hypoxia and the two normoxia conditions, respectively, $P = 0.004$). The ingestion of antioxidants reduced the glycolytic rate by 25% from 22.3 ± 6.8 to 16.9 ± 6.0 mmol.kg^{-1}. (30 s)$^{-1}$ ($P = 0.002$), while the reduction in the glycogenolytic rate did not reach statistical significance (from 27.2 ± 7.0 to 25.4 ± 10.3 mmol.kg^{-1}. (30 s)$^{-1}$, for the mean of the two placebo and the two antioxidants conditions, respectively, $P = 0.49$). Compared to placebo, 30 min after the end of the sprints preceded by antioxidants muscle lactate concentration was 74% greater (4.3 ± 3.0 vs. 8.1 ± 4.5 mmol.kg wet^{-1}, mean of the two placebo and the two antioxidants conditions, respectively, $P = 0.02$). The ratio ATP/ADP was similarly reduced after the sprints and recovered to pre-exercise levels 30 min later, regardless of the F_IO_2 and antioxidants ingestion (**Table 2**). Immediately after the sprints, the $NAD^+/NADH^+$ ratio was decreased more in hypoxia than normoxia (from 618 ± 355 to 42.5 ± 14.5 and from 452 ± 201 to 72.8 ± 28.6, mean of the two hypoxia and the two normoxia conditions, respectively, $P = 0.003$). The $NAD^+/NADH^+$ ratio was lower after the administration of antioxidants ($P = 0.03$, antioxidants main effect) (**Table 2**).

Serum glucose and insulin concentrations were increased after the sprints (**Figure 2**). Although the changes in serum glucose concentration were similar after the four conditions, the serum insulin concentration tended to be marginally greater (+15%) after the sprints preceded by the ingestion of antioxidants compared to the placebo conditions (ANOVA time effect, $P = 0.08$). After the sprints performed in hypoxia, the elevation of plasma insulin was marginally greater than in normoxia (F_IO_2 × time interaction, $P = 0.045$).

PDH Phosphorylation

Immediately after the sprint Ser^{293}-PDH-E1α phosphorylation was reduced to a similar level in all conditions (~66%, $P = 0.002$; **Figures 3A–C**). However, 30 min after the sprint preceded by the ingestion of antioxidants Ser^{293}-PDH-E1α phosphorylation reached pre-exercise values ($P = 0.86$). Ser^{293}-PDH-E1α phosphorylation was 93% greater after the ingestion of antioxidants than placebo (ANOVA antioxidants effect $P = 0.017$; **Figure 3E**). Ser^{293}-PDH-E1α was dephosphorylated to similar values immediately after the sprints in normoxia and hypoxia ($P = 0.68$, for the comparison between normoxia vs. hypoxia immediately after the sprints; **Figure 3G**).

Immediately after the sprints, Ser^{300}-PDH-E1α phosphorylation was reduced by 91% ($P < 0.001$), without significant differences between conditions (ANOVA antioxidants × F_IO_2 × time $P = 0.40$, **Figures 3A,B,D**). However, during the recovery period, the re-phosphorylation of Ser^{300} was slower than that of Ser^{293} (ANOVA phosphorylation type × time interaction $P = 0.012$), and 30 min after the end of the sprint Ser^{300}-PDH-E1α phosphorylation was still 44% below pre-exercise values ($P = 0.01$). Two hours after the end of the sprint Ser^{300}-PDH-E1α phosphorylation reached a value similar to that measured before the sprints ($P = 0.80$). The Ser^{300}-PDH-E1α phosphorylation values during the experiment preceded by the ingestion of antioxidants were 50% greater than after the intake of placebo. However, this difference was not statistically significant ($P = 0.14$; **Figure 3F**). Ser^{300}-PDH-E1α phosphorylation changes were similar in the normoxic and hypoxic sprints (ANOVA interaction: $P = 0.29$; **Figure 3H**).

The area under the curve (AUC) of Ser^{293}-PDH-E1α phosphorylation was 87% greater after the ingestion of antioxidants ($P = 0.01$), indicating a greater level of re-phosphorylation during the recovery period after the ingestion

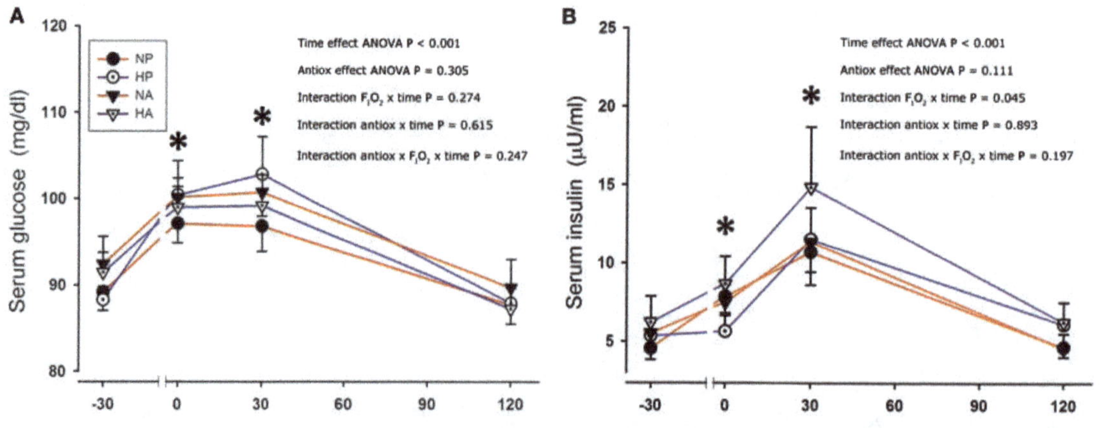

FIGURE 2 | Serum glucose and insulin. Serum glucose **(A)** and insulin concentration **(B)** before, immediately after, and 30 and 120 min after the end of a single 30-s all-out sprint (Wingate test) performed in normoxia placebo (black circles), hypoxia placebo (open circles, F_IO_2:0.105), normoxia antioxidants (black triangles) and hypoxia antioxidants (open triangles; F_IO_2:0.105). *$P < 0.05$ in comparison to resting (ANOVA, time main effect, $n = 9$).

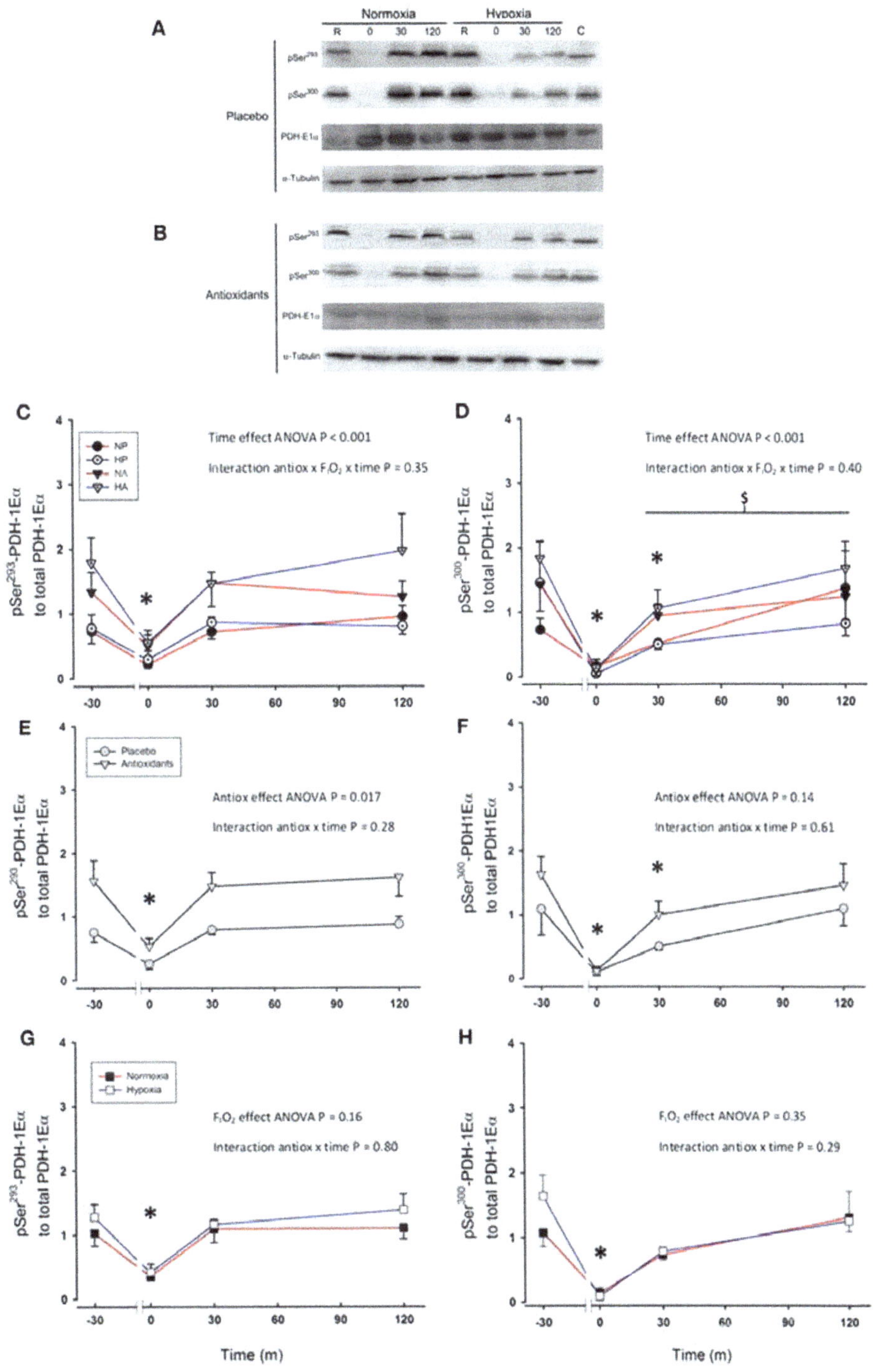

FIGURE 3 | Representative western blots for Ser^{293}-PDH-1Eα and Ser^{300}-PDH-1Eα phosphorylations and PDH-1Eα total protein expression in response to a single 30 s sprint after placebo **(A)** or antioxidants **(B)** intake. Levels of Ser^{293}-PDH-1Eα phosphorylation to PDH-1Eα total protein expression **(C,E,G)**, and Ser^{300}-PDH-1Eα phosphorylation to total PDH-1Eα total protein expression **(D,F,H)** before, immediately after, 30 and 120 min following the end of a single 30 s all-out sprint (Wingate test). **(C,D)** Responses to sprints performed in normoxia placebo (black circles), hypoxia placebo (open circles, F_IO_2: 0.105), normoxia antioxidants (black triangles) and hypoxia antioxidants (open triangles; F_IO_2: 0.105). **(E,F)** Represent the responses observed for two placebo conditions (gray circles) averaged compared to the average of the two antioxidants conditions (gray triangles). **(G,H)** Represent the responses for the average of the normoxic conditions (black squares) compared to the average of the hypoxic conditions (open squares; F_IO_2:0.105). $^*P < 0.05$ in comparison to resting (ANOVA, time main effect). $^\$P < 0.05$ compared to Ser^{293}-PDH-1Eα phosphorylation recovery. $n = 9$ for all variables.

of antioxidants. A similar trend was observed for the AUC of the Ser^{300}-PDH-E1α phosphorylation ($P = 0.061$).

There was an association between the changes in Ser^{293} and Ser^{300}-PDH-E1α phosphorylation observed from pre, to immediately after the sprints in the placebo conditions ($r = 0.74$, $P < 0.001$; $n = 18$), that was lost in the sprints preceded by the ingestion of antioxidants ($r = 0.35$, $P = 0.15$). There was also a negative association between the level of Ser^{300}-PDH-E1α phosphorylation at the end of the sprint and the mean and peak power during the sprint ($r = -0.81$, and $r = -86$, respectively, both $P < 0.01$, $n = 9$, each point representing the mean value of the four conditions for each subject). Likewise, a negative association was observed between the immediate post-exercise Ser^{293}-PDH-E1α phosphorylation and the corresponding $NAD^+/NADH^+$ ratio ($r = -0.80$, $P = 0.01$, $n = 9$, each point representing the mean value of the four conditions for each subject).

DISCUSSION

Compared to normoxia, during sprint exercise in severe acute hypoxia the glycolytic rate is increased leading to greater muscle lactate accumulation, acidification and oxidative stress (Morales-Alamo et al., 2012). Here we show that this increased accumulation of lactate is not due to a lower level of PDH activation during the sprint in hypoxia, pointing toward a mitochondrial limitation of the rate of pyruvate decarboxylation to acetyl-CoA and subsequent oxidation of acetyl groups. In addition, by administering a powerful antioxidant cocktail before the sprint we have demonstrated that antioxidants reduce the glycolytic rate and muscle lactate accumulation during the sprints by a mechanism independent of PDH activation, that seems unrelated to F_IO_2. We have also demonstrated that after the ingestion of antioxidants, PDH is re-phosphorylated to a higher level, which may facilitate a metabolic shift from carbohydrates to fat oxidation (Sjøberg et al., 2017) during the recovery period, at the expense of delaying the removal of muscle lactate. Our results confirm previous *in vitro* studies showing that the re-phosphorylation of Ser^{300}-PDH-E1α is slower than that of Ser^{293}-PDH-E1α (Yeaman et al., 1978), indicating a slightly different regulation of these two phosphorylation sites in human skeletal muscle or reflecting intrinsic differences between the two phosphorylations. This is also supported by the negative association observed between the level of Ser^{300}-PDH-E1α phosphorylation at the end of the sprint and the mean and peak power during the sprint, which was not observed in the case of Ser^{293}-PDH-E1α. The most plausible link between power output and Ser^{300}-PDH-E1α dephosphorylation is the increase of intracellular Ca^{2+}, which is a fundamental determinant of power output (Bakker et al., 2017).

PDH Dephosphorylation-Response to Sprint Exercise Is Not Modified by Antioxidants

The activity of PDH is regulated by phosphorylation/dephosphorylation of three serine residues (Ser^{232}, Ser^{293}, Ser^{300}) of the E1α subunit (Kolobova et al., 2001; Korotchkina and Patel, 2001) (**Figure 1**). Phosphorylation at any of the three sites leads to inhibition of the complex *in vitro* (Korotchkina and Patel, 1995). These phosphorylations are carried out by pyruvate dehydrogenase kinases, of which four isoforms have been identified (PDK1 to 4), while dephosphorylation is performed by PDH phosphatases, of which two isoforms have been identified (PDP1 and 2) (Teague et al., 1982; Huang et al., 1998). PDK1 is the only isoform reported to phosphorylate all three sites, while PDK2, PDK3, and PDK4 act on Ser^{293} and Ser^{300} *in vitro* (Kolobova et al., 2001; Korotchkina and Patel, 2001). The most abundant PDK in skeletal muscle is the isoform PDK4, followed by the isoform PDK2 and the less abundant is the isoform PDK1. Nevertheless, knockout mice for PDK2 and PDK4 have a constitutively active PDH in skeletal muscles (Rahimi et al., 2014).

Previous studies have shown that during sprint exercise in normoxia PDH activity is close to its maximum (Parolin et al., 1999), implying that in normoxia lactate accumulation is due to a limitation in the rate at which pyruvate is oxidized (Howlett et al., 1999). As a novelty, the present investigation shows that PDH is dephosphorylated to a similar extent in normoxia and hypoxia with or without antioxidants (**Figure 4**). Assuming that Ser^{293} and Ser^{300} PDH phosphorylations can be used to assess PDH activity indirectly (Linn et al., 1969; Pilegaard et al., 2006; Kiilerich et al., 2008, 2010), our data indicate similar levels of activation of PDH at the end of the sprint in all conditions. We have reported that during the sprints in severe acute hypoxia our subjects had higher oxidative stress than in normoxia, as shown by a 50% greater intramuscular protein carbonylation and more marked RNOS-mediated signaling (Morales-Alamo et al., 2012). Moreover, the $NAD^+/NADH^+$ ratio was decreased more after the sprints in hypoxia than normoxia (Morales-Alamo et al., 2012). $NADH^+$ is an activator of PDKs (Roche and Hiromasa, 2007), which inhibits PDH through serine phosphorylations (Hucho et al., 1972; Behal et al., 1993). However, PDH dephosphorylation was not greater immediately after the sprint in hypoxia than in normoxia, what is against a potentially greater level of PDK activity during the sprint in hypoxia than in normoxia.

Thus, both in normoxia and hypoxia, the main factor explaining the accumulation of lactate should relate to either an excessive stimulation of glycolysis and/or a limitation of mitochondrial disposal of pyruvate. Given the fact that leg O_2 delivery and leg O_2 uptake are reduced during sprint exercise in hypoxia compared to the same exercise in normoxia (Calbet et al., 2015), the greater accumulation of lactate in hypoxia than in normoxia likely reflects a mitochondrial limitation due to insufficient O_2 supply.

Nevertheless, our data could also indicate that during the sprints in severe acute hypoxia, and perhaps also in normoxia, the stimulation of glycolysis may be excessive in regard with the actual energy demand (Morales-Alamo et al., 2017). This possibility is supported by the fact that during sprint exercise in hypoxia mean power output was not reduced by the ingestion of antioxidants, despite a marked reduction of ATP provision by the glycolysis, that could not be compensated for by increasing

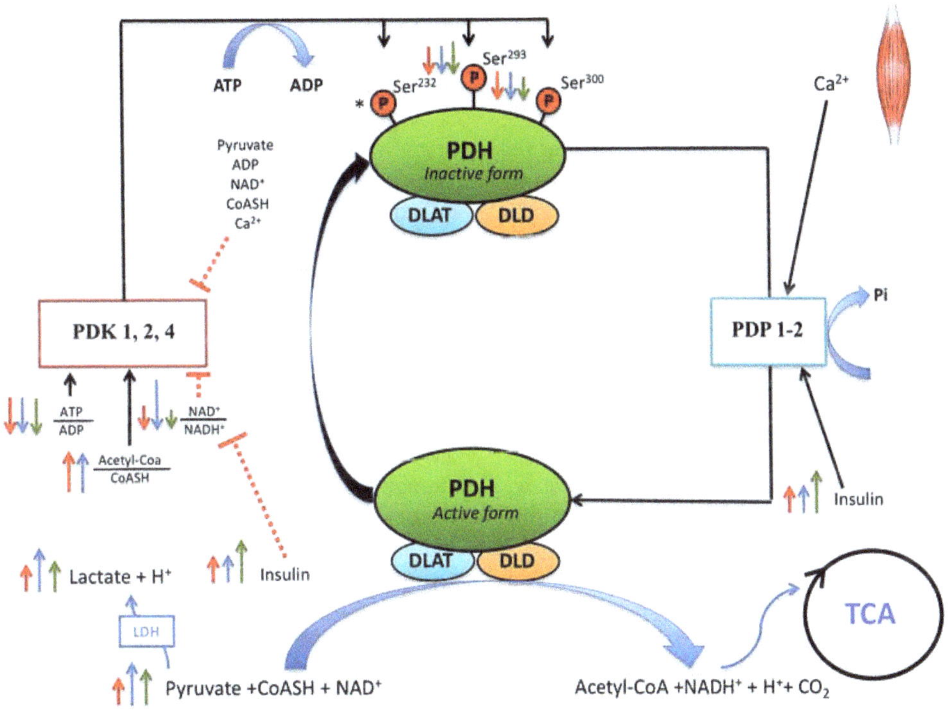

FIGURE 4 | Proposed regulation of PDH activity during sprint exercise and the early post-exercise recovery. During the sprint exercise muscle contractions elicit an immediate increase of sarcoplasmic (Ca^{2+}) which activates pyruvate dehydrogenase phosphatase (PDP, mainly PDP1 which is more expressed in skeletal muscle). PDPs dephosphorylate PDH in the serines 293 and 300, regardless of F_IO_2. While PDH dephosphorylation during sprint exercise is not modified by antioxidants, antioxidants facilitate Ser^{293}PDH-1Eα re-phosphorylation during the recovery period. This indicates that reactive nitrogen and oxygen species (RNOS) contribute maintaining PDH in its active form, or that RNOS slow-down re-phosphorylation during the recovery period. Several regulatory factors of PDKs activity are modified by sprint exercise. After the sprints, the ATP/ADP ratio is decreased to a similar extent in normoxia and hypoxia, regardless of the ingestion of antioxidants. The $NAD^+/NADH^+$ ratio is decreased to a greater extent in hypoxia than normoxia, with this effect being attenuated after the ingestion of antioxidants. Serum insulin increases after the sprint exercise, more when the sprints are performed in hypoxia than normoxia. Normoxia (red arrows), hypoxia (blue arrows), antioxidants (green arrows). The length of the arrow is representative of the magnitude of the change. *Indicates that Ser^{232}PDH-1Eα was not measured in the present investigation and, therefore, its regulation by F_IO_2 and RNOS during sprint exercise remains unknown.

VO_2, since during sprint exercise in hypoxia VO_2 was the same in the placebo and the antioxidants conditions. This finding contrasts with the reported reduction of muscle strength and muscle VO_2 after the intravenous administration of vitamin C and tempol in rats (Herspring et al., 2008). Moreover, the fact that mean power output was not reduced after the administration of antioxidants in acute hypoxia is intriguing because the glycolysis provides 50% or more of the overall energy expenditure during the Wingate test in normoxia (Bogdanis et al., 1996; Parolin et al., 1999) and even more during sprint exercise in hypoxia (Morales-Alamo et al., 2012). Therefore, our antioxidant cocktail should have contributed to reduce the energy demand by, for example, improving the P/O ratio and/or by lowering the energy cost of muscle contraction.

Mitochondria produces RNOS mainly at complexes I and III of the electron transport chain (Barja, 1999; Muller et al., 2004). Ascorbate prevents cytochrome *c* release from the mitochondrial inner membrane and stabilizes the mitochondrial membrane potential in response to hypoxia-reoxygenation (Dhar-Mascareño et al., 2005) and could improve the phosphorylation potential by increasing the proton motive force across the mitochondrial inner membrane (Brand and Nicholls, 2011). The presence of α-lipoic acid in our antioxidant cocktail could have amplified this effect (Cimolai et al., 2014). Moreover, in agreement with an improved mitochondrial efficiency, experiments in humans, have reported enhanced mitochondrial efficiency during exercise in moderate hypoxia (F_IO_2: 0.13) after nitrate supplementation (Vanhatalo et al., 2014). Antioxidants, like nitrates, increase NO bioavailability (Nyberg et al., 2012; Larsen et al., 2014), which can reduce proton back-leakage across the inner mitochondrial membrane increasing the P/O ratio (Clerc et al., 2007).

Antioxidants may also reduce the energy demand. One of the main contributors to energy expenditure during muscle contraction is the sarcoendoplasmic reticulum calcium pumps (SERCAs), which may account for ~50% of the overall energy expenditure at rest (Norris et al., 2010) and ~30–40% during muscle contractions (Barclay et al., 2007). SERCAs-energy expenditure can be lowered by reducing the amount of calcium efflux through the calcium channels [the ryanodine receptor and the inositol 1, 4, 5-trisphosphate receptors (IP3Rs)] and/or by decreasing Ca^{2+} leakage from the sarcoendoplasmic reticulum (Chernorudskiy and Zito, 2017). Both processes are increased by RNOS and attenuated by antioxidants (Xu et al., 1998;

Kang et al., 2008; Mazurek et al., 2014; Oda et al., 2015). Nevertheless, excessive oxidative stress may also reduce SERCAs activity (Chernorudskiy and Zito, 2017). Calcium transients were likely reduced during the sprints with antioxidants since CaMKII, a kinase that auto-phosphorylates depending on the magnitude of Ca^{2+} transients was less phosphorylated after the sprints preceded by the ingestion of antioxidants in our subjects (Morales-Alamo et al., 2013, 2017).

PDH Re-phosphorylation During the Recovery Period Is Increased by Antioxidants

The recovery of the resting PDH phosphorylation levels requires the activation of PDKs by acetyl-CoA, $NADH^+$ or ATP, which re-phosphorylate PDH favoring the oxidation of acetyl groups (Roche and Hiromasa, 2007; Rahimi et al., 2014). Here we show that antioxidants facilitate PDH re-phosphorylation during the recovery period, with faster re-phosphorylation of Ser^{293} than Ser^{300} (**Figure 4**), as previously shown with experiments *in vitro* (Yeaman et al., 1978). Cell-culture experiments have shown that antioxidants stimulate PDKs (Churchill et al., 2005). Although not measured here, PDK activity during the recovery period might have been stimulated by the lower $NAD^+/NADH^+$ ratio after the ingestion of antioxidants (**Figure 4**), as previously reported (Morales-Alamo et al., 2013, 2017). Cell-culture experiments have also shown that pyruvate dehydrogenase phosphatase 1 (PDP1) activity is stimulated by lipoic acid (Shan et al., 2014). Nevertheless, an enhanced α-lipoic acid-stimulated PDP1 activity after the ingestion of antioxidants is unlikely inasmuch PDH re-phosphorylation was facilitated during the recovery period after the ingestion of antioxidants. Although PDPs are stimulated by insulin (Thomas and Denton, 1986; Consitt et al., 2016), the insulin response to sprint exercise was not reduced after ingestion of antioxidants in the present study. Thus, the greater PDH re-phosphorylation during the recovery period after antioxidants cannot be attributed to an effect mediated by differences in the plasma insulin concentrations, since our results point toward higher insulin concentrations after the administration of antioxidants, which via PDP activation could delay, but not accelerate, PDH re-phosphorylation.

Another mechanism that could explain a faster re-phosphorylation of PDH during the recovery period after the ingestion of antioxidants is a reduction of the exercise-induced increase in insulin sensitivity by antioxidants (Trewin et al., 2015). Indeed, it has been reported that the increase of insulin sensitivity observed acutely after exercise is augmented in mice lacking the antioxidant enzyme Gpx1, an effect that was abolished by administration of the antioxidant N-acetylcysteine (Loh et al., 2009). This concurs with the lower post-exercise insulin sensitivity observed in humans who received N-acetylcysteine during exercise (Trewin et al., 2015).

As expected from a greater re-phosphorylation of PDH (i.e., inhibition of PDH) following the ingestion of antioxidants, muscle lactate concentration 30 min after the end of the sprints was almost twice as high after the ingestion of antioxidants. This likely reflects a lower rate of lactate oxidation during the recovery after the ingestion of antioxidants. Lactate oxidation must be preceded by the conversion of lactate into pyruvate and subsequently decarboxylated to acetyl-CoA by the PDH, which after the ingestion of antioxidants is less active (Gladden, 2006). Consequently, to maintain the flow of acetyl groups entering the Krebs cycle and the aerobic ATP resynthesis rate during the first 30–60 min after a sprint exercise preceded by the ingestion of antioxidants, fat oxidation should be increased.

Why Was Performance Not Improved by Antioxidants, Despite the Attenuation of Muscle Lactate Accumulation and Acidification?

Our findings are at odds with the current paradigm of muscle fatigue (Fitts, 1994; Bangsbo and Juel, 2006), but concur with alternative proposals based on human and animal experiments (Nielsen et al., 2001; Lamb and Stephenson, 2006; Morales-Alamo et al., 2015; Torres-Peralta et al., 2016a,b). Muscle fatigue during high-intensity exercise has been traditionally linked to the activation of glycolysis, the accumulation of lactate and the effects caused by the drop in muscle pH (Fitts, 1994). However, *in vitro* and animal experiments have shown that both intracellular acidification and lactate accumulation contribute to maintain muscle excitability attenuating fatigue (Westerblad et al., 1991; Allen et al., 1995; Pedersen et al., 2004, 2005). Specifically, lactate can inhibit ClC-1 Cl^- channels and increase the excitability and contractile function of depolarized rat muscles (de Paoli et al., 2010). More recently, the ergogenic effect of lactate accumulation has been confirmed in humans, which recovered partly from fatigue during 1 min of completed bilateral leg occlusion applied at the end of an incremental exercise to exhaustion, despite a 19–22% increase of muscle lactate during the ischemic recovery (Morales-Alamo et al., 2015). In the current investigation, peak power output was not affected by either hypoxia or antioxidants, while mean power output was only reduced by 5.3% in hypoxia (all conditions combined), despite a much greater accumulation of muscle lactate. The fact that muscle lactate could accumulate to higher levels with a minor impact on performance agrees with the idea that lactate and acidification is not as detrimental for muscle contraction as classically thought. However, the potential protective effect on muscle excitability by greater lactate accumulation during exercise in severe acute hypoxia was lost when the sprints were preceded by the intake of antioxidants, which reduced the glycolytic rate to values similar to those observed during the sprints performed in normoxia. This had a minor impact on performance and we think that our findings are compatible with mechanisms of task failure localized outside the active skeletal muscles (Calbet et al., 2015; Morales-Alamo et al., 2015; Torres-Peralta et al., 2016a,b).

In summary, this investigation shows that lactate accumulation during sprint exercise in severe acute hypoxia is not caused by reduced activation of the PDH, which dephosphorylates to similar levels in normoxia and hypoxia. The ingestion of antioxidants before sprint exercise reduces the glycolytic rate in normoxia and hypoxia without a negative impact on performance, implying that either the activation of glycolysis in hypoxia is excessive and/or the energy cost of muscle contraction is reduced by antioxidants. We have also shown that Ser^{293} re-phosphorylates a faster rate during the recovery period than Ser^{300}-PDH-E1α, suggesting slightly different regulatory mechanisms that remain to be identified. Finally, the ingestion of antioxidants is associated with increased PDH re-phosphorylation and slower elimination of muscle lactate during the recovery period.

AUTHOR CONTRIBUTIONS

JAC, DM-A, BG, and CD: Conception and design of the experiments; JAC, DM-A, BG, AS, and CD: Pre-testing, experimental preparation, and data collection; All co-authors: data analysis. The first draft of the manuscript was written by DM-A and JAC. All co-authors edited and proofread the manuscript and approved the final version.

ACKNOWLEDGMENTS

This study was supported by grants from the Ministerio de Educación y Ciencia (DEP2009-11638, DEP2010-21866, DEP2015-71171-R, and FEDER), FUNCIS (PI/10/07), Programa Innova Canarias 2020 (P.PE03-01-F08), Proyecto Estructurante de la ULPGC: ULPAPD-08/01-4, and Proyecto del Programa Propio de la ULPGC (ULPGC 2009-07 and ULPGC 2015/05), and III Convocatoria de Ayudas a la Investigación Cátedra Real Madrid-UEM (2010/01RM, Universidad Europea de Madrid). Special thanks are given to José Navarro de Tuero for his excellent technical assistance.

REFERENCES

Allen, D. G., Westerblad, H., and Lännergren, J. (1995). The role of intracellular acidosis in muscle fatigue. *Adv. Exp. Med. Biol.* 384, 57–68. doi: 10.1007/978-1-4899-1016-5_5

Bailey, D. M., Lawrenson, L., McEneny, J., Young, I. S., James, P. E., Jackson, S. K., et al. (2007). Electron paramagnetic spectroscopic evidence of exercise-induced free radical accumulation in human skeletal muscle. *Free Radic. Res.* 41, 182–190. doi: 10.1080/10715760601028867

Bakker, A. J., Cully, T. R., Wingate, C. D., Barclay, C. J., and Launikonis, B. S. (2017). Doublet stimulation increases Ca^{2+} binding to troponin C to ensure rapid force development in skeletal muscle. *J. Gen. Physiol.* 149, 323–334. doi: 10.1085/jgp.201611727

Bangsbo, J., and Juel, C. (2006). Counterpoint: lactic acid accumulation is a disadvantage during muscle activity. *J. Appl. Physiol.* 100, 1412–1413. discussion: 1413–1414.

Barclay, C. J., Woledge, R. C., and Curtin, N. A. (2007). Energy turnover for Ca^{2+} cycling in skeletal muscle. *J. Muscle Res. Cell Motil.* 28, 259–274. doi: 10.1007/s10974-007-9116-7

Barja, G. (1999). Mitochondrial oxygen radical generation and leak: sites of production in states 4 and 3, organ specificity, and relation to aging and longevity. *J. Bioenerg. Biomembr.* 31, 347–366. doi: 10.1023/A:1005427919188

Bass, J. J., Wilkinson, D. J., Rankin, D., Phillips, B. E., Szewczyk, N. J., Smith, K., et al. (2017). An overview of technical considerations for Western blotting applications to physiological research. *Scand. J. Med. Sci. Sports* 27, 4–25. doi: 10.1111/sms.12702

Behal, R. H., Buxton, D. B., Robertson, J. G., and Olson, M. S. (1993). Regulation of the pyruvate dehydrogenase multienzyme complex. *Annu. Rev. Nutr.* 13, 497–520. doi: 10.1146/annurev.nu.13.070193.002433

Bogdanis, G. C., Nevill, M. E., Boobis, L. H., and Lakomy, H. K. (1996). Contribution of phosphocreatine and aerobic metabolism to energy supply during repeated sprint exercise. *J. Appl. Physiol* 80, 876–884. doi: 10.1152/jappl.1996.80.3.876

Brand, M. D., and Nicholls, D. G. (2011). Assessing mitochondrial dysfunction in cells. *Biochem. J.* 435, 297–312. doi: 10.1042/BJ20110162

Brennan-Minnella, A. M., Won, S. J., and Swanson, R. A. (2015). NADPH oxidase-2: linking glucose, acidosis, and excitotoxicity in stroke. *Antioxid. Redox Signal.* 22, 161–174. doi: 10.1089/ars.2013.5767

Calbet, J. A., Chavarren, J., and Dorado, C. (1997). Fractional use of anaerobic capacity during a 30- and a 45-s Wingate test. *Eur. J. Appl. Physiol.* 76, 308–313. doi: 10.1007/s004210050253

Calbet, J. A., De Paz, J. A., Garatachea, N., Cabeza De Vaca, S., and Chavarren, J. (2003). Anaerobic energy provision does not limit Wingate exercise performance in endurance-trained cyclists. *J. Appl. Physiol.* 94, 668–676. doi: 10.1152/japplphysiol.00128.2002

Calbet, J. A., Losa-Reyna, J., Torres-Peralta, R., Rasmussen, P., Ponce-Gonzalez, J. G., Sheel, A. W., et al. (2015). Limitations to oxygen transport and utilization during sprint exercise in humans: evidence for a functional reserve in muscle O_2 diffusing capacity. *J. Physiol.* 593, 4649–4664. doi: 10.1113/JP270408

Calbet, J. A., Moysi, J. S., Dorado, C., and Rodríguez, L. P. (1998). Bone mineral content and density in professional tennis players. *Calcif. Tissue Int.* 62, 491–496. doi: 10.1007/s002239900467

Chasiotis, D., Sahlin, K., and Hultman, E. (1982). Regulation of glycogenolysis in human muscle at rest and during exercise. *J. Appl. Physiol. Respir. Environ. Exerc. Physiol.* 53, 708–715. doi: 10.1152/jappl.1982.53.3.708

Cheetham, M. E., Boobis, L. H., Brooks, S., and Williams, C. (1986). Human muscle metabolism during sprint running. *J. Appl. Physiol.* 61, 54–60. doi: 10.1152/jappl.1986.61.1.54

Chernorudskiy, A. L., and Zito, E. (2017). Regulation of calcium homeostasis by ER redox: a close-up of the ER/Mitochondria connection. *J. Mol. Biol.* 429, 620–632. doi: 10.1016/j.jmb.2017.01.017

Churchill, E. N., Murriel, C. L., Chen, C. H., Mochly-Rosen, D., and Szweda, L. I. (2005). Reperfusion-induced translocation of deltaPKC to cardiac mitochondria prevents pyruvate dehydrogenase reactivation. *Circ. Res.* 97, 78–85. doi: 10.1161/01.RES.0000173896.32522.6e

Cimolai, M. C., Vanasco, V., Marchini, T., Magnani, N. D., Evelson, P., and Alvarez, S. (2014). α-Lipoic acid protects kidney from oxidative stress and mitochondrial dysfunction associated to inflammatory conditions. *Food Funct.* 5, 3143–3150. doi: 10.1039/C4FO00489B

Clerc, P., Rigoulet, M., Leverve, X., and Fontaine, E. (2007). Nitric oxide increases oxidative phosphorylation efficiency. *J. Bioenerg. Biomembr.* 39, 158–166. doi: 10.1007/s10863-007-9074-1

Consitt, L. A., Saxena, G., Saneda, A., and Houmard, J. A. (2016). Age-related impairments in skeletal muscle PDH phosphorylation and plasma lactate are indicative of metabolic inflexibility and the effects of exercise training. *Am. J. Physiol. Endocrinol. Metab.* 311, E145–E156. doi: 10.1152/ajpendo.00452.2015

Cuevas, M. J., Almar, M., Garcia-Glez, J. C., García-López, D., De Paz, J. A., Alvear-Ordenes, I., et al. (2005). Changes in oxidative stress markers and NF-κB activation induced by sprint exercise. *Free Radic. Res.* 39, 431–439. doi: 10.1080/10715760500072149

de Paoli, F. V., Ørtenblad, N., Pedersen, T. H., Jørgensen, R., and Nielsen, O. B. (2010). Lactate *per se* improves the excitability of depolarized rat skeletal muscle by reducing the Cl-conductance. *J. Physiol.* 588, 4785–4794. doi: 10.1113/jphysiol.2010.196568

Dhar-Mascareño, M., Cárcamo, J. M., and Golde, D. W. (2005). Hypoxia-reoxygenation-induced mitochondrial damage and apoptosis in human endothelial cells are inhibited by vitamin C. *Free Radic. Biol. Med.* 38, 1311–1322. doi: 10.1016/j.freeradbiomed.2005.01.017

Dulhunty, A. F., Wei-LaPierre, L., Casarotto, M. G., and Beard, N. A. (2017). Core skeletal muscle ryanodine receptor calcium release complex. *Clin. Exp. Pharmacol. Physiol.* 44, 3–12. doi: 10.1111/1440-1681.12676

Fitts, R. H. (1994). Cellular mechanisms of muscle fatigue. *Physiol. Rev.* 74, 49–94. doi: 10.1152/physrev.1994.74.1.49

Gladden, L. B. (2006). Mammalian skeletal muscle can convert lactate to glycogen. *J. Appl. Physiol.* 100:2109. doi: 10.1152/japplphysiol.00163.2006

Gorostiaga, E. M., Navarro-Amézqueta, I., Cusso, R., Hellsten, Y., Calbet, J. A., Guerrero, M., et al. (2010). Anaerobic energy expenditure and mechanical efficiency during exhaustive leg press exercise. *PLoS ONE* 5:e13486. doi: 10.1371/journal.pone.0013486

Guerra, B., Gomez-Cabrera, M. C., Ponce-Gonzalez, J. G., Martinez-Bello, V. E., Guadalupe-Grau, A., Santana, A., et al. (2011). Repeated muscle biopsies through a single skin incision do not elicit muscle signaling, but IL-6 mRNA and STAT3 phosphorylation increase in injured muscle. *J. Appl. Physiol.* 110, 1708–1715. doi: 10.1152/japplphysiol.00091.2011

Guerra, B., Guadalupe-Grau, A., Fuentes, T., Ponce-González, J. G., Morales-Alamo, D., Olmedillas, H., et al. (2010). SIRT1, AMP-activated protein kinase phosphorylation and downstream kinases in response to a single bout of sprint exercise: influence of glucose ingestion. *Eur. J. Appl. Physiol.* 109, 731–743. doi: 10.1007/s00421-010-1413-y

Guerra, B., Santana, A., Fuentes, T., Delgado-Guerra, S., Cabrera-Socorro, A., Dorado, C., et al. (2007). Leptin receptors in human skeletal muscle. *J. Appl. Physiol.* 102, 1786–1792. doi: 10.1152/japplphysiol.01313.2006

Harris, R. C., Edwards, R. H., Hultman, E., Nordesjö, L. O., Nylind, B., and Sahlin, K. (1976). The time course of phosphorylcreatine resynthesis during recovery of the quadriceps muscle in man. *Pflugers Arch.* 367, 137–142. doi: 10.1007/BF00585149

Herspring, K. F., Ferreira, L. F., Copp, S. W., Snyder, B. S., Poole, D. C., and Musch, T. I. (2008). Effects of antioxidants on contracting spinotrapezius muscle microvascular oxygenation and blood flow in aged rats. *J. Appl. Physiol.* 105, 1889–1896. doi: 10.1152/japplphysiol.90642.2008

Howlett, R. A., Heigenhauser, G. J., and Spriet, L. L. (1999). Skeletal muscle metabolism during high-intensity sprint exercise is unaffected by dichloroacetate or acetate infusion. *J. Appl. Physiol.* 87, 1747–1751. doi: 10.1152/jappl.1999.87.5.1747

Huang, B., Gudi, R., Wu, P., Harris, R. A., Hamilton, J., and Popov, K. M. (1998). Isoenzymes of pyruvate dehydrogenase phosphatase. DNA-derived amino acid sequences, expression, and regulation. *J. Biol. Chem.* 273, 17680–17688. doi: 10.1074/jbc.273.28.17680

Hucho, F., Randall, D. D., Roche, T. E., Burgett, M. W., Pelley, J. W., and Reed, L. J. (1972). α-Keto acid dehydrogenase complexes. XVII. Kinetic and regulatory properties of pyruvate dehydrogenase kinase and pyruvate dehydrogenase phosphatase from bovine kidney and heart. *Arch. Biochem. Biophys.* 151, 328–340. doi: 10.1016/0003-9861(72)90504-8

Jackson, M. J. (2015). Redox regulation of muscle adaptations to contractile activity and aging. *J. Appl. Physiol.* 119, 163–171. doi: 10.1152/japplphysiol.00760.2014

Jackson, M. J., Pye, D., and Palomero, J. (2007). The production of reactive oxygen and nitrogen species by skeletal muscle. *J. Appl. Physiol.* 102, 1664–1670. doi: 10.1152/japplphysiol.01102.2006

Jones, N. L., McCartney, N., Graham, T., Spriet, L. L., Kowalchuk, J. M., Heigenhauser, G. J., et al. (1985). Muscle performance and metabolism in maximal isokinetic cycling at slow and fast speeds. *J. Appl. Physiol.* 59, 132–136. doi: 10.1152/jappl.1985.59.1.132

Kang, S., Kang, J., Kwon, H., Frueh, D., Yoo, S. H., Wagner, G., et al. (2008). Effects of redox potential and Ca^{2+} on the inositol 1,4,5-trisphosphate receptor L3-1 loop region: implications for receptor regulation. *J. Biol. Chem.* 283, 25567–25575. doi: 10.1074/jbc.M803321200

Katz, A., Sahlin, K., and Henriksson, J. (1986). Muscle ammonia metabolism during isometric contraction in humans. *Am. J. Physiol.* 250, C834–C840. doi: 10.1152/ajpcell.1986.250.6.C834

Kiilerich, K., Birk, J. B., Damsgaard, R., Wojtaszewski, J. F., and Pilegaard, H. (2008). Regulation of PDH in human arm and leg muscles at rest and during intense exercise. *Am. J. Physiol. Endocrinol. Metab.* 294, E36–E42. doi: 10.1152/ajpendo.00352.2007

Kiilerich, K., Gudmundsson, M., Birk, J. B., Lundby, C., Taudorf, S., Plomgaard, P., et al. (2010). Low muscle glycogen and elevated plasma free fatty acid modify but do not prevent exercise-induced PDH activation in human skeletal muscle. *Diabetes* 59, 26–32. doi: 10.2337/db09-1032

Kolobova, E., Tuganova, A., Boulatnikov, I., and Popov, K. M. (2001). Regulation of pyruvate dehydrogenase activity through phosphorylation at multiple sites. *Biochem. J.* 358, 69–77. doi: 10.1042/bj3580069

Korotchkina, L. G., and Patel, M. S. (1995). Mutagenesis studies of the phosphorylation sites of recombinant human pyruvate dehydrogenase. Site-specific regulation. *J. Biol. Chem.* 270, 14297–14304. doi: 10.1074/jbc.270.24.14297

Korotchkina, L. G., and Patel, M. S. (2001). Site specificity of four pyruvate dehydrogenase kinase isoenzymes toward the three phosphorylation sites of human pyruvate dehydrogenase. *J. Biol. Chem.* 276, 37223–37229. doi: 10.1074/jbc.M103069200

Lamb, G. D., and Stephenson, D. G. (2006). Point: lactic acid accumulation is an advantage during muscle activity. *J. Appl. Physiol.* 100, 1410–1412. discussion: 1414. doi: 10.1152/japplphysiol.00023.2006

Larsen, F. J., Schiffer, T. A., Ekblom, B., Mattsson, M. P., Checa, A., Wheelock, C. E., et al. (2014). Dietary nitrate reduces resting metabolic rate: a randomized, crossover study in humans. *Am. J. Clin. Nutr.* 99, 843–850. doi: 10.3945/ajcn.113.079491

Linn, T. C., Pettit, F. H., and Reed, L. J. (1969). Alpha-keto acid dehydrogenase complexes. X. Regulation of the activity of the pyruvate dehydrogenase complex from beef kidney mitochondria by phosphorylation and dephosphorylation. *Proc. Natl. Acad. Sci. U.S.A.* 62, 234–241. doi: 10.1073/pnas.62.1.234

Loh, K., Deng, H., Fukushima, A., Cai, X., Boivin, B., Galic, S., et al. (2009). Reactive oxygen species enhance insulin sensitivity. *Cell Metab.* 10, 260–272. doi: 10.1016/j.cmet.2009.08.009

Lowry, O. H., and Passonneau, J. V. (1972). *A Flexible System of Enzymatic Analysis*. New York, NY: Academic Press.

Mazurek, S. R., Bovo, E., and Zima, A. V. (2014). Regulation of sarcoplasmic reticulum Ca(2+) release by cytosolic glutathione in rabbit ventricular myocytes. *Free Radic. Biol. Med.* 68, 159–167. doi: 10.1016/j.freeradbiomed.2013.12.003

McLellan, T. M., Kavanagh, M. F., and Jacobs, I. (1990). The effect of hypoxia on performance during 30 s or 45 s of supramaximal exercise. *Eur. J. Appl. Physiol. Occup. Physiol.* 60, 155–161. doi: 10.1007/BF00846037

Morales-Alamo, D., and Calbet, J. A. (2014). Free radicals and sprint exercise in humans. *Free Radic. Res.* 48, 30–42. doi: 10.3109/10715762.2013.825043

Morales-Alamo, D., Guerra, B., Ponce-González, J. G., Guadalupe-Grau, A., Santana, A., Martin-Rincon, M., et al. (2017). Skeletal muscle signaling, metabolism, and performance during sprint exercise in severe acute hypoxia after the ingestion of antioxidants. *J. Appl. Physiol.* 123, 1235–1245. doi: 10.1152/japplphysiol.00384.2017

Morales-Alamo, D., Losa-Reyna, J., Torres-Peralta, R., Martin-Rincon, M., Perez-Valera, M., Curtelin, D., et al. (2015). What limits performance during whole-body incremental exercise to exhaustion in humans? *J. Physiol.* 593, 4631–4648. doi: 10.1113/JP270487

Morales-Alamo, D., Ponce-González, J. G., Guadalupe-Grau, A., Rodríguez-García, L., Santana, A., Cusso, M. R., et al. (2012). Increased oxidative stress and anaerobic energy release, but blunted Thr172-AMPKα phosphorylation, in response to sprint exercise in severe acute hypoxia in humans. *J. Appl. Physiol.* 113, 917–928. doi: 10.1152/japplphysiol.00415.2012

Morales-Alamo, D., Ponce-González, J. G., Guadalupe-Grau, A., Rodríguez-García, L., Santana, A., Cusso, R., et al. (2013). Critical role for free radicals on sprint exercise-induced CaMKII and AMPKα phosphorylation in human skeletal muscle. *J. Appl. Physiol.* 114, 566–577. doi: 10.1152/japplphysiol.01246.2012

Morgan, D., Cherny, V. V., Murphy, R., Katz, B. Z., and DeCoursey, T. E. (2005). The pH dependence of NADPH oxidase in human eosinophils. *J. Physiol.* 569, 419–431. doi: 10.1113/jphysiol.2005.094748

Muller, F. L., Liu, Y., and Van Remmen, H. (2004). Complex III releases superoxide to both sides of the inner mitochondrial membrane. *J. Biol. Chem.* 279, 49064–49073. doi: 10.1074/jbc.M407715200

Nielsen, O. B., de Paoli, F., and Overgaard, K. (2001). Protective effects of lactic acid on force production in rat skeletal muscle. *J. Physiol.* 536, 161–166. doi: 10.1111/j.1469-7793.2001.t01-1-00161.x

Norris, S. M., Bombardier, E., Smith, I. C., Vigna, C., and Tupling, A. R. (2010). ATP consumption by sarcoplasmic reticulum Ca^{2+} pumps accounts for 50% of resting metabolic rate in mouse fast and slow twitch skeletal muscle. *Am. J. Physiol. Cell Physiol.* 298, C521–C529. doi: 10.1152/ajpcell.00479.2009

Nyberg, M., Blackwell, J. R., Damsgaard, R., Jones, A. M., Hellsten, Y., and Mortensen, S. P. (2012). Lifelong physical activity prevents an age-related reduction in arterial and skeletal muscle nitric oxide bioavailability in humans. *J. Physiol.* 590, 5361–5370. doi: 10.1113/jphysiol.2012.239053

Oda, T., Yang, Y., Uchinoumi, H., Thomas, D. D., Chen-Izu, Y., Kato, T., et al. (2015). Oxidation of ryanodine receptor (RyR) and calmodulin enhance Ca release and pathologically alter, RyR structure and calmodulin affinity. *J. Mol. Cell. Cardiol.* 85, 240–248. doi: 10.1016/j.yjmcc.2015.06.009

Parolin, M. L., Chesley, A., Matsos, M. P., Spriet, L. L., Jones, N. L., and Heigenhauser, G. J. (1999). Regulation of skeletal muscle glycogen phosphorylase and PDH during maximal intermittent exercise. *Am. J. Physiol.* 277, E890–E900. doi: 10.1152/ajpendo.1999.277.5.E890

Parolin, M. L., Spriet, L. L., Hultman, E., Hollidge-Horvat, M. G., Jones, N. L., and Heigenhauser, G. J. (2000). Regulation of glycogen phosphorylase and PDH during exercise in human skeletal muscle during hypoxia. *Am. J. Physiol. Endocrinol. Metab.* 278, E522–E534. doi: 10.1152/ajpendo.2000.278.3.E522

Parra, J., Cadefau, J. A., Rodas, G., Amigó, N., and Cussó, R. (2000). The distribution of rest periods affects performance and adaptations of energy metabolism induced by high-intensity training in human muscle. *Acta Physiol. Scand.* 169, 157–165. doi: 10.1046/j.1365-201x.2000.00730.x

Pedersen, T. H., de Paoli, F., and Nielsen, O. B. (2005). Increased excitability of acidified skeletal muscle: role of chloride conductance. *J. Gen. Physiol.* 125, 237–246. doi: 10.1085/jgp.200409173

Pedersen, T. H., Nielsen, O. B., Lamb, G. D., and Stephenson, D. G. (2004). Intracellular acidosis enhances the excitability of working muscle. *Science* 305, 1144–1147. doi: 10.1126/science.1101141

Pilegaard, H., Birk, J. B., Sacchetti, M., Mourtzakis, M., Hardie, D. G., Stewart, G., et al. (2006). PDH-E1α dephosphorylation and activation in human skeletal muscle during exercise: effect of intralipid infusion. *Diabetes* 55, 3020–3027. doi: 10.2337/db06-0152

Putman, C. T., Jones, N. L., Lands, L. C., Bragg, T. M., Hollidge-Horvat, M. G., and Heigenhauser, G. J. (1995). Skeletal muscle pyruvate dehydrogenase activity during maximal exercise in humans. *Am. J. Physiol.* 269, E458–E468. doi: 10.1152/ajpendo.1995.269.3.E458

Radak, Z., Zhao, Z., Koltai, E., Ohno, H., and Atalay, M. (2013). Oxygen consumption and usage during physical exercise: the balance between oxidative stress and ROS-dependent adaptive signaling. *Antioxid. Redox Signal.* 18, 1208–1246. doi: 10.1089/ars.2011.4498

Rahimi, Y., Camporez, J. P., Petersen, M. C., Pesta, D., Perry, R. J., Jurczak, M. J., et al. (2014). Genetic activation of pyruvate dehydrogenase alters oxidative substrate selection to induce skeletal muscle insulin resistance. *Proc. Natl. Acad. Sci. U.S.A.* 111, 16508–16513. doi: 10.1073/pnas.1419104111

Richardson, R. S., Donato, A. J., Uberoi, A., Wray, D. W., Lawrenson, L., Nishiyama, S., et al. (2007). Exercise-induced brachial artery vasodilation: role of free radicals. *Am. J. Physiol. Heart Circ. Physiol.* 292, H1516–H1522. doi: 10.1152/ajpheart.01045.2006

Roche, T. E., and Hiromasa, Y. (2007). Pyruvate dehydrogenase kinase regulatory mechanisms and inhibition in treating diabetes, heart ischemia, and cancer. *Cell. Mol. Life Sci.* 64, 830–849. doi: 10.1007/s00018-007-6380-z

Shan, C., Kang, H. B., Elf, S., Xie, J., Gu, T. L., Aguiar, M., et al. (2014). Tyr-94 phosphorylation inhibits pyruvate dehydrogenase phosphatase 1 and promotes tumor growth. *J. Biol. Chem.* 289, 21413–21422. doi: 10.1074/jbc.M114.581124

Simchowitz, L. (1985). Intracellular pH modulates the generation of superoxide radicals by human neutrophils. *J. Clin. Invest.* 76, 1079–1089. doi: 10.1172/JCI112061

Sjøberg, K. A., Frøsig, C., Kjøbsted, R., Sylow, L., Kleinert, M., Betik, A. C., et al. (2017). Exercise increases human skeletal muscle insulin sensitivity via coordinated increases in microvascular perfusion and molecular signaling. *Diabetes* 66, 1501–1510. doi: 10.2337/db16-1327

Smith, P. K., Krohn, R. I., Hermanson, G. T., Mallia, A. K., Gartner, F. H., Provenzano, M. D., et al. (1985). Measurement of protein using bicinchoninic acid. *Anal. Biochem.* 150, 76–85. doi: 10.1016/0003-2697(85)90442-7

Tabatabaie, T., Potts, J. D., and Floyd, R. A. (1996). Reactive oxygen species-mediated inactivation of pyruvate dehydrogenase. *Arch. Biochem. Biophys.* 336, 290–296. doi: 10.1006/abbi.1996.0560

Teague, W. M., Pettit, F. H., Wu, T. L., Silberman, S. R., and Reed, L. J. (1982). Purification and properties of pyruvate dehydrogenase phosphatase from bovine heart and kidney. *Biochemistry* 21, 5585–5592. doi: 10.1021/bi00265a031

Thomas, A. P., and Denton, R. M. (1986). Use of toluene-permeabilized mitochondria to study the regulation of adipose tissue pyruvate dehydrogenase *in situ*. Further evidence that insulin acts through stimulation of pyruvate dehydrogenase phosphate phosphatase. *Biochem. J.* 238, 93–101. doi: 10.1042/bj2380093

Torres-Peralta, R., Losa-Reyna, J., Morales-Alamo, D., González-Izal, M., Pérez-Suárez, I., Ponce-González, J. G., et al. (2016a). Increased P_IO_2 at exhaustion in hypoxia enhances muscle activation and swiftly relieves fatigue: a placebo or a P_IO_2 dependent effect? *Front. Physiol.* 7:333. doi: 10.3389/fphys.2016.00333

Torres-Peralta, R., Morales-Alamo, D., Gonzalez-Izal, M., Losa-Reyna, J., Perez-Suarez, I., Izquierdo, M., et al. (2016b). Task failure during exercise to exhaustion in normoxia and hypoxia is due to reduced muscle activation caused by central mechanisms while muscle metaboreflex does not limit performance. *Front. Physiol.* 6:414. doi: 10.3389/fphys.2015.00414

Trewin, A. J., Lundell, L. S., Perry, B. D., Patil, K. V., Chibalin, A. V., Levinger, I., et al. (2015). Effect of N-acetylcysteine infusion on exercise-induced modulation of insulin sensitivity and signaling pathways in human skeletal muscle. *Am. J. Physiol. Endocrinol. Metab.* 309, E388–E397. doi: 10.1152/ajpendo.00605.2014

Vanhatalo, A., Jones, A. M., Blackwell, J. R., Winyard, P. G., and Fulford, J. (2014). Dietary nitrate accelerates postexercise muscle metabolic recovery and O_2 delivery in hypoxia. *J. Appl. Physiol.* 117, 1460–1470. doi: 10.1152/japplphysiol.00096.2014

Westerblad, H., Lee, J. A., Lännergren, J., and Allen, D. G. (1991). Cellular mechanisms of fatigue in skeletal muscle. *Am. J. Physiol.* 261, C195–C209. doi: 10.1152/ajpcell.1991.261.4.1-a

Wieland, O. H. (1983). The mammalian pyruvate dehydrogenase complex: structure and regulation. *Rev. Physiol. Biochem. Pharmacol.* 96, 123–170. doi: 10.1007/BFb0031008

Wu, C. A., Chao, Y., Shiah, S. G., and Lin, W. W. (2013). Nutrient deprivation induces the Warburg effect through ROS/AMPK-dependent activation of pyruvate dehydrogenase kinase. *Biochim. Biophys. Acta* 1833, 1147–1156. doi: 10.1016/j.bbamcr.2013.01.025

Xu, L., Eu, J. P., Meissner, G., and Stamler, J. S. (1998). Activation of the cardiac calcium release channel (ryanodine receptor) by poly-S-nitrosylation. *Science* 279, 234–237. doi: 10.1126/science.279.5348.234

Yeaman, S. J., Hutcheson, E. T., Roche, T. E., Pettit, F. H., Brown, J. R., Reed, L. J., et al. (1978). Sites of phosphorylation on pyruvate dehydrogenase from bovine kidney and heart. *Biochemistry* 17, 2364–2370. doi: 10.1021/bi00605a017

4

The Effect of Oxygen Enrichment on Cardiorespiratory and Neuropsychological Responses in Workers with Chronic Intermittent Exposure to High Altitude (ALMA, 5,050 m)

Fernando A. Moraga[1], Iván López[2], Alicia Morales[3], Daniel Soza[2] and Jessica Noack[3]*

[1] *Laboratorio de Fisiología, Hipoxia y Función Vascular, Departamento de Ciencias Biomédicas, Facultad de Medicina, Universidad Católica del Norte, Coquimbo, Chile,* [2] *Safety Group, Atacama Large Millimeter Submillimeter Array, Calama, Chile,* [3] *Departamento de Ciencias de la Salud, Escuela de Enfermería, Universidad Santo Tomás, Santiago, Chile*

Correspondence:
Fernando A. Moraga
fmoraga@ucn.cl

It is estimated that labor activity at high altitudes in Chile will increase from 60,000 to 120,000 workers by the year 2020. Oxygenation of spaces improves the quality of life for workers at high geographic altitudes (<5,000 m). The aim of this study was to determine the effect of a mobile oxygen module system on cardiorespiratory and neuropsychological performance in a population of workers from Atacama Large Millimeter/submillimeter Array (ALMA, 5,050 m) radiotelescope in the Chajnantor Valley, Chile. We evaluated pulse oximetry, systolic and diastolic arterial pressure (SAP/DAP), and performed neuropsychological tests (Mini-Mental State examination, Rey-Osterrieth Complex Figure test) at environmental oxygen conditions (5,050 m), and subsequently in a mobile oxygenation module that increases the fraction of oxygen in order to mimic the higher oxygen partial pressure of lower altitudes (2,900 m). The use of module oxygenation at an altitude of 5,050 m, simulating an altitude of 2,900 m, increased oxygen saturation from 84 ± 0.8 to $91 \pm 0.8\%$ ($p < 0.00001$), decreased heart rate from 90 ± 8 to 77 ± 12 bpm ($p < 0.01$) and DAP from 96 ± 3 to 87 ± 5 mmHg ($p < 0.01$). In addition, mental cognitive state of workers (Mini-Mental State Examination) shown an increased from 19 to 31 points ($p < 0.02$). Furthermore, the Rey-Osterrieth Complex Figure test (memory) shown a significant increase from 35 to 70 ($p < 0.0001$). The results demonstrate that the use of an oxygen module system at 5,050 m, simulating an altitude equivalent to 2,900 m, by increasing FiO_2 at 28%, significantly improves cardiorespiratory response and enhances neuropsychological performance in workers exposed to an altitude of 5,050 m.

Keywords: oxygen enrichment, neuropsychological impairment, oxygen saturation, heart rate, arterial pressure, chronic intermittent hypobaric hypoxia

INTRODUCTION

Exposure to high altitude has become an increasingly common event. As many as 140 million people live at altitudes over 2,500 m (Moore, 2001). However, mining activities at altitudes over 3,500 m are common in in the north of Chile and Peru. In Chile up until 1995, there were approximately 20,000 workers intermittently exposed to high altitudes for a long period of time (Jiménez, 1995), and this number is expected to increase to over 120,000 by the year 2020 (http://www.ccm.cl/wp-content/uploads/2016/06/fuerza_laboral_de_la_gran_mineria_chilena_2012_2020.pdf). In these conditions, chronic intermittent hypobaric hypoxia (CIHH) constitutes a model of hypobaric hypoxic exposure previously described by several authors (Jiménez, 1995; Richalet et al., 2002; Moraga et al., 2014).

The physiological consequences of the initial exposure to high altitude are widely known. For example, the incidence of acute mountain sickness depends on altitude reached, previous experience, velocity of ascent and is self-limited by exposure time (Davis and Hackett, 2017). Early studies showed the effect of acute exposure on neuropsychological performance. For instance, the reduction in oxygen at high altitude impairs mental and physical performance, and general well-being (Barcroft et al., 1923). In addition, studies performed in a population of miners at high altitude showed deterioration in cognition and motor function (Mc Farland, 1937). Exposure to high altitude resulted in impaired sleep quality with increased periodic breathing, increased awakenings and shorter stage 3 and 4 sleep, causing low productivity and altered general well-being (Gerard et al., 2000). All these effects were dependent on the altitude attained.

One way to avoid the consequences of high altitude hypoxemia is to reduce the equivalent altitude (altitude which provides the same PO_2 in moist inspired gas during ambient breathing). The first physiological response is given by an increase in ventilation and second by an artificial increase in oxygen supply. Therefore, we evaluated two different procedures that provide supplemental oxygen at high altitudes: an oxygen concentrator (West, 2016) and the use of liquid oxygen (Moraga et al., 2014). Both procedures mimic the higher oxygen partial pressure of a lower altitude by increasing in the oxygen fraction. The beneficial effects of this procedure enhancing sleep quality, neuropsychological function, and arterial oxygenation has been demonstrated in subjects exposed to conditions of simulated hypoxia at sea level, and subjects that have been acutely exposed to altitude hypoxia (West, 1995; Luks et al., 1998; Gerard et al., 2000; McElroy et al., 2000). Currently the only study performed during exposure to high altitude at 4,200 m, in miners acclimatized to CIHH, evaluated sleep quality and the nocturnal ventilation pattern, finding that they were significantly enhanced by oxygen administration (Moraga et al., 2014). However, no studies have evaluated a CIHH population at altitudes over 4,200 m. In addition, the ministry of health provided a technical guide for high altitude workers in 2014 that included a series of recommendations to reduce malaise during exposure to altitudes over 3,000 m. In regards to environmental oxygenation, the oxygen equivalent must be below 3,000 m with permanent control of temperature, relative humidity and room ventilation (web.minsal.cl/sites/default/files/guia_hipobaria_altitud.pdf). Therefore, our aim was probe a mobile module that reduced the equivalent altitude to values of 2,900 m, in an isolated sector at a very high altitude of 5,050 m in a population of workers from the Atacama Large Millimeter/ submillimeter Array (ALMA) radiotelescope in the Chajnantor valley, (Chile) and evaluate cardiorespiratory and neuropsychological on workers in both conditions.

SUBJECTS AND METHODS

Subjects

Thirteen voluntary subjects that lived at a low altitude ($<$1,000 m) and worked at ALMA (2,900 and 5,050 m) were studied. All subjects worked as antenna operators and had experience with CIHH for more than 4 years. Their shift pattern was 8 days of work at high altitude followed by 6 days rest at sea level. All subjects were free of cardiovascular, pulmonary, hematological, renal or hepatic diseases. All protocols and procedures performed in the present study were performed by following the Helsinki guidelines and have previously been approved by the Ethics Committee of the Facultad de Medicina of Universidad Católica del Norte and the ALMA Safety Department. A consent informed was obtained in written form each one of them previous being monitored.

Facilities

ALMA is located 30 Km from the town of San Pedro de Atacama. ALMA has two sectors: the first is located 16 kilometers from the town of San Pedro de Atacama and represents the base camp or Operations Support Facility (OSF) at 2,900 m; and the second sector is the Array Operation Site (AOS) where the antennas are located in the Chajnantor Valley. This valley is located 40 km from OSF at an altitude of 5,050 m. The full personnel capacity of ALMA (OSF and AOS) is close to 400 people, including scientists, operation specialists, and services that operate in chronic intermittent hypobaric hypoxia exposure.

Equipment

This study was performed at the AOS at 5,050 m where we designed a comfortable and mobile module (Oxymind™, INDURA, Chile) with facilities to increase the oxygen concentration (1 to 10%) and enhance the relative humidity and temperature (**Figure 1**). The oxygen concentration of the room air was controlled by a wide range oxygen sensor (0–50%, accuracy $\pm$ 2 ppm; Ultima XA, MSA, Pittsburg, USA) and maintained by a precise servo control system that allowed for an increase in oxygen concentration in 7% to reach 28 $\pm$ 0.5%, representing an equivalent altitude of 2,900 m with a lower low fire risk (West, 2001, 2003). In addition, precise control of CO_2, by using an infrared CO_2 sensor (ppm or % volume) (model Eagle 2, RKI Instruments Inc., Buffalo Grove, USA), was obtained by activating a fan (near 1400 m^3/h) in order to reduce the accumulation of CO_2 in the room (with a maintenance level of CO_2 $<$ 0.1%). Therefore, ventilation of the room was maintained by following the procedure described by West (1995) and Luks et al. (1998).

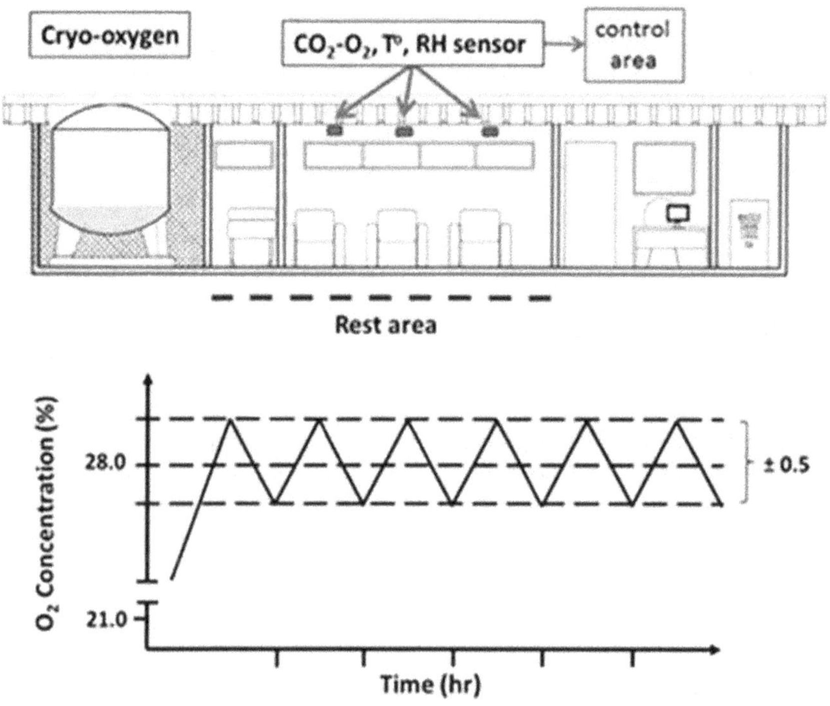

FIGURE 1 | The scheme represents a diagram of the mobile unit composed of three areas: cryo-oxygen, rest and control area. Control area measured concentration of gases (O_2 and CO_2), relative humidity (HR), and temperature (°C) and maintained these values at the established requirements. The bottom graph represents the oxygen level control pattern at 5,050 m.

Study Protocol

Cardiorespiratory responses and neuropsychological evaluations were performed in acclimatized workers 48 h after arrival to high altitude. All parameters were measured in two conditions: base camp (OSF, 2,900 m) and AOF (5,050 m) where voluntaries were evaluated breathing ambient air and breathing room air enriched with oxygen ($28 \pm 0.5\%$) at 5,050 m in order to reduce equivalent altitude to 2,900 m. The total exposure time in each condition was 20 min (20 min for cardiovascular and neuropsychological evaluations).

Cardiorespiratory Evaluations

Heart rate and oxygen saturation were continuously recorded in the subjects during the procedures with a pulse oximeter (Wristox 3100, Nonin, Minnesota, USA), all recordings were analyzed by nVision software (Nonin, Minnesota, USA). SpO_2 and heart rate values were extracted and analyzed min-min. Systolic arterial pressure (SAP), diastolic arterial pressure (DAP) and mean arterial pressure (MAP) were taken during the neuropsychological evaluation (model BM3, Bionet).

Neuropsychological Evaluation

In order to evaluate the effect of oxygen supply on cognitive function, a neuropsychological test was given to each volunteer. This test covered cognitive functions for memory and constructive praxis (Rey-Osterrieth Complex Figure test and Mini-Mental State Examination, MMSE).

Rey-Osterrieth Complex Figure Test

In our study, we use one of the most widely used test in both clinical and experimental settings to evaluate visuoconstructional abilities and nonverbal memory (Frank and Landeira-Fernandez, 2008). Subjects were given a blank paper to draw the figure best. They don't have of time for the copy or process to memory recall the draw. Afterward, the subjects were evaluated cardiorespiratory variables and MMSE, the time frame for this evaluation was approximately 10 min, and without warning each subject was given another blank sheet to recall the figure. The total time of evaluation, is don't was major than 15–20 min, in order to reduce the effects of fatigue produced by prolonged neurocognitive tests. Furthermore, time over 30 min the performance decay of this time (Loring et al., 1990). Each drawing was evaluated using a traditional scoring unit for the complex figure of 18 particular items of the complex figure (Loring et al., 1988), where each particular item was evaluated in accord to a two-point, with a total score of 36 points (**Table 1**). Considering that in our country we don't have a cut off values. However, empirical experience is accepted to copy values <27 points and memory values <17 points to both condition was considered such as deficiency visuoconstructional abilities and no verbal memory, respectively.

Mini-Mental State Examination (MMSE)

In our study we use the MMSE version of 35 points (Folstein et al., 1975). Each subject was examined in 5 mental state:

TABLE 1 | Traditional evaluation scoring for Rey-Osterrieth complex figure.

Criterias by each item	Score (0–2)
Placed and reproduced correctly	2
Reproduced incompletely placed incorrectly or presented some distortion	1
Placed or reproduced poorly	0.5
Absent or not recognized	0

Frank and Landeira-Fernandez (2000).

Orientation (10 points), Registration (3 points), Attention and calculation (8 points), Recall (3 points) and language (12 points). The presence of subject with values <24 points were considered cognitive alteration.

All analysis of each drawing of Rey-Osterrith Complex Figure test and MMSE were performed by blind evaluator at sea level. The lower neuropsychological test selection for our study was given by empirical experiences; these tests were significant at high altitude in workers with CIHH at 3,500 and 4,600 m (unpublished data).

Statistical Analysis

All results were expressed as mean ± standard deviation. Cardiorespiratory variables (SpO_2, HR, SAP, DAP) differences on means were analyzed using ANOVA followed by a Newman-Keuls test. Wilcoxon (Non-parametric test) to paired comparison was used to compare the difference of neuropsychological test. All differences were considered statistically significant when $p < 0.05$. Data analyses were performed using GraphPad Prism version 5.03 (GraphPad Software, Inc.).

RESULTS

Cardiorespiratory Variables at 2,900 and 5,050 m

Table 2 show a summary of the cardiorespiratory response obtained at camp base (OSF at 2,900 m) before ascending to the AOS at 5,050 m and cardiorespiratory values obtained in the AOS at 5,050 m. Pulse oximetry was decreased to values of 84 ± 0.8% ($p < 0.05$) that represent a fall approximately 9.7% in the arterial oxygenation and heart rate was increased to values of 90 ± 8 bpm ($p < 0.05$) that represented an increase of 16.8%, systolic arterial pressure was increased to values of 135 ± 18 mmHg that represented an increase of 11.6%, diastolic arterial pressure was increased to values of 96 ± 3 mmHg ($p < 0.05$) that represented an increase of 18.5% and mean arterial pressure was increased to values of 109 ± 8 mmHg ($p < 0.05$) that represented an increase of 15.9% was observed in all subjects when they arrived at 5,050 m, respect of values obtained in camp base (OSF, 2,900 m). During the protocol at 5,050 m when the subjects breathed room air, no modifications to the cardiorespiratory variables were observed. However, when subjects were placed in the module with an increase in FiO_2 to 28%, we observed a fast increase in the pulse oximetry to values of 91 ± 0.8 % ($p < 0.05$) that represented an increase of 8% arterial oxygenation and a fall in the cardiovascular response such as heart rate to values of 77 ± 12 bpm ($p < 0.05$) that represented a decreases by 14.4%, systolic arterial pressure to values of 128 ± 10 that represented a decreases 5.2%, diastolic arterial pressure to values of 87 ± 5 mmHg ($p < 0.05$) that represented a significant fall of 9.4% and mean arterial pressure to values of 101 ± 7 mmHg ($p < 0.05$) that represented a significant fall of 7.3%. No differences were observed in cardiorespiratory variables between OSF and AOS + O_2, reaching values similar to those observed at 2,900 m (OSF). **Figure 2** shows a typical pattern of oxygen saturation and heart rate recordings in a worker during a period of 40 min.

TABLE 2 | Cardiorespiratory response of workers exposed at 2,900 and 5,050 m.

	Altitude		
	2,900 m	5,050 m	
	Room air	Room air	Room air + 8 %O_2
SpO_2 (%)	93 ± 1	84 ± 0.8*	91 ± 0.8*
Heart rate (bpm)	77 ± 8	90 ± 8*	77 ± 12*
SAP (mmHg)	121 ± 6	135 ± 18	128 ± 10
DAP (mmHg)	81 ± 6	96 ± 3*	87 ± 5†
MAP (mmHg)	94 ± 8	109 ± 8*	101 ± 7†

*Values expressed as Mean ± SD. SpO_2, pulse oximetry; SAP, systolic arterial pressures; DAP, diastolic arterial pressure; MAP, mean arterial pressure. *$p < 0.001$ Room Air 2,900 vs. Room Air 5,050 m and 5,050 m + 8% O_2, †$p < 0.01$ Room air 5,050 m vs. Room Air 5,050 m + 8% O_2.*

Neuropsychological Assessment

Neuropsychological evaluations were performed with MMSE and revealed that when the subjects were tested in environmental oxygen conditions, 30% of the population presented disorders. However, upon entering the module with oxygen enrichment, this was reduced to 10% ($p < 0.05$). **Figure 3** represents the individual score obtained by MMSE.

When asked to evoke the Rey-Osterrieth Complex Figure test (memory), this capacity was significantly reduced in workers exposed to room air, with 50% of the patients meeting the criteria of a memory disorder (**Figures 4A,B**). However, when subjects were tested in the oxygen enriched module, the percentage of subjects below the cut off criteria was 10%, indicating a significant difference compared to subjects tested in environmental oxygen conditions.

DISCUSSION

This study is the first to assess the effect of environmental oxygen enrichment at 28% in very high altitude conditions (5,050 m) in a population of volunteers acclimatized to chronic and intermittent hypobaric hypoxia exposure for at least 4 years. Our results demonstrate that the mobile module that permits increased oxygen concentration, used to simulate an altitude equivalent to 2,900 m, significantly improved oxygen saturation and reduced heart rate and diastolic blood pressure, and enhanced neuropsychological performance in workers exposed to an altitude of 5,050 m.

Studies performed in CIHH models are scarce. Richalet et al. (2002) published results of a prospective study of workers exposed to CIHH for 2.5 years at an altitude of 4,500 m and described a developing acclimatization pattern along with emphasized health risks; right ventricular dilation and increased blood pressure. In addition, the incidence of acute mountain sickness is elevated on the first day, and is reduced, but does not disappear, with exposure time (Richalet et al., 2002). In addition, Brito et al. (2007) reported tachycardia, high blood pressure and low oxygen saturation after 12 years of CIHH exposure at 3,550 m. In addition, Siqués et al. (2009) found a significant increase in the diastolic pressure associated to lower oxygen saturation in young adults after 12 months of exposure at the same altitude. A study in acclimatized miners (1–14 years of CIHH exposure) showed the existence of periodic apnea breathing with episodes of arterial oxygen saturation reaching 67% (Moraga et al., 2014) at an altitude of 4,200 m. This severe level of hypoxemia triggers an increase in sympathetic tone. Previous studies support the observation that high altitude exposure promotes sympathetic activation and increases arterial pressure (Wolfel et al., 1994; Hansen and Sander, 2003). A preliminary study showed that 63% of people working at an altitude of 4,600 m had increased arterial pressure (>140/>90 mmHg) and oxygen saturation (<80%) (Moraga, unpublished results). In previous studies performed in our laboratory demonstrated that oxygen enrichment by 3–4% in a room at 4,200 m simulates an oxygen equivalent of 3,200 m, enhancing oxygen saturation, reducing heart rate, and inducing a general feeling of well-being in the morning. A better explanation of the effect of a decreased equivalent altitude with increased oxygen room is a decrease in the activation of the peripheral chemoreceptor as a consequence of reduced central neurosystem activation (see Dempsey et al., 2014). Previous studies support the role of carotid bodies in animal models where the carotid afferent was cut off, resulting in the abolishment of the sympathetic and hypertensive responses (see Prabhakar et al., 2012; Del Rio et al., 2016; Iturriaga et al., 2017).

In regard to the neuropsychological performance evaluated in our study, acute decreased oxygen availability at high altitudes is known to produce impaired mental and physical performance, increasing as the altitude also increases. The first studies performed in miners at 3,800 m, showed deterioration in cognition and motor function (Mc Farland, 1937). The first study that reported modifications in the neuropsychological response in miners exposed to CIHH, showed a decrease by

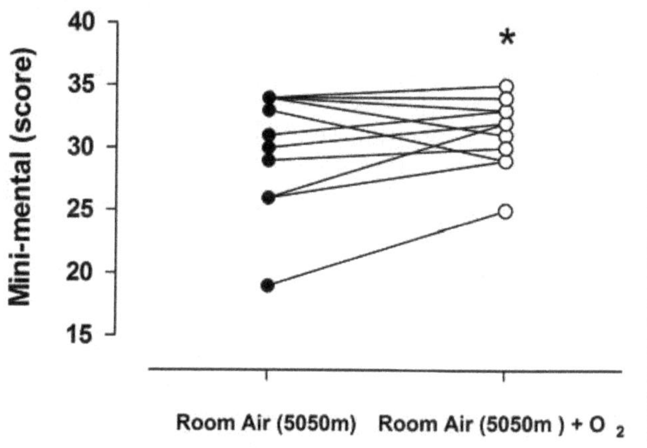

FIGURE 3 | Individual response on minimental score (MMscore) in 13 subjects breathing room air of 5,050 m (open circles) and room air of 5,050 m enriched with oxygen (closed circles). Values represent the score obtained of each subject in both condition. Lines represent the mean ± SD, asterisk $p < 0.001$.

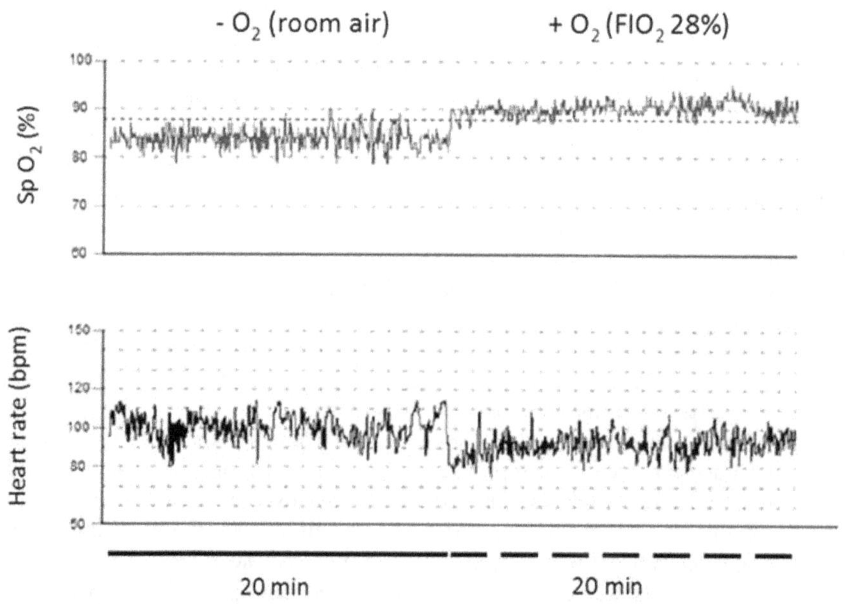

FIGURE 2 | Representative records of subjects tested at Chajnantor valley's (5,050 m) when breathing air alone (thin line pulse oximetry and thick line heart rate). The thick and segmented lines represent recording of 20 min without and with oxygen, respectively.

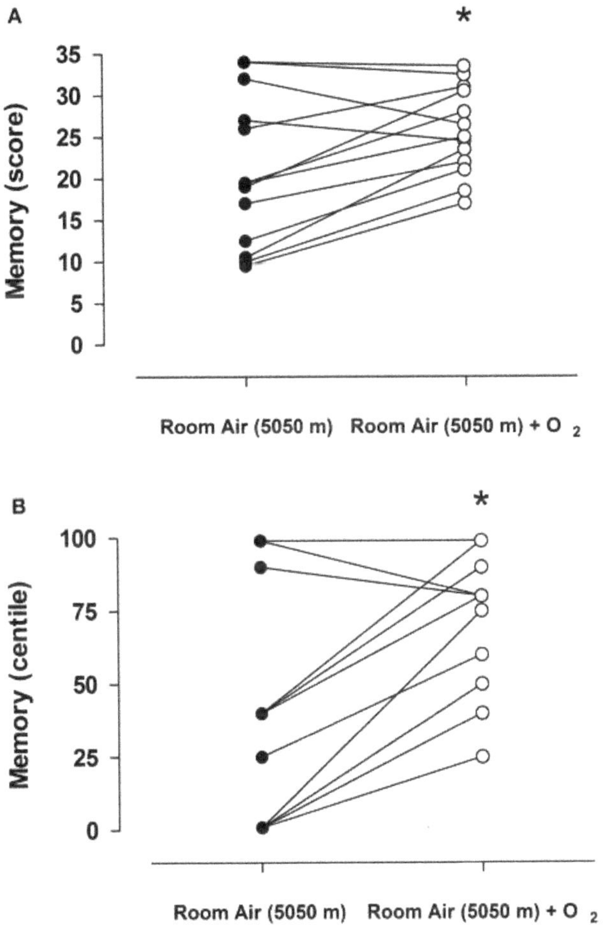

FIGURE 4 | Individual response to the Rey-Osterrieth Complex Figure (memory) in 13 subjects breathing room air of 5,050 m (open circles) and room air of 5,050 m enriched with oxygen (closed circles). **(A)** Represent absolute score obtained of each subject in both condition, and **(B)** represent values expressed in centile. The lines represent the mean ± SD, asterisk $p < 0.001$.

5% in the general cognitive aptitude on the 5th shift day at 4,500 m. The most affected elements were spatial aptitude (13% decrease) and mathematical reasoning (28% decrease) and neuropsychological attention (11% decrease) compared to evaluations performed at sea level (Jiménez, 1995). Additionally, in controlled hypobaric hypoxia conditions with an over imposed hypoxia of 5,000 m, neuropsychological function after increase of 6% percentage of oxygen on room, in no acclimatized voluntaries, reported an increase in oxygen saturation, quicker reaction times, improved hand-eye coordination, and more positive sense of well-being (Gerard et al., 2000). However, the study showed no significant improvement on neurophysiological function (Gerard et al., 2000). Therefore, our study is the first to assess neuropsychological performance in a population of acclimatized workers exposed to CIHH at a very high altitude (5,050 m) where room air levels were supplemented with oxygen at FiO_2 28% to obtain an equivalent altitude of 2,900 m. Exposure to high altitude decreased neuropsychological and cognitive functions for memory and constructive praxis (Rey-Osterrieth Complex Figure test, MMSE), however, this decreased response was reverted by increasing environmental oxygen at 28% in the room, supporting the notion that this response is due to low oxygen availability at very high altitudes, and our results suggest that this is a plastic response.

By other way, since the early work of Paul Bert in 1878, it has been assumed that the lower inspiratory pressure of oxygen is the primary stimulus for adaptation to hypoxia (See Conkin and Wessel, 2008). Later, Barcroft in 1925 showed that decreasing FIO_2 could produce a hypoxic condition (See Richard and Koehle, 2012). These studies were the starting point for the discussion about whether the physiological responses are equivalent in normobaric hypoxia and hypobaric hypoxia models (Savourey et al., 2003; Richard and Koehle, 2012) in order to predict susceptibility to suffer from acute mountain sickness (Savourey et al., 2003; Burtscher et al., 2008), optimal training for athletes (Levine and Stray-Gundersen, 2006) and others. In a recent review, evidence supported a difference in ventilation mechanisms between both hypoxia models (Coppel et al., 2015). In addition, the same study showed that the confounding factors such as time spent, temperature, humidity and statistical power, limit the conclusion of these finding (Coppel et al., 2015). However, a series of studies have shown that the hypobaric conditions of high altitude could have physiological effects that are independent of the fall in oxygen pressure (i.e., temperature, air density, fluid balance, the presence of a microbubble in pulmonary circulation, increased dead space, etc.) (Loeppky et al., 2005; Conkin and Wessel, 2008; Richard and Koehle, 2012; Coppel et al., 2015); but it is necessary to indicate that many of these studies were performed in simulated conditions (hypobaric or normobaric chambers). These conditions are very different to field studies, like that performed in our study since this evaluates workers acclimatized to CIHH at very high altitude (5,050 m), where increasing FiO_2 enhances well-being during their stay at high altitude. In a previous study, miners acclimatized to CIHH showed a different response to hemoconcentration during maximum exercise performed at sea level and high altitude (3,800 m), given by a mechanism mediated by a negative water balance (low intake, high loss) (Moraga et al., 2017), supporting the idea that the hypobaric condition of high altitude promotes a different response. Another, study evaluated heart rate and oxygen saturation during a hike at high altitude (Manua Kea, 4,205 m) and compared this with a simulate condition (normobaric hypoxia). The results showed that oxygen saturation was lower and heart rate was higher at high altitude compared with normobaric hypoxia (Netzer et al., 2017). More studies are necessary to improve our understanding of the mechanisms involved in tolerance and acclimatization to hypoxia, in all hypoxia exposure models (in our case, in miners exposed to CIHH).

LIMITATIONS

In our study it was impossible to perform a crossover long term study in the workers as they were only authorized by their supervisors to participate in the first evaluation, due to the high labor demand during the study period.

In conclusion, our study showed that the use of a mobile module oxygen system at 5,050 m, simulating an altitude equivalent to 2,900 m, significantly improves arterial oxygenation and heart rate, reduces diastolic blood pressure, and enhances neuropsychological performance. Our data support the requirements that the health ministry should implement to enhance the environmental work place; preventing and reducing the risk of labor at altitudes over 3,000 m.

AUTHOR CONTRIBUTIONS

FM conceived and designed the study. IL and AM supervises the overall the study. AM performed the statistical analysis. DS, AM, and JN contributed to sample and data collections. All authors drafted the report. All authors contributed to the interpretation of the results, critical revision of the manuscript and approved the final manuscript. FM is the guarantor.

FUNDING

This work was supported by the PI 537 I+D CORFO grant, Chile.

ACKNOWLEDGMENTS

We are grateful to all the volunteers from ALMA that participated in the study, and also for the facility support by the Safety Manager - ALMA.

REFERENCES

Barcroft, J., Binger, C. A., Bock, A. V., Doggart, J. H., Forbes, H. S., Harrop, G., et al. (1923). Observation upon the effects of high altitude on the physiological processes on the humans body, carried out in the Peruvian Andes, chiefly at Cerro de Pasco. *Phil. Trans. B* 211, 351–480. doi: 10.1098/rstb.1923.0008

Brito, J., Siqués, P., León-Velarde, F., De La Cruz, J. J., López, V., and Herruzo, R. (2007). Chronic intermittent hypoxia at high altitude exposure for over 12 years: assessment of hematological, cardiovascular, and renal effects. *High Alt. Med. Biol.* 8, 236–244. doi: 10.1089/ham.2007.8310

Burtscher, M., Szubski, C., and Faulhaber, M. (2008). Prediction of the susceptibility to AMS in simulated altitude. *Sleep Breath.* 12, 103–108. doi: 10.1007/s11325-007-0131-0

Conkin, J., and Wessel, J. H. (2008). Critique of the equivalent air altitude model. *Aviat Space Environ. Med.* 79, 975–982. doi: 10.3357/ASEM.2331.2008

Coppel, J., Hennis, P., Gilbert-Kawai, E., and Grocott, P. W. (2015). The physiological effect of hypoxia versus normobaric hypoxia: a systematic review of crossover trials. *Extrem. Physiol. Med.* 4:2. doi: 10.1186/s13728-014-0 021-6

Davis, C., and Hackett, P. (2017). Advances in the prevention and treatment of high altitude illness. *Emerg. Med. Clin. North Am.* 35, 241–260. doi: 10.1016/j.emc.2017.01.002

Del Rio, R., Andrade, D. C., Lucero, C., Arias, P., and Iturriaga, R. (2016). Carotid body ablation abrogates hypertension and autonomic alterations induced by intermittent hypoxia in rats. *Hypertension* 68, 436–445. doi: 10.1161/HYPERTENSIONAHA.116.07255

Dempsey, J. A., Powell, F. L., Bisgard, G. E., Blain, G. M., Poulin, M. J., and Smith, C. A. (2014). Role of chemoreception in cardiorespiratory acclimatization to, and deacclimatization from, hypoxia. *J. Appl. Physiol.* 116, 858–866. doi: 10.1152/japplphysiol.01126.2013

Folstein, M. F., Folstein, S. E., and McHugh, P. R. (1975). "Mini-mental state". A practical method for grading the cognitive state of patients for the clinician. *J. Psychiatr. Res.* 12, 189–198. doi: 10.1016/0022-3956(75)90026-6

Frank, J., and Landeira-Fernandez, J. (2008). Comparison between two scoring systems of the rey-osterrieth complex figures in left and right temporal lobe epileptic patients. *Arch. Clin. Neuropsycol.* 23, 839–845. doi: 10.1016/j.acn.2008.06.001

Gerard, A. B., McElroy, M. K., Taylor, M. J., Grant, I., Powell, F. L., Holverda, S., et al. (2000). Six percent oxygen enrichment of room air at simulated 5,000 m altitude improves neurological function. *High Alt. Med. Biol.* 1, 51–61. doi: 10.1089/152702900320685

Hansen, J., and Sander, M. (2003). Sympathetic neural overactivity in healthy humans after prolonged exposure to hypobaric hypoxia. *J. Physiol.* 546, 921–929. doi: 10.1113/jphysiol.2002.031765

Iturriaga, R., Oyarce, M. P., and Dias, A. C. R. (2017). Role of carotid body in intermittent hypoxia-related hypertension. *Curr. Hypertens. Rep.* 19:38. doi: 10.1007/s11906-017-0735-0

Jiménez, D. (1995). "High altitude intermittent chronic exposure: Andean miners," in *Hypoxia and the Brain*, eds J. R. Sutton, C. S. Houston, and G. Coates (Burlington: Queen City Printers), 284–291.

Levine, B. D., and Stray-Gundersen, J. (2006). Dose-response of altitude training: how much altitude is enough? *Adv. Exp. Med. Biol.* 588, 233–247. doi: 10.1007/978-0-387-34817-9_20

Loeppky, J. A., Roch, R. C., Maes, D., Hinghofer-Szalkay, H., Roessler, A., Gates, L., et al. (2005). Role of hypobaria in fluid balance response to hypoxia. *High Alt. Med. Biol.* 6, 60–71. doi: 10.1089/ham.2005.6.60

Loring, D. W., Lee, G. P., and Meador, K. J. (1988). Revising the Rey-Osterrieth: rating right hemisphere recall. *Arch. Clin. Neuropsychol.* 3, 239–247.

Loring, D. W., Martin, R. C., and Meador, K. J. (1990). Psychometric construction of the Rey-Osterrieth complex figure: methodological considerations and interrater reliability. *Arch. Clin. Neuropsychol.* 5, 1–14.

Luks, A. M., van Melick, H., Batarse, R. R., Powell, F. L., Grant, I., and West, J. B. (1998). Room oxygen enrichment improves sleep and subsequent day-time performance at high altitude. *Resp. Physiol.* 113, 247–258. doi: 10.1016/S0034-5687(98)00068-1

Mc Farland, R. A. (1937). Psychophysiological studies at high altitude in the Andes. *J. Comp. Psych.* 24, 189–220.

McElroy, M. K., Gerard, A. B., Powell, F. L., Pris, G. K., Sentse, N., Holverda, S., et al. (2000). Nocturnal O_2 enrichment of room air at high altitude increase daytime O_2 saturation without changing control of ventilation. *High Alt. Med. Biol.* 1, 197–206. doi: 10.1089/15270290050144190

Moore, L. G. (2001). Human genetic adaptation to high altitude. *High Alt. Med. Biol.* 2, 257–279. doi: 10.1089/152702901750265341

Moraga, F. A., Jiménez, D., Richalet, J. P., Vargas, M., and Osorio, J. (2014). Periodic breathing and oxygen supplementation in Chilean miners at high altitude (4200m). *Respir. Physiol. Neurobiol.* 203, 109–115. doi: 10.1016/j.resp.2014.09.001

Moraga, F. A., Osorio, J., Calderón-Jofré, R., and Pedreros, A. (2017). Hemoconcentration during maximum exercise in miners with chronic intermittent exposure to hypobaric hypoxia (3,800 m). *High Alt. Med. Biol.* doi: 10.1089/ham.2017.0011. [Epub ahead of print].

Netzer, N. C., Rausch, L., Eliasson, A. H., Gatterer, H., Friess, M. F., Burtscher, et al. (2017). SpO2 and heart rate during a real hike at altitude are significant different than at its simulation in normobaric hypoxia. *Front. Physiol.* 8:81. doi: 10.3389/fphys.2017.00081

Prabhakar, N. R., Kumar, G. K., and Peng, Y. J. (2012). Sympatho-adrenal activation by chronic intermittent hypoxia. *J. Appl. Physiol.* 113, 1304–1310. doi: 10.1152/japplphysiol.00444.2012

Richalet, J. P., Vargas, M., Jiménez, D., Antezana, A. M., Hudson, C., Cortès, G., et al. (2002). Chilean miners commuting from sea level to 4500 m: a prospective study. *High Alt. Med. Biol.* 3, 159–166. doi: 10.1089/15270290260131894

Richard, N. A., and Koehle, M. S. (2012). Differences in cardio-ventilatory response to hypobaric and normobaric hypoxia: a review. *Aviat Space Environ. Med.* 83, 677–684. doi: 10.3357/ASEM.3182.2012

Savourey, G., Launay, J. C., Besnard, Y., Guinet, A., and Travers, S. (2003). Normo- and hypobaric hypoxia: are there any physiological differences?. *Eur. J. Appl. Physiol.* 89, 122–126. doi: 10.1007/s00421-002-0789-8

Siqués, P., Brito, J., Banegas, J. R., León-Velarde, F., de la Cruz-Troca, J. J., López, V., et al. (2009). Blood pressure responses in young adults first exposed to high altitude for 12 months at 3550 m. *High Alt. Med. Biol.* 10, 329–335. doi: 10.1089/ham.2008.1103

West, J. B. (1995). Oxygen enrichment of room air to relieve the hypoxia of high altitude. *Resp. Physiol.* 99, 225–232. doi: 10.1016/0034-5687(94)00094-G

West, J. B. (2001). Safe upper limits for oxygen enrichment of room air at high altitude. *High Alt. Med. Biol.* 2,47–51. doi: 10.1089/152702901750067918

West, J. B. (2003). Improving oxygenation at high altitude: acclimatization and O2 enrichment. *High Alt. Med. Biol.* 4, 389–398. doi: 10.1089/152702903769192340

West, J. B. (2016). Oxygen conditioning: a new technique for improving living and working at high altitude. *Physiology* 31, 216–222. doi: 10.1152/physiol.00057.2015

Wolfel, E. E., Selland, M. A., Mazzeo, R. S., and Reeves, J. T.(1994). Systemic hypertension at 4,300 m is related to sympathoadrenal activity. *J. Appl. Physiol.* 76, 1643–1650. doi: 10.1152/jappl.1994.76.4.1643

5

Is Carotid Body Physiological O_2 Sensitivity Determined by a Unique Mitochondrial Phenotype?

*Andrew P. Holmes, Clare J. Ray, Andrew M. Coney and Prem Kumar**

Institute of Clinical Sciences, College of Medical and Dental Sciences, University of Birmingham, Birmingham, United Kingdom

Correspondence:
Prem Kumar
p.kumar@bham.ac.uk

The mammalian carotid body (CB) is the primary arterial chemoreceptor that responds to acute hypoxia, initiating systemic protective reflex responses that act to maintain O_2 delivery to the brain and vital organs. The CB is unique in that it is stimulated at O_2 levels above those that begin to impact on the metabolism of most other cell types. Whilst a large proportion of the CB chemotransduction cascade is well defined, the identity of the O_2 sensor remains highly controversial. This short review evaluates whether the mitochondria can adequately function as acute O_2 sensors in the CB. We consider the similarities between mitochondrial poisons and hypoxic stimuli in their ability to activate the CB chemotransduction cascade and initiate rapid cardiorespiratory reflexes. We evaluate whether the mitochondria are required for the CB to respond to hypoxia. We also discuss if the CB mitochondria are different to those located in other non-O_2 sensitive cells, and what might cause them to have an unusually low O_2 binding affinity. In particular we look at the potential roles of competitive inhibitors of mitochondrial complex IV such as nitric oxide in establishing mitochondrial and CB O_2-sensitivity. Finally, we discuss novel signaling mechanisms proposed to take place within and downstream of mitochondria that link mitochondrial metabolism with cellular depolarization.

Keywords: carotid body, hypoxia, mitochondria, nitric oxide, arterial chemoreceptor, O_2 sensor, metabolism, mitochondrial inhibitors

INTRODUCTION-THE CAROTID BODY AND HYPOXIA

The mammalian carotid body (CB) is a highly specialized sensory organ derived from the neural crest. The sensory units of the CB are the 'glomus' or 'type I' cells that respond to a variety of stimuli including hypoxia, hypercapnia, acidosis and hormones thereby allowing the CB to function as a polymodal receptor (Kumar and Bin-Jaliah, 2007; Ribeiro et al., 2013; Thompson et al., 2016). Type I cell activation leads to stimulation of adjacent chemoafferent fibers that relay sensory information into the central nervous system. The physiological consequence of CB stimulation is therefore the initiation of series of systemic protective reflexes characterized by increased ventilation, tachycardia, systemic vasoconstriction and adrenaline release from the adrenal medulla (Kumar, 2009).

There is now a general consensus that a series of key processes contribute to the CB hypoxic chemotransduction cascade. These include attenuation of outward K^+ current, type I cell depolarization, Ca^{2+} influx through L-type Ca^{2+} channels, neurosecretion and chemoafferent excitation (Kumar and Prabhakar, 2012; Lopez-Barneo et al., 2016). Single type I cells are exquisitely sensitive to O_2 and rapid (within ms) activation of the hypoxic chemotransduction cascade initiates at PO_2s of between 20–40 mmHg (Biscoe and Duchen, 1990; Buckler and Vaughan-Jones, 1994; Buckler and Turner, 2013); a level considerably greater than that at which cell metabolism is affected in O_2-insensitive cells.

What remains highly controversial is the molecular identity of the specific O_2 sensor within the type I cell. We would argue that the physiological O_2 sensor should exhibit certain key features: (1) expression in the type I cell permitting intrinsic O_2 sensitivity; (2) the ability to bind O_2; (3) its binding of O_2 occurs over the physiological range at which the type I cell is stimulated; (4) it is required for the CB to be stimulated by hypoxia; and (5) it is able to activate the CB transduction cascade within milliseconds. Many proposed sensors fit one or two of these criteria but few have been shown to adequately comply with all five.

In mammalian cells, O_2 is the terminal electron acceptor in the mitochondrial respiratory chain. Continuous binding and reduction of O_2 in the CuB/haem a_3 (cytochrome a_3) binuclear center of complex IV drives mitochondrial electron transport and promotes activation of the mitochondrial ATP synthase. The long-established, mitochondrial hypothesis for chemoreception proposes that CB excitation induced by hypoxia is initiated by a reduction in O_2 dependent mitochondrial energy respiration. This review will briefly critique the current evidence as to whether the mitochondria can be considered the functionally relevant O_2 sensors within the CB.

MITOCHONDRIAL INHIBITORS MIMIC ALL ASPECTS OF THE CAROTID BODY HYPOXIC CHEMOTRANSDUCTION CASCADE

All mitochondrial poisons induce chemoafferent excitation (Krylov and Anichkov, 1968; Mulligan et al., 1981; Obeso et al., 1989; Donnelly et al., 2014; Holmes et al., 2016, 2017) leading to rapid increases in ventilation (Owen and Gesell, 1931), heart rate and arterial blood glucose (Alvarez-Buylla and de Alvarez-Buylla, 1988). Chemoafferent responses are rapid, dose dependent and reversible (Donnelly et al., 2014; Holmes et al., 2016) and the magnitude of the rise in chemoafferent frequency caused by saturating concentrations is consistent with those evoked by severe hypoxia or anoxia (Krylov and Anichkov, 1968; Mulligan et al., 1981; Obeso et al., 1989). Furthermore, mitochondrial inhibitors and uncouplers augment neurotransmitter secretion, confirming an action through the type I cell rather than the afferent nerve endings (Obeso et al., 1989; Rocher et al., 1991). Despite the strong consistency between all of the different types of mitochondrial poisons (both in the older and more recent studies), it should be noted that some of the pharmacological agents used may not have acted selectively on the mitochondria and so the conclusions should be viewed with a certain degree of caution.

Mitochondrial poisons cause fast (within ms) type I cell depolarization and increases in $[Ca^{2+}]_i$. The size and timing of the $[Ca^{2+}]_i$ rise observed using many different mitochondrial inhibitors or uncouplers closely resembles that seen in hypoxia (Biscoe et al., 1989; Biscoe and Duchen, 1990; Wyatt and Buckler, 2004; Buckler, 2011). As with hypoxia (Buckler and Vaughan-Jones, 1994; Urena et al., 1994), the increases in $[Ca^{2+}]_i$ are dependent on cellular depolarization and extracellular Ca^{2+} influx through voltage gated Ca^{2+} channels (Wyatt and Buckler, 2004). TASK1/3, TREK-1, BK_{Ca}, $K_v4.1$, and $K_v4.3$, have all been shown to be expressed in the CB and inhibited by hypoxia (Buckler et al., 2000; Sanchez et al., 2002; Williams et al., 2004; Yamamoto and Taniguchi, 2006; Kim et al., 2009; Kreneisz et al., 2009; Turner and Buckler, 2013; Wang et al., 2017b). Of these, TASK1/3 and TASK-like K^+ currents are diminished by a multitude of mitochondrial inhibitors leading to membrane depolarization (Barbe et al., 2002; Wyatt and Buckler, 2004; Buckler, 2011; Turner and Buckler, 2013; Kim D. et al., 2015).

Recent evidence has revealed the presence of TRP and other non-selective Ca^{2+}-activated cation currents in type I cells that are activated by hypoxia (Kumar et al., 2006; Kang et al., 2014; Kim I. et al., 2015; Wang et al., 2017a). Although intriguing, the full functional relevance of these currents in type I cell O_2-sensing remains to be further characterized, and in particular whether these currents can be upregulated to preserve O_2 sensing in the absence of TASK channels (Turner and Buckler, 2013). Current evidence suggests that mitochondrial inhibitors are also capable of increasing these inward depolarizing currents (Kim I. et al., 2015; Wang et al., 2017a).

MITOCHONDRIA ARE NECESSARY FOR THE CAROTID BODY TO RESPOND TO HYPOXIA

The presence of functional mitochondria does appear necessary for the CB to respond fully to hypoxia. For instance, cyanide, rotenone and FCCP all attenuate TASK channel currents in such a way that prevents any further reduction by hypoxia (Wyatt and Buckler, 2004). In intact CB preparations oligomycin, cyanide and azide all reduce or abolish subsequent chemoafferent responses to hypoxia (Mulligan et al., 1981; Donnelly et al., 2014). Some of the attenuation observed in these experiments may have been due to impairment of oxidative phosphorylation in the chemoafferent fibers, limiting their excitability. Any such impairment is not apparent in response to physiological levels of hypoxia, since the PO_2 that activates the type I cells occurs at a much higher level than those which would decrease mitochondrial function in the chemoafferent fibers. As such, chemoafferent responses to sustained hypoxia are better maintained than those in response to sustained high doses of mitochondrial inhibitors (Mulligan et al., 1981).

In a recent study the importance of mitochondrial complex I was tested by developing mice deficient in *Ndufs2* (a gene coding for NADH dehydrogenase [ubiquinone] iron-sulfur protein 2- a component of complex I that participates in ubiquinone binding) in tyrosine hydroxylase positive cells (Fernandez-Aguera et al., 2015). Type I cells isolated from these mice were insensitive to hypoxia; they lacked any hypoxia-induced K^+ current attenuation, $[Ca^{2+}]_i$ elevation or neurotransmitter release. Furthermore, these mice failed to increase respiratory frequency when breathing 10% O_2. This work supported a previous study in which type I cell hypoxic chemosensitivity was abolished in the presence of rotenone (Ortega-Saenz et al., 2003). The authors propose a mechanism whereby exposure to hypoxia promotes reverse electron transport and ROS/NADH generation via complex I which is driven by a high rate of succinate oxidation at complex II. Accordingly, they have recently shown that genetic and pharmacological deactivation of complex II completely blocks type I cell hypoxic sensitivity (Gao et al., 2017).

This intriguing and elegant hypothesis does, however, show some discrepancies with evidence from earlier reports. For instance, similar experiments performed on CBs with heterozygous *Sdhd* knock out displayed an augmented, rather than depressed basal activity and had a completely preserved hypoxic response (Piruat et al., 2004). Furthermore, when rat type I cells were exposed to tetramethyl-*p*-phenylenediamine (TMPD) and ascorbate in the presence of rotenone, there was still a robust elevation in Ca^{2+} upon hypoxic stimulation (Wyatt and Buckler, 2004). This would suggest that feeding electrons into cytochrome c is sufficient to sustain type I cell hypoxic sensitivity even when complex I activity (and ROS generation) is inhibited. Complex IV activity rather than complex I and II may therefore be necessary for hypoxic chemotransduction. The same report also showed that application of H_2O_2 was unable to excite the type I cell directly. This observation is consistent with the lack of effect of multiple anti-oxidants used in other CB preparations and animal species (Sanz-Alfayate et al., 2001; Agapito et al., 2009; Gomez-Nino et al., 2009). Interestingly, using novel *ex vivo* CB culture techniques combined with FRET based ROS sensors, Bernardini et al. (2015) deduced that type I cell ROS actually decreases in hypoxia due to reduction in NADPH oxidase activity (an alternative ROS source). Clearly there is a need for reconciliation between these findings.

THE CAROTID BODY MITOCHONDRIA ARE UNIQUE AND HAVE A LOW THRESHOLD FOR O_2

The evidence that mitochondria are required for CB O_2 chemotransduction and that mitochondrial inhibitors can cause chemoexcitation, is not enough to define them as the O_2-sensors in the CB. Clearly, mitochondria are able to bind O_2. However, the K_m of the cytochrome a_3 for O_2 is reported to be <1 mmHg in isolated mitochondria and between 1–5 mmHg in dissociated cells and tissue preparations, with little variation existing between different cell types (Wilson et al., 1988; Tamura et al., 1989). This is far lower than the PO_2 at which the CB type I cells begin to be activated and, for this reason, is a common argument against the mitochondrial hypothesis.

However, there is now a substantial body of evidence indicating that the CB type I cell mitochondria are unique. Experiments performed by Mills and Jobsis (1970, 1972), were the first to identify an unusually low affinity cytochrome a_3 within the CB. Using absorbance spectra, they estimated that 43–67.5% of total cytochrome a_3 within the intact CB preparation had a remarkably low O_2 affinity. This fraction was reported to be almost 100% reduced at PO_2s between 7–9 mmHg and 50% reduced at a PO_2 as high as 90 mmHg. In contrast, the remaining fraction was only 50% reduced at a PO_2 of approximately 0.8 mmHg, comparable to cytochrome a_3 found in other tissues (Gnaiger, 2001). Thus, the CB appeared to express both low and high affinity subtypes of cytochrome a_3. At that time, the specific cellular location(s) of each was unclear. Later experiments utilized the photolabile binding of CO, to deduce that saturation of cytochrome a_3 with CO prevented any additional chemoafferent excitation during hypoxia, implying that not only was the cytochrome a_3 in the CB unusual, it was also required for O_2-sensing (Wilson et al., 1994; Lahiri et al., 1999). It should be pointed out that the concentrations of CO used in these studies could have directly modified the activity of the BK_{Ca} channel (Williams et al., 2004, 2008) and the generation of H_2S (Yuan et al., 2015) and as such some of the observations could be related to mechanisms independent of the mitochondria.

In dissociated rabbit type I cell clusters, mitochondrial electron transport begins to be inhibited at a high PO_2 value of approximately 40 mmHg (Duchen and Biscoe, 1992a). PO_2-NADH response curves demonstrate a significant 'right shift' in type I cells compared to sensory neurons, indicative of a heightened and distinctive O_2 sensitivity. In addition, mitochondrial depolarization occurs at higher PO_2s compared to O_2-insensitive cells (Duchen and Biscoe, 1992b). More recent work has verified the "right shifts" in both PO_2-NADH and PO_2-rh-123 response curves in rat type I cells, confirming that the unusually low mitochondrial O_2 affinity is conserved in multiple species (Turner and Buckler, 2013). By isolating complex IV activity with a cocktail of mitochondrial inhibitors plus TMPD and ascorbate, the authors were able to reveal that complex IV activity is a component of the mitochondria with the exceptionally low O_2 affinity. Importantly, type I cell hypoxic response curves for electron transport inhibition, mitochondrial depolarization and complex IV run-down display considerable overlap with the rise in Ca^{2+}, indicating that these processes are intimately linked. Therefore, it does appear that type I cell mitochondria have a highly specialized *low affinity* for O_2 due to an altered function/subtype of cytochrome a_3 in complex IV that predisposes CB energy metabolism to being impaired at high O_2 tensions. It is likely that the high affinity cytochrome a_3 in the CB described by Mills & Jöbsis is located in the non-O_2 sensing tissue such as the, nerve endings, blood vessels and type II cells.

Understanding the mechanism linking a fall in mitochondrial O_2 consumption with K^+ channel inhibition (or cation channel activation) is contentious. As previously mentioned, there could be a role for elevated mitochondrial ROS generation but this is still to be validated (Fernandez-Aguera et al., 2015). Another possibility is an alteration in cytosolic nucleotides. Switching from a cell attached to inside-out patch configuration diminishes background K^+ channel activity, suggesting that a basal level of an intracellular factor(s) activates TASK channels in normoxia (Varas et al., 2007). Addition of 5 mM MgATP in the inside-out configuration can restore about 50% of this background K^+ channel activity. Both mitochondrial inhibition and hypoxia also significantly elevate free Mg^{2+}, consistent with a decrease in MgATP. Thus, the fall in MgATP during hypoxia is likely to attenuate a significant proportion of TASK-current leading to depolarization. However, the remaining modulators that account for the other 50% of TASK current are still to be identified.

Another proposed mediator of TASK channel activity that is sensitive to changes in cytosolic nucleotide concentrations is AMPK (Wyatt et al., 2007). However, initial favorable studies based on pharmacological evidence have since been challenged by the finding that the AMPK-$\alpha_1\alpha_2$ deficient CB retains complete O_2-sensitivity (Mahmoud et al., 2016). Other groups have also shown that pharmacological targeting of AMPK does not impact on the hypoxia-induced K^+ channel inhibition (Kim et al., 2014). Discrepancies may arise from the non-selectivity of the drugs used to evaluate AMPK function and potential redundancy mechanisms known to develop in genetic animal models (Nowak et al., 1997). A final hypothesis is that a build-up in lactate upon mitochondrial inhibition in hypoxia activates the olfactory receptor Olfr78 (Chang et al., 2015). However, the concentration of lactate necessary to elevate Ca^{2+} in an intact CB preparation appears to be quite high (30 mM) and whether local levels reach this threshold during hypoxia is uncertain. We await a mechanism demonstrating how activation of Olfr78 (a G-protein-coupled receptor) modulates TASK or cation channel activity. A summary of the proposed O_2-sensitive mitochondrial signaling pathways in the CB is presented in **Figure 1**.

WHAT DETERMINES THE LOW O_2 AFFINITY OF THE CAROTID BODY MITOCHONDRIA?

We propose that there are 2 potential means to account for the extraordinary O_2 sensitivity of type I cell mitochondria. First, there could be a high level of production of a cytosolic factor that is able to freely diffuse into the mitochondria and then compete with O_2 binding in complex IV (**Figure 2**). We predict that this competition would render mitochondrial electron transport more susceptible to subsequent falls in O_2. We recently tested this by applying exogenous nitrite to CBs and subsequently measuring hypoxic sensitivity (Holmes et al., 2016). Nitrite is reduced within the mitochondria to generate local NO, a recognized competitive inhibitor of complex IV (Brown and Cooper, 1994; Cleeter et al., 1994; Castello et al.,

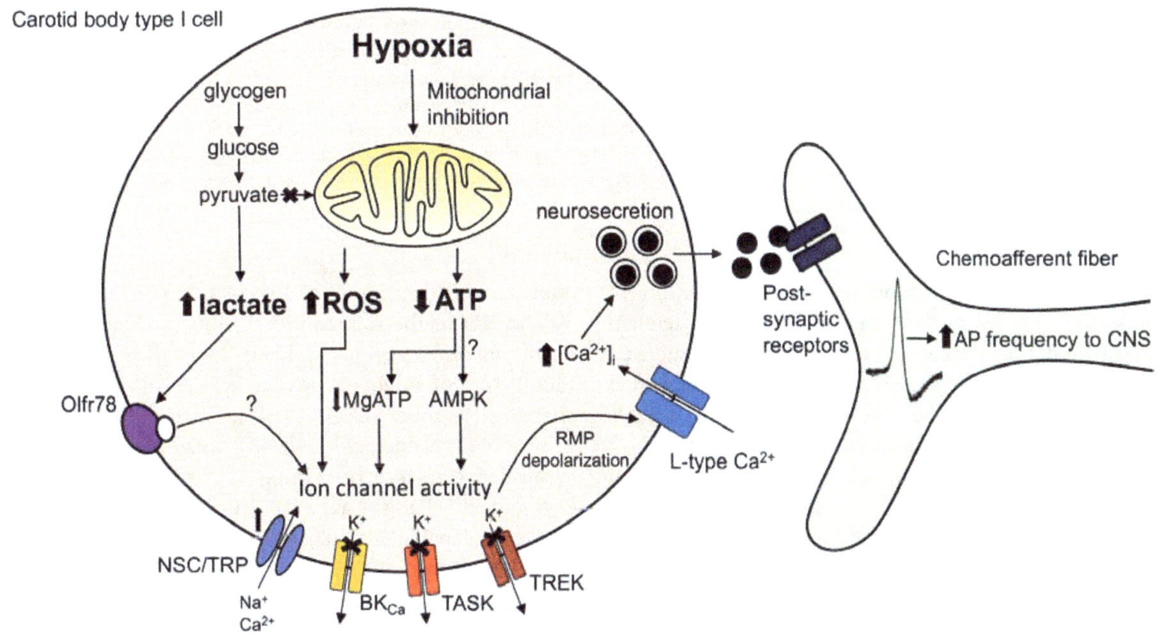

FIGURE 1 | Carotid body mitochondrial signaling mechanisms activated during hypoxia. Hypoxia-induced mitochondrial inhibition is proposed to increase lactate generation (Chang et al., 2015), augment mitochondrial complex I reactive oxygen species (ROS) production (Fernandez-Aguera et al., 2015) or reduce mitochondrial ATP synthesis (Buckler and Turner, 2013). These changes are proposed to directly or indirectly (e.g., via Olf78 receptor activation, reduced MgATP concentration or stimulation of AMP-activated protein kinase; AMPK) modify ion channel function leading to resting membrane potential (RMP) depolarization. This causes opening of L-type Ca^{2+} channels, neurosecretion and an increase in discharge frequency of the adjacent chemoafferent fibers. TRP, transient receptor potential channel; NSC, non-selective cation channel; BK_{Ca}, large conductance Ca^{2+}-activated K^+ channel; TASK, TWIK-related acid-sensitive K^+ channel; TREK, TWIK-related K^+ channel; AP, action potential.

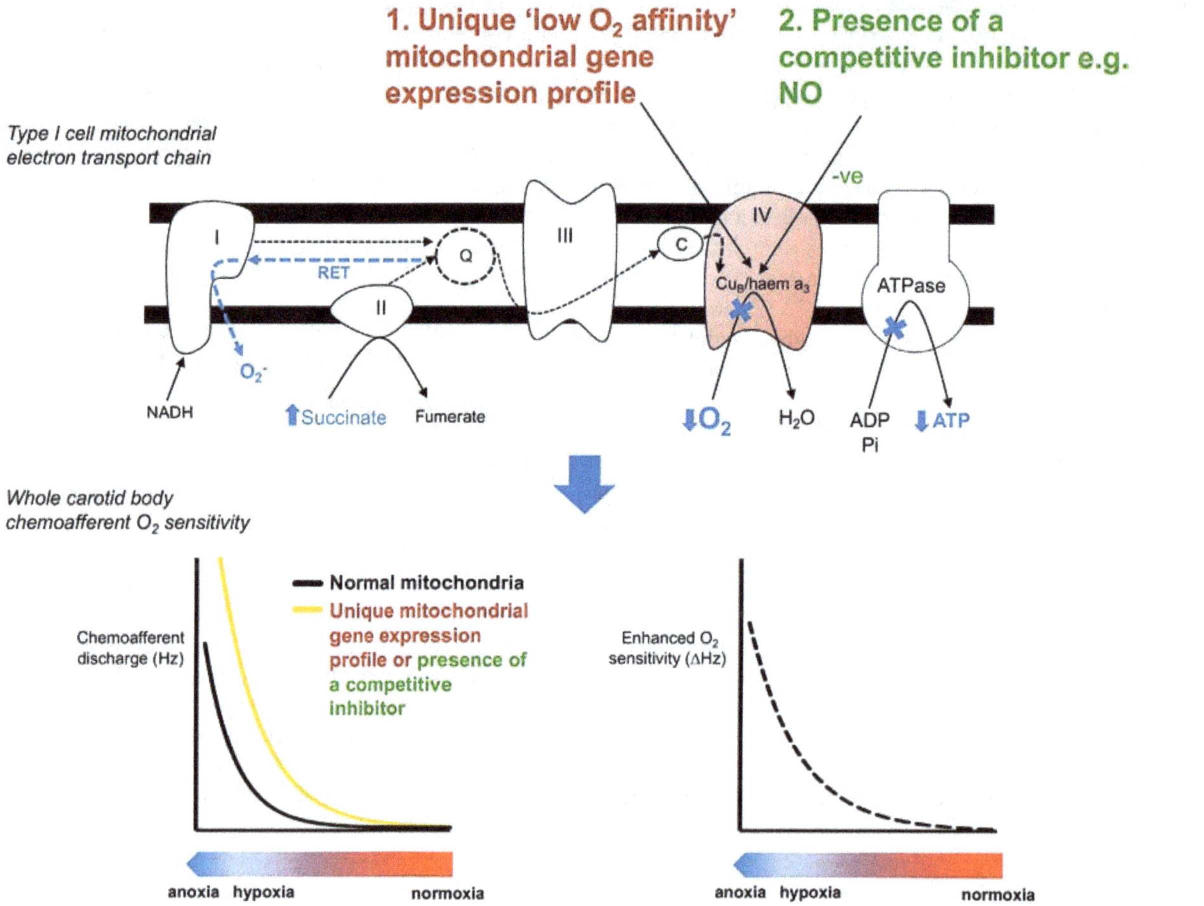

FIGURE 2 | Potential mechanisms underlying the unique low O_2 affinity mitochondria in the carotid body. Inhibition of mitochondrial function in the carotid body type I cell occurs at PO_2 values well above those that inhibit metabolism in other O_2 insensitive cells. This activates a number of proposed signaling pathways (shown in blue). The unique low O_2 affinity of the carotid body mitochondria could be due to (1) a unique mitochondrial gene expression profile or (2) the presence of a competitive inhibitor such as NO (Holmes et al., 2016). The impact of lower mitochondrial O_2 affinity is to cause a right-shift in the PO_2-chemoafferent response curve, thereby enhancing the functional O_2 sensitivity and allowing the carotid body to respond over a more physiological range of arterial PO_2s. RET, reverse electron transport.

2006, 2008; Basu et al., 2008). Moderate basal inhibition of the CB mitochondria by nitrite exaggerated the subsequent chemoafferent excitation during hypoxia signifying an increase in CB O_2 sensitivity. Therefore, we validated the idea that CB hypoxic sensitivity could be adjusted by a factor capable of competing with O_2 in the mitochondria and suggested a physiological role for endogenous NO in establishing type I cell mitochondrial O_2-sensitivity. Measurable amounts of NO have been detected in mitochondrial of type I cells (Yamamoto et al., 2006). A possible source is nitric oxide synthase 3 (NOS-3) given its location within the type I cell (Yamamoto et al., 2006). Interestingly, mice with reduced NOS-3 have a dampened hypoxic ventilatory response and a depressed CB function (Kline et al., 2000). One explanation for this is an adaptation to chronic hypoxia brought about by reduced CB blood flow. However, this is unlikely as there is no significant type I cell hyperplasia/hypertrophy (McGregor et al., 1984; Tatsumi et al., 1991). Instead, the blunted CB activity could be due to the lack of NO acting on the CB mitochondria. Consideration of the precise compartmentalization of NO should also be taken into account. Whilst NO in the mitochondria induces chemostimulation, its action in other regions is likely to have opposing effects via modulation of soluble guanylate cyclase and L-type Ca^{2+}/BK_{Ca} channels (Summers et al., 1999; Iturriaga et al., 2000; Silva and Lewis, 2002; Valdes et al., 2003). In addition, other diffusible cytosolic factors have been implicated in CB O_2 sensing including H_2S and CO (Peng et al., 2010; Yuan et al., 2015). Both of these gasses are capable of inhibiting type I cell mitochondria (Wilson et al., 1994; Lahiri et al., 1999; Buckler, 2011). Future experiments are required to evaluate if these substances act by setting type I cell mitochondrial O_2 sensitivity.

A second explanation for the low O_2-affinity of the type I cell mitochondria is that it has a unique gene expression profile (**Figure 2**). Exploring gene expression in the CB is challenging due to its relatively small size and heterogeneity. However, advances in molecular biology techniques now make it possible to perform whole genome analysis using just micrograms of tissue or even single cells. RNA-sequencing analysis has now revealed a number of mitochondrial related genes that have a particularly high expression in the type I cell (Zhou et al., 2016). Of these *Ndufa4l2* and *Cox4i2* have been shown to be more highly expressed in the CB compared with tissue from the superior cervical ganglion (Gao et al., 2017). Whether these two genes contribute to the low mitochondrial O_2 affinity remains to be determined but these findings do support the idea that CB mitochondria have a unique genetic signature encoding their mitochondrial complexes. We would expect many more genetic studies to probe this further until the type I cell mitochondria can be accurately modeled to pinpoint the structural conformation underlying its low O_2 affinity. An interesting comparator may be the mitochondria isolated from guinea pig CB which does not appear to have any inherent O_2 sensitivity (Gonzalez-Obeso et al., 2017).

CONCLUSION

On current evidence, it is very hard to disprove the mitochondrial hypothesis of CB O_2 sensing. The mitochondria seem to fulfill all five criteria that we have proposed for adequate O_2-sensors. What is less clear is a mechanistic understanding of how the low O_2 sensitivity of the CB mitochondria is achieved and if mitochondria are involved in establishing pathological changes in CB function.

AUTHOR CONTRIBUTIONS

AH, CR, AC, and PK all contributed to the writing and editing of the manuscript.

REFERENCES

Agapito, M. T., Sanz-Alfayate, G., Gomez-Nino, A., Gonzalez, C., and Obeso, A. (2009). General redox environment and carotid body chemoreceptor function. *Am. J. Physiol. Cell Physiol.* 296, C620–C631. doi: 10.1152/ajpcell.00542.2008

Alvarez-Buylla, R., and de Alvarez-Buylla, E. R. (1988). Carotid sinus receptors participate in glucose homeostasis. *Respir. Physiol.* 72, 347–359. doi: 10.1016/0034-5687(88)90093-X

Barbe, C., Al-Hashem, F., Conway, A. F., Dubuis, E., Vandier, C., and Kumar, P. (2002). A possible dual site of action for carbon monoxide-mediated chemoexcitation in the rat carotid body. *J. Physiol.* 543(Pt 3), 933–945. doi: 10.1113/jphysiol.2001.015750

Basu, S., Azarova, N. A., Font, M. D., King, S. B., Hogg, N., Gladwin, M. T., et al. (2008). Nitrite reductase activity of cytochrome c. *J. Biol. Chem.* 283, 32590–32597. doi: 10.1074/jbc.M806934200

Bernardini, A., Brockmeier, U., Metzen, E., Berchner-Pfannschmidt, U., Harde, E., Acker-Palmer, A., et al. (2015). Type I cell ROS kinetics under hypoxia in the intact mouse carotid body ex vivo: a FRET-based study. *Am. J. Physiol. Cell Physiol.* 308, C61–C67. doi: 10.1152/ajpcell.00370.2013

Biscoe, T. J., and Duchen, M. R. (1990). Responses of type I cells dissociated from the rabbit carotid body to hypoxia. *J. Physiol.* 428, 39–59. doi: 10.1113/jphysiol.1990.sp018199

Biscoe, T. J., Duchen, M. R., Eisner, D. A., O'Neill, S. C., and Valdeolmillos, M. (1989). Measurements of intracellular Ca2+ in dissociated type I cells of the rabbit carotid body. *J. Physiol.* 416, 421–434. doi: 10.1113/jphysiol.1989.sp017769

Brown, G. C., and Cooper, C. E. (1994). Nanomolar concentrations of nitric oxide reversibly inhibit synaptosomal respiration by competing with oxygen at cytochrome oxidase. *FEBS Lett.* 356, 295–298. doi: 10.1016/0014-5793(94)01290-3

Buckler, K. J. (2011). Effects of exogenous hydrogen sulphide on calcium signalling, background (TASK) K channel activity and mitochondrial function in chemoreceptor cells. *Pflugers Arch.* 463, 743–754. doi: 10.1007/s00424-012-1089-8

Buckler, K. J., and Turner, P. J. (2013). Oxygen sensitivity of mitochondrial function in rat arterial chemoreceptor cells. *J. Physiol.* 591(Pt 14), 3549–3563. doi: 10.1113/jphysiol.2013.257741

Buckler, K. J., and Vaughan-Jones, R. D. (1994). Effects of hypoxia on membrane potential and intracellular calcium in rat neonatal carotid body type I cells. *J. Physiol.* 476, 423–428. doi: 10.1113/jphysiol.1994.sp020143

Buckler, K. J., Williams, B. A., and Honore, E. (2000). An oxygen-, acid- and anaesthetic-sensitive TASK-like background potassium channel in rat arterial chemoreceptor cells. *J. Physiol.* 525(Pt 1), 135–142. doi: 10.1111/j.1469-7793.2000.00135.x

Castello, P. R., David, P. S., McClure, T., Crook, Z., and Poyton, R. O. (2006). Mitochondrial cytochrome oxidase produces nitric oxide under hypoxic conditions: implications for oxygen sensing and hypoxic signaling in eukaryotes. *Cell Metab.* 3, 277–287. doi: 10.1016/j.cmet.2006.02.011

Castello, P. R., Woo, D. K., Ball, K., Wojcik, J., Liu, L., and Poyton, R. O. (2008). Oxygen-regulated isoforms of cytochrome c oxidase have differential effects on its nitric oxide production and on hypoxic signaling. *Proc. Natl. Acad. Sci. U.S.A.* 105, 8203–8208. doi: 10.1073/pnas.0709461105

Chang, A. J., Ortega, F. E., Riegler, J., Adison, D. V. M., and Krasnow, M. A. (2015). Oxygen regulation of breathing through an olfactory receptor activated by lactate. *Nature* 527, 240–244. doi: 10.1038/nature15721

Cleeter, M. W., Cooper, J. M., Darley-Usmar, V. M., Moncada, S., and Schapira, A. H. (1994). Reversible inhibition of cytochrome c oxidase, the terminal enzyme of the mitochondrial respiratory chain, by nitric oxide. Implications for neurodegenerative diseases. *FEBS Lett.* 345, 50–54. doi: 10.1016/0014-5793(94)00424-2

Donnelly, D. F., Kim, I., Mulligan, E. M., and Carroll, J. L. (2014). Non-additive interactions between mitochondrial complex IV blockers and hypoxia in rat carotid body responses. *Respir. Physiol. Neurobiol.* 190, 62–69. doi: 10.1016/j.resp.2013.09.009

Duchen, M. R., and Biscoe, T. J. (1992a). Mitochondrial function in type I cells isolated from rabbit arterial chemoreceptors. *J. Physiol.* 450, 13–31.

Duchen, M. R., and Biscoe, T. J. (1992b). Relative mitochondrial membrane potential and [Ca2+]i in type I cells isolated from the rabbit carotid body. *J. Physiol.* 450, 33–61.

Fernandez-Aguera, M. C., Gao, L., Gonzalez-Rodriguez, P., Pintado, C. O., Arias-Mayenco, I., Garcia-Flores, P., et al. (2015). Oxygen sensing by arterial chemoreceptors depends on mitochondrial complex I Signaling. *Cell Metab.* 22, 825–837. doi: 10.1016/j.cmet.2015.09.004

Gao, L., Bonilla-Henao, V., Garcia-Flores, P., Arias-Mayenco, I., Ortega-Saenz, P., and Lopez-Barneo, J. (2017). Gene expression analyses reveal metabolic specifications in acute O-2-sensing chemoreceptor cells. *J. Physiol.* 595, 6091–6120. doi: 10.1113/jp274684

Gnaiger, E. (2001). Bioenergetics at low oxygen: dependence of respiration and phosphorylation on oxygen and adenosine diphosphate supply. *Respir. Physiol.* 128, 277–297. doi: 10.1016/s0034-5687(01)00307-3

Gomez-Nino, A., Agapito, M. T., Obeso, A., and Gonzalez, C. (2009). Effects of mitochondrial poisons on glutathione redox potential and carotid body chemoreceptor activity. *Respir. Physiol. Neurobiol.* 165, 104–111. doi: 10.1016/j.resp.2008.10.020

Gonzalez-Obeso, E., Docio, I., Olea, E., Cogolludo, A., Obeso, A., Rocher, A., et al. (2017). Guinea Pig oxygen-sensing and carotid body functional properties. *Front. Physiol.* 8:12. doi: 10.3389/fphys.2017.00285

Holmes, A. P., Ray, C. J., Pearson, S. A., Coney, A. M., and Kumar, P. (2017). Ecto-5′-nucleotidase (CD73) regulates peripheral chemoreceptor activity and cardiorespiratory responses to hypoxia. *J. Physiol.* doi: 10.1113/JP274498 [Epub ahead of print].

Holmes, A. P., Turner, P. J., Buckler, K. J., and Kumar, P. (2016). Moderate inhibition of mitochondrial function augments carotid body hypoxic sensitivity. *Pflugers Arch.* 468, 143–155. doi: 10.1007/s00424-015-1745-x

Iturriaga, R., Villanueva, S., and Mosqueira, M. (2000). Dual effects of nitric oxide on cat carotid body chemoreception. *J. Appl. Physiol.* 89, 1005–1012. doi: 10.1152/jappl.2000.89.3.1005

Kang, D., Wang, J., Hogan, J. O., Vennekens, R., Freichel, M., White, C., et al. (2014). Increase in cytosolic Ca2+ produced by hypoxia and other depolarizing stimuli activates a non-selective cation channel in chemoreceptor cells of rat carotid body. *J. Physiol.* 592(Pt 9), 1975–1992. doi: 10.1113/jphysiol.2013.266957

Kim, D., Cavanaugh, E. J., Kim, I., and Carroll, J. L. (2009). Heteromeric TASK-1/TASK-3 is the major oxygen-sensitive background K+ channel in rat carotid body glomus cells. *J. Physiol.* 587(Pt 12), 2963–2975. doi: 10.1113/jphysiol.2009.171181

Kim, D., Kang, D., Martin, E. A., Kim, I., and Carroll, J. L. (2014). Effects of modulators of AMP-activated protein kinase on TASK-1/3 and intracellular Ca(2+) concentration in rat carotid body glomus cells. *Respir. Physiol. Neurobiol.* 195, 19–26. doi: 10.1016/j.resp.2014.01.020

Kim, D., Kim, I., Wang, J., White, C., and Carroll, J. L. (2015). Hydrogen sulfide and hypoxia-induced changes in TASK (K2P3/9) activity and intracellular Ca(2+) concentration in rat carotid body glomus cells. *Respir. Physiol. Neurobiol.* 215, 30–38. doi: 10.1016/j.resp.2015.04.012

Kim, I., Fite, L., Donnelly, D. F., Kim, J. H., and Carroll, J. L. (2015). "Possible role of TRP channels in rat glomus cells," in *Arterial Chemoreceptors in Physiology and Pathophysiology*, eds C. Peers, P. Kumar, C. N. Wyatt, E. Gauda, C. A. Nurse, and N. Prabhakar (Berlin: Springer-Verlag), 227–232. doi: 10.1007/978-3-319-18440-1_25

Kline, D. D., Yang, T., Premkumar, D. R., Thomas, A. J., and Prabhakar, N. R. (2000). Blunted respiratory responses to hypoxia in mutant mice deficient in nitric oxide synthase-3. *J. Appl. Physiol.* 88, 1496–1508. doi: 10.1152/jappl.2000.88.4.1496

Kreneisz, O., Benoit, J. P., Bayliss, D. A., and Mulkey, D. K. (2009). AMP-activated protein kinase inhibits TREK channels. *J. Physiol.* 587(Pt 24), 5819–5830. doi: 10.1113/jphysiol.2009.180372

Krylov, S. S., and Anichkov, S. V. (1968). "The effect of metabolic inhibitors on carotid chemoreceptors," in *Arterial Chemoreceptors*, ed. R. W. Torrance (Oxford: Blackwell), 103–109.

Kumar, P. (2009). Systemic effects resulting from carotid body stimulation-invited article. *Adv. Exp. Med. Biol.* 648, 223–233. doi: 10.1007/978-90-481-2259-2_26

Kumar, P., and Bin-Jaliah, I. (2007). Adequate stimuli of the carotid body: more than an oxygen sensor? *Respir. Physiol. Neurobiol.* 157, 12–21. doi: 10.1016/j.resp.2007.01.007

Kumar, P., Pearson, S., and Gu, Y. C. (2006). A role for TRP channels in carotid body chemotransduction? *FASEB J.* 20, A1229–A1229. doi: 10.1007/978-3-319-18440-1_25

Kumar, P., and Prabhakar, N. R. (2012). Peripheral chemoreceptors: function and plasticity of the carotid body. *Compr. Physiol.* 2, 141–219. doi: 10.1002/cphy.c100069

Lahiri, S., Ehleben, W., and Acker, H. (1999). Chemoreceptor discharges and cytochrome redox changes of the rat carotid body: role of heme ligands. *Proc. Natl. Acad. Sci. U.S.A.* 96, 9427–9432. doi: 10.1073/pnas.96.16.9427

Lopez-Barneo, J., Gonzalez-Rodriguez, P., Gao, L., Fernandez-Aguera, M. C., Pardal, R., and Ortega-Saenz, P. (2016). Oxygen sensing by the carotid body: mechanisms and role in adaptation to hypoxia. *Am. J. Physiol. Cell Physiol.* 310, C629–C642. doi: 10.1152/ajpcell.00265.2015

Mahmoud, A. D., Lewis, S., Juricic, L., Udoh, U. A., Hartmann, S., Jansen, M. A., et al. (2016). AMP-activated protein kinase deficiency blocks the hypoxic ventilatory response and thus precipitates hypoventilation and Apnea. *Am. J. Respir. Crit. Care Med.* 193, 1032–1043. doi: 10.1164/rccm.201508-1667OC

McGregor, K. H., Gil, J., and Lahiri, S. (1984). A morphometric study of the carotid body in chronically hypoxic rats. *J. Appl. Physiol.* 57, 1430–1438. doi: 10.1152/jappl.1984.57.5.1430

Mills, E., and Jobsis, F. F. (1970). Simultaneous measurement of cytochrome a3 reduction and chemoreceptor afferent activity in the carotid body. *Nature* 225, 1147–1149. doi: 10.1038/2251147a0

Mills, E., and Jobsis, F. F. (1972). Mitochondrial respiratory chain of carotid body and chemoreceptor response to changes in oxygen tension. *J. Neurophysiol.* 35, 405–428. doi: 10.1152/jn.1972.35.4.405

Mulligan, E., Lahiri, S., and Storey, B. T. (1981). Carotid body O2 chemoreception and mitochondrial oxidative phosphorylation. *J. Appl. Physiol.* 51, 438–446. doi: 10.1152/jappl.1981.51.2.438

Nowak, M. A., Boerlijst, M. C., Cooke, J., and Smith, J. M. (1997). Evolution of genetic redundancy. *Nature* 388, 167–171. doi: 10.1038/40618

Obeso, A., Almaraz, L., and Gonzalez, C. (1989). Effects of cyanide and uncouplers on chemoreceptor activity and ATP content of the cat carotid body. *Brain Res.* 481, 250–257. doi: 10.1016/0006-8993(89)90801-9

Ortega-Saenz, P., Pardal, R., Garcia-Fernandez, M., and Lopez-Barneo, J. (2003). Rotenone selectively occludes sensitivity to hypoxia in rat carotid body glomus cells. *J. Physiol.* 548(Pt 3), 789–800. doi: 10.1113/jphysiol.2003.039693

Owen, H., and Gesell, R. (1931). Peripheral and central chemical control of pulmonary ventilation. *Proc. Soc. Exp. Biol. Med.* 28, 0765–0766. doi: 10.3181/00379727-28-5523

Peng, Y. J., Nanduri, J., Raghuraman, G., Souvannakitti, D., Gadalla, M. M., Kumar, G. K., et al. (2010). H2S mediates O2 sensing in the carotid body. *Proc. Natl. Acad. Sci. U.S.A.* 107, 10719–10724. doi: 10.1073/pnas.1005866107

Piruat, J. I., Pintado, C. O., Ortega-Saenz, P., Roche, M., and Lopez-Barneo, J. (2004). The mitochondrial SDHD gene is required for early embryogenesis, and its partial deficiency results in persistent carotid body glomus cell activation with full responsiveness to hypoxia. *Mol. Cell. Biol.* 24, 10933–10940. doi: 10.1128/MCB.24.24.10933-10940.2004

Ribeiro, M. J., Sacramento, J. F., Gonzalez, C., Guarino, M. P., Monteiro, E. C., and Conde, S. V. (2013). Carotid body denervation prevents the development of insulin resistance and hypertension induced by hypercaloric diets. *Diabetes Metab. Res. Rev.* 62, 2905–2916. doi: 10.2337/db12-1463

Rocher, A., Obeso, A., Gonzalez, C., and Herreros, B. (1991). Ionic mechanisms for the transduction of acidic stimuli in rabbit carotid body glomus cells. *J. Physiol.* 433, 533–548. doi: 10.1113/jphysiol.1991.sp018442

Sanchez, D., Lopez-Lopez, J. R., Perez-Garcia, M. T., Sanz-Alfayate, G., Obeso, A., Ganfornina, M. D., et al. (2002). Molecular identification of Kvalpha subunits that contribute to the oxygen-sensitive K+ current of chemoreceptor cells of the rabbit carotid body. *J. Physiol.* 542(Pt 2), 369–382.

Sanz-Alfayate, G., Obeso, A., Agapito, M. T., and Gonzalez, C. (2001). Reduced to oxidized glutathione ratios and oxygen sensing in calf and rabbit carotid body chemoreceptor cells. *J. Physiol.* 537(Pt 1), 209–220. doi: 10.1111/j.1469-7793.2001.0209k.x

Silva, J. M., and Lewis, D. L. (2002). Nitric oxide enhances Ca(2+)-dependent K(+) channel activity in rat carotid body cells. *Pflugers Arch.* 443, 671–675. doi: 10.1007/s00424-001-0745-1

Summers, B. A., Overholt, J. L., and Prabhakar, N. R. (1999). Nitric oxide inhibits L-type Ca2+ current in glomus cells of the rabbit carotid body via a cGMP-independent mechanism. *J. Neurophysiol.* 81, 1449–1457. doi: 10.1152/jn.1999.81.4.1449

Tamura, M., Hazeki, O., Nioka, S., and Chance, B. (1989). In vivo study of tissue oxygen metabolism using optical and nuclear magnetic resonance spectroscopies. *Annu. Rev. Physiol.* 51, 813–834. doi: 10.1146/annurev.ph.51.030189.004121

Tatsumi, K., Pickett, C. K., and Weil, J. V. (1991). Attenuated carotid body hypoxic sensitivity after prolonged hypoxic exposure. *J. Appl. Physiol.* 70, 748–755. doi: 10.1152/jappl.1991.70.2.748

Thompson, E. L., Ray, C. J., Holmes, A. P., Pye, R. L., Wyatt, C. N., Coney, A. M., et al. (2016). Adrenaline release evokes hyperpnoea and an increase in ventilatory CO2 sensitivity during hypoglycaemia: a role for the carotid body. *J. Physiol.* 594, 4439–4452. doi: 10.1113/jp272191

Turner, P. J., and Buckler, K. J. (2013). Oxygen and mitochondrial inhibitors modulate both monomeric and heteromeric TASK-1 and TASK-3 channels in mouse carotid body type-1 cells. *J. Physiol.* 591(Pt 23), 5977–5998. doi: 10.1113/jphysiol.2013.262022

Urena, J., Fernandez-Chacon, R., Benot, A. R., Alvarez, de Toledo, G. A., and Lopez-Barneo, J. (1994). Hypoxia induces voltage-dependent Ca2+ entry and quantal dopamine secretion in carotid body glomus cells. *Proc. Natl. Acad. Sci. U.S.A.* 91, 10208–10211. doi: 10.1073/pnas.91.21.10208

Valdes, V., Mosqueira, M., Rey, S., Del Rio, R., and Iturriaga, R. (2003). Inhibitory effects of NO on carotid body: contribution of neural and endothelial nitric oxide synthase isoforms. *Am. J. Physiol. Lung Cell Mol. Physiol.* 284, L57–L68. doi: 10.1152/ajplung.00494.2001

Varas, R., Wyatt, C. N., and Buckler, K. J. (2007). Modulation of TASK-like background potassium channels in rat arterial chemoreceptor cells by intracellular ATP and other nucleotides. *J. Physiol.* 583(Pt 2), 521–536. doi: 10.1113/jphysiol.2007.135657

Wang, J. J., Hogan, J. O., and Kim, D. (2017a). Voltage- and receptor-mediated activation of a non-selective cation channel in rat carotid body glomus cells. *Respir. Physiol. Neurobiol.* 237, 13–21. doi: 10.1016/j.resp.2016.12.005

Wang, J. J., Hogan, J. O., Wang, R., White, C., and Kim, D. (2017b). Role of cystathionine-gamma-lyase in hypoxia-induced changes in TASK activity, intracellular Ca2+ and ventilation in mice. *Respir. Physiol. Neurobiol.* 246, 98–106. doi: 10.1016/j.resp.2017.08.009

Williams, S. E., Brazier, S. P., Baban, N., Telezhkin, V., Muller, C. T., Riccardi, D., et al. (2008). A structural motif in the C-terminal tail of slo1 confers carbon monoxide sensitivity to human BK(Ca) channels. *Pflugers Arch. Eur. J. Physiol.* 456, 561–572. doi: 10.1007/s00424-007-0439-4

Williams, S. E., Wootton, P., Mason, H. S., Bould, J., Iles, D. E., Riccardi, D., et al. (2004). Hemoxygenase-2 is an oxygen sensor for a calcium-sensitive potassium channel. *Science* 306, 2093–2097. doi: 10.1126/science.1105010

Wilson, D. F., Mokashi, A., Chugh, D., Vinogradov, S., Osanai, S., and Lahiri, S. (1994). The primary oxygen sensor of the cat carotid body is cytochrome a3 of the mitochondrial respiratory chain. *FEBS Lett.* 351, 370–374. doi: 10.1016/0014-5793(94)00887-6

Wilson, D. F., Rumsey, W. L., Green, T. J., and Vanderkooi, J. M. (1988). The oxygen dependence of mitochondrial oxidative phosphorylation measured by a new optical method for measuring oxygen concentration. *J. Biol. Chem.* 263, 2712–2718.

Wyatt, C. N., and Buckler, K. J. (2004). The effect of mitochondrial inhibitors on membrane currents in isolated neonatal rat carotid body type I cells. *J. Physiol.* 556(Pt 1), 175–191. doi: 10.1113/jphysiol.2003.058131

Wyatt, C. N., Mustard, K. J., Pearson, S. A., Dallas, M. L., Atkinson, L., Kumar, P., et al. (2007). AMP-activated protein kinase mediates carotid body excitation by hypoxia. *J. Biol. Chem.* 282, 8092–8098. doi: 10.1074/jbc.M608742200

Yamamoto, Y., Konig, P., Henrich, M., Dedio, J., and Kummer, W. (2006). Hypoxia induces production of nitric oxide and reactive oxygen species in glomus cells of rat carotid body. *Cell Tissue Res.* 325, 3–11. doi: 10.1007/s00441-006-0178-4

Yamamoto, Y., and Taniguchi, K. (2006). Expression of tandem P domain K+ channel, TREK-1, in the rat carotid body. *J. Histochem. Cytochem.* 54, 467–472. doi: 10.1369/jhc.5A6755.2005

Yuan, G., Vasavda, C., Peng, Y. J., Makarenko, V. V., Raghuraman, G., Nanduri, J., et al. (2015). Protein kinase G-regulated production of H2S governs oxygen sensing. *Sci. Signal.* 8:ra37. doi: 10.1126/scisignal.2005846

Zhou, T., Chien, M.-S., Kaleem, S., and Matsunami, H. (2016). Single cell transcriptome analysis of mouse carotid body glomus cells. *J. Physiol.* 594, 4225–4251. doi: 10.1113/jp271936

6

AMPK-α1 or AMPK-α2 Deletion in Smooth Muscles does not Affect the Hypoxic Ventilatory Response or Systemic Arterial Blood Pressure Regulation during Hypoxia

*Sandy MacMillan and A. Mark Evans**

Centre for Discovery Brain Sciences and Centre for Cardiovascular Science, College of Medicine and Veterinary Medicine, University of Edinburgh, Edinburgh, United Kingdom

***Correspondence:**
A. Mark Evans
mark.evans@ed.ac.uk

The hypoxic ventilatory response (HVR) is markedly attenuated by AMPK-α1 deletion conditional on the expression of Cre-recombinase in tyrosine hydroxylase (TH) expressing cells, precipitating marked increases in apnea frequency and duration. It was concluded that ventilatory dysfunction caused by AMPK deficiency was driven by neurogenic mechanisms. However, TH is transiently expressed in other cell types during development, and it is evident that central respiratory depression can also be triggered by myogenic mechanisms that impact blood supply to the brain. We therefore assessed the effect on the HVR and systemic arterial blood pressure of AMPK deletion in vascular smooth muscles. There was no difference in minute ventilation during normoxia. However, increases in minute ventilation during severe hypoxia (8% O_2) were, if affected at all, augmented by AMPK-α1 and AMPK-α2 deletion in smooth muscles; despite the fact that hypoxia (8% O_2) evoked falls in arterial SpO_2 comparable with controls. Surprisingly, these mice exhibited no difference in systolic, diastolic or mean arterial blood pressure during normoxia or hypoxia. We conclude that neither AMPK-α1 nor AMPK-α2 are required in smooth muscle for the regulation of systemic arterial blood pressure during hypoxia, and that AMPK-α1 deficiency does not impact the HVR by myogenic mechanisms.

Keywords: AMPK, hypoxia, ventilation, blood pressure, smooth muscle

INTRODUCTION

The AMP-activated protein kinase (AMPK) is a cellular energy sensor that maintains cell-autonomous energy homeostasis. From its 2 α (catalytic), 2 β and 3 γ (regulatory) subunits 12 AMPK heterotrimers may be formed, each harboring different sensitivities to activation by increases in cellular AMP and ADP, and the capacity to directly phosphorylate and thus regulate different targets (Ross et al., 2016). AMPK is coupled to mitochondrial oxidative phosphorylation by two discrete albeit cooperative pathways, involving liver kinase B1 (LKB1) and changes in the cellular AMP:ATP and ADP:ATP ratios. Binding of AMP to the AMPK γ subunit increases activity 10-fold by allosteric activation alone, while AMP or ADP binding delivers increases in LKB1-dependent phosphorylation and reductions in dephosphorylation of Thr172 on the α

subunit that confer 100-fold further activation. All of these effects are inhibited by ATP (Gowans et al., 2013). LKB1 is, therefore, the principal pathway for AMPK activation during metabolic stresses such as hypoxia. However, there are alternative Ca^{2+}-dependent pathways to AMPK activation that are governed by the calmodulin-dependent protein kinase CaMKK2, which delivers increases in Thr172 phosphorylation and thus AMPK activation independent of changes in cellular AM(D)P:ATP ratios.

Classically AMPK regulates cell-autonomous pathways of energy supply by phosphorylating targets that switch off non-essential anabolic processes that consume ATP and switch on catabolic pathways that generate ATP, thereby compensating for deficits in ATP supply or availability (Ross et al., 2016). Recently, however, we demonstrated (Mahmoud et al., 2016) that the role of AMPK in metabolic homeostasis is not limited to such cell autonomous pathways, but extends to the hypoxic ventilatory response (HVR) (Teppema and Dahan, 2010; Wilson and Teppema, 2016) and thus O_2 and energy (ATP) supply to the body as a whole. In doing so AMPK acts to oppose central respiratory depression during hypoxia and thus resists hypoventilation and apnea.

However, the HVR could well be affected by AMPK deficiency in cell systems other than catecholaminergic neurons due to off-target AMPK deletion through "leakage" of Cre beyond those cells targeted by the conditional deletion strategy we employed. This possibility is highlighted by the fact that transient developmental expression of TH occurs in disparate cell groups that do not express TH in the adult (Lindeberg et al., 2004), including, for example, a subset of heart wall cells. Therefore, there remains the possibility that AMPK deficiency might somehow affect ventilatory control mechanisms through myogenic rather than neurogenic mechanisms. This is evident from the fact that systemic arteries dilate in response to tissue hypoxemia in order to match local perfusion to local metabolism (Roy and Sherrington, 1890), and evidence suggests a role for AMPK in this response (Goirand et al., 2007; Schneider et al., 2015). With "leakage" of Cre, off-target deletion of AMPK in arterial myocytes could attenuate arterial dilation and thus impact O_2 supply to the brain during hypoxia and the HVR. This possibility is highlighted by the fact that respiratory failure can be triggered through the Cushing reflex consequent to marked increases in blood pressure (Guyenet, 2000; Paton et al., 2009).

We therefore assessed the impact of AMPK deficiency in smooth muscles on blood pressure control and the HVR. Our data show that AMPK does not contribute to the HVR or blood pressure control during hypoxia through myogenic mechanisms.

MATERIALS AND METHODS

Experiments were performed in accordance with the regulations of the United Kingdom Animals (Scientific Procedures) Act of 1986. All studies and breeding were approved by the University of Edinburgh and performed under UK Home Office project licenses. Both male and female mice were used, and all were on a C57/Bl6 background. Numbers of mice ($\geq$3 per measure) used are indicated for each experiment. Global, dual knockout of the genes encoding AMPK-α1 (*Prkaa1*) and AMPK-α2 (*Prkaa2*) is embryonic lethal. We therefore employed conditional deletion of the genes for the AMPK-α1 or AMPK-α2 subunits, using mice in which the sequence encoding the catalytic site of either or both of the α subunits was flanked by loxP sequences (Lantier et al., 2014). To direct AMPK deletion to cells of the smooth muscle lineage, these were crossed with mice in which Cre recombinase was under the control of the transgelin (smooth muscle protein 22α) promoter (The Jackson Laboratory, Bar Harbor, ME, United States [stock number 017491, Tg(Tagln-cre)1Her/J in C57BL/6:129SJL background]). The presence of wild-type or floxed alleles and CRE recombinase were detected by PCR. We used four primers for Cre (Transgene 5′-GCGGTCTGGCAGTAAAAACTATC-3′ and 5′-GTGAAACAGCATTGCTGTCACTT-3′; internal positive control 5′-CTAGGCCACAGAATTGAAAGATCT-3′ and 5′-GTAGGTGGAAATTCTAGCATCATCC-3′; expected size WT = 324 bp, Cre = 100 bp). Two primers were used for each AMPK catalytic subunit: α1-forward 5′-TATTGCTGCCATTAGGCTAC-3′, α1-reverse: 5′-GACCTGAC AGAATAGGATATGCCCAACCTC-3′ (WT = 588 bp, Floxed = 682 bp); α2-forward 5′-GCTTAGCACGTTACCC TGGATGG-3′, α2-reverse: 5′-GTTATCAGCCCAACTAATT ACAC-3′ (WT = 204 bp, Floxed = 250 bp). 10 μl samples were run on 2% agarose gels with 0.01% v/v SYBR®Safe DNA Gel Stain (Invitrogen) in TBE buffer against a 100 bp DNA ladder (GeneRuler™, Fermentas) using a Model 200/2.0 Power Supply (Bio-Rad). Gels were imaged using a Genius Bio Imaging System and GeneSnap software (Syngene).

End-Point and Quantitative RT-PCR

For qPCR analysis, 2 μl of cDNA in RNase free water was made up to 20 μl with 10 μl FastStart Universal SYBR Green Master (ROX, Roche), 6.4 μl Ultra Pure Water (SIGMA) and forward and reverse primers for AMPK-α1 and AMPK-α2. The sample was then centrifuged and 20 μl added to a MicroAmpTM Fast Optical 96-Well Reaction Plate (Greiner bio-one), the reaction plate sealed with an optical adhesive cover (Applied Biosystems) and the plate centrifuged. The reaction was then run on a sequence detection system (Applied Biosystems) using AmpliTaq Fast DNA Polymerase, with a 2 min initial step at 50°C, followed by a 10 min step at 95°C, then 40x 15 s steps at 95°C. This was followed by a dissociation stage with 15 s at 95°C, 20 s at 60°C, and 15 s at 95°C. Negative controls included control cell aspirants for which no reverse transcriptase was added, and aspiration of extracellular medium and PCR controls. None of the controls produced any detectable amplicon, ruling out genomic or other contamination.

Plethysmography

As described previously (Mahmoud et al., 2016), we used a whole-body unrestrained plethysmograph, incorporating a Halcyon™ low noise pneumatochograph (Buxco Research Systems, United Kingdom) coupled to FinePointe acquisition and analysis software (Data Science International, United States). Following acclimation and baseline measurements (awake but quiet, undisturbed periods of breathing) under normoxia (room air), mice were exposed to hypoxia (8% O_2, with 0.05% CO_2, balanced with N_2) for 10 min. The FinePointe software automatically calculated the respiratory parameters assessed after application of exclusion criteria due to non-ventilatory artifacts (movement, sniffing, etc.). Data were acquired as 2 s averages and 2 to 4 data points of undisturbed breathing were selected for each time point of the HVR. Apneas were defined as a period of cessation of breathing that was greater than the average duration, including interval, of two successive breaths (~600 ms) of control mice during normoxia with a detection threshold of 0.25 mmHg (SD of noise).

Blood Pressure Measurements

Blood pressure was recorded using a CODA non-invasive blood pressure system (Kent Scientific, United States). Following five consecutive days of habituation "training," mice were restrained using a pre-warmed mouse holder and placed on a warming platform (Kent Scientific, United States). Resting blood pressure was measured 32 times per session and only stable readings throughout each session were considered for analysis. On separate days hypoxic blood pressure was measured using the following protocol: 13 cycles of normoxia, 16 cycles of hypoxia (8% O_2, with 0.05% CO_2, balanced with N_2; approximately 10 min) and finally eight cycles of recovery (approximately 5 min). Hypoxic gas originating from a pre-mixed gas cylinder (BOC, United Kingdom) was delivered at a flow rate of 2 L/min via a head cone that inserts into the mouse holder.

Measurement of Arterial Oxygen Saturation and Heart Rate

Arterial SpO_2 measurements of mice were obtained using the MouseSTAT^{TM} Pulse Oximeter (Kent Scientific, United States) and an infrared Y-style tail sensor at a sampling rate of 0.5 Hz. As above, mice were restrained using a pre-warmed mouse holder and placed on a warming platform (Kent Scientific, United States). Following 5 min of acclimation, baseline SpO_2 and heart rates were measured for 2 min immediately preceding a 10-min period of hypoxia (8% O_2, with 0.05% CO_2, balanced with N_2), followed by 3–5 min of recovery. Hypoxic gas originating from a pre-mixed gas cylinder (BOC, United Kingdom) was delivered at a flow rate of 2 L/min via a head cone that inserts into the mouse holder.

Statistical Analysis

Statistical comparison was completed using GraphPad Prism 6 for the following: plethysmography, two-way ANOVA with Bonferroni multiple comparison's test; blood pressure, one-way ANOVA with Bonferroni multiple comparison's test, SpO_2, two-way ANOVA with Bonferroni multiple comparison's test. $p < 0.05$ was considered significant.

RESULTS

We investigated the possibility that AMPK-α1 or AMPK-α2 subunits might support myogenic responses to hypoxia and thus impact the HVR and blood pressure control. To achieve this goal we developed mice with conditional deletion in smooth muscles of the gene encoding AMPK-α1 (*Prkaa1*) and AMPK-α2 (*Prkaa2*), respectively. Critical exons of the AMPK-α1 and -α2 subunit genes were flanked by loxP sequences (Lantier et al., 2014), and each floxed mouse line was crossed with mice expressing Cre recombinase under the control of the transgelin promoter (smooth muscle protein 22α) (El-Bizri et al., 2008). Previous studies have shown that transgelin-Cre mice do not exhibit Cre expression in endothelial cells, and therefore provide for selective gene deletion in smooth muscle versus endothelial cells (**Supplementary Figure S1**). It should be noted, however, that transient developmental expression of transgelin has been observed in atrial and ventricular myocytes. Consequently, genomic recombination will also occur in these cells despite the fact that they do not express transgelin in the adult (El-Bizri et al., 2008). Therefore, while imperfect, the use of transgelin-Cre mice provided us with the necessary level of specificity to determine the role of smooth muscle AMPK in myogenic responses to hypoxia that impact the HVR and blood pressure control.

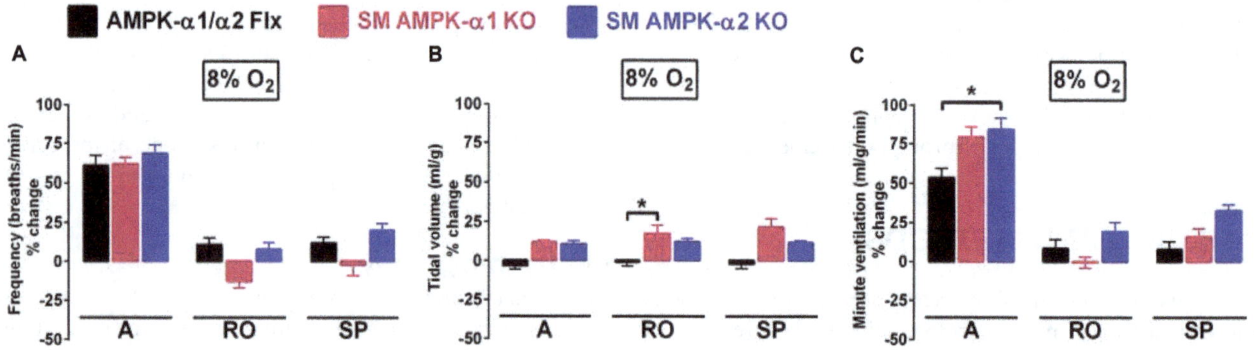

FIGURE 1 | The hypoxic ventilatory response (HVR) is not attenuated by conditional deletion of AMPK-α1 and AMPK-α2 subunits in smooth muscles. Bar charts show mean ± SEM for changes in **(A)** respiratory frequency, **(B)** tidal volume, and **(C)** minute ventilation for AMPK-α1/α2 floxed mice (Flx; black, $n = 12$), and for mice with AMPK-α1 ($n = 4$; magenta) and AMPK-α2 ($n = 4$; blue) deletion in smooth muscles (transgelin expressing cells) during the peak of the Augmenting phase (A), after approximately 100s of Roll Off (RO) and the plateau of the Sustained Phase (SP) of the response to hypoxia; *$p < 0.05$.

The Hypoxic Ventilatory Response Is Not Attenuated by AMPK-α1 or AMPK-α2 Deficiency in Smooth Muscles

Mice with conditional deletion of AMPK-α1 or AMPK-α2 subunits in smooth muscles exhibited no obvious phenotype and no ventilatory dysfunction or deficiency was evident during normoxia (not shown). Most significantly in the context of the present investigation, we identified no significant attenuation of the HVR relative to controls (AMPK-α1/α2 floxed; **Figure 1** and **Supplementary Figure S2A**). That said, we did observe subtle differences between genotypes.

For smooth muscle AMPK-α1 knockouts alone, there appeared to be an insignificant yet noticeable lowering, relative to controls, of breathing frequency during hypoxia following Roll-Off (≈100 s; −13 ± 4 and 11 ± 4%, respectively) that was maintained for the duration of the Sustained Phase (2–5 min; −2 ± 7 and 12 ± 4%, respectively) of the HVR (**Figure 1A**). By contrast, in both AMPK-α1 and AMPK-α2 knockouts larger increases in tidal volume were observed when compared to controls (**Figure 1B** and **Table 1**), which reached significance for AMPK-α1 knockouts, but only at the peak of Roll-Off (17 ± 6 versus −1 ± 3%, respectively; $p < 0.05$). Increases in minute ventilation during hypoxia also showed a tendency to be greater for AMPK-α1 and AMPK-α2 knockouts than for controls (AMPK-α1/α2 floxed). However this only reached significance during the initial Augmenting Phase of the HVR (**Figure 1C**; $p < 0.05$), which primarily results from increases in carotid body afferent input responses (Day and Wilson, 2007; Teppema and Dahan, 2010; Wilson and Teppema, 2016).

Perhaps most striking was the fact that deletion of neither the AMPK-α1 nor AMPK-α2 catalytic subunits in smooth muscles had any discernible effect on hypoxia-evoked apneas (**Figure 2**, **Table 1**, and **Supplementary Figure S2B**), when compared to controls (AMPK-α1/α2 floxed). This is evident from the fact that there was no difference in either the apnea frequency (**Figure 2A**), duration (**Figure 2B**), or apnea duration index (**Figure 2C**) in mice lacking AMPK-α1 or AMPK-α2 subunits in smooth muscles.

The aforementioned findings are in complete contrast to our observations on mice with AMPK-α1 deletion in catecholaminergic neurons (driven by TH-Cre) which exhibited marked attenuation of the HVR and pronounced increases in apnea frequency, duration and apnea duration index (Mahmoud et al., 2016).

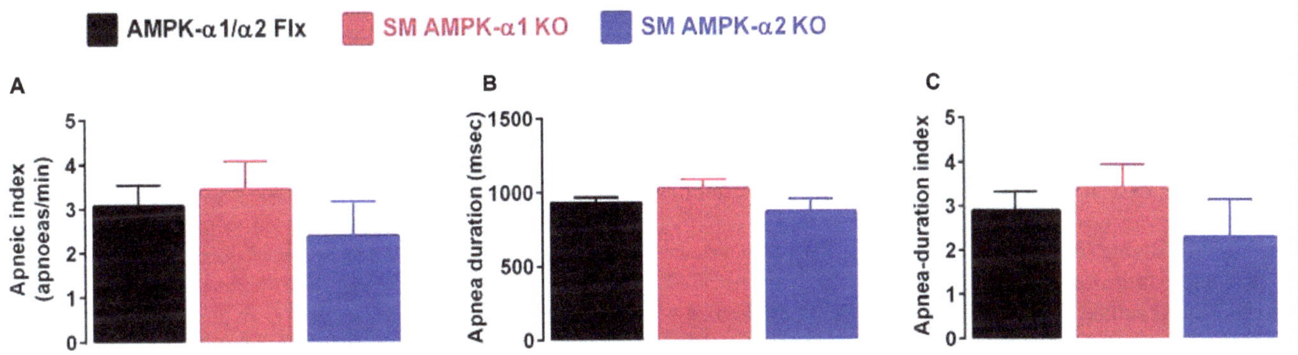

FIGURE 2 | Deletion of AMPK-α1 and AMPK-α2 subunits in smooth muscles does not affect apnea frequency or duration during hypoxia. Bar charts show mean ± SEM for the **(A)** apneic index (per minute), **(B)** apnea duration, and **(C)** apnea duration index (frequency × duration) of AMPK-α1/α2 floxed mice (Flx; black, *n* = 12), and for mice with AMPK-α1 (*n* = 4; magenta) and AMPK-α2 (*n* = 4; blue) deletion in smooth muscles (transgelin expressing cells).

TABLE 1 | Means ± SEM of percentage changes in breathing frequency, tidal volume, and minute ventilation and values for apnea frequency, apnea duration and apnea duration index during exposures to hypoxia (8%O_2) across all genotypes.

Genotype	Frequency	Tidal volume	Minute ventilation	Apnea frequency (min^{-1})	Apnea duration (ms)	Apnea duration index
AMPK-α1/α2 floxed	A 61 ± 7%	A -3 ± 2%	A 53 ± 6%	3.0 ± 0.5	936 ± 40	2.9 ± 0.5
	RO 11 ± 4%	RO -1 ± 3%	RO 8 ± 6%			
	SP 12 ± 4%	SP -2 ± 3%	SP 8 ± 5%			
SM AMPK-α1 knockouts	A 62 ± 4%	A 12 ± 1%	A 79 ± 7%	3.4 ± 1	1021 ± 86	3.4 ± 1
	RO -13 ± 4%	RO 17 ± 6%	RO -1 ± 4%			
	SP -2 ± 7%	SP 22 ± 5%	SP 16 ± 5%			
SM AMPK-α2 knockouts	A 68 ± 6%	A 10 ± 2%	A 84 ± 7%	2.4 ± 0.9	900 ± 90	2.3 ± 1
	RO 7 ± 5%	RO 12 ± 2%	RO 19 ± 6%			
	SP 20 ± 4%	SP 11 ± 1%	SP 33 ± 4%			

A, Augmenting Phase; RO, Roll-Off; SP, Sustained Phase.

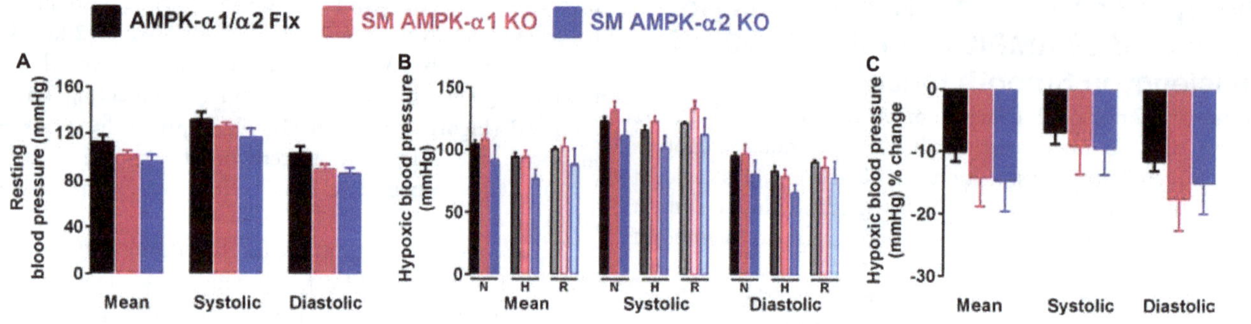

FIGURE 3 | Deletion of AMPK-α1 and AMPK-α2 subunits in smooth muscles has no effect on systemic arterial blood pressure during normoxia or hypoxia. **(A)** Bar charts show (mean ± SEM) the mean, systolic and diastolic blood pressure of control mice [AMPK-α1/α2 floxed (Flx); *n* = 4; black] and mice with AMPK-α1 (*n* = 4; magenta) and AMPK-α2 (*n* = 4; blue) deletion in smooth muscles (transgelin expressing cells). **(B)** Bar charts show the same measures of blood pressure during normoxia (N), after 10 min to hypoxia (H; 8% O_2) and following recovery to normoxia (R). **(C)** Bar charts show the percentage change in blood pressure during hypoxia.

Cardiovascular Responses to Hypoxia Remain Unaltered Following Deletion of AMPK-α1 and AMPK-α2 in Smooth Muscle Cells

We next assessed the effect of AMPK deficiency on cardiovascular function during hypoxia by monitoring systemic blood pressure during hypoxia. Deleting either AMPK-α1 or AMPK-α2 subunits in smooth muscle cells had little or no effect on resting blood pressure (**Figure 3A** and **Supplementary Figure S2C**). Furthermore neither smooth muscle AMPK-α1 nor -α2 deficiency affected hypoxia-evoked falls in systemic blood pressure in mice (**Figures 3B,C**, **Table 2**, and **Supplementary Figures S2Cii,iii**), which were comparable to the range of responses reported previously (Campen et al., 2005; Mahmoud et al., 2016).

That comparable levels of arterial hypoxia were achieved in all mice was confirmed by pulse oximetry, which demonstrated significant and similar falls in SpO_2 for all genotypes (**Figure 4** and **Supplementary Figure S2D**, $p < 0.0001$). Moreover there was no difference with respect to post-hypoxic recovery of arterial SpO_2 upon return to room air.

DISCUSSION

The present investigation demonstrates that the HVR is, if anything, slightly augmented rather than attenuated by AMPK-α1 or AMPK-α2 deficiency in smooth muscles (driven by transgelin-Cre). This outcome is in marked contrast to our previously reported finding that AMPK-α1 deficiency in catecholaminergic neurons (driven by TH-Cre) markedly attenuates the HVR and precipitates hypoventilation and apnea during hypoxia (Mahmoud et al., 2016). Therefore, outcomes are consistent with our previously proposed model of central oxygen-sensing by catecholaminergic neurons of the brainstem respiratory network. Briefly, we proposed that these neurons deliver increases in respiratory drive during hypoxia in a manner supported by AMPK heterotrimers incorporating the catalytic α1 subunit, the activity of which we hypothesized to be determined by integration of local hypoxic stress at the brainstem with carotid body afferent input responses that provide an index of peripheral hypoxia. Notably, natural selection in high-altitude (Andean) populations has led to single nucleotide polymorphisms in PRKAA1 (Bigham et al., 2014).

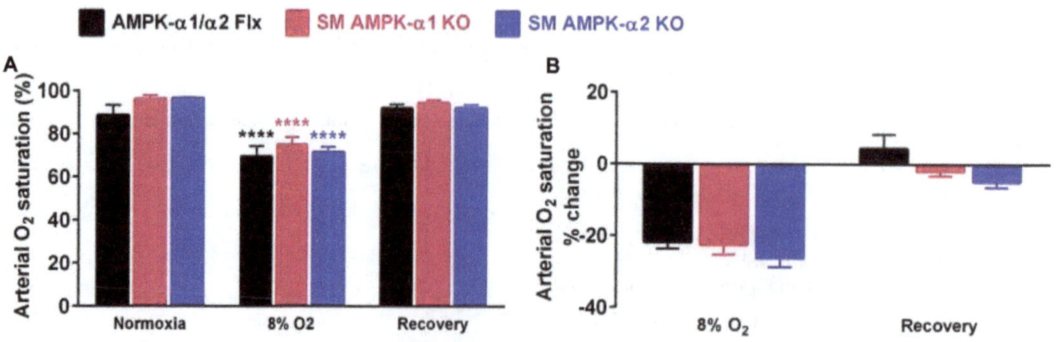

FIGURE 4 | Comparable falls in arterial oxygen saturation were evoked in all genotypes during hypoxia. **(A)** Bar charts show mean ± SEM for the arterial oxygen saturation (SpO_2) during normoxia, after 10 min of hypoxia (8% O_2) and following recovery to normoxia. **(B)** Percentage change in SpO_2. AMPK-α1/α2 floxed (Flx; black, *n* = 3), smooth muscle AMPK-α1 KO (magenta, *n* = 4) and smooth muscle AMPK-α2 KO (blue, *n* = 4) mice; ****$p < 0.001$.

TABLE 2 | Means ± SEM of values obtained by tail cuff blood pressure measurements and percentage changes in arterial SpO_2 before, during, and after exposures to hypoxia (8%O_2) across all genotypes.

Genotype	Resting BP (mmHg)	Mean BP (mmHg)	Sys BP (mmHg)	Dias BP (mmHg)	SpO_2
AMPK-α1/α2 floxed	M 112 ± 6	N 104 ± 3	N 123 ± 4	N 95 ± 3	N 89 ± 5%
	Sys 131 ± 7	H 94 ± 3.5	H 116 ± 3.5	H 84 ± 4	H 69 ± 5%
	Dias 103 ± 6	R 100 ± 2	R 121 ± 1	R 91 ± 2	R 92 ± 2%
AMPK-α1 knockouts	M 101 ± 4	N 108 ± 8	N 132 ± 7.5	N 97 ± 8	N 96 ± 2%
	Sys 126 ± 3	H 94 ± 5	H 123 ± 5	H 79 ± 6	H 75 ± 4%
	Dias 89 ± 4	R 89 ± 12	R 133 ± 7	R 87 ± 7.5	R 94 ± 1%
AMPK-α2 knockouts	M 96 ± 6	N 91 ± 12	N111 ± 13	N 81 ± 11	N 97 ± 0.5%
	Sys 117 ± 8	H 77 ± 7	H 102 ± 9.5	H 66 ± 6.5	H 71 ± 3%
	Dias 86 ± 5	R 102 ± 7	R 112 ± 13	R 79 ± 12	R 92 ± 2%

M, mean blood pressure; Sys, systolic blood pressure; Dias, diastolic blood pressure; N, normoxia (room air); H, hypoxia (8% O_2); R, recovery (room air).

The significance of our present findings lies in the fact that reduced cerebral arterial dilation could affect O_2 supply to the brain during hypoxia and thus the HVR through consequent respiratory depression, because the activity of brainstem respiratory networks is ultimately reliant on O_2 delivery via the vasculature that could be modulated systemically and locally through myogenic responses. Respiratory failure may also be triggered through the Cushing reflex consequent to increases in blood pressure (Guyenet, 2000; Paton et al., 2009), which would be exacerbated by block of arterial dilation consequent to AMPK deletion in arterial myocytes. Such system-specific responses could well be affected by a number of mechanisms through which AMPK has been proposed to regulate myocyte function, rendering outcomes susceptible to off-target AMPK deletion due to "leakage" of Cre beyond those cells targeted by conditional deletion strategies. This was a distinct possibility, given that transient developmental expression of TH occurs in disparate cell groups that do not express TH in the adult (Lindeberg et al., 2004), including, for example, a subset of heart wall cells.

The outcomes of our present investigation indicate that while AMPK has been shown to mediate *ex vivo* arterial dilation in some circumstances (Goirand et al., 2007; Schneider et al., 2015), neither the expression of AMPK-α1 nor AMPK-α2 catalytic subunits in smooth muscles is a pre-requisite for *in vivo* arterial dilation during hypoxia sufficient enough to impact systemic arterial blood pressures. This is evident because we observed little or no difference in peripheral hypoxic vasodilation between genotypes tested here. Moreover, systemic arterial pressures during normoxia and hypoxia were within the typical range previously reported for wild-type mice (Campen et al., 2004). Our findings do not, however, rule out a role for AMPK in maintaining resting vascular tone locally, or in governing organ-/tissue-specific perfusion and oxygen supply. Indeed, studies on other vascular beds have already revealed that AMPK might adjust local perfusion during hypoxia. For example, AMPK may mediate hypoxic pulmonary vasoconstriction (Evans et al., 2005, 2006; Evans, 2006), and thus assist ventilation-perfusion matching by diverting blood from oxygen deprived to oxygen rich areas of the lung (Bradford and Dean, 1894; von Euler and Liljestrand, 1946). Furthermore, evidence suggests that AMPK supports dilation of systemic arteries, such as the aorta and mesenteric arteries, at the level of smooth muscles that may counter tissue hypoxemia (Schneider et al., 2015; Moral-Sanz et al., 2016). Accordingly, AMPK has also been implicated in the regulation of uterine artery reactivity during hypoxia (Skeffington et al., 2015), perhaps linking maternal metabolic and cardiovascular responses during pregnancy and governing oxygen and nutrient supply to the fetus.

The mechanisms involved in systemic arterial dilation during hypoxia include AMPK-dependent activation of SERCA and BK_{Ca} channels in systemic arterial myocytes (Schneider et al., 2015), while AMPK exerts its effects on pulmonary arterial smooth muscle cells, at least in part, through direct phosphorylation and inhibition of the voltage-gated potassium channel $K_V1.5$ (Moral-Sanz et al., 2016). Significant to the context of our study, $K_V1.5$ availability has been proposed to impact cerebral myogenic responses (Koide et al., 2018), which could equally well be affected by loss of capacity for AMPK-dependent activation of SERCA and BK_{Ca} channels. Either way, our data argue strongly against the possibility that the HVR is influenced by AMPK-dependent mechanisms within smooth muscles that might affect local myogenic responses, irrespective of the tissue- and circulation-specific function they might impact. Nevertheless, it would be interesting to determine whether AMPK contributes to local autoregulatory mechanisms in the cerebral vasculature during hypoxia, even though we find no evidence of a significant contribution to the HVR or peripheral control of systemic blood pressures, which was the focus of this investigation. That said, we cannot rule out the possibility that the outcome of our previous studies using TH-Cre driven AMPK deletion might have been affected through off-target effects at the level of the vascular endothelium, because the conditional deletion strategy used here does not produce Cre expression in endothelial cells (El-Bizri et al., 2008). However, this seems unlikely given the outcomes of our present investigation. Therefore, hypoxic ventilatory dysfunction precipitated by AMPK-α1 deletion conditional on Cre expression in catecholaminergic neurons does not result, in whole or in part, from AMPK-α1 or AMPK-α2 deficiency in smooth muscles and consequent changes in systemic arterial blood pressure during hypoxia.

In short, AMPK likely supports the HVR through neurogenic but not myogenic mechanisms as previously proposed, by supporting increased respiratory drive (Mahmoud et al., 2016) and perhaps functional hyperemia (Bucher et al., 2014), each of which may be coordinated by catecholaminergic neurons of the brainstem cardiorespiratory network.

AUTHOR CONTRIBUTIONS

AME and SM wrote the manuscript. AME developed the conditonal *AMPK* knockout mice. AME and SM bred and genotyped the mice, performed plethysmography, blood pressure, and arterial oxygen saturation measurements, and analyzed the data.

FUNDING

This work was funded by the Wellcome Trust (WT081195MA) and the British Heart Foundation (RG/12/14/29885).

SUPPLEMENTARY MATERIAL

FIGURE S1 | End-point RT-PCR confirms AMPK deletion. End-point RT-PCR amplicons for transgelin and the catalytic α1 and α2 subunits of AMPK from lungs (right) and primary cultures of pulmonary arterial smooth muscle cells (PASMC, left) obtained from transgelin-Cre, C57BL6 (WT), AMPK-α1 and AMPK-α2 knockout mice.

FIGURE S2 | Deletion of AMPK-α1 or AMPK-α2 subunits in smooth muscles does not attenuate the HVR and has no effect on either apnea duration index or systemic arterial blood pressures during hypoxia. Box plots show the median (solid line), 25th to 75th percentiles (boxes), mean (+) and whiskers according to Tukey's method for: the % change of the ventilatory components of **(Ai)** breathing frequency, **(Aii)** tidal volume, and **(Aiii)** minute ventilation during the initial Augmenting Phase (A), the Roll-Off (RO), and the Sustained Phase (SP) of the hypoxic ventilatory response; **(Bi)** the apneic index (per minute), **(Bii)** apnea durations (in msec) and (Biii) apnea duration index (frequency x duration); Mean, Systolic and Diastolic blood pressures (in mmHg) measured **(Ci)** at rest, **(Cii)** before, during, and after a 10 min hypoxic challenge, and **(Ciii)** as % change during hypoxia; arterial oxygen saturation (in %) during **(Di)** normoxia, 10 min hypoxia, and recovery, and **(Dii)** as % change during hypoxia and recovery. $^*p < 0.05$; $^{***}p < 0.001$.

REFERENCES

Bigham, A. W., Julian, C. G., Wilson, M. J., Vargas, E., Browne, V. A., Shriver, M. D., et al. (2014). Maternal PRKAA1 and EDNRA genotypes are associated with birth weight, and PRKAA1 with uterine artery diameter and metabolic homeostasis at high altitude. *Physiol. Genomics* 46, 687–697. doi: 10.1152/physiolgenomics.00063.2014

Bradford, J. R., and Dean, H. P. (1894). The pulmonary circulation. *J. Physiol.* 16, 34–158. doi: 10.1113/jphysiol.1894.sp000493

Bucher, E. S., Fox, M. E., Kim, L., Kirkpatrick, D. C., Rodeberg, N. T., Belle, A. M., et al. (2014). Medullary norepinephrine neurons modulate local oxygen concentrations in the bed nucleus of the stria terminalis. *J. Cereb. Blood Flow Metab.* 34, 1128–1137. doi: 10.1038/jcbfm.2014.60

Campen, M. J., Shimoda, L. A., and O'Donnell, C. P. (2005). Acute and chronic cardiovascular effects of intermittent hypoxia in C57BL/6J mice. *J. Appl. Physiol.* 99, 2028–2035. doi: 10.1152/japplphysiol.00411.2005

Campen, M. J., Tagaito, Y., Li, J., Balbir, A., Tankersley, C. G., Smith, P., et al. (2004). Phenotypic variation in cardiovascular responses to acute hypoxic and hypercapnic exposure in mice. *Physiol. Genomics* 20, 15–20. doi: 10.1152/physiolgenomics.00197.2003

Day, T. A., and Wilson, R. J. (2007). Brainstem PCO2 modulates phrenic responses to specific carotid body hypoxia in an in situ dual perfused rat preparation. *J. Physiol.* 578, 843–857. doi: 10.1113/jphysiol.2006.119594

El-Bizri, N., Guignabert, C., Wang, L., Cheng, A., Stankunas, K., Chang, C. P., et al. (2008). SM22alpha-targeted deletion of bone morphogenetic protein receptor 1A in mice impairs cardiac and vascular development, and influences organogenesis. *Development* 135, 2981–2991. doi: 10.1242/dev.017863

Evans, A. M. (2006). AMP-activated protein kinase and the regulation of Ca^{2+} signalling in O2-sensing cells. *J. Physiol.* 574, 113–123. doi: 10.1113/jphysiol.2006.108381

Evans, A. M., Hardie, D. G., Galione, A., Peers, C., Kumar, P., and Wyatt, C. N. (2006). AMP-activated protein kinase couples mitochondrial inhibition by hypoxia to cell-specific Ca^{2+} signalling mechanisms in oxygen-sensing cells. *Novartis Found. Symp.* 272, 234–252.

Evans, A. M., Mustard, K. J., Wyatt, C. N., Peers, C., Dipp, M., Kumar, P., et al. (2005). Does AMP-activated protein kinase couple inhibition of mitochondrial oxidative phosphorylation by hypoxia to calcium signaling in O2-sensing cells? *J. Biol. Chem.* 280, 41504–41511. doi: 10.1074/jbc.M510040200

Goirand, F., Solar, M., Athea, Y., Viollet, B., Mateo, P., Fortin, D., et al. (2007). Activation of AMP kinase alpha1 subunit induces aortic vasorelaxation in mice. *J. Physiol.* 581, 1163–1171. doi: 10.1113/jphysiol.2007.132589

Gowans, G. J., Hawley, S. A., Ross, F. A., and Hardie, D. G. (2013). AMP is a true physiological regulator of AMP-activated protein kinase by both allosteric activation and enhancing net phosphorylation. *Cell Metab.* 18, 556–566. doi: 10.1016/j.cmet.2013.08.019

Guyenet, P. G. (2000). Neural structures that mediate sympathoexcitation during hypoxia. *Respir. Physiol.* 121, 147–162. doi:10.1016/S0034-5687(00)00125-0

Koide, M., Moshkforoush, A., Tsoukias, N. M., Hill-Eubanks, D. C., Wellman, G. C., Nelson, M. T., et al. (2018). The yin and yang of KV channels in cerebral small vessel pathologies. *Microcirculation* 25:e12436. doi: 10.1111/micc.12436

Lantier, L., Fentz, J., Mounier, R., Leclerc, J., Treebak, J. T., Pehmoller, C., et al. (2014). AMPK controls exercise endurance, mitochondrial oxidative capacity, and skeletal muscle integrity. *FASEB J.* 28, 3211–3224. doi: 10.1096/fj.14-250449

Lindeberg, J., Usoskin, D., Bengtsson, H., Gustafsson, A., Kylberg, A., Soderstrom, S., et al. (2004). Transgenic expression of Cre recombinase from the tyrosine hydroxylase locus. *Genesis* 40, 67–73. doi: 10.1002/gene.20065

Mahmoud, A. D., Lewis, S., Juricic, L., Udoh, U. A., Hartmann, S., Jansen, M. A., et al. (2016). AMP-activated protein kinase deficiency blocks the hypoxic ventilatory response and thus precipitates hypoventilation and apnea. *Am. J. Respir. Crit. Care Med.* 193, 1032–1043. doi: 10.1164/rccm.201508-1667OC

Moral-Sanz, J., Mahmoud, A. D., Ross, F. A., Eldstrom, J., Fedida, D., Hardie, D. G., et al. (2016). AMP-activated protein kinase inhibits Kv 1.5 channel currents of pulmonary arterial myocytes in response to hypoxia and inhibition of mitochondrial oxidative phosphorylation. *J. Physiol.* 594, 4901–4915. doi: 10.1113/JP272032

Paton, J. F., Dickinson, C. J., and Mitchell, G. (2009). Harvey Cushing and the regulation of blood pressure in giraffe, rat and man: introducing 'Cushing's mechanism'. *Exp. Physiol.* 94, 11–17. doi: 10.1113/expphysiol.2008.043455

Ross, F. A., MacKintosh, C., and Hardie, D. G. (2016). AMP-activated protein kinase: a cellular energy sensor that comes in 12 flavours. *FEBS J.* 283, 2987–3001. doi: 10.1111/febs.13698

Roy, C. S., and Sherrington, C. S. (1890). On the regulation of the blood-supply of the brain. *J. Physiol.* 11, 85–158. doi: 10.1113/jphysiol.1890.sp000321

Schneider, H., Schubert, K. M., Blodow, S., Kreutz, C. P., Erdogmus, S., Wiedenmann, M., et al. (2015). AMPK dilates resistance arteries via activation of SERCA and BKCa channels in smooth muscle. *Hypertension* 66, 108–116. doi: 10.1161/HYPERTENSIONAHA.115.05514

Skeffington, K. L., Higgins, J. S., Mahmoud, A. D., Evans, A. M., Sferruzzi-Perri, A. N., Fowden, A. L., et al. (2015). Hypoxia, AMPK activation and uterine artery vasoreactivity. *J. Physiol.* 594, 1357–1369. doi: 10.1113/JP270995

Teppema, L. J., and Dahan, A. (2010). The ventilatory response to hypoxia in mammals: mechanisms, measurement, and analysis. *Physiol. Rev.* 90, 675–754. doi: 10.1152/physrev.00012.2009

von Euler, U. S., and Liljestrand, G. (1946). Observations on the pulmonary arterial blood pressure in the cat. *Acta Physiol. Scand.* 12, 301–320. doi: 10.1111/j.1748-1716.1946.tb00389.x

Wilson, R. J., and Teppema, L. J. (2016). Integration of central and peripheral respiratory chemoreflexes. *Compr. Physiol.* 6, 1005–1041. doi: 10.1002/cphy.c140040

7

Chronic Hypobaric Hypoxia Modulates Primary Cilia Differently in Adult and Fetal Ovine Kidneys

*Kiumars Shamloo[1], Juan Chen[1], Jasmine Sardar[1], Rinzhin T. Sherpa[1], Rajasekharreddy Pala[1], Kimberly F. Atkinson[1], William J. Pearce[2], Lubo Zhang[2] and Surya M. Nauli[1,3]**

[1] Department of Biomedical and Pharmaceutical Sciences, Chapman University, Irvine, CA, United States, [2] Departments of Basic Sciences, Physiology and Pharmacology, Lawrence D. Longo MD Center for Perinatal Biology, Loma Linda University School of Medicine, Loma Linda, CA, United States, [3] Division of Nephrology and Hypertension, Department of Medicine, University of California, Irvine, Irvine, CA, United States

***Correspondence:**
Surya M. Nauli
nauli@chapman.edu;
snauli@uci.edu

Hypoxic environments at high altitude have significant effects on kidney injury. Following injury, renal primary cilia display length alterations. Primary cilia are mechanosensory organelles that regulate tubular architecture. The effect of hypoxia on cilia length is still controversial in cultured cells, and no corresponding *in vivo* study exists. Using fetal and adult sheep, we here study the effect of chronic hypobaric hypoxia on the renal injury, intracellular calcium signaling and the relationship between cilia length and cilia function. Our results show that although long-term hypoxia induces renal fibrosis in both fetal and adult kidneys, fetal kidneys are more susceptible to hypoxia-induced renal injury. Unlike hypoxic adult kidneys, hypoxic fetal kidneys are characterized by interstitial edema, tubular disparition and atrophy. We also noted that there is an increase in the cilia length as well as an increase in the cilia function in the hypoxic fetal proximal and distal collecting epithelia. Hypoxia, however, has no significant effect on primary cilia in the adult kidneys. Increased cilia length is also associated with greater flow-induced intracellular calcium signaling in renal epithelial cells from hypoxic fetuses. Our studies suggest that while hypoxia causes renal fibrosis in both adult and fetal kidneys, hypoxia-induced alteration in cilia length and function are specific to more severe renal injuries in fetal hypoxic kidneys.

Keywords: cilium, kidney injury, mechanosensor, pO_2, sheep, shear-stress, renal fibrosis

INTRODUCTION

Hypoxic environments in humans can result in the high-altitude renal syndrome (HARS) (Arestegui et al., 2011). HARS is characterized by reduced renal plasma flow (Becker et al., 1957), microalbuminuria (Becker et al., 1957), proteinuria (Jefferson et al., 2002; Chen et al., 2011), hyperuricemia (Jefferson et al., 2002) and systemic hypertension (Jefferson et al., 2002; Gilbert-Kawai et al., 2016). The kidneys have a fundamental role in adaption to regulate body fluids, electrolyte and acid-base homeostasis during acclimatization to high altitude and in mountain sickness syndromes. Kidneys also respond to hypoxic diuresis and natriuresis through inhibition of renal tubular sodium reabsorption, in addition to erythropoietin production (Haditsch et al., 2015).

Kidneys are very susceptible to lowered oxygen tensions (Mayer, 2011; Fu et al., 2016). In acute hypoxia, kidneys exhibit defense mechanisms centered around the activation of hypoxia-inducible factor (HIF) (Minet et al., 2000; Rosenberger et al., 2006). HIF up-regulates pro-angiogenic factors that protect against capillary rarefaction. HIF also increases expression of matrix metalloproteinases that effect repair and protect against fibrosis by degrading extracellular matrix. In chronic hypoxia, however, HIF mRNA is destabilized, shutting-down the kidney's initial protective mechanisms (Uchida et al., 2004). The expression of pro-angiogenic factors is repressed, and the expression of dys-angiogenic factors is increased. This may thus result in capillary rarefaction and potential fibrosis.

Primary cilia are sensory organelles that sense extracellular milieu along the tubule of a nephron. Abnormal cilia length and function result in polycystic kidneys (Nauli et al., 2003, 2006; Xu et al., 2007). Renal cilia also display length and function alterations following kidney injury. Primary cilia play a crucial role in cisplatin-induced tubular apoptosis by regulating tubular apoptotic pathway (Wang et al., 2013). Primary cilia also undergo abnormal changes in renal transplant biopsies with acute tubular injury (Hayek et al., 2013). During injury, renal cilia decrease in length in both humans and mice (Verghese et al., 2008, 2011). The shortened cilia length serves to attenuate cilia-mediated signaling pathways in response to extracellular stress, which promotes infiltration of neutrophils and macrophages in the kidney (Prodromou et al., 2012). However, the effects of chronic hypobaric hypoxia on primary cilia have yet to be investigated.

Changes in fluid-shear stress generated by urine movement can also contribute to kidney injury if the primary cilia are not functioning normally. Thus, the change in urinary flow associated with nephropathies has been proposed to be a potential insult for tubular cells leading to disorganization of the tubular epithelium (Maggiorani et al., 2015).

Based on the evidence above, it has been proposed that cilia play important roles in sensing environmental cues caused by injury and in the repair process for reestablishing a new epithelial layer of differentiated cells (Bell et al., 2011; Wang and Dong, 2013). By using a series of human renal transplant biopsies, it was found that acute tubular necrosis is associated with more than two-fold longer cilia 1-week after kidney injury, and normalization of cilium length occurred at a later stage. These results indicate that cilia function could be a clinically relevant indicator of kidney injury and repair in patients with kidney transplantation (Wang and Dong, 2013).

Despite the fact that hypoxic environment at high altitude may have significant effects on the kidneys, the histological analysis of renal architecture has never been examined especially in the fetus. Given the background information, our premises indicate that hypoxia causes renal injury/damage and that renal injury often includes altered cilia structure/function. Thus, our hypothesis is that hypoxia causes altered cilia structure/function. Here, we examined the effects of hypoxic high-altitude on the kidneys in adult and fetal sheep. We also took this opportunity to study cilia length-function relationship in response to chronic hypobaric hypoxia, because it has been reported that HIF could alter the structural length of primary cilia in hypoxic *in vitro* models (Verghese et al., 2011; Ding et al., 2015; Lavagnino et al., 2016; Resnick, 2016).

METHODS

The sheep were purchased from Nebeker Ranch, Inc. (Lancaster, CA). The normoxic control animals were maintained at sea level throughout the gestation period (300 m). To induce chronic high-altitude hypoxia, the animals were then transported at 30 days of gestation to the Barcroft Laboratory, White Mountain Research Station at Bishop, CA (3,801 m). The hypoxic animals stayed in Bishop for 110 days. Both normoxic control and hypoxic animals were fed Alfalfa hay in a "keyhole" feeder in addition to providing a mineral block *ad libitum*. The animals were transported from Bishop to the laboratory immediately before the studies (Dasgupta et al., 2012; Thorpe et al., 2013).

Two-years-old pregnant sheep and near-term 146 gestational day fetal lambs were used. Please note that sheep gestation typically lasts ~150 days. The sheep were anesthetized with thiamylal (10 mg/kg, i.v.) followed by inhalation of 1.5–2.0% halothane. An incision was made in the abdomen, and kidneys were isolated and immediately placed in either 10% buffer formalin or the phosphate-buffered sucrose solution (30% sucrose, 137 mM NaCl, 2.7 mM KCl, 10 mM Na_2HPO_4, 1.8 KH_2PO_4, 1 mM $CaCl_2 \bullet 2H_2O$ and 0.5 mM $MgCl_2 \bullet 6H_2O$ at pH 7.4). All procedures and protocols were conducted in full compliance with the Animal Welfare Act, followed the guidelines by the National Institutes of Health Guide for the Care and Use of Laboratory Animals, and were approved by the Institutional Animal Care and Use Committee at Loma Linda University, CA.

Tissue Processing

Kidney cross-sections of the cortex and medulla were dehydrated with isopropyl alcohol and infiltrated with paraffin in a tissue processor (Excelsior AS, Thermo Scientific, Inc.). Tissues were allowed to solidify in a base mold and then snapped into plastic tissue cassettes using a paraffin molding processor (HistoStar, Thermo Scientific, Inc.). Samples were cut to 5 μm thickness sections with a microtome (HM 355 S, Thermo Scientific, Inc.), and continuous "ribbon" of the sections were formed. Sections were carefully transferred onto a 40°C water dish for about 3–5 min to flatten and avoid wrinkles in the sectioned tissues.

Tissue slices were placed on the charged microscope slides, and deparaffinization was performed by placing the slides in a 60°C oven for 30 min in order to melt any extra paraffin. Slides were rinsed twice with a xylene solution for 5 min each, followed by hydration through a series of washing for 1 min each in decreasing alcohol concentrations (100, 95, 80, 70%). Slides were then submerged in the distilled water for 3 min for the staining process.

Tissue Staining

For H&E staining, tissues were stained with hematoxylin for 5 min, rinsed with tap water for 1 min and dipped for 1 sec in acid alcohol (200 ml of 50% alcohol containing 500 μL HCl 5N). Tissues were then stained with Eosin for 2 min and rinsed with distilled water for 1 min followed by dehydration with 95% and 100% alcohol each for 1 min and cleaning with xylene for 2 min. Coverslip was mounted onto a slide with xylene compatible mounting media.

For periodic acid Schiffs (PAS) staining, staining kit (*Polysciences, Inc.*) was used and experiments were performed based on the Company's protocol. Briefly, tissues were oxidized in 0.5% periodic acid for 5 min. After washing with deionized (DI) water, tissue sections were placed in Schiff's reagent for 15 min then rinsed with 0.55% potassium metabisulfite. Slides were washed in tap water for 10 min to allow the color to develop in the tissues, which were then counterstained with acidified Harris Hematoxylin for 30 s. Slides were washed with tap water until the tissues turned to a blue color. After dehydration with 95 and 100% alcohol each for 1 min and clearing with xylene for 2 min, the coverslips were mounted onto the slides with a xylene compatible mounting media.

For Masson's Trichrome staining, a staining kit (*Polysciences, Inc.*) was used according to the manufacture's instructions. Briefly, tissues were incubated in Bouin's fixative solution at 60°C for 1 h and rinsed with warm tap water for 2–3 min until the yellow color disappeared. Fresh Weigert's iron hematoxylin working solution was prepared by mixing Weigert's hematoxylin A and Weigert's hematoxylin B in a 1:1 ratio. Tissues were incubated in the working solution for 20 min and rinsed for 5 min with distilled water. Tissues were then stained with Biebrich Scarlet-Acid Fuchsin solution for 15 min and rinsed with tap water to remove any extra solution-residue. After rinsing with distilled water, the tissues were soaked in Phosphotungstic / Phosphomolibdic acid for 10 min, transferred to Aniline Blue for 7 min and washed with distilled water until the slides were clear. Tissues were then soaked in 1% acetic acid for 1 min and washed with distilled water for 1 min. After dehydration with 95 and 100% alcohol each for 1 min followed by cleaning with xylene for 2 min, the coverslips were mounted onto the slides with a xylene compatible mounting media.

For immunofluorescence staining, heat-induced epitope retrieval was performed using a pressure cooker and Tris-EDTA buffer (10 mM Tris base, 1 mM EDTA solution, 0.05% Tween 20, pH 9.0). Tris-EDTA buffer was first boiled in the pressure cooker to 100°C. Tissues were then maintained in the pressure cooker at about 121°C and 15 psi for 8 min. The pressure cooker and slides were then chilled quickly with cold tap water. The slides were rinsed three times with phosphate buffer saline (PBS) and blocked in PBS solution containing 5% bovine serum albumin for 15 min in a humidifying chamber. Using our standard protocol (Loghman-Adham et al., 2003; Nauli et al., 2003, 2006), tissues were stained with the ciliary marker acetylated-α-tubulin (1:1,000 dilution; Sigma-Aldrich, Inc.), distal tubular marker bolichos biflorus agglutinin (DBA; 4:1,000 dilution; Vector Laboratory, Inc.), proximal tubular marker lotus tetragonolobusl lectin (LTL; 4:1,000 dilution; Vector Laboratory, Inc.), and nucleus marker DAPI (Vector Laboratory, Inc.).

Primary Cell Culture

Isolation of renal epithelia from fresh tissues has been previously described in detail (Loghman-Adham et al., 2003; Nauli et al., 2003, 2006). After extensive washing in phosphate-buffered sucrose solution, the cortex and medullary regions of kidney were dissected into pieces and incubated with collagenase followed by 0.05% trypsin/0.53 mM EDTA at 37°C for 15–20 min. After vortexing vigorously for 5 min, ice-cold HBSS containing 10% FBS was added to inactivate the trypsin. The cells were further released from the fibrous basement membrane by trituration, washed twice with HBSS. Cells were then sorted based on their surface markers for DBA or LTL and resuspended in fresh culture medium. To allow attachment, the cells was grown in DMEM containing 10% FBS and supplemented with 5 μg/ml insulin, 5 μg/ml transferrin, 5 ng/ml selenium, 36 ng/ml (10^{-7} M) hydrocortisone, 10^{-8} M triiodothyronine, 10 ng/ml EGF, and 50 ng/ml PGE1, as well as 100 U/ml penicillin, and 100 μg/ml streptomycin in a 37°C humidified incubator ventilated with 5% CO_2—95% O_2. The culture medium was changed every 2–3 days until confluency was reached.

Cilia Function and Length Measurements

Bending primary cilia with fluid-flow activates the cilium and increases cytoplasmic calcium in renal epithelial cells (Praetorius and Spring, 2001; Liu et al., 2005; Jin et al., 2014). Thus, intracellular calcium was measured with Fura2-AM [to study cilia function] as previously described (Nauli et al., 2013). Briefly, after pre-incubation with 5 μM Fura2-AM for 30 min at 37°C, the tissues were equilibrated for at least a minute. The optimal shear-stress of 0.8 dyne/cm^2 was used to monitor changes in cytosolic calcium as previously described (Nauli et al., 2013). Ionomycin (1 μM) was used at the end of each experiment to confirm Fura-2 loading and determine minimal and maximal ratiometric fluorescence signals. Cells were then analyzed for cilia length by staining with the ciliary marker acetylated-α-tubulin by staining with the ciliary marker acetylated-α-tubulin as previously described (Loghman-Adham et al., 2003; Nauli et al., 2003, 2006).

Data Analysis

All images represent the extracted information from the digital pictures. Images were captured through a Nikon Ti-E microscope. The Nikon NIS Elements for Advanced Research software was used for image capture and analysis, including automatic object recognition, image scanning and color binary segmentation. Scale bars were provided in all figures to indicate the actual image reduction size. All morphometric data were reported as mean ± SEM. Distribution analyses were performed and presented on all data sets to verify normal data distributions. After distribution and variance analyses, data comparisons for more than two groups were performed using ANOVA test followed by a Tukey *post-hoc* analysis. The correlation between cilia length and cilia function was analyzed with the ordinary least squares (OLS) regression of y on x, because the ordinary least products (OLP) would not allow analysis of covariance as a technique for testing the equality of slopes or intercepts in linear regressions (Ludbrook, 2012). Pearson correlation coefficients were therefore used to analyze the significance of differences in the coefficients correlating primary cilia length and function. Asterisks (*) denote with statistical significance differences at $p <$ 0.05 relative to corresponding control groups as indicated in the figures.

A total of 12 sheep and 12 lambs was used; for each normoxic or hypoxic group, 6 sheep and 6 lambs were used ($N = 6$ sheep and $N = 6$ lambs for normoxia; $N = 6$ sheep and $N = 6$ lambs for hypoxia). From each animal, both kidneys were collected for different studies. Each pair of kidneys were randomly selected for an immediate fixation in formalin or trypsinization for cell culture. From each kidney, a minimum of 10 experimental replicates was sampled. All statistical analysis was done with *GraphPad Prism*, version 5.0b.

RESULTS

The normoxic control animals had maternal and fetal arterial PO_2 (PaO_2) of 102 ± 2 and 25 ± 1 mmHg, respectively. The hypoxic maternal and hypoxic fetal PaO_2 were 60 ± 2 and 19 ± 1 mmHg, respectively.

Fetal Hypoxic Kidneys Were Characterized by Interstitial Medullary Edema

Representative images of H&E stained renal tissue sections from normoxic and hypoxic kidneys are presented (**Figure 1A**). In all kidney sections, light microscopy analysis indicated that the cortex regions of the kidneys had normal glomeruli. There were no significant differences in glomerulus size between normoxic and hypoxic kidneys (**Figure 1B**). Capillary loops of the glomeruli were also normal, and the number and morphology of endothelial cells were comparable between normoxic and hypoxic tissues.

In normoxic fetal kidneys, all tubules were closely spaced in the interstitium. Tubules were lined with a single layer of epithelia and well-organized nuclei. In hypoxic fetuses, the renal cortex demonstrated some evidence of mesangial and intercapillary cell proliferation. The renal medulla showed apparent atrophic tubules, interstitial fibrosis and edema, and tubular disparition characterized by greater inter-tubular spaces and separation of tubules filled with edema (**Figure 1C**).

While all tubules in adult sheep were closely spaced in the interstitium and lined by a single layer of cells with well-organized nuclei, some abnormalities were observed in the chronically hypoxic kidney. The hypoxic kidneys showed some proliferation of mesangial cells in the cortex and slight tubular edema in the medullary region. Otherwise, the surrounding tubules appeared normal in both normoxic and hypoxic adult kidneys.

Hypoxia Modulated Medullary Tubular Basement Membrane Thickness

PAS staining was done to highlight basement membranes of glomerular capillary loops and tubular epithelia. Renal tissue sections from normoxic and hypoxic kidneys are shown in the representative images (**Figure 2A**). There were no significant differences in basement membranes thicknesses of glomerular capillary loops between normoxic and hypoxic adult kidneys.

Basement membrane thicknesses of the tubules were significantly less in hypoxic fetal kidneys compared to normoxic fetal kidneys (**Figure 2B**). Although a reverse trend was

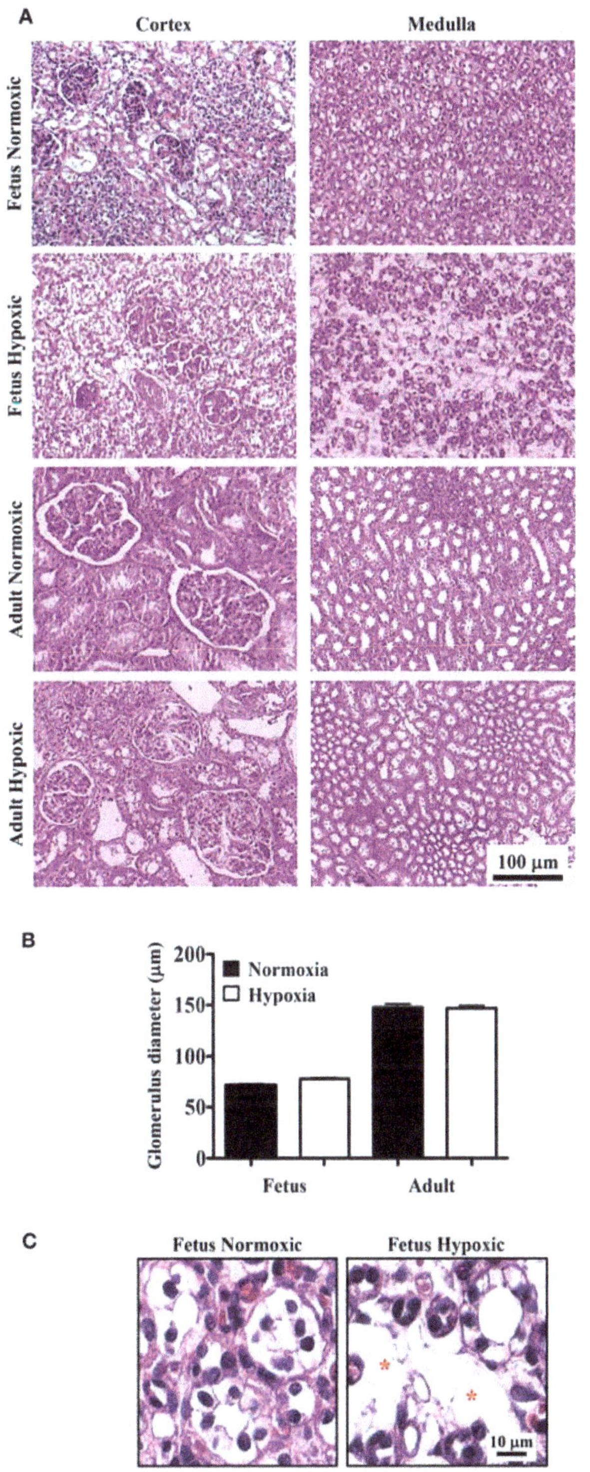

FIGURE 1 | Haemotoxylin and Eosin (H&E) staining to study effects of long-term hypoxia. **(A)** Kidneys were stained with H&E, and representative images were taken at the cortex and medullary regions of the kidneys. **(B)** Glomerular diameters were measured and quantified. **(C)** Representative images show that in fetal hypoxic kidney, tubules are separated by interstitial medullary edema as denoted by asterisks. $N = 6$ animals for each group; statistical analysis was performed with ANOVA followed by the Tukey *post-hoc* test.

observed in adult kidneys, it was not statistically significant in adult normoxic or hypoxic kidneys. To refine the statistical analysis, tubular membrane thicknesses were re-measured by discriminating the tubular origins. In proximal tubules, no significant difference in tubular membrane thickness was observed (**Figure 2C**). In distal collecting tubules, tubular membranes were significantly thicker in hypoxic than normoxic adult kidneys. As expected, tubular membrane thicknesses were significantly less in hypoxic compared to normoxic fetal kidneys.

As observed in the H&E staining, hypoxic fetal kidneys showed interstitial medullary edema, fibrosis, tubular disparition and atrophy characterized by greater inter-tubular space (**Figure 2D**).

Long-Term Hypoxia Induced Renal Fibrosis

To examine potential fibrosis in the kidneys, Masson's Trichrome staining was performed to highlight deposition of collagen and fibrin fibers. Renal tissue sections from normoxic and hypoxic kidneys are shown in representative images (**Figure 3A**). The percentage of blue-stained area was calculated using a binary threshold program, which indicated significant fibrosis in hypoxic compared to normoxic kidney tissues (**Figure 3B**). In normoxic tissues, there was some collagen fibers that were normally distributed around renal tubules. In hypoxic tissues, normal distributions of collagen fibers were observed, but abnormal depositions of collagen/fibrin fibers were also observed throughout tubular epithelia and interstitial spaces.

As observed in the H&E and PAS staining, hypoxic fetal kidney showed interstitial medullary edema characterized by more inter-tubular space (**Figure 3C**). As also seen in previous staining, hypoxia modulated lumen size of distal tubules in both fetal and adult kidneys (**Figure 3D**). No significant changes in lumen size were observed in proximal tubules.

Fetal Hypoxic Kidney Was Characterized by Longer Renal Epithelial Primary Cilia

It remains uncertain if hypoxia can maintain and stabilize the primary cilia or it would inhibit primary cilia formation (Verghese et al., 2011; Ding et al., 2015; Lavagnino et al., 2016; Resnick, 2016). To investigate the effect of chronic hypoxia, primary cilia were labeled with the cilia marker acetylated-α-tubulin. Representative images of renal tissue sections from normoxic and hypoxic kidneys are shown for staining of cilia and tubular markers. Distal collecting (**Figure 4A**) and proximal (**Figure 4B**) tubular markers were used to identify cilia length in respective tubules. Cilia measurements were the represented in the bar graphs to compare the distributions of the cilia length (**Figure 4C**). While hypoxia did not significantly alter cilia length in adult kidneys, fetal kidneys were very susceptible to hypoxia (**Figure 4D**). Cilia length was significantly longer in hypoxic fetal kidneys than normoxic fetal kidneys.

Of note, that the distal collecting tubules had larger lumen sizes in adult than fetal kidneys. This may be associated with longer cilia in adult than fetal distal collecting tubules. For the first time, our studies show that the length of primary cilia in distal collecting tubules become longer during maturation, while

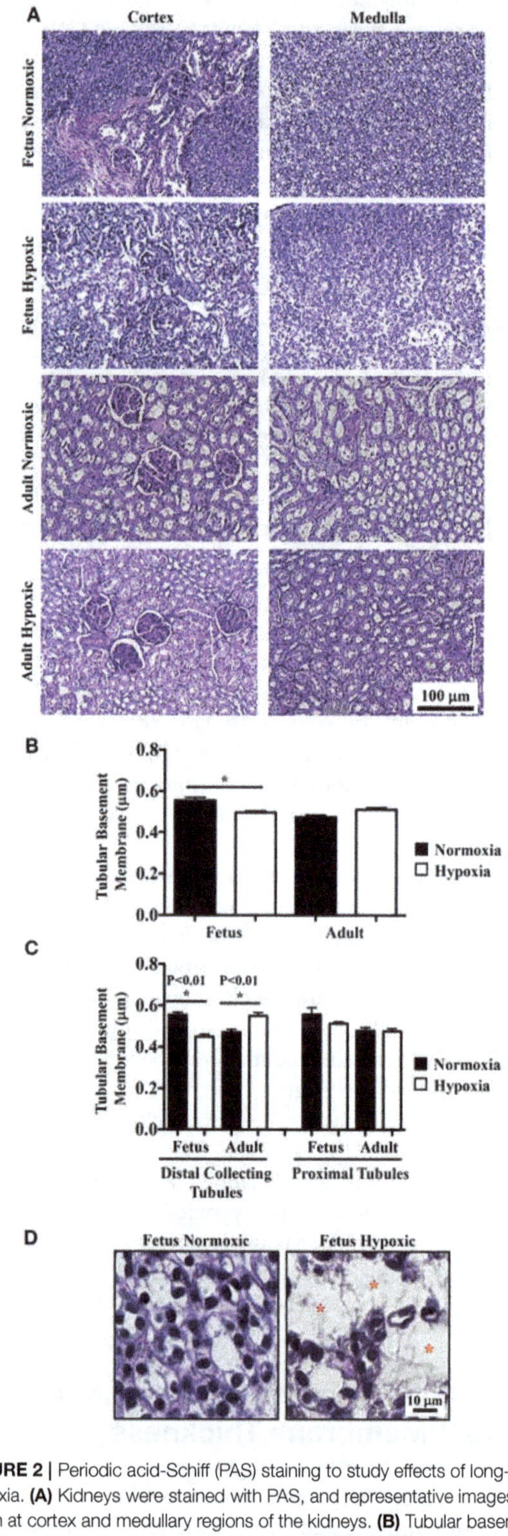

FIGURE 2 | Periodic acid-Schiff (PAS) staining to study effects of long-term hypoxia. **(A)** Kidneys were stained with PAS, and representative images were taken at cortex and medullary regions of the kidneys. **(B)** Tubular basement membrane thickness was measured and quantified. **(C)** More detail analysis of basement membrane was achieved by separation between distal collecting and proximal tubules. **(D)** Representative images show that in fetal hypoxic kidney, tubules were separated by interstitial medullary edema as denoted by red asterisks. *Indicates significant differences between normoxic and hypoxic groups. $N = 6$ animals for each group; statistical analysis was performed with ANOVA followed by the Tukey *post-hoc* test.

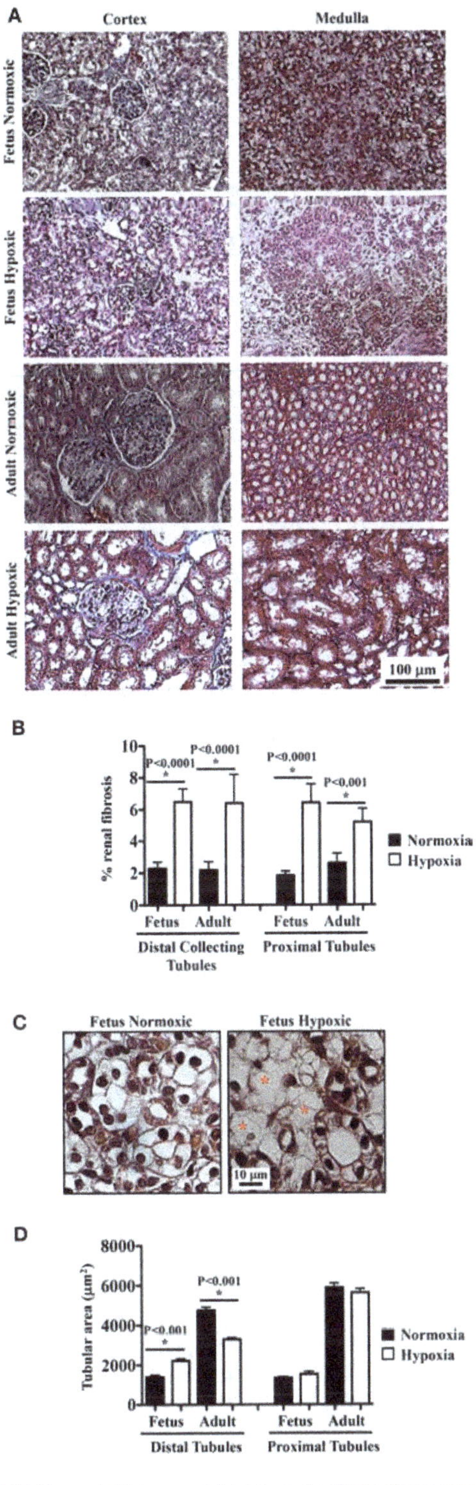

FIGURE 3 | Masson's Trichrome staining to study effects of long-term hypoxia. **(A)** Kidneys were stained with Masson's Trichrome, and representative images were taken at cortex and medullary regions of the kidneys. **(B)** Interstitial renal fibrosis was measured and quantified. **(C)** Representative images show that in fetal hypoxic kidney, tubules were separated by interstitial medullary edema as denoted by red asterisks. **(D)** Tubular areas were measured, quantified and compared. *Indicates significant differences between normoxic and hypoxic groups. $N = 6$ animals for each group; statistical analysis was performed with ANOVA followed by the Tukey *post-hoc* test.

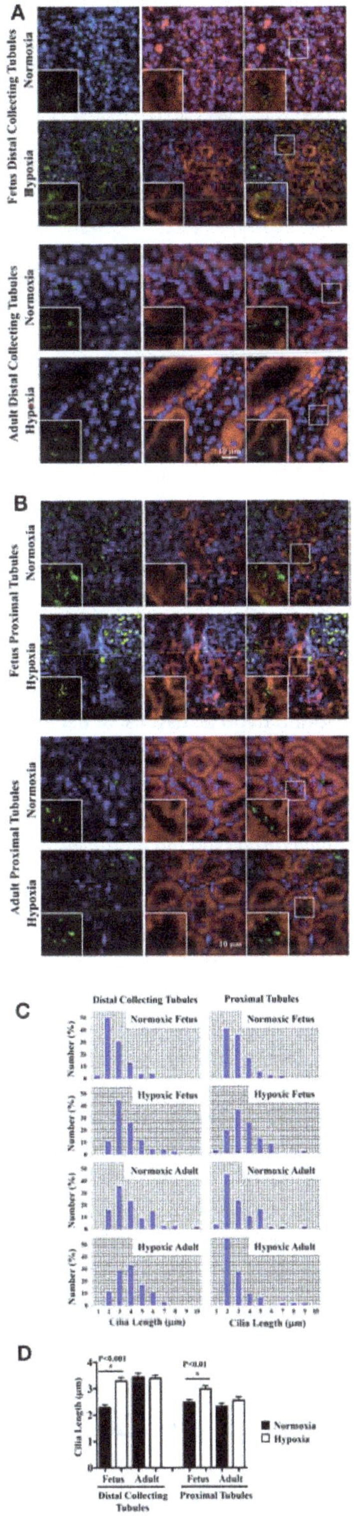

FIGURE 4 | Immunofluorescence staining to study effects of long-term hypoxia on cilia length *in vivo*. **(A)** Kidneys were stained with ciliary marker (acetylated-α-tubulin; green), distal collecting marker (DBA; red) and nucleus marker (DAPI; blue). **(B)** Instead of DBA, kidneys were stained with proximal tubular marker (LTL; red). White boxes show enlargement of the images to

(Continued)

FIGURE 4 | Continued
depict the magnified view of primary cilia. **(C)** The length of primary cilia was measured and represented in the bar graph to depict length distribution within each group. **(D)** Cilia length was quantified. *Indicates significant differences between normoxic and hypoxic groups. $N = 6$ animals for each group; statistical analysis was performed with ANOVA followed by the Tukey *post-hoc* test.

there is no change in proximal tubule cilia length from fetuses to adults.

Fetal Hypoxic Kidney Had Greater Sensitivity in Response to Fluid-Shear Stress

Renal primary cilia are mechanosensory organelles that sense filtrate moving within the tubules. To examine the possibility that hypoxia could alter mechanosensory of cellular responses, renal epithelia were isolated, cultured, stained with a cilia marker and challenged with shear-stress. Representative images of these cells from normoxic and hypoxic kidneys reveal changes in cilia length (**Figure 5A**). On average about 80% of cells had cilia, and there were no apparent differences in cilia formation between normoxic and hypoxic tissues, or between fetal and adult kidneys. Cilia measurements were then tabulated to compare their distributions (**Figure 5B**). Cilia measurements were also tabulated to analyze the impact of hypoxia on cilia lengths (**Figure 5C**). While hypoxia did not significantly alter cilia length in adult cells, cilia length was significantly longer in hypoxic than normoxic fetal cells. Interestingly, trend in cilia length changes was similar for *in vitro* and *in vivo* preparations. When the overall cilia length *in vivo* kidney (**Figure 4**) or *in vitro* cell culture (**Figure 5**) were averaged, it was apparent that the *in vitro* cell culture produced much longer cilia than observed *in vivo* (6.35 ± 0.28 μm vs. 2.84 ± 0.12 μm; $p < 0.00005$).

To examine the effect of chronic hypoxia on mechanosensory cilia function, cells were challenged with 0.8 dyne/cm^2 shear-stress. Changes in cytosolic calcium were averaged and plotted in line graphs (**Figure 6A**). When peaks of cytosolic calcium were examined, hypoxia significantly enhanced mechanosensory function in fetal epithelial cells (**Figure 6B**). In contrast, hypoxia did not significantly alter mechanosensory sensitivity in adult cells.

Hypoxia-Induced Longer Cilia Were Associated with Greater Cilia Function

It has been hypothesized that longer cilia are more sensitive to fluid-shear stress (Abdul-Majeed et al., 2012; Upadhyay et al., 2014). To examine the effect of hypoxia on cilia length-function relationship, both *in vivo* (**Figure 4**) and *in vitro* (**Figure 5**) cilia lengths were used to assess changes in cilia function. When *in vivo* cilia length was plotted against cilia function, no apparent length-function association was observed (**Figure 7A**; $R^2 = 0.42$). Because hypoxia did not alter cilia length in adult kidneys, length-function relationship was next analyzed only in

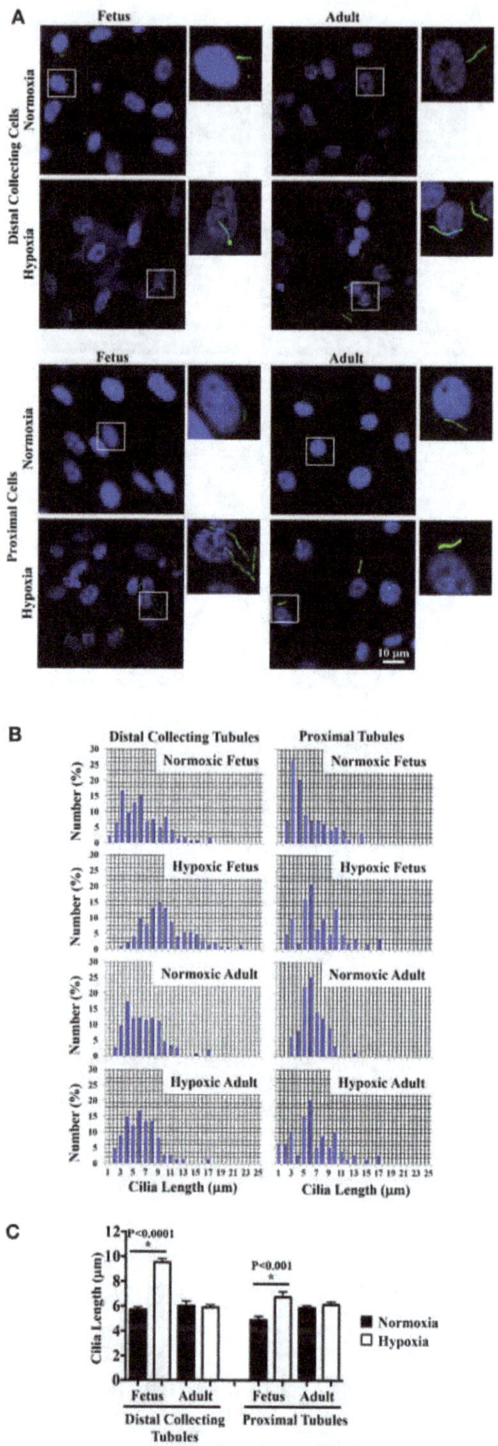

FIGURE 5 | Immunofluorescence staining to study effects of long-term hypoxia on cilia length in *in vitro* cultures. **(A)** Ovine renal epithelia were isolated and stained with ciliary marker (acetylated-α-tubulin; green) and nucleus marker (DAPI; blue). White boxes show enlargement of the images to depict the presence of primary cilia. **(B)** The length of primary cilia was measured and tabulated in the bar graph to depict length distribution within each group. **(C)** Cilia length was quantified. *Indicates significant differences between normoxic and hypoxic groups. $N = 6$ animals for each group; statistical analysis was performed with ANOVA followed by the Tukey *post-hoc* test.

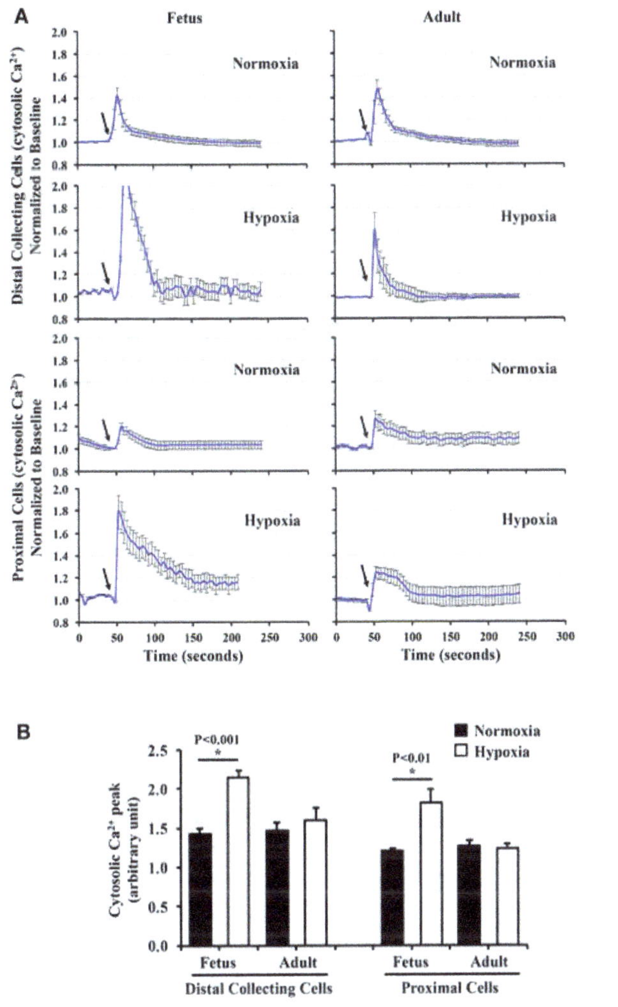

FIGURE 6 | Cytosolic calcium measurement to study effects of long-term hypoxia. **(A)** Cytosolic calcium was measured with Fura-2AM. After equilibration for 30 min, baseline calcium signal was taken for 50 s. Cells were challenged with fluid-shear stress (arrows), and averaged changes in cytosolic calcium for each group were presented in line graphs. **(B)** The peak of calcium changes was selected to depict the function of primary cilia. The bar graph shows the averaged calcium peak in response to fluid-shear stress. $N = 6$ animals for each group; statistical analysis was performed with ANOVA followed by the Tukey *post-hoc* test.

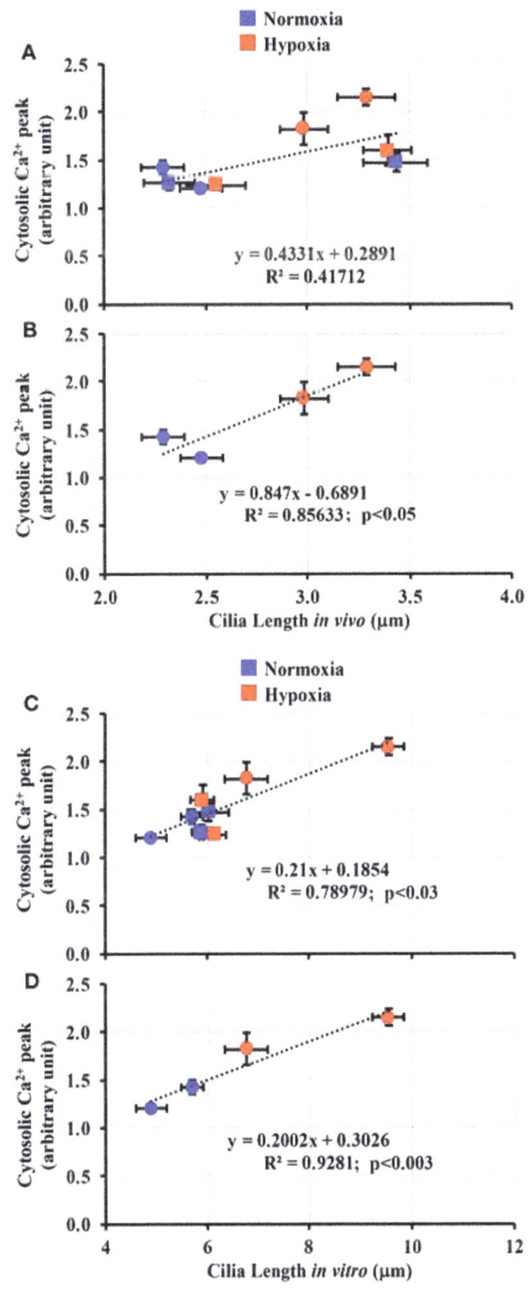

FIGURE 7 | Correlation between cilia length-function. **(A)** Cilia length-function relation was plotted in a dot plot from both fetal and adult groups *in vivo*. **(B)** Because hypoxia affected mainly on fetal renal cilia, the length-function relation showed a greater correlation when plotted only for fetus. **(C)** Cilia length was next taken from the *in vitro* measurement. Cilia length-function relation was plotted in a dot plot from both fetal and adult groups. **(D)** Because hypoxia affected mainly on fetal renal cilia, the length-function relation showed a greater correlation when plotted only for fetus. $N = 6$ animals for each group; statistical analysis was performed with the Pearson correlation coefficient test.

fetal kidneys. This revealed significant correlation within length-function relationships (**Figure 7B**; $R^2 = 0.86$). When *in vitro* cilia length was analyzed, the cilia function was significantly correlated with cilia length following either inclusion (**Figure 7C**; $R^2 = 0.79$) or exclusion (**Figure 7D**; $R^2 = 0.93$) of adult kidneys.

DISCUSSION

Although kidneys are important for regulation of body fluid, pH, electrolyte, hormone and overall metabolism, the effects of chronic hypobaric hypoxia on fetal kidneys have never been examined. We therefore study the effects of chronic hypoxia on fetal and adult sheep kidneys within the cortex and medullary regions. Effects of hypoxia on mechanosensory primary cilia are also evaluated. Our studies suggest that: (1) there are no significant differences in glomerulus size between normoxic and hypoxic kidneys; (2) the hypoxic kidneys show proliferation

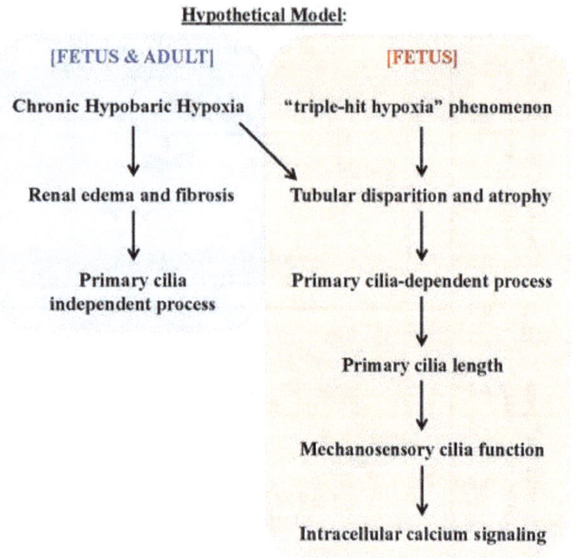

FIGURE 8 | Hypothetical model on the effects of chronic hypoxia-induced renal injury on primary cilia. The chronic hypobaric hypoxia induces kidney injuries, such (as) renal edema and fibrosis. Such injuries may be considered "mild" that does not alter primary cilia length and function. The triple-hit hypoxia, compounding the chronic hypoxia, is a phenomenon independently observed in fetus. The tripe-hit hypoxia is characterized by 1) chronic hypoxia-induced maladaptation of uteroplacental vasoconstriction, 2) redistribution of blood flow away from the fetal kidneys and 3) the unique oxygen-poor blood circulation in the fetal kidneys. This triggers cilia length increase, which in turn improves cilia function. The overall response will result in changes of intracellular calcium signaling.

of mesangial cells, medullary edema and fibrosis; (3) hypoxia modulates changes in tubular basement membranes; and (4) compared to adult kidneys, fetal kidneys are more susceptible to hypoxia-induced tubular disparition and atrophy, characterized by alterations in primary cilia and function.

A previous study has demonstrated enlargement of renal glomeruli in hypoxic children (Naeye, 1965). However, our studies do not support glomerulus enlargement in the hypoxic fetal or adult sheep kidneys. This discrepancy could potentially be due to an age-specific effect. For example, glomerular enlargement only occurs after the first month of life, while the size of glomeruli is normal at birth in those hypoxic children (Naeye, 1965). Since all of these children die as a result of unknown illness, it is also possible that other genetic and environmental factors contributed to the glomerulus enlargement. For example, an oxonic acid diet in rats is known to cause hyperuricemia through elevated plasma renin activity (Eraranta et al., 2008). Glomerular hypertrophy is observed in oxonic acid-induced hyperuricemia and can be prevented by ACE inhibitor therapy in the rats (Nakagawa et al., 2003).

Abnormal mesangial cells, edema and fibrosis are observed in our hypoxic kidneys. This is possibly a result from interstitial renal injury due to chronic hypobaric hypoxia. Of note, the deposition of collagen and fibrin fiber that functions as a by-product of a reparative process, is commonly used as an index of various renal injury (Ma et al., 1998; Kaissling and Le Hir, 2008; Forbes et al., 2012). Although hypoxia is one of the stimuli that drives chronic kidney disease (Fu et al., 2016), our studies further reveal that hypoxia could alter the thickness of tubular basement membranes. Interestingly, hypoxia only induces changes in basement membranes of distal collecting tubules. This could be due to medullary regions that operate within a relatively lower range of pO_2, and it is therefore more susceptible to hypoxic injury than proximal regions (Heyman et al., 1997; El Sabbahy and Vaidya, 2011). Greater susceptibility of medullary regions to hypoxia might thus contribute to an increase in collecting distal tubular basement membrane of adult kidneys. Unlike adult medullary tissues, however, hypoxia actually causes a decrease in medullary basement membrane in fetal kidney. This could possibly be due to tubular disparition and atrophy, which are very apparent in the fetal medulla. The thinning in basement membrane in medullary tissues might therefore be associated with a degeneration of tubular structure, as observed in fetal hypoxic kidneys.

Based on the histological analyses, fetal kidneys are more susceptible to hypoxia, possibly due to a "triple-hit hypoxia" phenomenon. In addition to the hypobaric hypoxia in the atmosphere, fetal kidneys are impacted by three additional factors (triple-hit). First, chronic hypoxia induces vasoconstriction in sheep uterine arteries during gestation (Hu et al., 2012; Xiao et al., 2013). This maladaptation of the uteroplacental circulation can result in reduced tissue perfusion and further exacerbate the effects of hypoxia. Second, in hypoxic fetal sheep there is a rapid drop in fetal heart rate and a rise in mean arterial blood pressure that redistributes blood flow to the heart and brain at the expense of the renal circulation. Hypoxia therefore reduces renal blood flow, resulting in renal hypoperfusion (Robillard et al., 1986; Green et al., 1997). Third, the unique fetal circulation system allows oxygen-rich blood from the aorta to mix with oxygen-poor blood before reaching renal circulation (Nakamura et al., 1987). Thus, the fetal circulation system reduces oxygenation support to the kidneys.

Our results also indicate that greater susceptibility to hypoxia in fetal kidneys could be associated with changes in primary cilia length and function throughout the nephrons. Primary cilia are sensory organelles rising from the apical surface of most mammalian cells. Cilia are activated during bending by fluid-flow, which in turn initiates an intracellular calcium response (Praetorius and Spring, 2001; Liu et al., 2005; Nauli et al., 2013). Previous studies demonstrate a link between cilia length and hypoxia-inducible mechanisms. In tendon cells, hypoxia inhibits primary cilia formation and cellular mechano-responsiveness (Lavagnino et al., 2016). However, studies in different hypoxic models using renal epithelial cells indicate that primary cilia are longer and that expression of HIF maintains primary cilia length (Verghese et al., 2011; Ding et al., 2015). Interestingly, the renal epithelial cilia become more flexible during hypoxia (Resnick, 2016), and it thus might alter cilia function. Consistent with this view, a correlation between cilia length and function in response to chronic hypoxia is observed in our studies. Interestingly, greater cilia length in hypoxic fetal kidney *in vivo* are maintained as measured in *in vitro* cell culture. This could be due to epigenetic changes occurring during hypoxia. Of note, long-term hypoxia during gestation has been reported to cause epigenetic adaptation in the sheep (Dasgupta et al., 2012; Chen et al., 2014).

Our studies indicate that chronic hypobaric hypoxia could induce renal injury (**Figure 8**). Renal hypoperfusion as a result from the "triple-hit hypoxia" phenomenon seen in fetus would further induce tubular disparition and atrophy, a process that modulated changes in cilia length and function. This, in turn, induces an increase in intracellular calcium fluxes in response to fluid-shear stress. Our results potentially point to a complex renal injury caused by chronic hypoxia with regards to primary cilia.

It has been reported that kidney compensation induced by a reduction of renal mass results in primary cilia elongation, and this elongation is associated with an increased production of reactive oxygen species (Han et al., 2016). In addition, renal primary cilia lengthens after acute tubular necrosis (Verghese et al., 2009). The contribution of primary cilia from acute to chronic injury is also confirmed when a ciliary protein is inactivated. In this case, renal damages are more pronounced following ischemia/reperfusion, and this induces microcyst formation (Bastos et al., 2009). In addition to the association of human renal carcinoma and primary cilia (Ding et al., 2015), acute injury can induce chronic kidney disease through cyst formation in the absence of normal renal cilia (Patel et al., 2008). Furthermore, mechanosensory function of cilia is abnormal in chronic kidney disease patients (Nauli et al., 2006; Xu et al., 2007). Based on these findings, we speculate that the increases in hypoxia-induced cilia-related calcium signaling in hypoxic fetal kidneys serves a potential mechanism associated with renal injury. Without doubt, future studies on the hypoxia-induced changes in intracellular calcium are warranted.

AUTHOR CONTRIBUTIONS

KS analyzed data, contributed to drafting the manuscript and oversaw the entire progress. JC and RS performed the calcium studies. JS and RP performed cilia measurements and kidney staining. KA assisted in sample collections. WP and LZ provided the kidney samples. LZ and SMN finalized the manuscript and oversaw the research project.

FUNDING

The project is funded in part by Congressionally Directed Medical Research Program PR130153 (SMN) and National Institutes of Health Grants HD083132 (LZ).

ACKNOWLEDGMENTS

Authors would like to acknowledge and thank Alisz Demecs and Maki Takahashi for their editing and technical support.

REFERENCES

Abdul-Majeed, S., Moloney, B. C., and Nauli, S. M. (2012). Mechanisms regulating cilia growth and cilia function in endothelial cells. *Cell. Mol. Life Sci.* 69, 165–173. doi: 10.1007/s00018-011-0744-0

Arestegui, A. H., Fuquay, R., Sirota, J., Swenson, E. R., Schoene, R. B., Jefferson, J. A., et al. (2011). High altitude renal syndrome (HARS). *J. Am. Soc. Nephrol.* 22, 1963–1968. doi: 10.1681/ASN.2010121316

Bastos, A. P., Piontek, K., Silva, A. M., Martini, D., Menezes, L. F., Fonseca, J. M., et al. (2009). Pkd1 haploinsufficiency increases renal damage and induces microcyst formation following ischemia/reperfusion. *J. Am. Soc. Nephrol.* 20, 2389–2402. doi: 10.1681/ASN.2008040435

Becker, E. L., Schilling, J. A., and Harvey, R. B. (1957). Renal function in man acclimatized to high altitude. *J. Appl. Physiol.* 10, 79–80.

Bell, P. D., Fitzgibbon, W., Sas, K., Stenbit, A. E., Amria, M., Houston, A., et al. (2011). Loss of primary cilia upregulates renal hypertrophic signaling and promotes cystogenesis. *J. Am. Soc. Nephrol.* 22, 839–848. doi: 10.1681/ASN.2010050526

Chen, M., Dasgupta, C., Xiong, F., and Zhang, L. (2014). Epigenetic upregulation of large-conductance Ca^{2+}-activated K^{+} channel expression in uterine vascular adaptation to pregnancy. *Hypertension* 64, 610–618. doi: 10.1161/HYPERTENSIONAHA.114.03407

Chen, W., Liu, Q., Wang, H., Chen, W., Johnson, R. J., Dong, X., et al. (2011). Prevalence and risk factors of chronic kidney disease: a population study in the Tibetan population. *Nephrol. Dial. Transplant* 26, 1592–1599. doi: 10.1093/ndt/gfq608

Dasgupta, C., Chen, M., Zhang, H., Yang, S., and Zhang, L. (2012). Chronic hypoxia during gestation causes epigenetic repression of the estrogen receptor-alpha gene in ovine uterine arteries via heightened promoter methylation. *Hypertension* 60, 697–704. doi: 10.1161/HYPERTENSIONAHA.112.198242

Ding, X. F., Zhou, J., Hu, Q. Y., Liu, S. C., and Chen, G. (2015). The tumor suppressor pVHL down-regulates never-in-mitosis A-related kinase 8 via hypoxia-inducible factors to maintain cilia in human renal cancer cells. *J. Biol. Chem.* 290, 1389–1394. doi: 10.1074/jbc.M114.589226

El Sabbahy, M., and Vaidya, V. S. (2011). Ischemic kidney injury and mechanisms of tissue repair. *Wiley Interdiscip. Rev. Syst. Biol. Med.* 3, 606–618. doi: 10.1002/wsbm.133

Eraranta, A., Kurra, V., Tahvanainen, A. M., Vehmas, T. I., Koobi, P., Lakkisto, P., et al. (2008). Oxonic acid-induced hyperuricemia elevates plasma aldosterone in experimental renal insufficiency. *J. Hypertens.* 26, 1661–1668. doi: 10.1097/HJH.0b013e328303205d

Forbes, M. S., Thornhill, B. A., Minor, J. J., Gordon, K. A., Galarreta, C. I., and Chevalier, R. L. (2012). Fight-or-flight: murine unilateral ureteral obstruction causes extensive proximal tubular degeneration, collecting duct dilatation, and minimal fibrosis. *Am. J. Physiol. Renal Physiol.* 303, F120–F129. doi: 10.1152/ajprenal.00110.2012

Fu, Q., Colgan, S. P., and Shelley, C. S. (2016). Hypoxia: the force that drives chronic kidney disease. *Clin. Med. Res.* 14, 15–39. doi: 10.3121/cmr.2015.1282

Gilbert-Kawai, E., Martin, D., Grocott, M., and Levett, D. (2016). High altitude-related hypertensive crisis and acute kidney injury in an asymptomatic healthy individual. *Extrem. Physiol. Med.* 5:10. doi: 10.1186/s13728-016-0051-3

Green, L. R., Bennet, L., Robson, S., and Hanson, M. A. (1997). The role of carotid chemoreceptors in the effects of hypoxia on renal blood flow in the late gestation sheep fetus. *Exp. Physiol.* 82, 183–192. doi: 10.1113/expphysiol.1997.sp004007

Haditsch, B., Roessler, A., Krisper, P., Frisch, H., Hinghofer-Szalkay, H. G., and Goswami, N. (2015). Volume regulation and renal function at high altitude across gender. *PLoS ONE* 10:e0118730. doi: 10.1371/journal.pone.0118730

Han, S. J., Jang, H. S., Kim, J. I., Lipschutz, J. H., and Park, K. M. (2016). Unilateral nephrectomy elongates primary cilia in the remaining kidney via reactive oxygen species. *Sci. Rep.* 6:22281. doi: 10.1038/srep22281

Hayek, S., Parasuraman, R., Desai, H. S., Samarapungavan, D., Li, W., Wolforth, S. C., et al. (2013). Primary cilia metaplasia in renal transplant biopsies with acute tubular injury. *Ultrastruct. Pathol.* 37, 159–163. doi: 10.3109/01913123.2013.768745

Heyman, S. N., Rosen, S., and Brezis, M. (1997). The renal medulla: life at the edge of anoxia. *Blood Purif.* 15, 232–242.

Hu, X. Q., Xiao, D., Zhu, R., Huang, X., Yang, S., Wilson, S. M., et al. (2012). Chronic hypoxia suppresses pregnancy-induced upregulation of large-conductance Ca^{2+}-activated K^+ channel activity in uterine arteries. *Hypertension* 60, 214–222. doi: 10.1161/HYPERTENSIONAHA.112.196097

Jefferson, J. A., Escudero, E., Hurtado, M. E., Kelly, J. P., Swenson, E. R., Wener, M. H., et al. (2002). Hyperuricemia, hypertension, and proteinuria associated with high-altitude polycythemia. *Am. J. Kidney Dis.* 39, 1135–1142. doi: 10.1053/ajkd.2002.33380

Jin, X., Mohieldin, A. M., Muntean, B. S., Green, J. A., Shah, J. V., Mykytyn, K., et al. (2014). Cilioplasm is a cellular compartment for calcium signaling in response to mechanical and chemical stimuli. *Cell. Mol. Life Sci.* 71, 2165–2178. doi: 10.1007/s00018-013-1483-1

Kaissling, B., and Le Hir, M. (2008). The renal cortical interstitium: morphological and functional aspects. *Histochem. Cell Biol.* 130, 247–262. doi: 10.1007/s00418-008-0452-5

Lavagnino, M., Oslapas, A. N., Gardner, K. L., and Arnoczky, S. P. (2016). Hypoxia inhibits primary cilia formation and reduces cell-mediated contraction in stress-deprived rat tail tendon fascicles. *Muscles Ligaments Tendons J.* 6, 193–197. doi: 10.11138/mltj/2016.6.2.193

Liu, W., Murcia, N. S., Duan, Y., Weinbaum, S., Yoder, B. K., Schwiebert, E., et al. (2005). Mechanoregulation of intracellular Ca^{2+} concentration is attenuated in collecting duct of monocilium-impaired orpk mice. *Am. J. Physiol. Renal Physiol.* 289, F978–F988. doi: 10.1152/ajprenal.00260.2004

Loghman-Adham, M., Nauli, S. M., Soto, C. E., Kariuki, B., and Zhou, J. (2003). Immortalized epithelial cells from human autosomal dominant polycystic kidney cysts. *Am. J. Physiol. Renal Physiol.* 285, F397–F412. doi: 10.1152/ajprenal.00310.2002

Ludbrook, J. (2012). A primer for biomedical scientists on how to execute model II linear regression analysis. *Clin. Exp. Pharmacol. Physiol.* 39, 329–335. doi: 10.1111/j.1440-1681.2011.05643.x

Ma, J., Nishimura, H., Fogo, A., Kon, V., Inagami, T., and Ichikawa, I. (1998). Accelerated fibrosis and collagen deposition develop in the renal interstitium of angiotensin type 2 receptor null mutant mice during ureteral obstruction. *Kidney Int.* 53, 937–944. doi: 10.1111/j.1523-1755.1998.00893.x

Maggiorani, D., Dissard, R., Belloy, M., Saulnier-Blache, J. S., Casemayou, A., Ducasse, L., et al. (2015). Shear stress-induced alteration of epithelial organization in human renal tubular cells. *PLoS ONE* 10:e0131416. doi: 10.1371/journal.pone.0131416

Mayer, G. (2011). Capillary rarefaction, hypoxia, VEGF and angiogenesis in chronic renal disease. *Nephrol. Dial. Transplant* 26, 1132–1137. doi: 10.1093/ndt/gfq832

Minet, E., Arnould, T., Michel, G., Roland, I., Mottet, D., Raes, M., et al. (2000). ERK activation upon hypoxia: involvement in HIF-1 activation. *FEBS Lett.* 468, 53–58. doi: 10.1016/S0014-5793(00)01181-9

Naeye, R. L. (1965). Children at high altitude: pulmonary and renal abnormalities. *Circ. Res.* 16, 33–38. doi: 10.1161/01.RES.16.1.33

Nakagawa, T., Mazzali, M., Kang, D. H., Kanellis, J., Watanabe, S., Sanchez-Lozada, L. G., et al. (2003). Hyperuricemia causes glomerular hypertrophy in the rat. *Am. J. Nephrol.* 23, 2–7. doi: 10.1159/000066303

Nakamura, K. T., Matherne, G. P., McWeeny, O. J., Smith, B. A., and Robillard, J. E. (1987). Renal hemodynamics and functional changes during the transition from fetal to newborn life in sheep. *Pediatr. Res.* 21, 229–234. doi: 10.1203/00006450-198703000-00003

Nauli, S. M., Alenghat, F. J., Luo, Y., Williams, E., Vassilev, P., Li, X., et al. (2003). Polycystins 1 and 2 mediate mechanosensation in the primary cilium of kidney cells. *Nat. Genet.* 33, 129–137. doi: 10.1038/ng1076

Nauli, S. M., Jin, X., AbouAlaiwi, W. A., El-Jouni, W., Su, X., and Zhou, J. (2013). Non-motile primary cilia as fluid shear stress mechanosensors. *Meth. Enzymol.* 525, 1–20. doi: 10.1016/B978-0-12-397944-5.00001-8

Nauli, S. M., Rossetti, S., Kolb, R. J., Alenghat, F. J., Consugar, M. B., Harris, P. C., et al. (2006). Loss of polycystin-1 in human cyst-lining epithelia leads to ciliary dysfunction. *J. Am. Soc. Nephrol.* 17, 1015–1025. doi: 10.1681/ASN.2005080830

Patel, V., Li, L., Cobo-Stark, P., Shao, X., Somlo, S., Lin, F., et al. (2008). Acute kidney injury and aberrant planar cell polarity induce cyst formation in mice lacking renal cilia. *Hum. Mol. Genet.* 17, 1578–1590. doi: 10.1093/hmg/ddn045

Praetorius, H. A., and Spring, K. R. (2001). Bending the MDCK cell primary cilium increases intracellular calcium. *J. Membr. Biol.* 184, 71–79. doi: 10.1007/s00232-001-0075-4

Prodromou, N. V., Thompson, C. L., Osborn, D. P., Cogger, K. F., Ashworth, R., Knight, M. M., et al. (2012). Heat shock induces rapid resorption of primary cilia. *J. Cell Sci.* 125, 4297–4305. doi: 10.1242/jcs.100545

Resnick, A. (2016). HIF stabilization weakens primary cilia. *PLoS ONE* 11:e0165907. doi: 10.1371/journal.pone.0165907

Robillard, J. E., Nakamura, K. T., and DiBona, G. F. (1986). Effects of renal denervation on renal responses to hypoxemia in fetal lambs. *Am. J. Physiol.* 250, F294–F301.

Rosenberger, C., Rosen, S., Shina, A., Bernhardt, W., Wiesener, M. S., Frei, U., et al. (2006). Hypoxia-inducible factors and tubular cell survival in isolated perfused kidneys. *Kidney Int.* 70, 60–70. doi: 10.1038/sj.ki.5000395

Thorpe, R. B., Stockman, S. L., Williams, J. M., Lincoln, T. M., and Pearce, W. J. (2013). Hypoxic depression of PKG-mediated inhibition of serotonergic contraction in ovine carotid arteries. *Am. J. Physiol. Regul. Integr. Comp. Physiol.* 304, R734–R743. doi: 10.1152/ajpregu.00212.2012

Uchida, T., Rossignol, F., Matthay, M. A., Mounier, R., Couette, S., Clottes, E., et al. (2004). Prolonged hypoxia differentially regulates hypoxia-inducible factor (HIF)-1alpha and HIF-2alpha expression in lung epithelial cells: implication of natural antisense HIF-1alpha. *J. Biol. Chem.* 279, 14871–14878. doi: 10.1074/jbc.M400461200

Upadhyay, V. S., Muntean, B. S., Kathem, S. H., Hwang, J. J., Aboualaiwi, W. A., and Nauli, S. M. (2014). Roles of dopamine receptor on chemosensory and mechanosensory primary cilia in renal epithelial cells. *Front. Physiol.* 5:72. doi: 10.3389/fphys.2014.00072

Verghese, E., Ricardo, S. D., Weidenfeld, R., Zhuang, J., Hill, P. A., Langham, R. G., et al. (2009). Renal primary cilia lengthen after acute tubular necrosis. *J. Am. Soc. Nephrol.* 20, 2147–2153. doi: 10.1681/ASN.2008101105

Verghese, E., Weidenfeld, R., Bertram, J. F., Ricardo, S. D., and Deane, J. A. (2008). Renal cilia display length alterations following tubular injury and are present early in epithelial repair. *Nephrol. Dial. Transplant* 23, 834–841. doi: 10.1093/ndt/gfm743

Verghese, E., Zhuang, J., Saiti, D., Ricardo, S. D., and Deane, J. A. (2011). *In vitro* investigation of renal epithelial injury suggests that primary cilium length is regulated by hypoxia-inducible mechanisms. *Cell Biol. Int.* 35, 909–913. doi: 10.1042/CBI20090154

Wang, S., and Dong, Z. (2013). Primary cilia and kidney injury: current research status and future perspectives. *Am. J. Physiol. Renal Physiol.* 305, F1085–F1098. doi: 10.1152/ajprenal.00399.2013

Wang, S., Wei, Q., Dong, G., and Dong, Z. (2013). ERK-mediated suppression of cilia in cisplatin-induced tubular cell apoptosis and acute kidney injury. *Biochim. Biophys. Acta* 1832, 1582–1590. doi: 10.1016/j.bbadis.2013.05.023

Xiao, D., Hu, X. Q., Huang, X., Zhou, J., Wilson, S. M., Yang, S., et al. (2013). Chronic hypoxia during gestation enhances uterine arterial myogenic tone via heightened oxidative stress. *PLoS ONE* 8:e73731. doi: 10.1371/journal.pone.0073731

Xu, C., Rossetti, S., Jiang, L., Harris, P. C., Brown-Glaberman, U., Wandinger-Ness, A., et al. (2007). Human ADPKD primary cyst epithelial cells with a novel, single codon deletion in the PKD1 gene exhibit defective ciliary polycystin localization and loss of flow-induced Ca^{2+} signaling. *Am. J. Physiol. Renal Physiol.* 292, F930–F945. doi: 10.1152/ajprenal.00285.2006

8

Postural Control in Lowlanders with COPD Traveling to 3100 m: Data from a Randomized Trial Evaluating the Effect of Preventive Dexamethasone Treatment

Lara Muralt[1,2], Michael Furian[1,2], Mona Lichtblau[1,2], Sayaka S. Aeschbacher[1,2], Ross A. Clark[3], Bermet Estebesova[2,4], Ulan Sheraliev[2,4], Nuriddin Marazhapov[2,4], Batyr Osmonov[2,4], Maya Bisang[1,2], Stefanie Ulrich[1,2], Tsogyal D. Latshang[1,2], Silvia Ulrich[1,2], Talant M. Sooronbaev[2,4] and Konrad E. Bloch[1,2,4]*

[1] *Department of Respiratory Medicine, University Hospital Zurich, Zurich, Switzerland,* [2] *Kyrgyz-Swiss High Altitude Clinic and Medical Research Center, Tuja-Ashu, Kyrgyzstan,* [3] *School of Health and Sports Science, University of the Sunshine Coast, Sunshine Coast, QLD, Australia,* [4] *Department of Respiratory Medicine, National Center for Cardiology and Internal Medicine, Bishkek, Kyrgyzstan*

***Correspondence:**
Konrad E. Bloch
konrad.bloch@usz.ch

Objective: To evaluate the effects of acute exposure to high altitude and preventive dexamethasone treatment on postural control in patients with chronic obstructive pulmonary disease (COPD).

Methods: In this randomized, double-blind parallel-group trial, 104 lowlanders with COPD GOLD 1-2 age 20–75 years, living near Bishkek (760 m), were randomized to receive either dexamethasone (2 × 4 mg/day p.o.) or placebo on the day before ascent and during a 2-day sojourn at Tuja-Ashu high altitude clinic (3100 m), Kyrgyzstan. Postural control was assessed with a Wii Balance Board^{TM} at 760 m and 1 day after arrival at 3100 m. Patients were instructed to stand immobile on both legs with eyes open during five tests of 30 s each, while the center of pressure path length (PL) was measured.

Results: With ascent from 760 to 3100 m the PL increased in the placebo group from median (quartiles) 29.2 (25.8; 38.2) to 31.5 (27.3; 39.3) cm ($P < 0.05$); in the dexamethasone group the corresponding increase from 28.8 (22.8; 34.5) to 29.9 (25.2; 37.0) cm was not significant ($P = 0.10$). The mean difference (95% CI) between dexamethasone and placebo groups in altitude-induced changes (treatment effect) was −0.3 (−3.2 to 2.5) cm, ($P = 0.41$). Multivariable regression analysis confirmed a significant increase in PL with higher altitude (coefficient 1.6, 95% CI 0.2 to 3.1, $P = 0.031$) but no effect of dexamethasone was shown (coefficient −0.2, 95% CI −0.4 to 3.6, $P = 0.925$), even when controlled for several potential confounders. PL changes were related more to antero-posterior than lateral sway. Twenty-two of 104 patients had an altitude-related increase in the antero-posterior sway velocity of >25%, what has been associated with an increased risk of falls in previous studies.

Conclusion: Lowlanders with COPD travelling from 760 to 3100 m revealed postural instability 24 h after arriving at high altitude, and this was not prevented by dexamethasone.

Trial Registration: clinicaltrials.gov Identifier: NCT02450968.

Keywords: chronic obstructive pulmonary disease, altitude, hypoxia, postural control, dexamethasone, acute mountain sickness

INTRODUCTION

Today many settlements worldwide are located at high altitudes (above 2500 m), with regular working places even above 3000 m. Moreover, mountain tourism and air travel are increasingly popular. Therefore, a large number of people, among them also patients with respiratory conditions, are exposed to hypobaric hypoxia. There are concerns that these patients may suffer from altitude-related adverse health effects including impaired postural control (PC), which may lead to falls or impaired performance during various tasks with consecutive accidents. In healthy individuals we have previously observed an impairment in PC already at altitudes of 1630 and 2590 m (Stadelmann et al., 2015). Other studies in healthy volunteers at a higher altitude (Mount Rosa, 4559 m) and in hypobaric chambers (Holness et al., 1982; Cymerman et al., 2001) have also demonstrated worsening of PC. The underlying mechanisms are poorly understood but it is presumed, that hypoxia affects different sensory functions (visual, somatosensory and vestibular) as well as the central nervous system that controls posture-regulating muscles especially in the lower limbs and trunk within a few minutes of exposure to altitudes of 2438 m (8000 ft) or higher (Wagner et al., 2011; Chiba et al., 2016). During sojourns of more than a few hours at high altitude PC may additionally be disturbed by acute mountain sickness (AMS), which causes headache, ataxia, weakness, dizziness, and decrements of alertness.

Chronic obstructive pulmonary disease (COPD) is associated with chronic inflammation and obstruction of the airways, parenchymal destruction of the lung with impaired gas exchange that promotes hypoxemia and increased pulmonary artery pressure (Vogelmeier et al., 2018). Given the high prevalence of COPD, it is expected that many affected patients are undertaking high altitude or air travel thereby suffering from impaired PC, although this has not been specifically studied. Previous observations suggest that elderly persons and patients with COPD suffer from an impaired PC already at sea level (Muir et al., 2010; Porto et al., 2015). Due to their pulmonary gas exchange impairment COPD patients may have more severe hypoxemia than healthy individuals at corresponding altitude. Thus, we reasoned that COPD patients may experience pronounced PC impairments during altitude or air travel with potentially grave consequences such as dangerous falls, and that measures to prevent or reduce this risk would be desirable.

The purpose of the current study was therefore twofold: (1) to test the hypothesis that lowlanders with COPD would experience impairments in PC during a stay at 3100 m and (2) that these impairments could be prevented by treatment with dexamethasone, a drug with potent glucocorticoid action. We selected dexamethasone for this study because glucocorticoids are used to treat COPD exacerbations and because it is effective in prevention and treatment of AMS in healthy mountaineers.

MATERIALS AND METHODS

Study Design and Setting

The current study was performed from June to August 2015 within the scope of a randomized, placebo controlled double blind parallel design trial evaluating effectiveness of dexamethasone in prevention of altitude-related adverse health effects (ARAHE) in lowlanders with COPD traveling to and staying for 2 days at the high altitude (3100 m) clinic of Tuja-Ashu, Kyrgyztan (clinicaltrials.gov Identifier: NCT02450968). The effects of altitude and of dexamethasone on AMS and various other clinical and physiologic outcomes have been reported recently (Furian et al., 2018).

Participants

Men and women, aged 20–75 years, living in the Bishkek area (Kyrgyz Republic, mean altitude 760 m) diagnosed with COPD according to GOLD guidelines, grades 1–2, $FEV_1/FVC < 0.7$ and $FEV_1 > 50\%$ predicted were invited to participate. Exclusion criteria were severe COPD with $FEV_1 < 50\%$ predicted, hypoxemia < 92% at 760 m measured by pulse oximetry, COPD exacerbation, reversible airflow obstruction, a history suggesting asthma or other respiratory disease, diabetes, uncontrolled cardiovascular disease (such as systemic arterial hypertension, coronary artery disease, previous stroke), history of obstructive sleep apnea, pneumothorax in the last 2 months, untreated or symptomatic peptic ulcer disease, or glaucoma and other conditions that might have interfered with protocol compliance including current heavy smoking (>20 cigarettes per day). Participants gave written informed consent. The study was approved by the Ethics Committee of the National Center of Cardiology and Internal Medicine, Bishkek, Kyrgyzstan(01-8/405) and was endorsed by the Cantonal Ethics Committee Zurich, Switzerland.

Interventions

Participants underwent baseline evaluation in Bishkek (760 m). One to three weeks later, they travelled to the Tuja-Ashu high altitude clinic (3100 m) by minibus within 3–5 h and stayed there for 2 days. On the day before ascent and while staying at 3100 m, participants took 4 mg capsules of oral dexamethasone twice daily or identical looking placebo capsules under the supervision of an investigator. During the study, participants continued their regular medication and no other treatment was allowed. For safety reasons, participants with clinically relevant AMS defined by an AMSc score ≥0.7 (see below), severe hypoxemia (SpO_2 < 75% for > 30 min, or < 70% for > 15 min), or any other condition requiring an intervention according to the decision of an independent physician were treated with supplemental oxygen and other appropriate means.

Assessments

A medical history and clinical examination were obtained. AMS was assessed by the environmental symptoms cerebral score (AMSc) comprising 11 questions on AMS symptoms each rated from 0 (not at all) to 5 (extreme) (Sampson et al., 1983). The weighted sum of responses ranges from 0 to 5. Scores ≥0.7 are considered to reflect clinically relevant AMS. Pulse oximetry during rest (SpO_2, Konica-Minolta PULSOX-300i) and spirometry (EasyOne; NDD, Zurich, Switzerland) were performed.

PC was assessed by a Wii Balance Board (WBB, Redmond, WA, United States), 30 cm × 50 cm in size, as previously described (Clark et al., 2010; Stadelmann et al., 2015). Examinations took place at 760 m and on the second day of the stay at 3100 m, within 20–26 h after arrival. The subjects stood on the WBB on both legs with eyes open and feet positioned in a 30° angle, 20 cm apart. They were instructed to focus on a black dot on the wall, 1.5 m in front of them at eye level, to keep their hands beside the body and stand as still as possible during five tests each lasting 30 s and separated by a resting period of 2–3 min. During the tests, the WBB recorded displacements of the center of gravity of the subject by 4 integrated sensors, using the sampling method and filtering technique described in detail previously (Clark et al., 2017). A customized software (Labview 8.5 National Instruments, Austin, TX, United States) was used to calibrate the WBB with standard weights and to compute the center of gravity path length (COPL), and the mean and SD sway amplitude and velocity in the antero-posterior (AP) and medio-lateral (ML) directions (Clark et al., 2010; Holmes et al., 2013).

Outcomes and Sample Size Estimation

The main outcome was the center of pressure path length (COPL) and additional outcomes were other variables from PC tests and from clinical and physiological examinations including clinically relevant AMS, severe hypoxemia, and other adverse effects that required an intervention as mentioned above. Since the minimal important difference for COPL and other indices of PC has not been established we based the sample size estimation for this study on previous studies in 51 healthy individuals who showed a significant change in indices of PC measured by the Wii balance board at 2590 m (Stadelmann et al., 2015). In addition, a sample size estimation was performed for the primary outcome of the main trial associated with the current study, the cumulative incidence of ARAHE during the stay at 3100 m. According to these calculations, a minimal number of 100 participants including drop-outs were required to detect a 50% reduction in ARAHE by dexamethasone (Furian et al., 2018).

Randomization and Blinding

Participants were randomized 1:1 to dexamethasone or placebo treatment by a computer algorithm minimizing for differences in sex, age ≤ or > 50 years, FEV_1 < or ≥ 80% predicted (Pocock and Simon, 1975).

Study drugs were dispensed by an independent pharmacist in sets of capsules labeled with a concealed code. Participants and investigators were blinded to the assigned treatment until the completion of data analysis.

Data Analysis

The primary data analysis was performed in the per protocol population of participants who had successful evaluations at both altitudes. In addition, an intention to treat analysis of the main outcome, the COPL, was performed including data from all randomized participants with missing data replaced by multiple imputations. A separate analysis restricted to data from patients >40 years of age was also performed excluding occasional younger participants fulfilling spirometric criteria of COPD but may not suffering from the classical form of the disease. To reduce effects of measurement variability, mean results from the five tests at each location are reported. Occasional individual missing data in one of the five tests were replaced by group medians of the corresponding altitude. Since most variables were non-normally distributed, data are summarized by medians and quartiles. Effect sizes were quantified by Cohen's d (i.e., d = the difference between two altitudes divided by the pooled standard); with values of d < 0.2 considered small, 0.5 to 0.8, medium, and > 0.8, strong (Cohen, 1977). The effects of altitude and of the drug were evaluated by computing mean differences and 95% confidence intervals (95% CI). Multivariable regression analysis was performed with the COPL or AP sway velocity as dependent variable and altitude or SpO_2, dexamethasone, body height, age, FEV_1 (% predicted) and presence of AMS as independent variables. A p-value < 0.05 was considered statistically significant.

RESULTS

A total of 118 patients with COPD fulfilled the inclusion criteria and participated in the study (**Figure 1**). In 2 patients in the dexamethasone group, balance tests at 3100 m could not be performed because of AMS; in 12 additional patients, balance tests were not available at both altitudes for various reasons. Datasets from 104 patients who successfully underwent balance tests at both locations could be included into the per protocol analysis (**Figure 1**). **Table 1** shows the demographic data of the study participants. 70 of the 104 participants (67%) suffered from mild airflow obstruction (GOLD grade 1) and 34 (33%) from moderate airflow obstruction (GOLD grade 2); 97 participants (93%) were >40 years old and 6 participants (7%) were <40 years old (31 to 38 years). 27 of the 118 patients (23%), 13 using dexamethasone, 14 using placebo (P = 0.749, Chi-square statistic) suffered from clinically relevant AMS, severe hypoxemia, or other altitude-related adverse health effects.

With ascent from 760 to 3100 m the COPL increased significantly in the placebo group from median (quartiles)

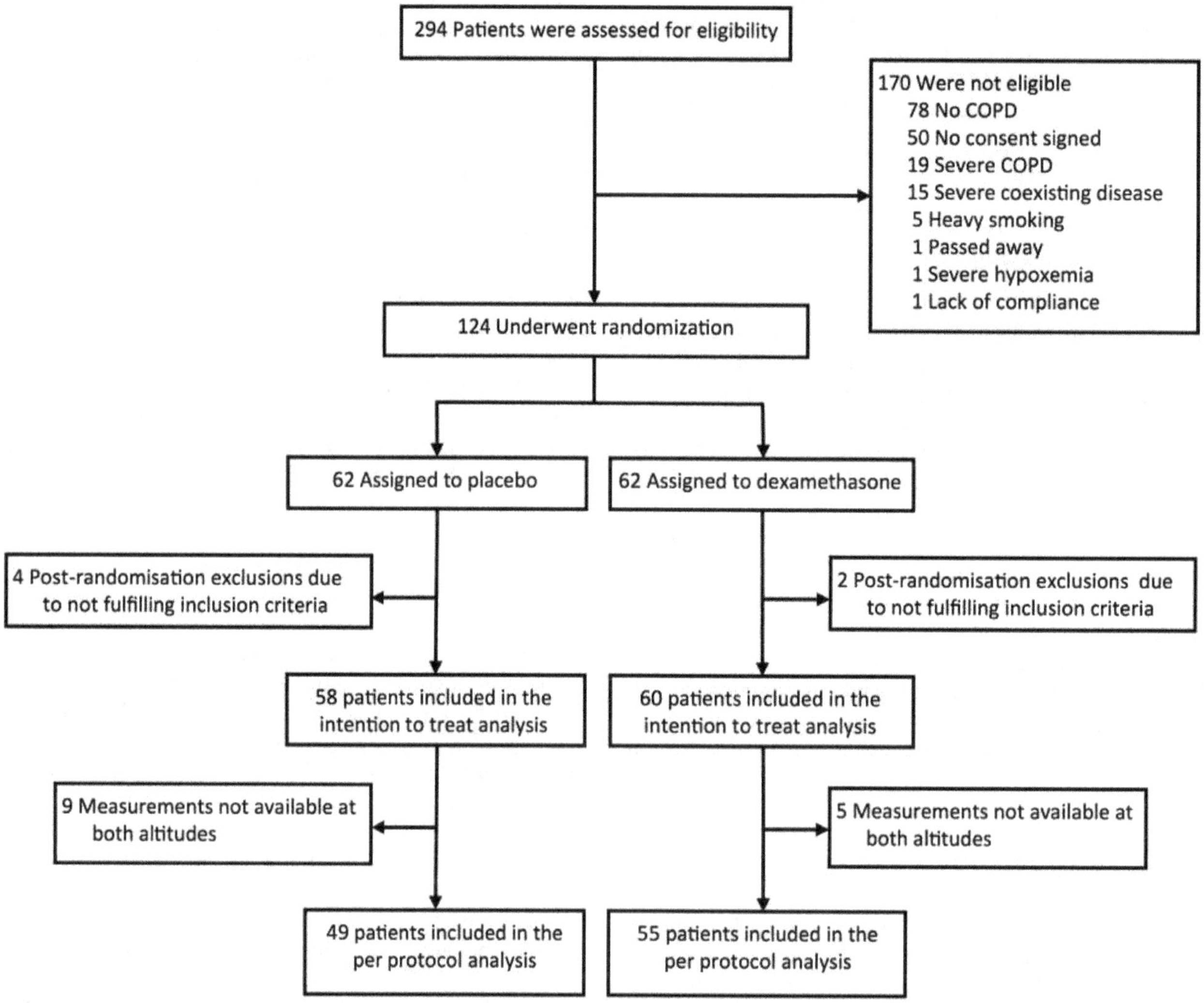

FIGURE 1 | Study flowchart. 124 patients were randomized to dexamethasone respectively placebo. 6 patients were excluded after randomization leaving 118 patients in the intention to treat analysis. In 14 patients, successful balance tests were not available because of altitude-related adverse health effects (2) or incomplete test series (12). 104 patients were included into the per protocol analysis.

29.2 cm (25.8; 38.2) to 31.5 cm (27.3; 39.3) ($P < 0.05$) but in the dexamethasone group the corresponding increase from 28.8 cm (22.8; 34.5) to 29.9 cm (25.2; 37.0) was not significant ($P = 0.10$) (**Table 2**). An example of COPL recordings in a representative individual is shown in **Figure 2**. Mean altitude-induced changes in COPL are shown in **Figure 3**. The mean (95% CI) effect size (Cohen's d) of the altitude-induced COPL change in the placebo group was $d = 0.2$ (0.02 to 0.39) and in the dexamethasone group 0.17 (−0.02 to 0.37).

Whereas the AP sway velocity increased significantly with ascent to 3100 m in both groups, the medio-lateral sway velocity did not change in any group. Dexamethasone had no significant effect on any index of the PC. The mean difference between dexamethasone and placebo groups in altitude-induced changes in COPL (treatment effect) was −0.3 cm (95% CI −3.2 to 2.5) ($P = 0.41$) (**Figures 3, 4**). The intention to treat analysis of the COPL revealed similar results as the per protocol analysis: the mean altitude-induced change in COPL in the placebo group was 2.1 cm (95% CI 0.2 to 3.9, $P = 0.028$) in the dexamethasone group the corresponding change was 1.8 cm (95% CI 0.01 to 3.7, $P = 0.049$) and the treatment effect was −0.2 cm (95% CI −2.8 to 2.4, $P = 0.869$).

Multivariable regression analysis confirmed a significant increase of 1.6 cm (0.2 to 3.1) [mean (95% CI)] in COPL and of 0.048 cm/s (0.009 to 0.087) in AP sway velocity when ascending form 760 m to 3100 m but no decrease with dexamethasone when controlled for several potential confounders (**Tables 3, 4**). The mean (95% CI) effect size of the altitude-induced change adjusted for potential confounders listed in **Table 3** was $d = 0.42$ (0.36 to 0.48) in the placebo group and $d = 0.49$ (0.41 to 0.58) in the dexamethasone group. Taking SpO_2 instead of altitude as the predictor in multivariable regression confirmed that hypoxemia was associated with impaired PC: for each percentage point of reduction in SpO_2 the COPL was elongated by 0.3 cm (95% CI

−0.5 to −0.05, $P = 0.017$) (Supplementary Table S1). A similar negative correlation was found among SpO_2 and AP sway velocity (Supplementary Table S2).

Dexamethasone had no significant effect in the multivariable regression on the COPL, AP- or ML-velocity (**Tables 3, 4** and Supplementary Tables S1, S2). However, age and body height were associated with increased COPL and AP-velocity.

The presence or absence of AMS during the whole stay at altitude had no significant influence on the COPL. However, the movements in AP-direction, which are more influenced by changes of altitude, were significantly increased in those participants suffering from AMS (Supplementary Tables S2, S3).

In a regression analysis including the ten consecutive performed tests (five tests at 760 m and the five at 3100 m) no learning effect was observed (Supplementary Table S4).

TABLE 1 | Demographic data.

	Placebo	Dexamethasone
N	49	55
Sex, male/female	43/6	45/10
Age, years	60 (55; 64)	57 (51; 62)
GOLD grade I/II, *n*	36/13	34/21
FEV_1, liters	2.7 (2.2; 2.9)	2.5 (1.9; 2.9)
FEV_1, % predicted	96 (78; 108)	84 (70; 102)
FVC, liters	4.3 (3.7; 4.9)	4.1 (3.3; 4.5)
FVC, % predicted	121 (107; 137)	115 (98; 125)
FEV_1/FVC	0.65 (0.6; 0.67)	0.63 (0.55; 0.66)
Cigarettes, pack years	25 (2; 38)	20 (0; 34)
BMI, kg/m^2	24.8 (22.4; 26.8)	25.1 (23.1; 28.0)
Weight, kg	72 (65; 78)	71 (63; 80)
Height, m	1.70 (1.66; 1.75)	1.68 (1.63; 1.73)
SpO_2 (760 m), %	95 (94; 96)	95 (94; 96)
SpO_2 (3100 m), %	90 (88; 91)	90 (89; 92)
Medication		
Inhaled bronchodilators, *n* (%)	2 (4%)	1 (2%)
Inhaled corticosteroids, *n* (%)	0 (0%)	0 (0%)
Antihypertensive drugs, *n* (%)	5 (10%)	7 (13%)
Beta-blocker, *n* (%)	3 (6%)	3 (5%)
Aspirin, *n* (%)	5 (10%)	5 (9%)
Antidiabetic drugs, *n* (%)	1 (2%)	0 (0%)

Values are shown in numbers or median (quartiles); FEV_1 = Forced expiratory volume in 1 second; FVC = Forced vital capacity; SpO_2 = arterial oxygen saturation. GOLD = Global Initiative for Chronic Obstructive Lung Disease.

Restricting the regression analysis to the 97 participants > 40 years old revealed similar results as those in **Tables 3, 4** including all 104 participants, i.e., there was a significant effect of altitude on COPL and AP sway velocity but no significant effect of dexamethasone (Supplementary Tables S5, S6).

DISCUSSION

We studied the effects of acute high altitude exposure (3100 m) and of preventive dexamethasone treatment on postural control (PC) in lowlanders with mild to moderate COPD (GOLD grade 1 - 2). Our randomized, placebo controlled, double-blind trial demonstrates that measures of PC, including AP sway velocity and COPL increased at the higher altitude, consistent with impaired PC during acute exposure to hypobaric hypoxia. The results further revealed that the altitude-induced postural instability was not prevented by treatment with dexamethasone.

The current study is the first evaluating PC in lowlanders with COPD ascending rapidly to high altitude. It is generally assumed that the adverse effects of altitude exposure are related to hypoxia in the nervous system and possibly muscles (Chiba et al., 2016). Consistently, multiple regression analyses taking several independent variables into account (dexamethasone, age, sex, FEV_1 in % predicted, body height) confirmed an independent negative effect of SpO_2 on COPL. Previous studies on PC in various simulated and real altitudes have included small numbers of mainly young, healthy volunteers and were conducted in various settings, with different protocols and devices. In the largest study, a randomized cross-over trial, performed in 51 healthy young men staying for 2 days each at 1630 and 2590 m in the Alps, an altitude-related increase in COPL mainly due to AP sway was observed (Stadelmann et al., 2015). Consistently, in the current study, as well as in other previous studies, postural stability was mainly impaired in the AP direction, while ML sway was unchanged at altitude. Other studies using different protocols and tests evaluated effects of much shorter exposures to normobaric hypoxia (minutes to a few hours) at altitude ranging from 2438 m to 5906 m and generally confirmed impairment of PC.

In one study, sensomotoric, visual, and vestibular components of hypoxia-induced impairment of PC were evaluated in combination and separately by varying experimental conditions such as visual inputs (eyes open/closed, sway-referenced visual

TABLE 2 | Center of pressure path length at 760 m and 3100 m with placebo and dexamethasone treatment.

	Placebo		Dexamethasone	
	760 m	3100 m	760 m	3100 m
Center of pressure path length, cm	29.2 (25.8; 38.2)	31.5* (27.3; 39.3)	28.8 (22.8; 34.5)	29.9 (25.2; 37.0)
Maximal AP amplitude, cm	2.362 (1.881; 2.806)	2.306 (2.083; 2.679)	2.535 (1.975; 3.113)	2.402 (1.848; 2.914)
AP velocity, cm/s	0.746 (0.645; 0.884)	0.797* (0.689; 1.030)	0.710 (0.570; 0.907)	0.760* (0.587; 1.011)
ML velocity, cm/s	0.500 (0.400; 0.665)	0.518 (0.469; 0.702)	0.509 (0.387; 0.598)	0.491 (0.413; 0.641)

*Values are shown in median (quartiles); AP, antero-posterior; ML, medio-lateral; *$p < 0.05$ vs. baseline 760 m, paired Wilcoxon rank sum test.*

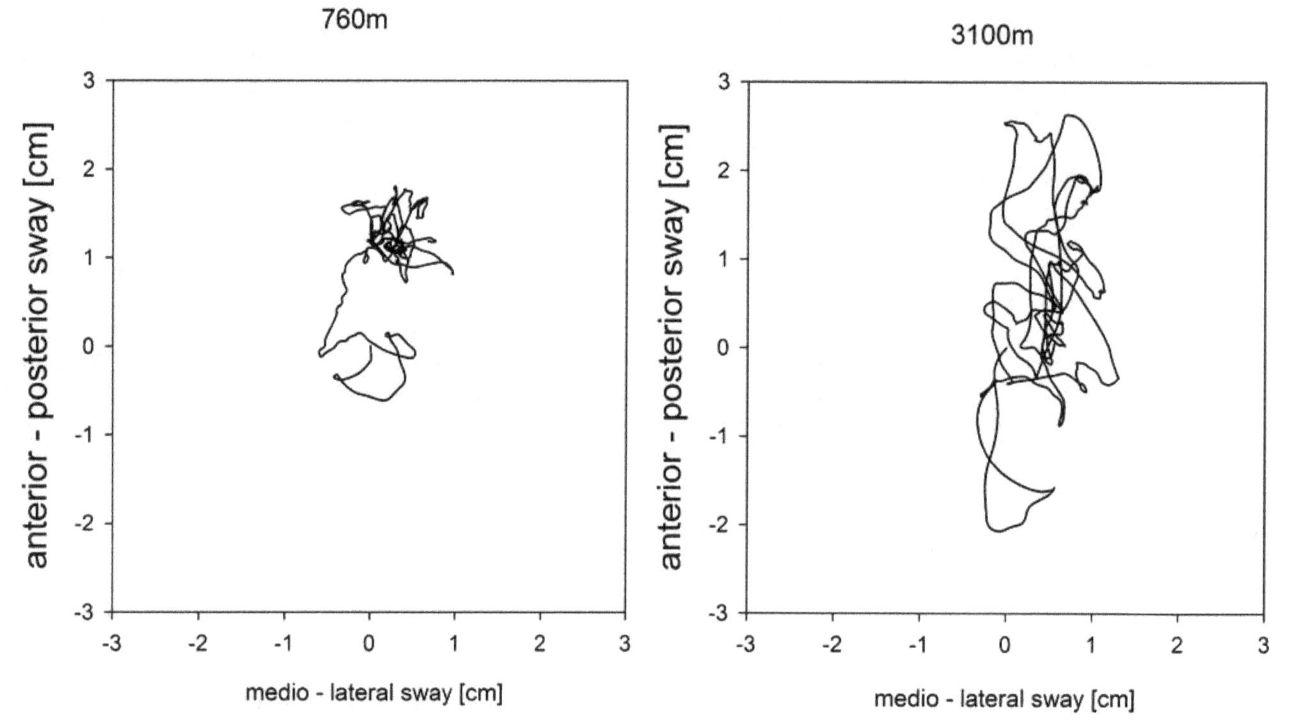

FIGURE 2 | Example of a center of pressure path in an individual COPD patient at 760 m **(left)** and at 3100 m **(right)**. Measurement at 760 m and 3100 m: center of pressure path length (COPL), 21.6 and 39.8 cm; antero-posterior sway velocity, 0.476 and 0.995 cm/s; medio-lateral sway velocity, 0.437 and 0.67 cm/s.

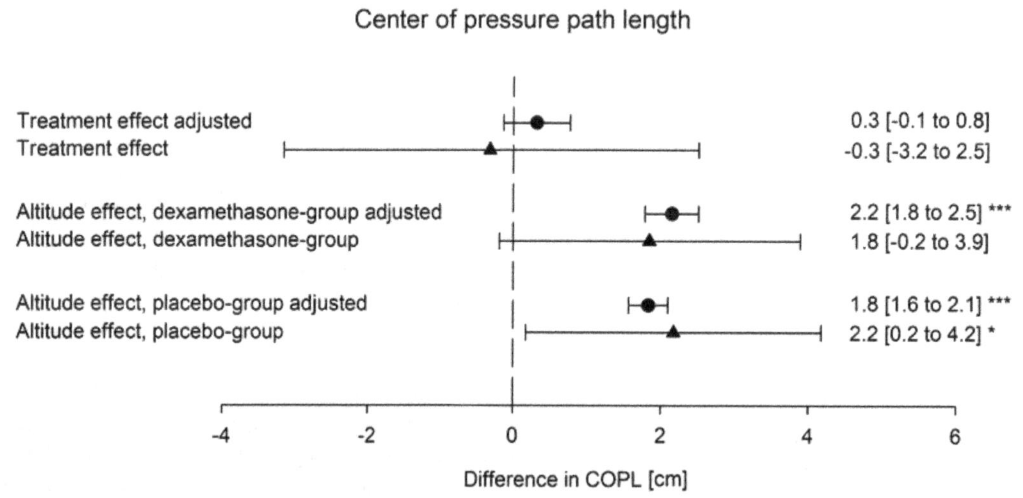

FIGURE 3 | Effect of altitude and of dexamethasone on the center of pressure path length. Altitude effect; difference between the center of pressure path length at 760 m and 3100 m; dexamethasone effect, difference of the altitude effect in the dexamethasone group minus the altitude effect in the placebo group. Mean values and 95% confidence intervals of altitude-induced changes and of differences between dexamethasone and placebo are shown. **p*-values < 0.05, ***p* < 0.01, ****p* < 0.001. Triangles represent raw values, circles represent values adjusted by multiple regression for age, height, weight, forced expiratory volume in 1 second and acute mountain sickness score.

field), resting and moving platform. The results of these investigations confirmed that static PC (eyes open) and reaction time to unexpected movements of the platform were impaired even during very short exposures of less than 1 h to altitudes equivalent to 2438 m and 3048 m (Wagner et al., 2011).

While most previous studies were performed in young volunteers between 21 and 56 years of age, Drum et al. (2016) evaluated the combined mild normobaric hypoxia (altitude equivalent 2600 m) and exercise (a 40 min treadmill walk) in a group of 37 healthy seniors (mean ± SD age 62 ± 4 years).

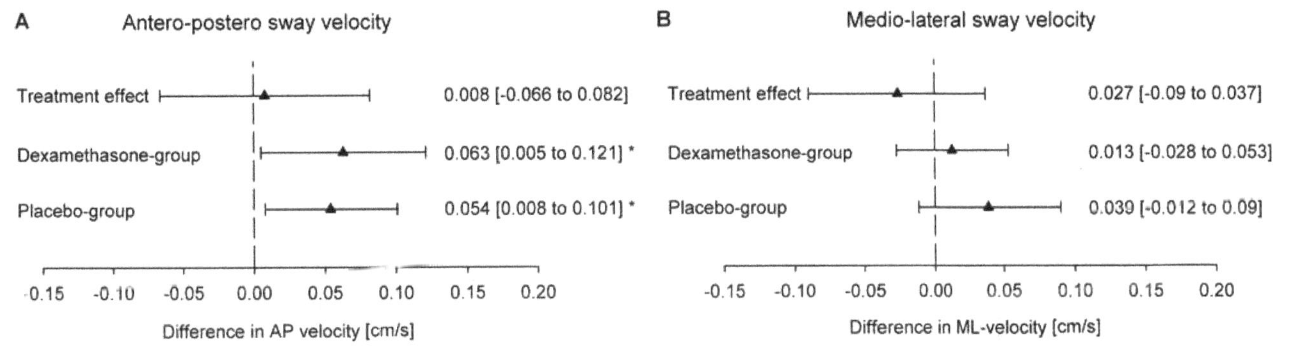

FIGURE 4 | Effect of the altitude and of dexamethasone on sway velocity in the **(A)** antero-posterior (AP) direction and **(B)** medio-lateral (ML) direction. Altitude effect, difference between the center of pressure path length at 760 m and 3100 m; dexamethasone effect, difference of the altitude effect in the dexamethasone group minus the altitude effect in the placebo group. Values are shown as mean (95% CI); $^*p < 0.05$.

TABLE 3 | Effect of high altitude exposure on the center of pressure path length: multivariable regression.

Dependent variable: Center of pressure path length, cm			
R^2 entire model = 0.180 $P < 0.001$	**Coefficient**	**95% CI**	***P*-Value**
Altitude (1 = 760 m; 2 = 3100 m)	1.6	0.2 to 3.1	0.031
Drug (1 = Plc; 2 = Dex)	−0.2	−4.0 to 3.6	0.925
Age, years	0.4	0.2 to 0.6	0.001
Sex (1 = men; 2 = women)	1.1	−6.1 to 8.4	0.760
Height, cm	0.5	0.2 to 0.8	0.003
FEV_1, % pred.	−0.1	−0.2 to 0.0	0.082
AMS (1 = No; 2 = Yes)	3.4	−1.3 to 8.8	0.144
Intercept	−61.7	−123.3 to −0.0	0.050

Plc, Placebo; Dex, Dexamethasone; FEV_1, % pred., Forced expiratory volume in 1 second in % of the predicted FEV_1; AMS, development of acute mountain sickness during altitude exposure assessed by the environmental symptoms score $\geq$0.7.

TABLE 4 | Effect of high altitude exposure on the antero-posterior sway velocity: multivariable regression.

Dependent variable: AP sway velocity, cm/s			
R^2 entire model = 0.180 $P < 0.001$	**Coefficient**	**[95% CI]**	***P*-Value**
Altitude (1 = 760 m; 2 = 3100 m)	0.048	0.009 to 0.087	0.016
Drug (1 = Plc; 2 = Dex)	0.006	−0.104 to 0.116	0.915
Age, years	0.011	0.004 to 0.018	0.001
Sex (1 = men; 2 = women)	−0.037	−0.231 to 0.157	0.708
Height, cm	0.012	0.003 to 0.020	0.009
FEV_1, % pred	−0.003	−0.007 to 0.000	0.078
AMS (1 = No; 2 = Yes)	0.099	−0.014 to 0.212	0.085
Intercept	−1.577	−3.385 to 0.230	0.087

Plc, Placebo; Dex, Dexamethasone; FEV_1, % pred., Forced expiratory volume in 1 second in % of the predicted FEV_1; AMS, development of acute mountain sickness during altitude exposure assessed by the environmental symptoms score $\geq$0.7.

Balance tests did not reveal an effect of simulated altitude at rest but COPL were larger immediately after exercise at near sea level conditions and even more so after exercise at simulated altitude, suggesting a combined effect of muscular fatigue and hypoxia on PC in these elderly individuals. The current study confirms and extends these observations in a different setting in COPD patients by demonstrating an independent negative effect of altitude and older age on PC even at rest without prior exercise (**Tables 3, 4**). Since COPD results from long-term cumulative noxious exposures it is most commonly observed in older individuals (>40 years). In the current study 7/104 (6%) participants were between 31 and 38 years old, an age that is not typically compatible with the classical form of COPD. We speculate that these individuals might have suffered from infections and exposure to smoke and indoor air pollution since early childhood. Such "disadvantage factors" may have promoted irreversible airflow obstruction at a relatively young age (Vogelmeier et al., 2018). Excluding data from participants <40 years of age from analysis confirmed a robust effect of altitude on PC in the 97 older COPD patients (>40 years old).

Since regression analysis of data in the current study indicates that altitude as well as age and body height adversely affects PC, it is important to take this into account when assessing PC. Moreover, the study by Drum et al. (2016) suggests that prior exercise may also affect PC, which may be particularly relevant for older individuals desiring to hike in the mountains.

Postural imbalance and ataxia are established diagnostic criteria for severe AMS and high altitude cerebral edema (HACE) (West, 1996; Hackett and Roach, 2004). The AMS questionnaire includes items like "dizziness/lightheadedness" or "my coordination is off" and the heel-to-toe walking as elements related to postural balance (Sampson et al., 1983; Sutton et al., 1992). However, studies on the relation among postural instability at altitude and AMS are controversial. Most studies could not show a relation between AMS and PC (Baumgartner et al., 2002; Cymerman et al., 2001). In the current investigation, multiple regression analysis did not reveal consistent results. Whereas AMS was not a significant predictor of the COPL, it was significantly correlated with the AP-velocity and AP-amplitude. We cannot exclude that the lack of a significant association between COPL and AMS was related to the low prevalence of AMS in our study. Further investigations are required to better define interactions among AMS and PC measured objectively by a Wii balance board and other techniques in order to determine clinically relevant changes in objective indices of PC at high altitude and their relation to altitude-related illnesses including AMS.

To date, data on prevention or treatment of impairment in PC at altitude are scant. Baumgartner and coworkers administered supplemental oxygen to volunteers at 4559 m but failed to detect a beneficial effect on PC although symptoms of AMS were reduced by the intervention (Baumgartner and Bartsch, 2002). These authors therefore suggested that postural ataxia at altitude resulted from different hypoxia-dependent mechanisms than AMS. In the current study we used dexamethasone to evaluate whether it might prevent impairments in PC, AMS, and other altitude-related adverse health effects such as insomnia and cognitive deficiencies in COPD patients. The reason for the lack of a protective effect of dexamethasone on PC remains unexplained. For safety reasons, the study protocol required that all participants suffering from clinically relevant AMS, severe hypoxemia or other adverse health effects were treated with supplemental oxygen and other appropriate means. These predefined precautions may have introduced a "survivor effect" preventing the observation of more severe PC impairments in the most susceptible persons and, thus, obscuring a significant effect of dexamethasone in the per protocol analysis. However, the intention to treat analysis with replacement of missing data by multiple imputation revealed similar altitude-induced changes in COPL and confirmed absence of a significant effect of dexamethasone thereby not supporting a relevant "survivor effect".

We cannot exclude that the applied dose of 2 mg × 4 mg dexamethasone/day was insufficient to prevent altitude-induced effects on PC. We selected this dose because it is recommended for AMS prevention in current guidelines and was effective in previous studies (Luks et al., 2014; Zheng et al., 2014). We did not want to use a higher dose of dexamethasone because of potential side effects including hypoglycemia. It is also possible that the only mild impairment of PC we found in the COPD patients reduced the sensitivity of our trial to detect a significant reduction in the altitude-induced impairment. The current results and those from previous studies (Stadelmann et al., 2015) suggest that the Wii balance board is a convenient technique to detect small to moderate altitude-related effect sizes of PC changes under field conditions. However, the accuracy of this simple and inexpensive tool was inferior compared to a laboratory-grade force platform in previous studies (Leach et al., 2014). Therefore, limitations in our measurement technique may have concealed minor effects of dexamethasone on PC even though we tried to minimize instrument-related inaccuracies by repeated calibrations, and by using the same board for all measurements in each individual. Moreover, we computed mean values from five tests in each individual in order to reduce variability in the outcomes.

A limitation of our study is the lack of a healthy, age-matched control group of Kyrgyz individuals, which would have allowed to better assess the independent effect of COPD on PC. The clinical relevance of the severity of PC impairment observed in the current study is uncertain as we were unable to correlate these findings directly to a clinical outcome. Kwok and coworkers have shown that elderly individuals, 60–85 years of age, with a greater (i.e., at the 75th percentile) baseline AP sway velocity measured by a Wii balance board had an approximately twofold greater risk of falls in the following year compared to controls with less (i.e., at the 25th percentile) postural sway at baseline. For comparison, 22 of the COPD patients in this current study had an altitude-related increase in the AP sway velocity of >25% – a change that was associated with a twofold risk of falls in the cited study (Kwok et al., 2015). Comparison of the current to the cited study is hampered by differences in protocol and setting. Nevertheless, it is conceivable that any measurable impairment of PC might increase the risk of falls with potentially grave consequences for mountain travelers.

CONCLUSION

This is the first study investigating PC in non-acclimatized patients with mild to moderate COPD travelling from their altitude of residence of around 760 m to a high altitude of 3100 m. The main findings were an impairment of PC at altitude as demonstrated by an increase in COPL and AP sway velocity. Dexamethasone in a dose of 2 mg × 4 mg per day did not prevent this impairment.

AUTHOR CONTRIBUTIONS

LM contributed to study design, data collection, analysis, and drafting the manuscript. MF, ML, SA, BE, US, NM, BO, MB, StU, TL, SiU, and TS contributed to study design, data collection, and critically revising the manuscript. RC contributed to analysis of data. KB contributed to study design, data analysis, and revision of the manuscript.

FUNDING

The study was supported by the Swiss National Science Foundation, the Lunge Zurich, and the Schweizerische Unfallversicherungsanstalt SUVA, Switzerland.

REFERENCES

Baumgartner, R. W., and Bartsch, P. (2002). Ataxia in acute mountain sickness does not improve with short-term oxygen inhalation. *High Alt. Med. Biol.* 3, 283–287. doi: 10.1089/152702902320604269

Baumgartner, R. W., Eichenberger, U., and Bartsch, P. (2002). Postural ataxia at high altitude is not related to mild to moderate acute mountain sickness. *Eur. J. Appl. Physiol.* 86, 322–326. doi: 10.1007/s00421-001-0534-8

Chiba, R., Takakusaki, K., Ota, J., Yozu, A., and Haga, N. (2016). Human upright posture control models based on multisensory inputs; in fast and slow dynamics. *Neurosci. Res.* 104, 96–104. doi: 10.1016/j.neures.2015.12.002

Clark, R. A., Bryant, A. L., Pua, Y., McCrory, P., Bennell, K., and Hunt, M. (2010). Validity and reliability of the Nintendo Wii Balance Board for assessment of standing balance. *Gait Posture* 31, 307–310. doi: 10.1016/j.gaitpost.2009.11.012

Clark, R. A., Seah, F. J., Chong, H. C., Poon, C. L., Tan, J. W., Mentiplay, B. F., et al. (2017). Standing balance post total knee arthroplasty: sensitivity to change analysis from four to twelve weeks in 466 patients. *Osteoarthritis Cartilage* 25, 42–45. doi: 10.1016/j.joca.2016.08.009

Cohen, J. (1977). *Statistical Power Analysis for the Behavioral Sciences*. New York, NY: Academic Press, 474.

Cymerman, A., Muza, S. R., Beidleman, B. A., Ditzler, D. T., and Fulco, C. S. (2001). Postural instability and acute mountain sickness during exposure to 24 hours of simulated altitude (4300 m). *High Alt. Med. Biol.* 2, 509–514. doi: 10.1089/152702901753397072

Drum, S. N., Faude, O., de Fay du Lavallaz, E., Allemann, R., Nève, G., and Donath, L. (2016). Acute effects of walking at moderate normobaric hypoxia on gait and balance performance in healthy community-dwelling seniors: a randomized controlled crossover study. *Arch. Gerontol. Geriatr.* 67, 74–79. doi: 10.1016/j.archger.2016.06.022

Furian, M., Lichtblau, M., Aeschbacher, S. S., Estebesova, B., Emilov, B., Sheraliev, U., et al. (2018). Efficacy of dexamethasone in preventing acute mountain sickness in COPD patients. Randomized Trial. *Chest* (in press).

Hackett, P. H., and Roach, R. C. (2004). High altitude cerebral edema. *High Alt. Med. Biol.* 5, 136–146. doi: 10.1089/1527029041352054

Holmes, J. D., Jenkins, M. E., Johnson, A. M., Hunt, M. A., and Clark, R. A. (2013). Validity of the Nintendo Wii(R) balance board for the assessment of standing balance in Parkinson's disease. *Clin. Rehabil.* 27, 361–366. doi: 10.1177/0269215512458684

Holness, D. E., Fraser, W. D., Eastman, D. E., Porlier, J. A., and Paul, M. A. (1982). Postural stability during slow-onset and rapid-onset hypoxia. *Aviat. Space Environ. Med.* 53, 647–651.

Kwok, B. C., Clark, R. A., and Pua, Y. H. (2015). Novel use of the Wii Balance Board to prospectively predict falls in community-dwelling older adults. *Clin. Biomech.* 30, 481–484. doi: 10.1016/j.clinbiomech.2015.03.006

Leach, J. M., Mancini, M., Peterka, R. J., Hayes, T. L., and Horak, F. B. (2014). Validating and calibrating the Nintendo Wii balance board to derive reliable center of pressure measures. *Sensors* 14, 18244–18267. doi: 10.3390/s141018244

Luks, A. M., McIntosh, S. E., Grissom, C. K., Auerbach, P. S., Rodway, G. W., Schoene, R. B., et al. (2014). Wilderness Medical Society practice guidelines for the prevention and treatment of acute altitude illness: 2014 update. *Wilderness Environ. Med.* 25(Suppl. 4), S4–S14. doi: 10.1016/j.wem.2014.06.017

Muir, S. W., Berg, K., Chesworth, B., Klar, N., and Speechley, M. (2010). Quantifying the magnitude of risk for balance impairment on falls in community-dwelling older adults: a systematic review and meta-analysis. *J. Clin. Epidemiol.* 63, 389–406. doi: 10.1016/j.jclinepi.2009.06.010

Pocock, S. J., and Simon, R. (1975). Sequential treatment assignment with balancing for prognostic factors in the controlled clinical trial. *Biometrics* 31, 103–115. doi: 10.2307/2529712

Porto, E. F., Castro, A. A., Schmidt, V. G., Rabelo, H. M., Kümpel, C., Nascimento, O. A., et al. (2015). Postural control in chronic obstructive pulmonary disease: a systematic review. *Int. J. Chron. Obstruct. Pulmon. Dis.* 10, 1233–1239. doi: 10.2147/COPD.S63955

Sampson, J. B., Cymerman, A., Burse, R. L., Maher, J. T., and Rock, P. B. (1983). Procedures for the measurement of acute mountain sickness. *Aviat. Space Environ. Med.* 54(12 Pt 1), 1063–1073.

Stadelmann, K., Latshang, T. D., Lo Cascio, C. M., Clark, R. A., Huber, R., Kohler, M., et al. (2015). Impaired postural control in healthy men at moderate altitude (1630 m and 2590 m): data from a randomized trial. *PLoS One* 10:e0116695. doi: 10.1371/journal.pone.0116695

Sutton, J. R., Coates, G., and Houston, C. S. (eds). (1992). *The Lake Louise Consensus on the Definition and Quantification of Altitude Illness, Hypoxia and Mountain Medicine*. Burlington, VT: Queen City Printers.

Vogelmeier, C. F., et al. (2018). *Global Strategy for the Diagnosis, Management and Prevention of Chronic Obstructive Pulmonary Disease 2018 Report*. Available at: www.goldcopd.org [accessed May 17, 2018].

Wagner, L. S., Oakley, S. R., Vang, P., Noble, B. N., Cevette, M. J., and Stepanek, J. P. (2011). Hypoxia-induced changes in standing balance. *Aviat. Space Environ. Med.* 82, 518–522. doi: 10.3357/ASEM.2885.2011

West, J. B. (1996). T.H. Ravenhill and his contributions to mountain sickness. *J. Appl. Physiol.* 80, 715–724. doi: 10.1152/jappl.1996.80.3.715

Zheng, C. R., Chen, G. Z., Yu, J., Qin, J., Song, P., Bian, S. Z., et al. (2014). Inhaled budesonide and oral dexamethasone prevent acute mountain sickness. *Am. J. Med.* 127, 1001.e2–1009.e2. doi: 10.1016/j.amjmed.2014.04.012

9

Physiological and Biological Responses to Short-Term Intermittent Hypobaric Hypoxia Exposure: From Sports and Mountain Medicine to New Biomedical Applications

Ginés Viscor[1], Joan R. Torrella[1], Luisa Corral[2], Antoni Ricart[2], Casimiro Javierre[2], Teresa Pages[1] and Josep L. Ventura[2]*

[1] Physiology Section, Department of Cell Biology, Physiology and Immunology, Faculty of Biology, Universitat de Barcelona, Barcelona, Spain, [2] Exercise Physiology Unit, Department of Physiological Sciences, Faculty of Medicine and Health Sciences, Universitat de Barcelona, L'Hospitalet de Llobregat, Barcelona, Spain

***Correspondence:**
Ginés Viscor
gviscor@ub.edu

In recent years, the altitude acclimatization responses elicited by short-term intermittent exposure to hypoxia have been subject to renewed attention. The main goal of short-term intermittent hypobaric hypoxia exposure programs was originally to improve the aerobic capacity of athletes or to accelerate the altitude acclimatization response in alpinists, since such programs induce an increase in erythrocyte mass. Several model programs of intermittent exposure to hypoxia have presented efficiency with respect to this goal, without any of the inconveniences or negative consequences associated with permanent stays at moderate or high altitudes. Artificial intermittent exposure to normobaric hypoxia systems have seen a rapid rise in popularity among recreational and professional athletes, not only due to their unbeatable cost/efficiency ratio, but also because they help prevent common inconveniences associated with high-altitude stays such as social isolation, nutritional limitations, and other minor health and comfort-related annoyances. Today, intermittent exposure to hypobaric hypoxia is known to elicit other physiological response types in several organs and body systems. These responses range from alterations in the ventilatory pattern to modulation of the mitochondrial function. The central role played by hypoxia-inducible factor (HIF) in activating a signaling molecular cascade after hypoxia exposure is well known. Among these targets, several growth factors that upregulate the capillary bed by inducing angiogenesis and promoting oxidative metabolism merit special attention. Applying intermittent hypobaric hypoxia to promote the action of some molecules, such as angiogenic factors, could improve repair and recovery in many tissue types. This article uses a comprehensive approach to examine data obtained in recent years. We consider evidence collected from different tissues, including myocardial capillarization, skeletal muscle fiber types and fiber size changes induced by intermittent hypoxia exposure, and discuss the evidence that points to beneficial interventions in applied fields such as sport science. Short-term intermittent hypoxia may not only be useful for healthy people, but could also be considered a promising tool to be applied, with due caution, to some pathophysiological states.

Keywords: **intermittent hypoxia, erythropoiesis, angiogenesis, cardioprotection, bronchial asthma, neuroprotection, circulating stem cells, regenerative medicine**

INTERMITTENT HYPOXIA: CONCEPT AND HISTORICAL BACKGROUND

The term "intermittent hypoxia" is widely used and applies to a wide spectrum of situations that range from alpine expeditions to obstructive sleep apnea (OSA). However, in physiological terms, there are often few similarities between these conditions (Viscor et al., 2014). Although the same physiological responses are elicited by the same sensors and signaling pathways, the varied intensity and duration of the hypoxia switches different mechanisms on and off at different times, thus making the final physiological changes induced in the whole organism highly variable. In addition, a high variability in human tolerance to hypoxia has been reported, and it is now known to vary throughout the lives of individuals (Canouï-Poitrine et al., 2014; Richalet and Lhuissier, 2015). As a consequence, specialists have engaged in an interesting discussion about how to measure and define hypoxic "dosage" (Serebrovskaya et al., 2008; Garvican-Lewis et al., 2016). In general, three different types of intermittent hypoxia can be considered:

a) Episodic intermittent hypoxia, which consists of successive short episodes of hypoxia with variable intensity. This may be present in permanent situations such as OSA, in transitory situations such as surgical ischemia-reperfusion (to one or several organs) and in some sporting activities such as parachuting and extreme skiing, in which the subject may not even notice the hypoxia.
b) Intervallic intermittent hypoxia, which is characterized by long periods of normoxia interspersed with periods of hypoxia, as seen in frequent alpine expeditions and trekking at altitude, mountain rescue teams, regular intercontinental commercial flight crews (when in flight, commercial airplane cabins are usually regulated at pressures equivalent to a moderate altitude of about 2,000 m above sea level), and even astronauts at the International Space Station or future extraplanetary missions.
c) Chronic intermittent hypoxia, which affects individuals who work under shift systems characterized by work at moderate or high altitudes alternating with periods of rest at sea level. This last model is common in the Andes region and in the Central Asian mining industry, but is also found in contractors for astronomical observatories, the military and customs, and police and border control personnel in many high-elevation countries.

The concept of "hypoxic training" was coined during the 1930s in the academic environment of the former Soviet Union, and was considered a useful therapeutic tool after it was shown to have beneficial effects on a number of different pathologies, even though the mechanisms involved in these favorable effects were unclear (Agadzhanyan and Torshin, 1986; Serebrovskaya, 2002). For instance, it was reported to have a beneficial effect on hypertension and cardiovascular diseases (Aleshin et al., 1993). Later, new experimental studies corroborated some of these findings and provided a fresh insight through enhanced plasma lipid profiles (Tin'kov and Aksenov, 2002). Nowadays in former Soviet States, hypoxic training is systematically applied as a non-pharmacological strategy for treating a wide range of alterations, including chronic lung disease, bronchial asthma, hypertension, diabetes mellitus, Parkinson's disease, emotional disorders and radiation toxicity, and for the prophylactic treatment of some occupational diseases (Ge et al., 1994; Xi and Serebrovskaya, 2012). In Western countries, intermittent hypoxia exposure programs were first applied in the field of sports medicine to improve aerobic capacity and for pre-acclimatization to altitude (Richalet et al., 1992; Levine and Stray-Gundersen, 1997; Rodríguez et al., 1999; Stray-Gundersen and Levine, 1999; Casas M. et al., 2000; Ricart et al., 2000).

Our group took an in-depth look at the physiological responses to intermittent exposure to hypobaric hypoxia (IEHH) in hypobaric (low barometric pressure) chambers. A detailed study of the precise mechanisms that underlie these adaptive responses (erythropoiesis, angiogenesis and the release of circulating stem cells) in humans and in an experimental rodent model encouraged us to explore the possibilities of applying IEHH programs with biomedical and therapeutic purposes (Panisello et al., 2007, 2008; Esteva et al., 2009; Viscor et al., 2009; Corral et al., 2014b). Thus, we recently demonstrated the efficacy of applying IEHH programs (passive exposure only or combined with exercise protocols) in the recovery of a range of injuries (Corral et al., 2014a; Núñez-Espinosa et al., 2014; Rizo-Roca et al., 2017a,b). These results are consistent with the new paradigm that proposes biphasic effects in the response to hypoxia (hormesis); that is, its harmful or beneficial effects depend on the frequency and severity of the hypoxic challenge to the organism or tissue in question (Navarrete-Opazo and Mitchell, 2014).

BIOLOGICAL EFFECTS OF INTERMITTENT HYPOXIA EXPOSURE

The molecular mechanisms involved in the response to hypoxia at the cellular level are relatively well understood (Fábián et al., 2016; Bhattarai et al., 2017; Koyasu et al., 2017). However, the complexity of the interactions between the divergent signaling pathways and the time frame of the various processes on different tissues and organs, together with the significant individual variability in humans' susceptibility to hypoxia (Rathat et al., 1992), pose formidable challenges to researching the potential benefits of regular programs involving exposure to real or simulated altitudes. This paper presents a series of examples of how intermittent exposure to hypoxia can benefit certain patients, although it is not intended to be an exhaustive list. Obviously, these programs must always be applied with due caution and under rigorous clinical controls, as with any pharmacological treatment.

Erythropoiesis

Table 1 lists several representative studies of the favorable effects of intermittent hypoxia exposure by increasing erythropoiesis. A detailed report on the rate of erythropoietin (EPO) formation and plasma lifetime in humans in response to acute hypobaric hypoxia exposure in a hypobaric chamber was first provided by the group led by Christian Bauer in Zurich (Eckardt et al., 1989). Later, the pivotal role of hypoxia-inducible factor 1 (HIF-1) in the transcriptional response of EPO to hypoxia was also described (Wang and Semenza, 1993). These seminal works and many subsequent studies sparked an interest in applying IEHH programs to increase erythrocyte mass as a way of improving the aerobic capacity of athletes. Recombinant human erythropoietin (rHuEPO) opened up a new chapter in the correction of uremic anemia due to chronic renal failure (Egrie et al., 1986; London et al., 1989; Najean et al., 1989), but also led to unethical use in sports medicine. The celebration of the 1968 Summer Olympics held in Mexico City (2,250 m above sea level) aroused interest in studying the effects of altitude on human performance. The reduced performance in sporting events with a high aerobic component was evident, while participants in competitions with a clear anaerobic character saw no decline in their performance, and some even beat their records (Di Prampero et al., 1970). As a consequence, stays at high altitude and other artificial hypoxia exposure strategies in athletes were subject to intense study; a wide range of strategies, from permanent stays at moderate or high geographic altitudes (Antezana et al., 1994; Richalet et al., 1994) to different patterns of intermittent exposure (Levine and Stray-Gundersen, 1997; Chapman et al., 1998; Rodríguez et al., 1999; Casas M. et al., 2000; Karlsen et al., 2001; Stray-Gundersen et al., 2001; Ge et al., 2002; Lundby et al., 2007; Richalet and Gore, 2008) were examined. Noticeable differences in protocols and hypoxia exposure methods led to intense debate on the usefulness of intermittent hypoxia exposure for elite athletes, given that hypoxic dose and interindividual variability represent two of the main constraints (Chapman et al., 1998; Casas H. et al., 2000; Julian et al., 2004; Gore et al., 2006; Wilber et al., 2007; Truijens et al., 2008; Rodríguez et al., 2015). In parallel, there was rising interest in understanding the non-erythropoietic effects of EPO. The discovery of multi-tissue erythropoietin receptor expression provided an insight into erythropoietin (EPO) activity that went beyond its role in the regulation of red blood cell production, including a key role in cardioprotection, brain development and neuroprotection, through a coordinated response against tissue oxygen shortage (Noguchi et al., 2007; Arcasoy, 2008; Burger et al., 2009; Chateauvieux et al., 2011; Jia et al., 2012; Zhang Y. et al., 2014b), thus contributing to ischemic preconditioning, an interesting and important property of organ survival that could also prove very useful for new biomedical applications.

Angiogenesis and Muscle Capillarization

In **Table 2**, some examples of the effects of intermittent hypoxia exposure on angiogenesis, vascular remodeling, muscle capillarization and hypertension are presented. In addition to its erythropoietic role, HIF-1 is the main mediator of angiogenesis in response to hypoxic conditions (Rey and Semenza, 2010) and has been considered a potential therapeutic target in many diseases. Two different strategies have been applied: HIF-1 upregulation for ischemic diseases (Li et al., 2014) and HIF-1 inhibition for cancer and endometriosis (Zhou et al., 2012; Bhattarai et al., 2017). Multiple angiogenic factors have been tested in the past; however, therapies that use only one proangiogenic agent to elicit angiogenesis were shown to be insufficient (Hirota and Semenza, 2006). Therefore, the addition of non-pharmacological treatments based on hypoxia-induced angiogenesis may be a successful strategy (Zimna and Kurpisz, 2015).

The physiological response elicited by hypoxia at moderate altitude exposure (1,800–3,000 m) is low, but increases when combined with exercise, with additional specific responses that are not observed when similar exercise levels are carried out in normoxia (Bärtsch et al., 2008). Moreover, even greater adaptations are obtained when the hypoxic intervention is accompanied by high-intensity training (Faiss et al., 2013; Sanchez and Borrani, 2018).

Although altitude is generally associated with increased health risks in most patients and elderly individuals, several studies have reported therapeutic benefits associated with exercising in mild hypoxia in a variety of alterations (Bailey et al., 2001; Burtscher et al., 2004; Wiesner et al., 2010). As exercising in moderate hypoxia seems to play a valuable role as an additional "therapeutic strategy," albeit one with both benefits and risks, new insights on this paradigm are now increasing. Some critical analysis and guidelines for hypertensive, obese and elderly individuals have recently been proposed (Millet et al., 2016). These concluded that intermittent hypoxic training seems to be well tolerated by most patients, in a similar way to healthy individuals, and that hypoxia and exercise may have additive or synergistic effects, probably mediated by several factors, including nitric oxide, angiogenesis and "altitude anorexia," thereby paving the way for researchers to identify the optimal individual combination of exercise and hypoxia.

Cardiac Remodeling

Aerobic exercise activities have traditionally been widely recommended for preventing disease and promoting health. Today, resistance training is usually included in physical activity counseling, even for older adults and people with a range of cardiac conditions (Haskell et al., 2007; Nelson et al., 2007; Heuschmann et al., 2010), and there is solid evidence of different echocardiographic repercussions (Kenney et al., 2012). The cardioprotective effects of chronic intermittent hypoxia have been extensively studied, and their positive effect has shown to be related to preservation of mitochondrial function and inhibition

TABLE 1 | Examples of the effects of intermittent hypoxia exposure on erythropoiesis.

Subjects	Hypoxia time	Hypoxia method	Hypoxia dosage	Outcome	References
Healthy men ($n = 6$)	5.5 h	HC	3,000–4,000 m	↑EPO	Eckardt et al., 1989
Alpinists ($n = 10$; 4 w + 6 m)	10 d	Altitude	6,542 m	↑Hct ↑[Hb]	Richalet et al., 1994
Competitive ($n = 13$; 4 w + 9 m)	4 h TL/d for 4 wk	Altitude (LH-TL) Altitude (LH-TH)	1,250/2,500 m	↑Hct ↑[Hb] ↑RBC_{mass}	Levine and Stray-Gundersen, 1997
Competitive ($n = 39$; 12 w + 27 m)	30 h (14 d)	Altitude (LH-TL) Altitude (LH-TH)	1,200–1,400 m/2,500–3,000 m	↑EPO	Chapman et al., 1998
Alpinists ($n = 17$; 3 w + 14 m)	3–5 h/d for 9 d	HC	4,000–5,500 m	↑Hct ↑[Hb] ↑RBC	Rodríguez et al., 1999
Elite alpinists ($n = 6$; 1 w + 5 m) Alpinists ($n = 17$; 3 w + 14 m) Novice men ($n = 8$)	3–5 h/d for 17 d 3–5 h/d for 9 d 1.5 h/d × 3 d/wk for 3 wk	HC	4,000–5,500 m	↑Hct ↑[Hb] ↑RBC (all protocols)	Casas H. et al., 2000
Elite runners ($n = 26$; 9 w + 17 m)	4 wk (4 h TL/d)	Altitude LH-TL	1,225/2,500 m	↑EPO ↑Hct ↑[Hb]	Stray-Gundersen et al., 2001
Healthy people ($n = 48$; 16 w + 32 m)	24 h	HC	1,780m 2,085m 2,454m 2,800m	↑EPO (6 h) ↓EPO (24 h) ↑EPO (6 h) ↓EPO (24 h) ↑EPO (6 h) ↑EPO (24 h ↑EPO (6 h) ↑EPO (24 h)	Ge et al., 2002
Competitive ($n = 17$; 3 w + 14 m)	(IHT 5:5) 70 min/d (5 d/wk) for 4 wk	NH	$FiO_2 = 0.12$ (≈4,400 m) $FiO_2 = 0.11$ (≈5,200 m) $FiO_2 = 0.10$ (≈5,800 m) $FiO_2 = 0.10$ (≈5,800 m)	No changes	Julian et al., 2004
Competitive ($n = 23$; 12 w + 11 m)	3 h/d × 5 d/wk for 4 wk	HC	4,000–5,500 m	↑EPO (3 h after)	Gore et al., 2006
Competitive ($n = 87$; 28 w + 59 m)	4 wk (≥22 h) 4 wk (12–16 h)	Altitude HC	2,000–2,500 m 2,500–3,000 m	↑EPO	Wilber et al., 2007
Elite athletes ($n = 41$) XC Skiers ($n = 11$) Swimmers ($n = 18$) Runners ($n = 12$)	18 nights 13 nights 18 nights	NH and Altitude (LH-TL)	1,200/ /2,500–3,500 m /2,500–3,000 m /2,500–3,000 m	↑[Hb] ↑Hct ↑[Hb] ↑[Hb]	Richalet and Gore, 2008
Trained rats	4 h/d × 5 d/wk for 2 wk	HC	4,000 m	↑[Hb]↑Hct ↑RBC	Núñez-Espinosa et al., 2014
Male trained triathletes ($n = 18$) -Normoxia ($n = 9$) -Hypoxia ($n = 9$)	1 h/d × 2 d/wk for 7 wk	NH	$FiO_2 = 0.145$-0.15 (≈2,800–2,500 m)	↑[Hb] ↑RBC	Ramos-Campo et al., 2015
Elite swimmers ($n = 54$; 30w+24m)	3 or 4 wk	Altitude LH-TH vs. LL-TL vs. LH-TH+TL	690/2,320 m	↑tHb_{mass} for LH-TH and LH-TH+TL	Rodríguez et al., 2015
Male well-trained triathletes ($n = 28$) -HH ($n = 11$) -NH ($n = 10$) -Normoxia ($n = 7$)	230 h for 18 d 238 h for 18 d	Altitude (LH-TL) NH (LH-TL)	<1,200/2,250m 1,150 m/(≈2,250 m)	↑Hb_{mass} (similar in NH & HH)	Hauser et al., 2016

Altitude, geographic altitude; EPO, serum or plasma erythropietin levels; FiO_2, Fraction of inspired oxygen; [Hb], Blood hemoglobin concentration; Hb_{mass}, whole body hemoglobin mass; HC, Hypobaric Chamber; Hct, Hematocrit; IHT(5:5), intermittent hypoxic training, alternating 5 min hypoxia with 5 min normoxia along the session; LH-TH, Living High-Training High; LH-TL, Living High-Training Low; NH, normobaric hypoxia; RBC, red blood cell count; RBC_{mass}, whole body erythrocytic mass.

of potassium channels sensitive to ATP (mitoKATP) present in the sarcoplasmic and mitochondrial membranes (Ostádal et al., 1989; Asemu et al., 1999, 2000; Chouabe et al., 2004; Ostadal and Kolar, 2007). Additional myocardial remodeling data were reported by our group using a model of IEHH (Panisello et al., 2007). Both chronic and intermittent exposure models supported the potential beneficial effects of acute exposure in coronary patients reported in pioneering studies conducted by Peruvian cardiologist Emilio Marticorena (Marticorena, 1993; Marticorena et al., 2001; Reynafarje and Marticorena, 2002; Valle et al., 2006). In rodents, it has been demonstrated that endurance exercise training and IEHH modulate cardiac mitochondria to a protective phenotype characterized by decreased induction of mitochondrial permeability transition pore and apoptotic signaling (Magalhães et al., 2013, 2014). However, there are no studies on humans on cardiac remodeling that combine

TABLE 2 | Examples of the effects of intermittent hypoxia exposure on angiogenesis, vascular remodeling, muscle capillarization, and hypertension.

Subjects	Time of hypoxia	Hypoxia method	Hypoxia dosage	Outcome	References
Healthy (*n* = 32 m) 14 normoxic (SL) 18 hypoxic (≈2,500 m)	3 cycling/wk for 4 wk	NH	FiO_2 = 0.16 (≈2,500 m)	↑Lipid peroxidation during hipoxia	Bailey et al., 2001
Males (*n* = 16) Double blind groups 8 healthy 8 prior myocardial infarction	IHT 3–4 × (3–5:3) 15 sessions in 3 wk	NH	FiO_2 = 0.14–0.10 (≈3,500–≈5,800 m)	↑Aerobic capacity ↑exercise tolerance (without differences in patients)	Burtscher et al., 2004
Sedentary male rats	4 h/d, 5 d/wk for 22 d	HC	5,000 m	↑Capillary density ↓Diffusion distances for slow fibres	Panisello et al., 2008
Overweight to obese subjects group (*n* = 24)	4 wk training under hypoxia at 65% VO_2max	NH	FiO_2 = 0.15 (≈2,760 m)	Better physical fitness, metabolic risk markers, and body composition	Wiesner et al., 2010
Male Wistar rats (hyperlipidemia induced by 8 wk high-fat diet)	3 × (10 s:10 s) ischemia/reperfusion preceding 180 min reperfusion	Ischemic postconditioning	Ischemia: 30 min LAD occlusion followed by 180 min of reperfusion	Up-regulation of HIF-1α can be cardioprotective	Li et al., 2014

FiO_2, Fraction of inspired oxygen; HC, Hypobaric Chamber; HIF, hypoxia inducible factor; NH, Normobaric hypoxia; IHT, Intermittent hypoxic training alternating hypoxia with normoxia along the session; LAD, left anterior descending coronary artery; VO_2max, maximal oxygen consumption capacity.

hypoxia and exercise, other than those dealing with OSA models. There have been extensive studies on patients suffering from this syndrome, and several pieces of evidence may be found in the literature: the progression and reversibility of atrial remodeling following stretch release may help prevent atrial fibrillation (Thanigaimani et al., 2017), the important prognostic information of right-sided heart dysfunction (Kusunose et al., 2016) and the evidence that OSA is associated independently with decreasing left ventricular systolic function and reduced right ventricular function (Korcarz et al., 2016). Nevertheless, this cardiac remodeling in OSA patients –individuals characterized by sustained systemic acidosis, hypercapnia and cerebral vasodilation– might not be present during intermittent hypoxia exposure in healthy subjects, in which alkalosis and hypocapnia, both induced by the hyperventilation caused by adrenergic drive, are evident and probably lead to cerebral vascular constriction and reduced effects of hypoxic insult (Viscor et al., 2014). Consequently, some of the changes and/or adaptive responses found in these pathological conditions must be interpreted with caution. In conclusion, there is no solid evidence for pernicious cardiac remodeling, but rather the opposite, after intermittent hypoxia in healthy individuals, whether accompanied by physical exercise or not. **Table 3** contrasts the deteriorated cardiac function in OSA patients in comparison to several studies demonstrating, both in experimental animal models and human coronary patients, the positive effects of intermittent hypoxia exposure on cardiac function.

Treatment of Bronchial Asthma

Despite modern advances in the treatments, bronchial asthma continues being a potentially severe illness. All treatments focus on the improvement of bronchial obstruction, but nowadays we do not have an etiological definitive treatment. Bronchial asthma generates great dependence on a variety of medications and therefore frequently submits the patient to derived complications (Chiu et al., 1981; Fairfax et al., 1999; van der Woude et al., 2001; Salpeter et al., 2006). The Experts Committee of the United States Food & Drug Administration published a consensus document about the risks of the antiasthma medications, some of them potentially lethal (DeNoon, 2008).

For that reason, every procedure that could diminish pharmacological dependence among asthmatic patients should be considered a benefit. IEHH programs represent a realistic possibility to apply a minimally aggressive non-pharmacological approach that would reduce bronchial obstruction and pharmacological dependence in these patients.

As early as the nineteenth century there was social wisdom and medical knowledge that respiratory illnesses may improve in the mountains. The sanatoriums for respiratory patients, traditionally, were located at moderate altitude in the mountains. Notable examples were the Dutch Asthma Center, Davos, Clavadel, at 1,686 m over the sea level (Switzerland) and the Istituto Pio XII, Misurina, Auronzo at 1,756 m (Italy) devoted to childhood bronchial asthma. The first medical reference we found about bronchial asthma and altitude is an inquiry between the doctors of Davos referring that 133 among their 143 patients with bronchial asthma that spent their holidays in this mountain town, did not present any acute episode of asthma and that 81% reported persistent improvement of the illness (Turban and Spengler, 1906).

Moreover, different epidemiological studies showed the beneficial effects of living at moderate altitude in the prevalence and severity of bronchial asthma (van Velzen et al., 1996; Yangzong et al., 2006; Droma et al., 2007; Kiechl-Kohlendorfer et al., 2007; Sy et al., 2007). However, acute hypoxia exposure, as occurs with acute altitude exposure, as in many other stress situations, can induce an asthmatic episode of bronchoconstriction. On the other hand, when the acclimatization process advances, the asthmatic illness improved or even disappeared (Allegra et al., 1995; Christie

TABLE 3 | Examples of the positive effects of intermittent hypoxia exposure on cardiac pathologies.

Subjects	Time of hypoxia	Hypoxia method	Hypoxia dosage	Outcome	References
Acclimatized rats (4 d–12 wk)	8 h/d × 5 d/wk (12 wk)	HC	Sea level – 7,000 m	↑Pulmonary hypertension	Ostádal et al., 1989
Coronary patients (n = 5)	8 walks (in 4 wk)	Progressive Altitude	900–5,200 m	↑Cardiac function	Marticorena, 1993
Rats	4 h/d (3 wk)	HC	5,000 m	↓Ischemia	Asemu et al., 1999
Rats	4 or 8 h/d (3 or 6 wk)	HC	5,000 or 7,000 m	"Dose dependent" opposite effects	Asemu et al., 2000
Coronary patients (n = 8)	4 h/wk (13 wk)	HC	4,000 m	↑Cardiac function ↑NO	Marticorena et al., 2001
Guinea pigs	Chronic vs. sea-level	Altitude	4,500 m	↑Efficiency in generate ATP	Reynafarje and Marticorena, 2002
Rats	20 d	HC	4,500 m	↓Aging remodeling	Chouabe et al., 2004
Coronary patients (n = 6)	4 h/wk (14 wk)	HC	2,400–4,000 m	↑Myocardial perfusion	Valle et al., 2006
Rats	4 h/d × 5 d/wk (22 d)	HC	5,000 m	↑Myocardial capillaries	Panisello et al., 2007
Rats	5 h/d (5 wk)	HC + exercise	6,000 m	↑Cardiac function	Magalhães et al., 2013
Rats	5 h/d (5 wk)	HC + exercise	6,000 m	↑Heart mitochondrial function after DOXO treatment	Magalhães et al., 2014
OSA patients	Chronic	OSA	OSA	↓Ventricular function	Korcarz et al., 2016
OSA patients	Chronic	OSA	OSA	↓Ventricular function	Kusunose et al., 2016

Altitude, geographic altitude; DOXO, Doxorubicin treatment; HC, Hypobaric Chamber; NO, nitric oxide; OSA, Obstructive sleep apnea.

et al., 1995; Cogo et al., 1997, 2004; Gourgoulianis et al., 2001; Karagiannidis et al., 2006; Schultze-Werninghaus, 2006, 2008). Regrettably, this improvement vanished upon returning to the sea level.

The triad altitude exposure-hypoxia-acclimatization produces a number of physiological changes, some of which are accepted as related to the improvement of bronchial asthma: (a) a different breathing control pattern (Harrison et al., 2002; Serebrovskaya et al., 2003), (b) mitochondrial changes that optimize oxygen metabolism during the normal acclimatization process (Levett et al., 2012), and (c) the decrease in free radicals and the associated anti-inflammatory and immunosuppressive effects (Meehan, 1987; Simon et al., 1994; Serebrovskaya et al., 2003; Ohta et al., 2011; Oliver et al., 2013).

Since bronchial asthma improves with acclimatization to altitude and IEHH stimulates the acclimatization process (Rodríguez et al., 1999, 2000; Casas H. et al., 2000; Casas M. et al., 2000; Ibáñez et al., 2000; Ricart et al., 2000), it could be hypothesized that IEHH improves bronchial asthma. In fact, some medical studies have shown the usefulness of intermittent hypoxia exposure as a treatment for bronchial asthma (Harrison et al., 2002; Serebrovskaya et al., 2003). However, due to the different techniques and protocols used to produce the hypoxia and the wide dispersion of data, further research is required to design more effective protocols for intermittent hypoxia exposure that could prove useful in treating this disease. The ultimate objective of such treatments must be to reduce bronchial obstruction and the dependence on potentially dangerous drugs. Moreover, if protocols demonstrate a good response in bronchial asthma mitigation, they could also be useful for treating other illnesses with inflammatory backdrop. **Table 4** summarizes some of the results that demonstrate a favorable effect of exposure to hypoxia on the symptoms of bronchial asthma.

Neurological Impact of Hypoxic Exposure

Hypobaric hypoxic exposure at altitude, usually long-term, results in several pathophysiological and psychological conditions associated with the nervous system. The term high altitude deterioration (HAD) was first used by members of early Mount Everest expeditions to denote the deterioration in mental and physical condition due to prolonged time spent at high altitudes (Ward, 1954). It is well known among climbers that staying at extreme altitudes for long periods is deleterious (Milledge, 2003). Manifestations vary depending on the altitude reached and the individual's hypoxia tolerance, but include acute and chronic mountain sickness, memory loss and high-altitude cerebral edema (Lieberman et al., 1994; Hornbein, 2001; West et al., 2013). Acute mountain sickness generally occurs 6 to 12 h after an unacclimatized person ascends to 2,500 m or higher (Bärtsch and Swenson, 2013). As a result, cognitive function may be impaired under hypoxia (Virués-Ortega et al., 2006), although the physiological changes that occur during acclimatization prevent mountain sickness. Given the acclimatization-like responses triggered by intermittent hypoxic exposure, it offers protection against severe hypoxia exposure damage and has been reported to produce beneficial effects (Kushwah et al., 2016). Our group reported how short-term (3-h sessions on three consecutive days) IEHH with surface muscle electrostimulation increased the concentration of circulating progenitor cells in the peripheral blood of humans (Viscor et al., 2009). However, we were unable to reproduce these results later in healthy patients and those with traumatic brain injuries (Corral et al., 2014a,b), thus raising doubts about the potential role of hypoxia exposure in the release of stem cells to circulation and its involvement in the tissue regeneration process. In any case, the translation of the physiological effects of IEHH to humans is not straightforward in the field of neurology.

TABLE 4 | Examples of the application of intermittent hypoxia exposure on bronchial asthma patients.

Subjects	Time of hypoxia	Hypoxia method	Hypoxia dosage	Outcome	References
Asthmatic (*n* = 143)	1–3 mo (living at Davos)	Altitude	1,686 m	Improvement in 133 patients	Turban and Spengler, 1906
Asthmatic (*n* = 14)	5 weeks (living at Davos)	Altitude	1,686 m	Improvement in patients with HDM IgE-meditated allergy	Simon et al., 1994
Asthmatic (*n* = 11)	Mt Rosa & near Mt Everest BC (after 3–6 d trekking)	Altitude	4,559 and 5,050 m	↓Bronchial responsiveness to hypoosmolar aerosol 72 h after arrival	Allegra et al., 1995
Asthmatic (*n* = 14)	1 mo (living at Davos)	Altitude	1,686 m	↑Airway responsiveness to histamine after return to SL in children with atopic asthma at altitude	Christie et al., 1995
Asthmatic (*n* = 16)	1 mo (living at Davos)	Altitude	1,560 m	↓Airways inflammation	van Velzen et al., 1996
Asthmatic (*n* = 11)	3 d trekking from 2,800 to 5,050 m	Altitude	5,050 m	↓Bronchial response	Cogo et al., 1997
Children (*n* = 874) Epidemiologic study	Chronic	Altitude	SL - 1,200 m	↓Prevalence ↓morbidity of bronchial asthma in children at altitude	Gourgoulianis et al., 2001
Athletes (*n* = 40; 20 asthmatic)	IHT 6 × (5:5) 15 sessions in 3 wk	NH	≈6,800 m	Improvement in symptoms ↓Medication use	Harrison et al., 2002
Central Tibet epidemiologic study	Permanent stay	Altitude	3,000–4,500 m	↓Prevalence ↑Risk due to western lifestyle	Yangzong et al., 2006
Asthmatics (*n* = 11)	3 wk (living at Davos)	Altitude	1,686 m	↓local airway inflammation	Karagiannidis et al., 2006
Asmathics (*n* = 296) Retrospective review	2 wk–9 mo	Altitude	1,500–1,800 m	Beneficial effect, in particular in steroid-dependent patients	Schultze-Werninghaus, 2006
Epidemiologic ISAAC–HWO study 13–14 y old children (*n* = 3,196)	Chronic (living in Lhasa)	Altitude	3,658 m	↓Prevalence (Asthma prevalence in Lhasa was the lowest worldwide in ISAAC study)	Droma et al., 2007
Epidemiologic study Hospitalized asthmatic children 6–11 y old (*n* = 305)	Chronic	Altitude	450–1,800 m	↓Risk of hospitalization for atopic asthma	Kiechl-Kohlendorfer et al., 2007
Epidemiologic study (*n* = 9984)	Chronic	Altitude	1,500 m	↓Prevalence ↓Asthma-like symptoms	Sy et al., 2007
Asthmatics (*n* = 428) Retrospective review	3 wk–9 mo	Altitude	1,500 m	Beneficial effects beyond the effects of allergen avoidance	Schultze-Werninghaus, 2008
Mice (*in vivo*; lymphoid organs)	2 h	NH	$FiO_2 = 0.08$ $FiO_2 = 0.21$ $FiO_2 = 1$	↓T cell activation T cell activation *in vivo* is dependent on localization and decrease with hypoxia	Ohta et al., 2011
Mountaineers (*n* = 27)	Alpine activities 11–18 d over 3,777 m	Altitude	3,777 m	↓Development of new immunity in humans	Oliver et al., 2013

Altitude, geographic altitude; BC, Base camp; FiO_2, Fraction of inspired oxygen; HC, Hypobaric Chamber; HDM, house dust mite; IHT, Intermittent hypoxic training alternating hypoxia with normoxia along the session; ISSAC, International Study of Asthma and Allergies in Childhood; WHO, World Health Organization.

The brain's protective mechanisms involved in intermittent exposure to hypoxia have been widely studied using experimental animal models, and numerous beneficial effects have been reported. Intermittent hypoxia facilitates the proliferation of neural stem cells *in situ* in the subventricular zone and dentate gyrus of rat brains (Zhu et al., 2005; Ross et al., 2012). Xu et al. (2007) described a time-dependent migration of neural progenitor cells (NPC), promoted by hypoxia-induced astrocytes, thereby suggesting a role for astrocytes in NPC replacement therapy in the central nervous system. Intermittent hypoxia stimulated hippocampal angiogenesis and neurogenesis and improved short-term memory indices in control mice; and, in brain-injured mice, it reduced injury size and prevented memory impairments (Bouslama et al., 2015). It was recently reported that activation of HIF-1 is involved in hyperglycemia-aggravated blood-brain barrier disruption in an ischemic stroke model (Zhang et al., 2016b). Moreover, glycemic control by insulin abolished HIF-1α upregulation in diabetic animals and reduced blood-brain barrier permeability and brain infarction (Zhang et al., 2016b). Acute intermittent hypoxia can trigger spinal plasticity associated with sustained increases in respiratory, somatic and/or autonomic motor output (Streeter et al., 2017).

In rats, intermittent hypobaric hypoxia preconditioning caused a reduction in the degree of brain injury following ischemia-reperfusion by reducing hippocampal neuronal apoptosis by local upregulation of neuroglobin and Bcl-2 expression (Wu et al., 2015). Neuroglobin is an intracellular monomer hemoprotein that was discovered by Burmester et al. (2000) and is expressed in the central and peripheral nervous system, cerebrospinal fluid, retina and some endocrine areas of the brain (Burmester and Hankeln, 2004). It reversibly binds oxygen with a higher affinity than normal adult hemoglobin, and plays a critical role in brain tissue protection facing a possible oxygen delivery shortage (Ascenzi et al., 2016). Bcl-2 is an anti-apoptotic protein localized in the outer membrane of the mitochondria; overexpression of Bcl-2 in neurons can inhibit neuron apoptosis induced by ischemia-reperfusion injury by maintaining the integrity of mitochondria (Xing et al., 2008; Zhang et al., 2008).

Kushwah et al. (2016) also explored the ameliorating potential of intermittent hypoxia against the detrimental effects of unpredictable chronic mild stress (UCMS) on anxiety and depression-like behavior in rats, through the enhancement of neurogenesis in the hippocampus, a response mediated by brain derived neurotrophic factor (BDNF). In the postischemic rat brain, intermittent hypoxia intervention rescued ischemia-induced spatial learning and memory impairment by inducing hippocampal neurogenesis and functional synaptogenesis via BDNF expression (Tsai et al., 2013).

Nowadays, intermittent hypoxia exposure is known to enhance neurogenesis at multiple stages. Notch1 is a transcription factor in the neuron's membrane that regulates several stages of neurogenesis and promotes differentiation of progenitor cells into astroglia. Notch1 is activated by hypoxia *in vivo*, and such activation has been shown to be required for hypoxia-induced neurogenesis (Zhang K. et al., 2014a). Chronic IEHH pretreatment can reduce cerebral ischemic injury, which, as similarly reported for myocardium (see above), is mediated through upregulation of the expression and activity of mitochondrial membrane ATP-sensitive potassium channel (mitoKATP) (Zhang et al., 2016a). As is well known, hypoxia inducible factor-1 (HIF-1) is the key transcription factor that controls early adaptive responses to the lack of oxygen in mammalian cells. HIF-1α and HIF-1β expression was measured during acclimatization to hypobaric hypoxia in the rat cerebral cortex, and neurons, astrocytes, ependymal cells and possibly endothelial cells were the cell types that expressed HIF-1α (Chávez et al., 2000). Thus, the vascular remodeling and metabolic changes triggered during prolonged hypoxia may restore normal oxygen delivery levels to brain tissue (Agani et al., 2002; Chavez and LaManna, 2002).

Finally, there is solid evidence of the beneficial effects of intermittent hypoxia exposure on spinal cord neural tissue repair. Complete or incomplete spinal cord injuries are characterized by spared synaptic pathways below the level of the injury. Intermittent hypoxia elicits plasticity in the spinal cord and strengthens these spared synaptic pathways, expressed as respiratory and somatic functional recovery in both experimental animals and humans with traumatic spinal cord injury (Navarrete-Opazo et al., 2015, 2017a,b; Dougherty et al., 2017; Trumbower et al., 2017). **Table 5** lists studies reporting beneficial neurological impact after a wide range of intermittent hypoxia exposure protocols.

Other Pathological Conditions Where the Use of Intermittent Hypoxia Exposure Has Potential Therapeutic Value

Since the altitude-hypoxia-acclimatization triad is known to have some antioxidant, anti-inflammatory and immunosuppressive effects (Meehan, 1987; Meehan et al., 1988; Ohta et al., 2011; Oliver et al., 2013), a benefit in some other pathologies related to immune response, such as psoriasis, atopy, arthritis or autoimmune pneumonitis can be expected. This is still a controversial field with no extensive clinical studies available, although some medical descriptive studies point to potential future research opportunities (Singh et al., 1977; Vocks et al., 1999; Engst and Vocks, 2000; Steiner, 2009).

Intermittent exposure to both normobaric and hypobaric hypoxia has been related to some protective effects (Cai et al., 2003; Costa et al., 2013) and beneficial outcomes in several pathological conditions, especially in those related to metabolic syndrome (Marquez et al., 2013; Leone and Lalande, 2017; Serebrovska et al., 2017). The possible role of intermittent hypoxia on body weight control has also attracted considerable attention. In addition to improving exercise performance and diet control, intermittent exposure protocols to normobaric and hypobaric hypoxia have been applied in an attempt to potentiate weight loss, showing in some cases positive short-term results (Haufe et al., 2008; Netzer et al., 2008; Lippl et al., 2010; Wiesner et al., 2010; Cabrera-Aguilera et al., in press). However, a long-term study failed to demonstrate permanent body weight reduction after IEHH (Gatterer et al., 2015), suggesting that additional research is needed to clarify the discrepancies reported in this field.

In summary, recent reports call for increased attention to the potential benefits of the application of intermittent hypoxia protocols in several clinical areas (Dale et al., 2014; Mateika et al., 2015). It is likely that future studies will yield important new information regarding potential therapeutic uses of intermittent hypoxia. **Table 6** lists a non-exhaustive but representative sample of studies reporting favorable impact of intermittent hypoxia exposure in other pathological conditions.

INTERMITTENT HYPOXIA IN SPORT

The benefits of intermittent hypoxia programs in competitive sport are still a subject of scientific debate. **Table 7** shows several examples of intermittent hypoxia exposure effect on the improvement of human physical performance. A prior consideration to bear in mind when dealing with this topic is that two inherent factors justify the diversity of results in the field of elite sport: (a) the narrow margin of improvement detectable in elite athletes; and (b) the limitation in the sample size when performing studies with this population. Both factors contribute to reduced statistical power in most of these studies.

Other sources of variability are the wide range of exposure patterns, differing hypoxic doses (or altitude), and the kind of hypoxia (hypobaric or normobaric), as is discussed below. The

TABLE 5 | Examples of the effects of intermittent hypoxia exposure with favorable neurological impact.

Subjects	Time of hypoxia	Hypoxia method	Hypoxia dosage	Outcome	References
Rats	6 h, 12 h, or 1, 4, 7, 14, or 21 d	HC	BP = 380 Torr (≈5,500 m)	↑Hct ↑GLUT-1 ↑VEGF ↑brain HIF-1α until 14 d ↓brain HIF-1α at 21 d	Chávez et al., 2000
Cell culture	4 h	NH	1%O_2 + 5%CO_2 + N_2	↑HIF-1α (NO interferes expression)	Agani et al., 2002
Rats (male)	11–13 min	Ischemia	Ischemia after cardiac arrest	↑HIF-1α 12 h–7 d ↑IGF-1	Chavez and LaManna, 2002
Rats (male) (3 groups)	4 h/d for 2 wk	HC	3,000 m 5,000 m Control normoxic	↑BrdU-labeled cells in SVZ and DG (NPC) in rat brain	Zhu et al., 2005
Astrocytes and NPC culture from brain cortex of newborn rats	6, 12, 18, and 24 h	NH	1%O_2 + 5%CO_2 + N_2 (astrocytes)	↑Migration of NPC by hypoxia-induced astrocytes (maximal at 18 h)	Xu et al., 2007
Neuronal cultures of 16–18 days old fetuses of Sprague–Dawley rats	6 h "ischemia" 48 h "reperfusion"	NH	Anoxic atmosphere (5%CO_2 + 95%N_2)	Mitochondrial dysfunction & ER stress ⇒ neuronal apoptosis ↑Bcl-2 ⇒ ↓Apoptosis	Zhang et al., 2008
Rats (n = 122) -Ischemia MCA n = 42 -Ischemia MCA + post-cond n = 42 -Control group n = 40	60 min MCA ischemia post-cond (60 min after reperfusion): reperfusion for 30 s, MCA occluded for 5 cycles × 30 s	Ischemia (MCA occlusion)	Unknown (ischemia)	↑Bcl-2 ↑Hsp70 ↓Cytochrome *c* ↓Bax translocation to the mitochondria ↓Caspase-3 ↓Infarct volume ↓Oxidative stress ↑Neurologic scores	Xing et al., 2008
Neonatal mice: acute IH and control group	40 min 20 × (1:1)	NH	FiO_2 = 0.10 (10% O_2)	↑SVZ derived NPC *in vitro*	Ross et al., 2012
Rats (n = 55) Groups: with or without MCAO and/or IH, and/or zidovudine	4 h/d for 7 d	NH	FiO_2 = 0.12 (12% O_2)	Post brain ischemia: ↑Synaptogenesis via BDNF ↑Neurogenesis ↑Spatial learning and memory	Tsai et al., 2013
TBI medical history human males. 4 groups: -Exercise and SES (n = 5) -Cycling (n = 5) -IHH and SES (n = 6) -Control (n = 5)	2 h/d × 3 d/wk for 12 wk	HC	4,500 m	↑CPC No changes in psychological tests ↑Aerobic capacity or workload	Corral et al., 2014a
Mice (wildtype vs. Notch1 KO)	4 h/d during consecutive 28 d	HC	2,000 m	↑Notch1 ↑Hypoxia induced neurogenesis	Zhang K. et al., 2014a
Newborn mice with brain injury 3 Groups (n = 373) -Hypoxia separated from the mother -Normoxia separated from the mother Control with mother	20 events/h, 6 h/d from postnatal day 6 (P6) to P10	NH	FiO_2 = 0.08 (8% O_2)	Control mice: ↑Hippocampal angiogenesis ↑Neurogenesis ↑Short-term memory indices Brain-injured mice: ↓Injury size ↓Memory impairments	Bouslama et al., 2015
Rats (n = 48) hypocampal CA1 region. 4 groups with or without ischemia-reperfusion and IHH	Hypoxia for 4 d once a day I/R 8 min	*In vivo* I/R	Unknown (ischemia)	↑Surviving cells in the hippocampal CA1 in IHH+IR ↑Bcl-2	Wu et al., 2015
Rats with C2 medular hemisection (n = 32)	IHT 10 × (5:5) intervals (total 95 min) for 7 d	NH	FiO_2 = 0.105 (10.5% O_2)	↑Breathing capacity ↑Contralateral diaphragm (adenosine dependent) –2° intercostal muscle (adenosine independent)	Navarrete-Opazo et al., 2015
Rats (male) with Chronic Mild Stress induced depression (n = 60) and controls (n = 20)	4 h/d for 2 wk	HC	5,000 m	Avoid neuronal loss ↑Neurogenesis ↑BDNF–TrkB signaling	Kushwah et al., 2016

(Continued)

TABLE 5 | Continued

Subjects	Time of hypoxia	Hypoxia method	Hypoxia dosage	Outcome	References
Rats (*n* = 195) 6 groups with chronic 5 wk stress and/or IHH or IMIP or antagonist of mitoKATP	6 h/d for 28 days	HC	5,000 m	↑Expression and activity of $mitoK_{ATP}$ ↓Cerebral ischemia injury ↓UCMS	Zhang et al., 2016a
Rats with C2 medular hemisection (*n* = 27) with or without hypoxia + adenosine inhibitor	8 wk post-lesion 5 min hypoxia, 5-min normoxic 10 times (95 min) 7 d, AIH 3/wk 8 wk	NH	$FiO_2 = 0.105$ (10.5% O_2)	↑Tidal volume and bilateral diaphragm activity (enhanced by adenosine receptor inhibitor) for 4 wk	Navarrete-Opazo et al., 2017b
Rats with spinal C2 hemisection. 1) 7d after lesion 2) 7wk after lesion + serotonin receptor antagonist	IHT 10 × (5:5) intervals (total 110 min)	NH	$FiO_2 = 0.105$ (10.5% O_2)	↑Breathing capacity Serotonin independent in acute (2wk) and serotonin dependent in chronic (8wk)	Dougherty et al., 2017
Humans incomplete spinal cord injured (*n* = 35): IH + BWSTT (*n* = 18) NX + BWSTT (*n* = 17)	IHT 15 × (1.5:1.5) intervals for 5 consecutive d + 3 d/wk for 3 wk	NH	$FiO_2 = 0.09$ (9% O_2)	↑Walking recovery and endurance (up to 5wk)	Navarrete-Opazo et al., 2017a
Rats (*n* =12)	IHT 3 × (5:5)	NH	$FiO_2 = 0.11$ (11% O_2) alternating with hyperoxia $FiO_2 = 0.5$ (O_2 50%)	↑or↓in firing rate of midcervical interneurons altering connectivity	Streeter et al., 2017
Men with chronic incomplete spinal cord injury (*n* = 6) (double-blind, crossover study)	IHT 15 × (1.5:1) intervals for 5 consecutive d + hand opening practice	NH	$FiO_2 = 0.09$ (9% O_2)	↑Hand dexterity, function, or opening in all participants	Trumbower et al., 2017

In IHT protocols hypoxia was alternated with room air ($FiO_2 = 0.209$) if nothing else is indicated. AIH, acute intermittent hypoxia; BDNF, brain derived neurotrophic factor; Bcl-2, B cell lymphoma/leukemia-2; BP, barometric pressure; BrdU, 5-Bromo-2-deoxyuridine-5-monophosphate; BWSTT, body weight-supported treadmill training; CAO, carotid artery occlusion; CIHH, chronic intermittent hypobaric hypoxia; CPC, circulating progenitor cells; DG, dentate gyrus; FiO_2, Fraction of inspired oxygen; GLUT-1, glucose transporter-1; HC, Hypobaric Chamber; Hct, hematocrit; HIF, Hypoxia inducible factor; Hsp70, heat shock protein70; IGF-1, insulin-like growth factor-1; IH, intermittent hypoxia; IHH, intermittent hypobaric hypoxia; IHT, intervallic hypoxic training alternating hypoxia and normoxia along the session; IMIP, imipramine; I/R, ischemia-reperfusion; KO, knockout mutant; MCA, medium cerebral artery; MCAO, middle cerebral artery occlusion; NH, normobaric hypoxia; NO, nitric oxide; NPC, neural progenitor cells; NX, normoxia (placebo); ER, endoplasmic reticulum; TBI, traumatic brain injury; UCMS, Unpredictable Chronic Mild Stress; VEGF, vascular endothelial growth factor; SES, surface electrical stimulation; SVZ, subventricular zone.

living high-training low (LH-TL) pattern (Levine and Stray-Gundersen, 1997) is the most widespread training schedule, although sometimes the reverse model, living low-training-high (LL-TH), is also applied, especially when artificial hypoxia is used. Moreover, studies evaluating training at altitude during permanent stays are also very usual.

In addition to other reports cited in precedent sections, a high number of studies have consistently found positive effects of IEHH programs to improve exercise performance. Thus, 4 weeks of LH-TL improved sea-level running performance in trained runners (Levine and Stray-Gundersen, 1997). Short-term intermittent hypobaric hypoxia (in a hypobaric chamber) improved the aerobic performance capacity in healthy subjects (Rodríguez et al., 1999). Intermittent hypobaric hypoxia combined with low-intensity exercise induced altitude acclimation, improved lactate threshold and ventilatory anaerobic threshold in healthy subjects (Casas M. et al., 2000). Normobaric hypoxia increased the growth hormone response to maximal resistance exercise in trained men (Filopoulos et al., 2017). Finally, a reduction in the severity of acute mountain sickness was also reported after several intermittent normobaric hypoxia protocols (Schommer et al., 2010; Wille et al., 2012; Dehnert et al., 2014).

In contrast, other studies did not detect significant improvements in exercise performance. Four weeks of IEHH did not improve oxygen transport in trained swimmers and runners (Rodríguez et al., 2007) nor did it change the submaximal economy in a group of well-trained athletes (Truijens et al., 2008). Seven weeks of normobaric hypoxia training in triathletes, caused an improvement in hematological parameters but not in the aerobic performance (Ramos-Campo et al., 2015). Finally, a recent systematic review and meta-analysis did not reveal a significant benefit of resistance training in hypoxia compared to the same training in normoxia (Ramos-Campo et al., 2018).

In general, it is commonly accepted that the application of intermittent hypoxia exposure has beneficial effects for competitive sport in the same way as for the biomedical field. As discussed above, the wide difference in effects that have been reported in the literature can be explained by individual susceptibility and the diversity of intermittent hypoxia patterns applied (Debevec and Mekljavic, 2013). The adaptive or maladaptive responses can be due to differences in the

TABLE 6 | Examples of the effects of intermittent hypoxia exposure with favorable impact in other pathological conditions.

Subjects	Time of hypoxia	Hypoxia method	Hypoxia dosage	Outcome	References
Epidemiological study (1965–1972) in 20,000 altitude native men vs. to 130,700 lowlanders (760 m)	Chronic	Altitude	3,692–5,538 m	↓Diseases ↓Morbidity rates	Singh et al., 1977
Rats ($n = 24$)	8 h/d for 30 d	HC	5,000 m	↑Resistance to epileptogenic action of penicillin	Agadzhanyan and Torshin, 1986
Healthy men ($n = 7$) (operation Everest II)	40 d	HC	7,620 m	↓T cell function ↓PHA-stimulated thymidine uptake	Meehan, 1987
Healthy men ($n = 8$) (operation Everest II)	4 weeks 5 d at 2,286m 28 d at 7,620 m (gradually) peaks 1–4 h at 8,839 m	HC	2,286 m 7,620 m 8,839 m	↓Phytohemagglutinin-stimulated thymidine uptake and protein synthesis in mononuclear cells ↑Monocytes ↑Plasma IgM & IgA ↓T-cell activation	Meehan et al., 1988
Essential hypertension patients	30 min/d, 5 d/wk for 3 wks	HC	3,500 m	↓BP ↓Blood vol ↓[Na]serum ↑Microcirculation ↑PO_2 tissue ↓cholesterol	Aleshin et al., 1993
Tibetan natives at moderate (M) and high (H) altitudes	Chronic	Altitude	M: 2,000–3,000 m H: 4,000–4,700 m	↓HR ↓HVR ↓$V_E$max in group at H altitude	Ge et al., 1994
Psoriasis affected patients ($n = 76$)	4 wk	Altitude	1,560 m	↓Psoriasis no changes in plasma cortisol	Vocks et al., 1999
Neurodermitis patients ($n = 31,438$)	4 wk	Altitude	1,560 m	↓Dermatosis ↓Psoriasis ↓ECP	Engst and Vocks, 2000
Coronary patients ($n = 46$)	22 sessions 3 h/d	HC	3,500 m	↓Total cholesterol ↑HDL ↓LDL ↓VLDL ↓TG	Tin'kov and Aksenov, 2002
Mice ($n = 9$)	IHT 5 × (6:6)	NH	$FiO_2 = 0.06$	↑EPO; ↑heart HIF-1α	Cai et al., 2003
Obese subjects (BMI > 27) ($n = 20$) -Hypoxia ($n = 10$; 8 w + 2 m) -Sham ($n = 10$; 8 w + 2 m)	1.5 h/d, 3 d/wk for 8 wk exercising at 60% VO_2max	NH	$FiO_2 = 0.15$ (≈2,500 m) $FiO_2 = 0.201$ (≈450 m)	↓BMI and ↑BW loss ↓cholesterol ↓TG and ↓LDL	Netzer et al., 2008
Healthy men ($n = 20$) -Hypoxia ($n = 10$) -Normoxia ($n = 10$)	1 h/d, 3 d/wk for 4 wk exercising at 3 mmol/L Lac HR	NH	$FiO_2 = 0.15$ (≈2,760 m) $FiO_2 = 0.21$ (≈SL)	↓Body fat content ↓TG ↓HOMA-Index fasting insulin and ↓AUCins	Haufe et al., 2008
Atopic dermatitis and psoriasis patients (mini-review)	12 d–4 wk	Altitude	1,560 m	↓Symptoms	Steiner, 2009
Obese men ($n = 20$)	1 week	Altitude	2,650 m	↓BW ↑BMR ↓Food intake ↑Basal leptin ↓diastolic BP	Lippl et al., 2010
Overweight to obese subjects ($n = 24$)	4 wk training under hypoxia at 65% VO_2max	NH	$FiO_2 = 0.15$ (≈2,760 m)	↑Physical fitness ↓Metabolic risk markers ↑Body composition	Wiesner et al., 2010
Mice (*in vivo*; lymphoid organs)	Acute 2 h exposure	NH	$FiO_2 = 0.08$ $FiO_2 = 0.21$ $FiO_2 = 1$ (variable in organs: thymus < lymphoid nodes < spleen)	↑T-cell activation in better oxygenated tissues. T-cell activation *in vivo* is dependent on localization and decrease with hypoxia	Ohta et al., 2011
Mice (WT vs. KO)	Myoblast cell culture	NH	5 vs. 21%	Endogenous EPO promotes satellite activation and functional recovery after muscle injury	Jia et al., 2012
Rats ($n = 8$)	3 h/d for 6 d	HC	5,500 m	Injured excitotoxic brain: ↑EPO ↓Lipid peroxidation ↓Apoptotic cell death	Costa et al., 2013
Healthy adult sedentary men ($n = 28$)	2 × 20 min/d × 3 d/wk for 10 weeks	HC (CVAC) 5 fluctuations/min	Progressive: SL - 3,048 m (wk 1) SL - 6,096 m (wk 5–10)	No changes in Hct, [Hb], cholesterol and insulin ↓Fasting plasma glucose ↓Plasma glucose in response to oral glucose tolerance test	Marquez et al., 2013
Recreationally active mountaineers ($n = 10$; 3 w + 7 m)	28 h	Altitude	3,777 m	↓Immune response	Oliver et al., 2013

(Continued)

TABLE 6 | Continued

Subjects	Time of hypoxia	Hypoxia method	Hypoxia dosage	Outcome	References
Obese patients (BMI > 30 kg/m^2) (*n* = 16; 4 w + 12 m)	52 sess of 90 min (8 mo)	NH	Exercise: 3,500 m Rest: 4,500 m	No added effects by hypoxia to those provoked by moderate intensity exercise	Gatterer et al., 2015
Prediabetic adult patients (*n* = 11; 6 w + 5 m)	3 sess/wk for 3 wk	NH (IHT 5:5)	FiO_2 = 0.12 (≈4,400 m)	↑mRNA expression of HIF-1α and target genes ↓Fasting plasma glucose ↓Plasma glucose response to 2 h post-oral glucose tolerance test	Serebrovska et al., 2017
Trained rats (*n* = 78) -Basal (*n* = 6) -Hypoxia (*n* = 24) -Hypoxia + LAE (*n* = 24) -Normoxia (*n* = 24)	4 h/d for 14 d	HC	4,000 m	m. soleus: ↑Histological muscle damage recovery No change in fiber types ↓Fiber size ↑Capillarisation ↑VEGF expression ↑Citrate synthase activity ↑PGC-1α	Rizo-Roca et al., 2017a
Trained Rats (*n* = 78) -Basal (*n* = 6) -Hypoxia (*n* = 24) -Hypoxia + LAE (*n* = 24) -Normoxia (*n* = 24)	4 h/d for 14 d	HC	4,000 m	m. soleus: ↑Mitochondrial biogenesis markers ↑Mitochondrial dynamics markers ↓Oxidative stress ↓Apoptotic signalling	Rizo-Roca et al., 2017b
Rats (*n* = 28) -Normoxia sedentary (*n* = 7) -Normoxia + EET (*n* = 7) -Hypoxia sedentary (*n* = 7) -Hypoxia + EET (*n* = 7)	5 h/d for 4 wk	HC	6,000 m	↓Food intake ↓Body weight gain ↓Oxygen consumption Additive effect of IHH+EET	Cabrera-Aguilera et al., in press

3 mmol/L Lac HR, heart rate corresponding to the 3 mmol/L lactate value in the FiO_2-specific incremental test; Altitude, geographic altitude; AMS, acute mountain sickness; AUCins, Insulin response (area under curve) to oral glucose tolerance test; BMI, body mass index; BMR, basal metabolic rate; BP, arterial blood pressure; BW; body weight; CVAC, Cyclic Variations in Altitude Conditioning; ECP, eosinophil cationic protein; EET, endurance exercise training; EPO, Erythropietin; FiO_2, Fraction of inspired oxygen; [Hb], Blood hemoglobin concentration; HC, Hypobaric Chamber; Hct, Hematocrit; HDL, high density lipoproteins; IHT, Intermittent hypoxic training alternating hypoxia with normoxia along the exposure protocol; HOMA-Index, homeostatic model assessment index of insulin resistance; HR, Heart rate; HVR, hypoxic ventilatory response; IHH, intermittent hypobaric hypoxia; IHT (6:6), intermittent hypoxic training, alternating 6 min hypoxia with 6 min normoxia along the session; LAE, light aerobic exercise; LDL, low density lipoproteins; NH, normobaric hypoxia; TG, plasma triglycerides; $V_E$max; maximal exercise pulmonary ventilation; VLDL, very low density lipoproteins.

frequency, severity or duration of hypoxic episodes (Serebrovska et al., 2016). Factors such as age, sex or genotypic variability may also contribute to varying results (Almendros et al., 2014). A review of relevant publications between 1980 and 2015 concluded that evidence regarding the effects of altitude training on athletic performance is weak but that the natural stay at altitude combined with a live high-train low training strategy may provide the best protocol for enhancing endurance performance in elite and subelite athletes (Khodaee et al., 2016), thus confirming similar findings in a previous study (Bonetti and Hopkins, 2009). Finally, a recently published meta-analysis on the effect of natural or simulated altitude training in team-sport athletes conclude that hypoxic intervention appears to be a worthwhile training strategy for improvement in team-sport athletes, with enhanced performance over control groups persisting for at least 4 weeks post-intervention (Hamlin et al., 2018). Also, our recent data indicate that contractile activity seems to be necessary to trigger in skeletal muscle the adaptive responses induced by intermittent exposure to hypoxia (Rizo-Roca et al., 2018).

Although most of the expected effects of altitude training and IEHH programs have been mainly aimed at improving aerobic capacity (Stray-Gundersen and Levine, 1999; Wilber, 2004), some reports also have described benefits for strength training at moderate hypoxia levels (Nummela and Rusko, 2000; Manimmanakorn et al., 2013; Álvarez-Herms et al., 2015b, 2016). The underlying mechanism of these responses remain to be clarified, but potential psychological benefits may be derived of the perception of increased effort during hypoxic training (Álvarez-Herms et al., 2016). In addition, training during hypoxia may result in a greater increase in muscular endurance than the same training load performed in normoxia, probably because of increased angiogenesis in skeletal muscle level (Kon et al., 2014), can be involved in those improvements.

NORMOBARIC VS. HYPOBARIC HYPOXIA: THE SAME STIMULUS?

When artificial methods of producing hypoxia exposure were first developed, no attention was paid to the differences between hypobaric (low barometric pressure) and normobaric (low oxygen content in an inhaled gas mixture) hypoxia. It seems evident that the same physiological effects are expected for

TABLE 7 | Examples of the intermittent hypoxia exposure on the improvement of human physical performance.

Subjects	Time of hypoxia	Hypoxia method	Hypoxia dosage	Outcome	References
Elite alpinists ($n = 5$; 1 w + 4 m)	1 wk chronic + 38 h for 4 d	Altitude + HC	4,350–4,807 m (1 wk at Mt Blanc) 5,000–8,500 m (4 d at HC)	↑SaO_2 during HT ↑Altitude acclimatization	Richalet et al., 1992
Competitive ($n = 39$, 12 w + 27 m)	4 wk	Altitude	LH-TL 1,250/2,500 m	↑VO_2max	Levine and Stray-Gundersen, 1997
Competitive ($n = 39$; 12 w + 27 m)	14 d	LH-TL LH-TH	1,200–1,400 m/2,500–3,000 m	↑VO_2max ↑VO_2max	Chapman et al., 1998
Alpinists ($n = 17$)	3–5 h/d for 9 d	HC	4,000–5,500 m	Vo_2max ↑Lact/Vel	Rodríguez et al., 1999
Competitive ($n = 126$, 37 w + 89 m)	4 wk	Altitude	LH-TL 1,250/2,500 m	↑Vo_2max in responders	Stray-Gundersen and Levine, 1999
Alpinists ($n = 9$)	2 h/d 14 d	HC	5,000 m	↑V_E ↑SaO_2 during exercise at 5,000m	Ricart et al., 2000
Elite athletes ($n = 18$; 2 w + 16 m) -Hypoxia ($n = 8$; 2 w + 6 m) -Control ($n = 10$; 10 m)	10 d	NH (LH-TL)	$FiO_2 = 0.158$ (≈2,200 m)	↓400-m race time ↑resting blood pH	Nummela and Rusko, 2000
Elite alpinists ($n = 6$)	3–5 h/d for 17 d	HC	4,000–5,500 m	↑TtE ↑Lact/Vel	Casas M. et al., 2000
Competitive ($n = 23$; 11 w + 12 m) -Hypoxia ($n = 11$) -Normoxia ($n = 12$)	3 h/d, 5 d/wk for 4 wk	HC	4,000–5,500 m	Marginal ↑VO_2max ($p < 0.07$) but only in swimmers	Rodríguez et al., 2007
Elite athletes ($n = 41$) -XC Skiers ($n = 11$) -Swimmers ($n = 18$) -Runners ($n = 12$)	18 nights 13 nights 18 nights	NH and Altitude (LH-TL)	1,200m/ /2,500–3,500 m /2,500–3,000 m /2,500–3,000 m	↑VO_2max ↑VO_2max ↑VO_2max	Richalet and Gore, 2008
Competitive ($n = 28$; 11 w + 17 m)	3 h/d, 5 d/wk for 4 wk	HC	4,000–5,500 m	No changes in submaximal economy	Truijens et al., 2008
Meta-Analysis of 51 studies on elite and sub-elite athletes	Diverse	Natural vs. artificial altitude (no discrimination between artificial NH or HH)	Diverse	↑Maximal endurance power output after natural and brief intermittent artificial LH-TL	Bonetti and Hopkins, 2009
Randomized, placebo-controlled, double-blind study ($n = 40$; 18 w + 22 m)	3 × 70 min/wk for 3 wk exercising + 4 × 90 min passive for 1 wk	NH	2,500 m (wk-1) 3,000 m (wk-2) 3,500 m (wk-3) 4,500 m (wk-4)	↓AMS 1st d at 3,611 m ≅AMS 2nd d at 4,559 m	Schommer et al., 2010
Healthy men ($n = 26$) Randomized, placebo-controlled, double-blind study	1 h/d for 1 wk	NH	$FiO_2 = 0.126$ (≈4,500 m)	↓AMS after 8 h at $FIo_2 = 0.113$ (≈5,300 m)	Wille et al., 2012
Female netballer players ($n = 30$) -Hypoxic training -Vascular occlusion training -Control	0–90° bilateral knee extension and flexion 3 sess/wk for 5 wk	NH	FiO_2 = variable to maintain SpO_2≈80%	↑MVC_3 ↑MVC_{30} ↑$Reps_{20}$	Manimmanakorn et al., 2013
USARIEM Retrospective review ($n = 170$; 37 w + 133 m)	Several	Altitude, HC and NH	4,300 m	HC or altitude much more effective than NH for ↓AMS and ↑performance during acute altitude exposure	Fulco et al., 2013
Healthy unacclimatized men ($n = 42$) -Hypoxia ($n = 21$) -Normoxia ($n = 21$)	Sleep for 14 consecutive nights	NH	FiO_2≈0.145 (≈2,600 m)	↓AMS after 20 h at $FIo_2 = 0.12$ (≈4,500 m)	Dehnert et al., 2014
Healthy men ($n = 16$) -Hypoxia ($n = 9$) -Normoxia ($n = 7$)	Resistance training 2 sess/wk for 8 wk (16 sessions in total)	NH	$FiO_2 = 0.144$ (≈3,000 m)	↑Muscular endurance ↑VEGF ↑Capillary-to-fiber ratio	Kon et al., 2014

(Continued)

TABLE 7 | Continued

Subjects	Time of hypoxia	Hypoxia method	Hypoxia dosage	Outcome	References
Male elite athletes (n = 12) -Hypoxia (n = 6) -Normoxia (n = 6)	CST 3 sess/wk for 4 wk (27 h in total)	HC	3,000 m	↑Anaerobic performance	Álvarez-Herms et al., 2015a
Elite swimmers (n = 54; 30 w + 24 m)	3 or 4 wk	Altitude LH-TH vs. LL-TL vs. LH-TH+TL	690/2,320 m	↓TT for LH-TH+TL	Rodríguez et al., 2015
Male trained triathletes (n = 18) -Hypoxia (n = 9) -Normoxia (n = 9)	1 h/d × 2 d/wk for 7 wk	NH	FiO_2 = 0.145–0.15 (≈2,800–2,500 m)	No differences in aerobic performance	Ramos-Campo et al., 2015
Male well-trained triathletes (n = 16)	18 d	NH and Altitude LH-TL	1,100/2,250 m	↑VO_2max ↓3-km run time	Saugy et al., 2016
Well-trained (n = 16)	Acute exposure during HIIE jump test	NH	FiO_2 = 0.165 (≈1,900 m) FiO_2 = 0.135 (≈3,500 m)	↑Effort perception	Álvarez-Herms et al., 2016
Well-trained men (n = 16)	Acute exposure during 5 × 3 45° leg press and bench press at 85% 1RM test	NH	FiO_2 = 0.165 (≈1,900 m)	Serum ↑Lactate ↑GH	Filopoulos et al., 2017
Male endurance-trained (n = 15) -Hypoxia (n = 9) -Normoxia (n = 6)	IHT 6 × (5:5) at 80–85% of vVO_2max 3 sess/wk for 6 wk	NH	FiO_2 = 0.106 (≈5,000 m) (wk 1–2) FiO_2 = 0.114 (≈5,500 m) (wk 3–6)	↑TtE at 95% VO_2max	Sanchez and Borrani, 2018

1RM, one repetition maximum; Altitude, geographical altitude; AMS, acute mountain sickness; CST, circuit strength training; FiO_2, Fraction of inspired oxygen; HC, Hypobaric Chamber; HIIE, high intensity intervallic exercise; HT, hypoxic test (at 4,800 m equivalent attitude); IHT, Intermittent hypoxic training alternating hypoxia during exercise with normoxia during recovery between sets; Lact/Vel, Lactate/Velocity curve (up-arrow means right shift); LH-TL, Living High-Training Low; LH-TH, Living High-Training High; MVC_3, 3 s maximal voluntary contraction; MVC_{30}, 30 s maximal voluntary contraction; NH, Normobaric hypoxia; TtE, Time to exhaustion; $Reps_{20}$, maximal number of repetitions at 20% 1RM; TT, time trial; USARIEM, United States Army Research Institute of Environmental Medicine; VO_2max, maximal oxygen consumption capacity.

a determined alveolar oxygen partial pressure, regardless of the technical means used. However, data in the literature present consistent discrepancies after applying hypobaric and normobaric hypoxia, which could be attributed to alterations in other environmental parameters that affect alveolar gas composition, such as carbon dioxide partial pressure, humidity and temperature. For instance, even for the same level of oxygen partial pressure, the atmospheric composition in a small hypoxic tent with low air turnover (limited by the flow capacity of the hypoxic device) can be very different from the air composition in a hypobaric chamber. Generally, the use of powerful vacuum pumps in hypobaric chamber systems guarantees sufficient renewal of the air inside the room, thus preventing carbon dioxide accumulation and a rise in air temperature and humidity, factors that could become unbalanced in small volume hypoxic tents, especially with exercising subjects inside. In a comparative study of hypobaric (low pressure chamber) and normobaric hypoxia (hypoxic tent) during a submaximal exercise test in the same subjects, differences were observed in some cardiorespiratory and heart rate variability parameters between the two artificial hypoxia systems used (Basualto-Alarcón et al., 2012).

An interesting and dynamic debate, which is beyond the scope of this review, is currently under way among altitude researchers concerning whether or not hypobaric hypoxia induces different responses from normobaric hypoxia (Girard, 2012; Millet et al., 2012; Hauser et al., 2016; Saugy et al., 2016). Some evidences demonstrate that there are different physiological responses and outcomes between exposure to normobaric and hypobaric hypoxia conditions (Savourey et al., 2003; Fulco et al., 2013; Millet et al., 2013; Beidleman et al., 2014; Debevec and Millet, 2014; Boos et al., 2016; DiPasquale, 2017). For instance, it has been reported that the decrease in air density that accompanies the partial pressure drop of oxygen at geographic altitude affects the way in which explosive actions are executed and increases movement velocity and power during force-velocity bench presses in comparison to normobaric hypoxia (Feriche et al., 2014).

CONCLUSIONS

A growing body of knowledge supports the beneficial effects of natural or simulated altitude techniques on health outcomes (Navarrete-Opazo and Mitchell, 2014; Millet et al., 2016; Lizamore and Hamlin, 2017). Future research should be oriented to: (1) gain more in-depth knowledge of the subcellular mechanisms involved in the hypoxic response at different tissue levels, (2) standardize hypoxia exposure methods and establish a universal method for measuring, and repeatedly applying, hypoxic dosage, (3) improve predictions of individual hypoxia tolerance to prevent possible negative consequences, (4) apply this new knowledge to the selection and education of altitude workers, (5) improve altitude acclimatization, altitude training camps and altitude competition events to benefit mountaineers, athletes and coaches, and finally (6) cautiously explore the application of IEHH in pathological conditions.

AUTHOR CONTRIBUTIONS

GV, JV, AR, and LC contributed to the initial draft of the manuscript; GV and JT edited the document after contributions from all authors; All authors reviewed and approved the final version.

ACKNOWLEDGMENTS

This study was supported in part by research grants DEP2010-22205-C02-01, DEP2010-2205-C02-02, DEP2013 48334-C2-1P, and DEP2013-48334-C2-2-P from the Plan Nacional de I+D+i (Spain's Ministry of Economy, Industry and Competitiveness). The authors thank Christopher Evans and Paula Weiss (Language Advisory Service, Universitat de Barcelona) for their help editing the manuscript.

REFERENCES

Agadzhanyan, N. A., and Torshin, V. I. (1986). Effect of adaptation to hypoxia on resistance of rats to the epileptogenic action of penicillin. *Bull. Exp. Biol. Med.* 102, 1669–1671. doi: 10.1007/BF00840791

Agani, F. H., Puchowicz, M., Chavez, J. C., Pichiule, P., and LaManna, J. (2002). Role of nitric oxide in the regulation of HIF-1α expression during hypoxia. *Am. J. Physiol. Cell Physiol.* 283, C178–C186. doi: 10.1152/ajpcell.00381.2001

Aleshin, I. A., Kots, I. I., Tverdokhlib, V. P., Galiautdinov, G. S., Vdovenko, L. G., Zabirov, M. R., et al. (1993). [The nondrug treatment of hypertension patients by their adaptation to periodic hypoxia in a barochamber]. *Ter. Arkh.* 65, 23–29.

Allegra, L., Cogo, A., Legnani, D., Diano, P. L., Fasano, V., and Negretto, G. G. (1995). High altitude exposure reduces bronchial responsiveness to hypo-osmolar aerosol in lowland asthmatics. *Eur. Respir. J.* 8, 1842–1846. doi: 10.1183/09031936.95.08111842

Almendros, I., Wang, Y., and Gozal, D. (2014). The polymorphic and contradictory aspects of intermittent hypoxia. *Am. J. Physiol. Lung Cell. Mol. Physiol.* 307, L129–L140. doi: 10.1152/ajplung.00089.2014

Álvarez-Herms, J., Julià-Sánchez, S., Corbi, F., Pagès, T., and Viscor, G. (2015a). A program of circuit resistance training under hypobaric hypoxia conditions improves the anaerobic performance of athletes. *Sci. Sports* 31, 78–87. doi: 10.1016/j.scispo.2015.08.005

Álvarez-Herms, J., Julià-Sánchez, S., Gatterer, H., Blank, C., Corbi, F., Pagès, T., et al. (2016). Anaerobic training in hypoxia: A new approach to stimulate the rating of effort perception. *Physiol. Behav.* 163, 37–42. doi: 10.1016/j.physbeh.2016.04.035

Álvarez-Herms, J., Julià-Sánchez, S., Hamlin, M., and Viscor, G. (2015b). Strength training under hypoxic conditions. *Physiol. Rep.* 3:e12227. doi: 10.14814/phy2.12227

Antezana, A. M., Kacimi, R., Le Trong, J. L., Marchal, M., Abousahl, I., Dubray, C., et al. (1994). Adrenergic status of humans during prolonged exposure to the altitude of 6,542 m. *J. Appl. Physiol.* 76, 1055–1059. doi: 10.1152/jappl.1994.76.3.1055

Arcasoy, M. O. (2008). The non-haematopoietic biological effects of erythropoietin. *Br. J. Haematol.* 141, 14–31. doi: 10.1111/j.1365-2141.2008.07014.x

Ascenzi, P., di Masi, A., Leboffe, L., Fiocchetti, M., Nuzzo, M. T., Brunori, M., et al. (2016). Neuroglobin: From structure to function in health and disease. *Mol. Aspects Med.* 52, 1–48. doi: 10.1016/j.mam.2016.10.004

Asemu, G., Neckár, J., Szárszoi, O., Papousek, F., Ostádal, B., and Kolar, F. (2000). Effects of adaptation to intermittent high altitude hypoxia on ischemic ventricular arrhythmias in rats. *Physiol. Res.* 49, 597–606. Available online at: http://www.biomed.cas.cz/physiolres/pdf/49/49_597.pdf

Asemu, G., Papousek, F., Ostádal, B., and Kolár, F. (1999). Adaptation to high altitude hypoxia protects the rat heart against ischemia-induced arrhythmias. Involvement of mitochondrial K(ATP) channel. *J. Mol. Cell. Cardiol.* 31, 1821–1831. doi: 10.1006/jmcc.1999.1013

Bailey, D. M., Davies, B., and Young, I. S. (2001). Intermittent hypoxic training: implications for lipid peroxidation induced by acute normoxic exercise in active men. *Clin. Sci.* 101, 465–475. doi: 10.1042/cs1010465

Bärtsch, P., and Swenson, E. R. (2013). Clinical practice: acute high-altitude illnesses. *N. Engl. J. Med.* 368, 2294–2302. doi: 10.1056/NEJMcp1214870

Bärtsch, P., Dehnert, C., Friedmann-Bette, B., and Tadibi, V. (2008). Intermittent hypoxia at rest for improvement of athletic performance. *Scand. J. Med. Sci. Sports* 18(Suppl. 1), 50–56. doi: 10.1111/j.1600-0838.2008.00832.x

Basualto-Alarcón, C., Rodas, G., Galilea, P. A., Riera, J., Pagés, T., Ricart, A., et al. (2012). Cardiorespiratory parameters during submaximal exercise under acute exposure to normobaric and hypobaric hypoxia. *Apunt. Med. l'Esport* 47, 65–72. doi: 10.1016/j.apunts.2011.11.005

Beidleman, B. A., Fulco, C. S., Staab, J. E., Andrew, S. P., and Muza, S. R. (2014). Cycling performance decrement is greater in hypobaric versus normobaric hypoxia. *Extrem. Physiol. Med.* 3:8. doi: 10.1186/2046-7648-3-8

Bhattarai, D., Xu, X., and Lee, K. (2017). Hypoxia-inducible factor-1 (HIF-1) inhibitors from the last decade (2007 to 2016): A "structure-activity relationship" perspective. *Med. Res. Rev.* 38, 1–39. doi: 10.1002/med.21477

Bonetti, D. L., and Hopkins, W. G. (2009). Sea-level exercise performance following adaptation to hypoxia: a meta-analysis. *Sports Med.* 39, 107–127. doi: 10.2165/00007256-200939020-00002

Boos, C. J., O'Hara, J. P., Mellor, A., Hodkinson, P. D., Tsakirides, C., Reeve, N., et al. (2016). A four-way comparison of cardiac function with normobaric normoxia, normobaric hypoxia, hypobaric hypoxia and genuine high altitude. *PLoS ONE* 11:e0152868. doi: 10.1371/journal.pone.0152868

Bouslama, M., Adla-Biassette, H., Ramanantsoa, N., Bourgeois, T., Bollen, B., Brissaud, O., et al. (2015). Protective effects of intermittent hypoxia on brain and memory in a mouse model of apnea of prematurity. *Front. Physiol.* 6:313. doi: 10.3389/fphys.2015.00313

Burger, D., Xenocostas, A., and Feng, Q. P. (2009). Molecular basis of cardioprotection by erythropoietin. *Curr. Mol. Pharmacol.* 2, 56–69. doi: 10.2174/1874467210902010056

Burmester, T., and Hankeln, T. (2004). Neuroglobin: a respiratory protein of the nervous system. *News Physiol. Sci.* 19, 110–113. doi: 10.1152/nips.01513.2003

Burmester, T., Weich, B., Reinhardt, S., and Hankeln, T. (2000). A vertebrate globin expressed in the brain. *Nature* 407, 520–523. doi: 10.1038/35035093

Burtscher, M., Pachinger, O., Ehrenbourg, I., Günther, M., Faulhaber, M., Reinhard, P., et al. (2004). Intermittent hypoxia increases exercise tolerance in elderly men with and without coronary artery disease. *Int J Cardiol.* 96, 247–254. doi: 10.1016/j.ijcard.2003.07.021

Cabrera-Aguilera, I., Rizo-Roca, D., Marques, E., Santocildes, G., Pagès, T., Viscor, G., et al. (in press). Additive effects of intermittent hypobaric hypoxia and endurance training on body weight, food intake, and oxygen consumption in rats. *High Alt. Med. Biol.* doi: 10.1089/ham.2018.0013

Cai, Z., Manalo, D. J., Wei, G., Rodriguez, E. R., Fox-Talbot, K., Lu, H., et al. (2003). Hearts from rodents exposed to intermittent hypoxia or erythropoietin are protected against ischemia-reperfusion injury. *Circulation* 108, 79–85. doi: 10.1161/01.CIR.0000078635.89229.8A

Canouï-Poitrine, F., Veerabudun, K., Larmignat, P., Letournel, M., Bastuji-Garin, S., and Richalet, J.-P. (2014). Risk prediction score for severe high altitude illness: a cohort study. *PLoS ONE* 9:e100642. doi: 10.1371/journal.pone.0100642

Casas, H., Casas, M., Ricart, A., Rama, R., Ibáñez, J., Palacios, L., et al. (2000). Efectiveness of three short intermittent hypobaric hypoxia protocols: hematological responses. *J. Exerc. Physiol.* 3, 38–45. Available online at: http://www.asep.org/asep/asep/PAGES.PDF

Casas, M., Casas, H., Pagés, T., Rama, R., Ricart, A., Ventura, J. L., et al. (2000). Intermittent hypobaric hypoxia induces altitude acclimation and improves the lactate threshold. *Aviat. Space. Environ. Med.* 71, 125–30.

Chapman, R. F., Stray-Gundersen, J., and Levine, B. D. (1998). Individual variation in response to altitude training. *J. Appl. Physiol.* 85, 1448–1456. doi: 10.1152/jappl.1998.85.4.1448

Chateauvieux, S., Grigorakaki, C., Morceau, F., Dicato, M., and Diederich, M. (2011). Erythropoietin, erythropoiesis and beyond. *Biochem. Pharmacol.* 82, 1291–1303. doi: 10.1016/j.bcp.2011.06.045

Chávez, J. C., Agani, F., Pichiule, P., and LaManna, J. C. (2000). Expression of hypoxia-inducible factor-1alpha in the brain of rats during chronic hypoxia. *J. Appl. Physiol.* 89, 1937–1942. doi: 10.1152/jappl.2000.89.5.1937

Chavez, J. C., and LaManna, J. C. (2002). Activation of hypoxia-inducible factor-1 in the rat cerebral cortex after transient global ischemia: potential role of insulin-like growth factor-1. *J. Neurosci.* 22, 8922–8931. doi: 10.1523/JNEUROSCI.22-20-08922.2002

Chiu, J. T., Wells, I., and Novey, H. S. (1981). Incidence of fungal precipitins in patients treated with beclomethasone dipropionate aerosol. *Ann. Allergy* 46, 137–9.

Chouabe, C., Ricci, E., Amsellem, J., Blaineau, S., Dalmaz, Y., Favier, R., et al. (2004). Effects of aging on the cardiac remodeling induced by chronic high-altitude hypoxia in rat. *Am. J. Physiol. Heart Circ. Physiol.* 287, H1246–H1253. doi: 10.1152/ajpheart.00199.2004

Christie, P. E., Yntema, J. L., Tagari, P., Ysselstijn, H., Ford-Hutchinson, A. W., and Lee, T. H. (1995). Effect of altitude on urinary leukotriene (LT) E4 excretion and airway responsiveness to histamine in children with atopic asthma. *Eur. Respir. J.* 8, 357–363. doi: 10.1183/09031936.95.08030357

Cogo, A., Basnyat, B., Legnani, D., and Allegra, L. (1997). Bronchial asthma and airway hyperresponsiveness at high altitude. *Respiration.* 64, 444–449. doi: 10.1159/000196721

Cogo, A., Fischer, R., and Schoene, R. (2004). Respiratory diseases and high altitude. *High Alt. Med. Biol.* 5, 435–444. doi: 10.1089/ham.2004.5.435

Corral, L., Conde, L., Guillam,ó, E., Blasi, J., Juncadella, M., Javierre, C., et al. (2014a). Circulating progenitor cells during exercise, muscle electro-stimulation and intermittent hypobaric hypoxia in patients with traumatic brain injury: a pilot study. *NeuroRehabilitation* 35, 763–769. doi: 10.3233/NRE-141172

Corral, L., Javierre, C., Blasi, J., Viscor, G., Ricart, A., and Ventura, J. L. (2014b). Combined intermittent hypobaric hypoxia and muscle electro-stimulation: a method to increase circulating progenitor cell concentration? *J. Transl. Med.* 12:174. doi: 10.1186/1479-5876-12-174

Costa, D. C., Alva, N., Trigueros, L., Gamez, A., Carbonell, T., and Rama, R. (2013). Intermittent hypobaric hypoxia induces neuroprotection in kainate-induced oxidative stress in rats. *J. Mol. Neurosci.* 50, 402–410. doi: 10.1007/s12031-012-9945-8

Dale, E. A., Ben Mabrouk, F., and Mitchell, G. S. (2014). Unexpected benefits of intermittent hypoxia: enhanced respiratory and nonrespiratory motor function. *Physiology (Bethesda).* 29, 39–48. doi: 10.1152/physiol.00012.2013

Debevec, T., and Mekljavic, I. B. (2013). Short intermittent hypoxia for improvement of athletic performance: reality or a placebo? / Kratkotrajna intermitentna hipoksija za izboljsanje sportne sposobnosti: realnost ali placebo? *Kinesiol. Slov.* 19, 5–28. Available online at: https://search.proquest.com/openview/22ce1795696590210cf7a98ba0253a14/1?

Debevec, T., and Millet, G. (2014). Discerning normobaric and hypobaric hypoxia: significance of exposure duration. *J. Appl. Physiol.* 116:1255. doi: 10.1152/japplphysiol.00319.2013.5

Dehnert, C., Böhm, A., Grigoriev, I., Menold, E., and Bärtsch, P. (2014). Sleeping in moderate hypoxia at home for prevention of acute mountain sickness (AMS): a placebo-controlled, randomized double-blind study. *Wilderness Environ. Med.* 25, 263–271. doi: 10.1016/j.wem.2014.04.004

DeNoon, D. J. (2008). FDA panel asks: are asthma drugs safe? *Medscape WebMD*, December 10th. Available online at: https://www.medscape.com/viewarticle/585129 [Accessed December 27, 2017]

Di Prampero, P. E., Piñera Limas, F., and Sassi, G. (1970). Maximal muscular power, aerobic and anaerobic, in 116 athletes performing at the XIXth olympic games in Mexico. *Ergonomics* 13, 665–674. doi: 10.1080/00140137008931192

DiPasquale, D. M. (2017). Moving the debate forward: are normobaric and hypobaric hypoxia interchangeable in the study of altitude? *Curr. Sports Med. Rep.* 16, 68–70. doi: 10.1249/JSR.0000000000000337

Dougherty, B. J., Terada, J., Springborn, S. R., Vinit, S., MacFarlane, P. M., and Mitchell, G. S. (2017). Daily acute intermittent hypoxia improves breathing function with acute and chronic spinal injury via distinct mechanisms. *Respir. Physiol. Neurobiol.* doi: 10.1016/j.resp.2017.05.004. [Epub ahead of print].

Droma, Y., Kunii, O., Yangzom, Y., Shan, M., Pingzo, L., and Song, P. (2007). Prevalence and severity of asthma and allergies in schoolchildren in Lhasa, Tibet. *Clin. Exp. Allergy* 37, 1326–1333. doi: 10.1111/j.1365-2222.2007.02781.x

Eckardt, K. U., Boutellier, U., Kurtz, A., Schopen, M., Koller, E. A., and Bauer, C. (1989). Rate of erythropoietin formation in humans in response to acute hypobaric hypoxia. *J Appl Physiol.* 66, 1785–1788. doi: 10.1152/jappl.1989.66.4.1785

Egrie, J. C., Strickland, T. W., Lane, J., Aoki, K., Cohen, A. M., Smalling, R., et al. (1986). Characterization and biological effects of recombinant human erythropoietin. *Immunobiology* 172, 213–224. doi: 10.1016/S0171-2985(86)80101-2

Engst, R., and Vocks, E. (2000). [High-mountain climate therapy for skin diseases and allergies - Mode of action, therapeutic results, and immunologic effects]. *Rehabilitation* 39, 215–222. doi: 10.1055/s-2000-5897

Esteva, S., Panisello, P., Torrella, J. R., Pagés, T., and Viscor, G. (2009). Blood rheology adjustments in rats after a program of intermittent exposure to hypobaric hypoxia. *High Alt. Med. Biol.* 10, 275–281. doi: 10.1089/ham.2008.1086

Fábián, Z., Taylor, C. T., and Nguyen, L. K. (2016). Understanding complexity in the HIF signaling pathway using systems biology and mathematical modeling. *J. Mol. Med. (Berl).* 94, 377–390. doi: 10.1007/s00109-016-1383-6

Fairfax, A. J., David, V., and Douce, G. (1999). Laryngeal aspergillosis following high dose inhaled fluticasone therapy for asthma. *Thorax* 54, 860–861. doi: 10.1136/thx.54.9.860

Faiss, R., Girard, O., and Millet, G. P. (2013). Advancing hypoxic training in team sports: from intermittent hypoxic training to repeated sprint training in hypoxia. *Br. J. Sports Med.* 47 (Suppl. 1), i45–i50. doi: 10.1136/bjsports-2013-092741

Feriche, B., García-Ramos, A., Calderón-Soto, C., Drobnic, F., Bonitch-Góngora, J. G., Galilea, P. A., et al. (2014). Effect of acute exposure to moderate altitude on muscle power: hypobaric hypoxia vs. *normobaric hypoxia. PLoS ONE* 9:e114072. doi: 10.1371/journal.pone.0114072

Filopoulos, D., Cormack, S. J., and Whyte, D. G. (2017). Normobaric hypoxia increases the growth hormone response to maximal resistance exercise in trained men. *Eur. J. Sport Sci.* 17, 821–829. doi: 10.1080/17461391.2017.1317834

Fulco, C. S., Beidleman, B. A., and Muza, S. R. (2013). Effectiveness of preacclimatization strategies for high-altitude exposure. *Exerc. Sport Sci. Rev.* 41, 55–63. doi: 10.1097/JES.0b013e31825eaa33

Garvican-Lewis, L. A., Sharpe, K., and Gore, C. J. (2016). Time for a new metric for hypoxic dose? *J. Appl. Physiol.* 121, 352–355. doi: 10.1152/japplphysiol.00579.2015

Gatterer, H., Haacke, S., Burtscher, M., Faulhaber, M., Melmer, A., Ebenbichler, C., et al. (2015). Normobaric Intermittent Hypoxia over 8 Months Does Not Reduce Body Weight and Metabolic Risk Factors-a Randomized, Single Blind, Placebo-Controlled Study in Normobaric Hypoxia and Normobaric Sham Hypoxia. *Obes. Facts* 8, 200–209. doi: 10.1159/000431157

Ge, R. L., Chen, Q. H., and He, L. G. (1994). [Characteristics of hypoxic ventilatory response in Tibetan living at moderate and high altitudes]. *Zhonghua Jie He He Hu Xi Za Zhi* 17, 364–6, 384.

Ge, R., Witkowski, S., Zhang, Y., Alfrey, C., Sivieri, M., Karlsen, T., et al. (2002). Determinants of erythropoietin release in response to short-term hypobaric hypoxia. *J. Appl. Physiol.* 92, 2361–2367. doi: 10.1152/japplphysiol.00684.2001

Girard, O. (2012). Comments on point:counterpoint: hypobaric hypoxia induces / does not induce different responses from normobaric hypoxia - Reduced air resistance with terrestrial altitude alters run sprint performance. *J. Appl. Physiol. (Bethesda, MD* 1985) 112:1788. doi: 10.1152/japplphysiol.00356.2012

Gore, C. J., Rodríguez, F. A., Truijens, M. J., Townsend, N. E., Stray-Gundersen, J., and Levine, B. D. (2006). Increased serum erythropoietin but not red cell production after 4 wk of intermittent hypobaric hypoxia (4,000-5,500 m). *J. Appl. Physiol.* 101, 1386–1393. doi: 10.1152/japplphysiol.00342.2006

Gourgoulianis, K. I., Brelas, N., Hatziparasides, G., Papayianni, M., and Molyvdas, P. A. (2001). The influence of altitude in bronchial asthma. *Arch. Med. Res.* 32, 429–431. doi: 10.1016/S0188-4409(01)00302-2

Hamlin, M. J., Lizamore, C. A., and Hopkins, W. G. (2018). The effect of natural or simulated altitude training on high-intensity intermittent running performance in team-sport athletes: a meta-analysis. *Sports Med.* 48, 431–446. doi: 10.1007/s40279-017-0809-9

Harrison, C. C., Fleming, J. M., and Giles, L. C. (2002). Does interval hypoxic training affect the lung function of asthmatic athletes. *New Zeal. J. Sport. Med.* 30, 64–67. Available online at: http://blm-altitude.com/blm/uploads/images/Gallery/Applications/Health-and-Wellness/Lung-Function-Asthmatic-Athletes.pdf

Haskell, W. L., Lee, I.-M., Pate, R. R., Powell, K. E., Blair, S. N., Franklin, B. A., et al. (2007). Physical activity and public health: updated recommendation for adults from the American College of Sports Medicine and the American Heart Association. *Med. Sci. Sports Exerc.* 39, 1423–1434. doi: 10.1161/CIRCULATIONAHA.107.185649

Haufe, S., Wiesner, S., Engeli, S., Luft, F. C., and Jordan, J. (2008). Influences of normobaric hypoxia training on metabolic risk markers in human subjects. *Med. Sci. Sports Exerc.* 40, 1939–1944. doi: 10.1249/MSS.0b013e31817f1988

Hauser, A., Schmitt, L., Troesch, S., Saugy, J. J., Cejuela-Anta, R., Faiss, R., et al. (2016). Similar hemoglobin mass response in hypobaric and normobaric hypoxia in athletes. *Med. Sci. Sports Exerc.* 48, 734–741. doi: 10.1249/MSS.0000000000000808

Heuschmann, P., Hoffmann, U., Piepoli, M. F., Verschuren, M., Halcox, J., Reviewers, D., et al. (2010). Secondary prevention through cardiac rehabilitation : physical activity counselling and exercise training Key components of the position paper from the Cardiac rehabilitation section of the European Association of Cardiovascular Prevention and Rehabilitation. *Eur Heart J.* 31, 1967–1976. doi: 10.1093/eurheartj/ehq236

Hirota, K., and Semenza, G. L. (2006). Regulation of angiogenesis by hypoxia-inducible factor 1. *Crit. Rev. Oncol. Hematol.* 59, 15–26. doi: 10.1016/j.critrevonc.2005.12.003

Hornbein, T. F. (2001). The high-altitude brain. *J. Exp. Biol.* 204, 3129–3132. Available online at: http://jeb.biologists.org/content/204/18/3129.full.pdf

Ibáñez, J., Casas, H., Casas, M., Rama, R., Ricart, A., Ventura, J. L., et al. (2000). L'exposition intermittente à l'hypoxie en caisson hypobarique: effets physiologiques et applications. *Médecine du Sport* 74, 32–34

Jia, Y., Suzuki, N., Yamamoto, M., Gassmann, M., and Noguchi, C. T. (2012). Endogenous erythropoietin signaling facilitates skeletal muscle repair and recovery following pharmacologically induced damage. *FASEB J.* 26, 2847–2858. doi: 10.1096/fj.11-196618

Julian, C. G., Gore, C. J., Wilber, R. L., Daniels, J. T., Fredericson, M., Stray-Gundersen, J., et al. (2004). Intermittent normobaric hypoxia does not alter performance or erythropoietic markers in highly trained distance runners. *J. Appl. Physiol.* 96, 1800–1807. doi: 10.1016/j.obhdp.2010.11.002

Karagiannidis, C., Hense, G., Rueckert, B., Mantel, P. Y., Ichters, B., Blaser, K., et al. (2006). High-altitude climate therapy reduces local airway inflammation and modulates lymphocyte activation. *Scand. J. Immunol.* 63, 304–310. doi: 10.1111/j.1365-3083.2006.01739.x

Karlsen, T., Resaland, G. K., Ri-Li, G., Sivieri, M., Witowski, S., Yates, R., et al. (2001). Epo response to 24 hrs of artificial hypobaric hypoxia predicts epo response to natural altitude. *Med. Sci. Sport. Exerc.* 33:S98. Available online at: https://journals.lww.com/acsm-msse/Fulltext/2001/05001/EPO_RESPONSE_TO_24_HRS_OF_ARTIFICIAL_HYPOBARIC.556.aspx

Kenney, W. L., Wilmore, J. H., Costill, D. L., and Wilmore, J. H. (2012). *Physiology of Sport and Exercise. 5th Edn.* Champaign IL: Human Kinetics

Khodaee, M., Grothe, H. L., Seyfert, J. H., and VanBaak, K. (2016). Athletes at high altitude. *Sports Health* 8, 126–132. doi: 10.1177/1941738116630948

Kiechl-Kohlendorfer, U., Horak, E., Mueller, W., Strobl, R., Haberland, C., Fink, F. M., et al. (2007). Living at high altitude and risk of hospitalisation for atopic asthma in children: results from a large prospective birth-cohort study. *Arch. Dis. Child.* 92, 339–342. doi: 10.1136/adc.2006.106278

Kon, M., Ohiwa, N., Honda, A., Matsubayashi, T., Ikeda, T., Akimoto, T., et al. (2014). Effects of systemic hypoxia on human muscular adaptations to resistance exercise training. *Physiol. Rep.* 2, 1–13. doi: 10.14814/phy2.12033

Korcarz, C. E., Peppard, P. E., Young, T. B., Chapman, C. B., Hla, K. M., Barnet, J. H., et al. (2016). Effects of obstructive sleep apnea and obesity on cardiac remodeling: the wisconsin sleep cohort study. *Sleep* 39, 1187–1195. doi: 10.5665/sleep.5828

Koyasu, S., Kobayashi, M., Goto, Y., Hiraoka, M., and Harada, H. (2017). Regulatory mechanisms of hypoxia-inducible factor 1 activity: two decades of knowledge. *Cancer Sci.* 109, 560–571. doi: 10.1111/cas.13483

Kushwah, N., Jain, V., Deep, S., Prasad, D., Singh, S. B., and Khan, N. (2016). Neuroprotective role of intermittent hypobaric hypoxia in unpredictable chronic mild stress induced depression in rats. *PLoS ONE* 11:e0149309. doi: 10.1371/journal.pone.0149309

Kusunose, K., Phelan, D., Seicean, S., Seicean, A., Collier, P., Boden, K. A., et al. (2016). Relation of echocardiographic characteristics of the right-sided heart with incident heart failure and mortality in patients with sleep-disordered breathing and preserved left ventricular ejection fraction. *Am. J. Cardiol.* 118, 1268–1273. doi: 10.1016/j.amjcard.2016.07.024

Leone, R. J., and Lalande, S. (2017). Intermittent hypoxia as a means to improve aerobic capacity in type 2 diabetes. *Med. Hypotheses* 100, 59–63. doi: 10.1016/j.mehy.2017.01.010

Levett, D. Z., Radford, E. J., Menassa, D. A., Graber, E. F., Morash, A. J., Hoppeler, H., et al. (2012). Acclimatization of skeletal muscle mitochondria to high-altitude hypoxia during an ascent of Everest. *FASEB J.* 26, 1431–1441. doi: 10.1096/fj.11-197772

Levine, B. D., and Stray-Gundersen, J. (1997). "Living high-training low": effect of moderate-altitude acclimatization with low-altitude training on performance. *J. Appl. Physiol.* 83, 102–112. doi: 10.1152/jappl.1997.83.1.102

Li, X., Zhao, H., Wu, Y., Zhang, S., Zhao, X., Zhang, Y., et al. (2014). Up-regulation of hypoxia-inducible factor-1alpha enhanced the cardioprotective effects of ischemic postconditioning in hyperlipidemic rats. *Acta Biochim Biophys Sin* 46, 112–118. doi: 10.1093/abbs/gmt132

Lieberman, P., Protopapas, A., Reed, E., Youngs, J. W., and Kanki, B. G. (1994). Cognitive defects at altitude. *Nature* 372:325. doi: 10.1038/372325a0

Lippl, F. J., Neubauer, S., Schipfer, S., Lichter, N., Tufman, A., Otto, B., et al. (2010). Hypobaric hypoxia causes body weight reduction in obese subjects. *Obesity* 18, 675–681. doi: 10.1038/oby.2009.509

Lizamore, C. A., and Hamlin, M. J. (2017). The use of simulated altitude techniques for beneficial cardiovascular health outcomes in nonathletic, sedentary, and clinical populations: a literature review. *High Alt. Med. Biol.* 18, 305–321. doi: 10.1089/ham.2017.0050

London, G. M., Zins, B., Pannier, B., Naret, C., Berthelot, J. M., Jacquot, C., et al. (1989). Vascular changes in hemodialysis patients in response to recombinant human erythropoietin. *Kidney Int.* 36, 878–882. doi: 10.1038/ki.1989.274

Lundby, C., Calbet, J. A. L., Sander, M., Van Hall, G., Mazzeo, R. S., Stray-Gundersen, J., et al. (2007). Exercise economy does not change after acclimatization to moderate to very high altitude. *Scand. J. Med. Sci. Sport.* 17, 281–291. doi: 10.1111/j.1600-0838.2006.00530.x

Magalhães, J., Falcão-Pires, I., Gonçalves, I. O., Lumini-Oliveira, J., Marques-Aleixo, I., Dos Passos, E., et al. (2013). Synergistic impact of endurance training and intermittent hypobaric hypoxia on cardiac function and mitochondrial energetic and signaling. *Int. J. Cardiol.* 168, 5363–5371. doi: 10.1016/j.ijcard.2013.08.001

Magalhães, J., Gonçalves, I. O., Lumini-Oliveira, J., Marques-Aleixo, I., Passos, E., Rocha-Rodrigues, S., et al. (2014). Modulation of cardiac mitochondrial permeability transition and apoptotic signaling by endurance training and intermittent hypobaric hypoxia. *Int. J. Cardiol.* 173, 40–45. doi: 10.1016/j.ijcard.2014.02.011

Manimmanakorn, A., Manimmanakorn, N., Taylor, R., Draper, N., Billaut, F., Shearman, J. P., et al. (2013). Effects of resistance training combined with vascular occlusion or hypoxia on neuromuscular function in athletes. *Eur. J. Appl. Physiol.* 113, 1767–1774. doi: 10.1007/s00421-013-2605-z

Marquez, J. L., Rubinstein, S., Fattor, J. A., Shah, O., Hoffman, A. R., and Friedlander, A. L. (2013). Cyclic hypobaric hypoxia improves markers of glucose metabolism in middle-aged men. *High Alt. Med. Biol.* 14, 263–272. doi: 10.1089/ham.2012.1057

Marticorena, E. A. (1993). Montañismo médico: Rehabilitación de pacientes coronarios con by-pass. *Rev. Peru. Cardiol.* 19, 25–29.

Marticorena, E. A., Marticorena, J. A., Gutierrez, I., Rodríguez, V., Fernández-Dávila, L., Oyola, L., et al. (2001). Factor relajante del endotelio (ON) en rehabilitación coronaria con cámara hipobárica. *Rev. Peru. Cardiol.* 27, 148–149. Avavilable online at: http://sisbib.unmsm.edu.pe/bvrevistas/cardiologia/anteriores.htm

Mateika, J. H., El-Chami, M., Shaheen, D., and Ivers, B. (2015). Intermittent hypoxia: a low-risk research tool with therapeutic value in humans: Fig. 1. *J. Appl. Physiol.* 118, 520–532. doi: 10.1152/japplphysiol.00564.2014

Meehan, R. T. (1987). Immune suppression at high altitude. *Ann. Emerg. Med.* 16, 974–979. doi: 10.1016/S0196-0644(87)80743-6

Meehan, R., Duncan, U., Neale, L., Taylor, G., Muchmore, H., Scott, N., et al. (1988). Operation Everest II: alterations in the immune system at high altitudes. *J. Clin. Immunol.* 8, 397–406. doi: 10.1007/BF00917156

Milledge, J. S. (2003). "Altitude deterioration," in *Health and Height* (Barcelona: Publicacions Universitat de Barcelona), 173–180. Available online at: http://www.publicacions.ub.edu/ficha.aspx?cod=06036

Millet, G. P., Debevec, T., Brocherie, F., Malatesta, D., and Girard, O. (2016). Therapeutic use of exercising in hypoxia : promises and limitations. *Front. Physiol.* 7:224. doi: 10.3389/fphys.2016.00224

Millet, G. P., Faiss, R., and Pialoux, V. (2012). Point: Counterpoint: Hypobaric hypoxia induces/does not induce different responses from normobaric hypoxia. *J. Appl. Physiol.* 112, 1783–1784. doi: 10.1152/japplphysiol.00067.2012

Millet, G. P., Faiss, R., and Pialoux, V. (2013). Evidence for differences between hypobaric and normobaric hypoxia is conclusive. *Exerc. Sport Sci. Rev.* 41:133. doi: 10.1097/JES.0b013e318271a5e1

Najean, Y., Moynot, A., Deschryver, F., Zins, B., Naret, C., Jacquot, C., et al. (1989). Kinetics of erythropoiesis in dialysis patients receiving recombinant erythropoietin treatment. *Nephrol. Dial. Transplant* 4, 350–355. doi: 10.1093/oxfordjournals.ndt.a091889

Navarrete-Opazo, A., Alcayaga, J., Sepúlveda, O., Rojas, E., and Astudillo, C. (2017a). Repetitive intermittent hypoxia and locomotor training enhances walking function in incomplete spinal cord injury subjects: a randomized, triple-blind, placebo-controlled clinical trial. *J. Neurotrauma* 34, 1803–1812. doi: 10.1089/neu.2016.4478

Navarrete-Opazo, A., and Mitchell, G. S. (2014). Therapeutic potential of intermittent hypoxia: a matter of dose. *Am. J. Physiol. Regul. Integr. Comp. Physiol.* 307, R1181–R1197. doi: 10.1152/ajpregu.00208.2014

Navarrete-Opazo, A., Dougherty, B. J., and Mitchell, G. S. (2017b). Enhanced recovery of breathing capacity from combined adenosine 2A receptor inhibition and daily acute intermittent hypoxia after chronic cervical spinal injury. *Exp. Neurol.* 287, 93–101. doi: 10.1016/j.expneurol.2016.03.026

Navarrete-Opazo, A., Vinit, S., Dougherty, B. J., and Mitchell, G. S. (2015). Daily acute intermittent hypoxia elicits functional recovery of diaphragm and inspiratory intercostal muscle activity after acute cervical spinal injury. *Exp. Neurol.* 266, 1–10. doi: 10.1016/j.expneurol.2015.02.007

Nelson, M. E., Rejeski, W. J., Blair, S. N., Duncan, P. W., Judge, J. O., King, A. C., et al. (2007). Physical activity and public health in older adults: recommendation from the American College of Sports Medicine and the American Heart Association. *Med. Sci. Sports Exerc.* 39, 1435–1445. doi: 10.1249/mss.0b013e3180616aa2

Netzer, N. C., Chytra, R., and Küpper, T. (2008). Low intense physical exercise in normobaric hypoxia leads to more weight loss in obese people than low intense physical exercise in normobaric sham hypoxia. *Sleep Breath.* 12, 129–134. doi: 10.1007/s11325-007-0149-3

Noguchi, C. T., Asavaritikrai, P., Teng, R., and Jia, Y. (2007). Role of erythropoietin in the brain. 64, 159–171 doi: 10.1016/j.critrevonc.2007.03.001

Nummela, A., and Rusko, H. (2000). Acclimatization to altitude and normoxic training improve 400-m running performance at sea level. *J. Sports Sci.* 18, 411–419. doi: 10.1080/02640410050074340

Núñez-Espinosa, C., Douziech, A., Ríos-Kristjánsson, J. G., Rizo, D., Torrella, J. R., Pagès, T., et al. (2014). Effect of intermittent hypoxia and exercise on blood rheology and oxygen transport in trained rats. *Respir. Physiol. Neurobiol.* 192, 112–117. doi: 10.1016/j.resp.2013.12.011

Ohta, A. A., Diwanji, R., Kini, R., Subramanian, M., Ohta, A. A., and Sitkovsky, M. (2011). *In vivo* T cell activation in lymphoid tissues is inhibited in the oxygen-poor microenvironment. *Front. Immunol.* 2:27. doi: 10.3389/fimmu.2011.00027

Oliver, S. J., Macdonald, J. H., Harper Smith, A. D., Lawley, J. S., Gallagher, C., a., Di Felice, U., et al. (2013). High altitude impairs *in vivo* immunity in humans. *High Alt. Med. Biol.* 14, 144–149. doi: 10.1089/ham.2012.1070

Ostadal, B., and Kolar, F. (2007). Cardiac adaptation to chronic high-altitude hypoxia: beneficial and adverse effects. *Respir. Physiol. Neurobiol.* 158, 224 236. doi: 10.1016/j.resp.2007.03.005

Ostádal, B., Kolár, F., Pelouch, V., Bass, A., Samánek, M., and Procházka, J. (1989). The effect of chronic hypoxia on the developing cardiopulmonary system. *Biomed. Biochim. Acta* 48, S58–62.

Panisello, P., Torrella, J. R., Esteva, S., Pagés, T., and Viscor, G. (2008). Capillary supply, fibre types and fibre morphometry in rat tibialis anterior and diaphragm muscles after intermittent exposure to hypobaric hypoxia. *Eur. J. Appl. Physiol.* 103, 203–213. doi: 10.1007/s00421-008-0691-0

Panisello, P., Torrella, J. R., Pagés, T., and Viscor, G. (2007). Capillary supply and fiber morphometry in rat myocardium after intermittent exposure to hypobaric hypoxia. *High Alt. Med. Biol.* 8, 322–330. doi: 10.1089/ham.2007.1030

Ramos-Campo, D. J., Martínez-Sánchez, F., Esteban-García, P., Rubio-Arias, J. A., Clemente-Suarez, V. J., and Jiménez-Díaz, J. F. (2015). The effects of intermittent hypoxia training on hematological and aerobic performance in triathletes. *Acta Physiol. Hung.* 102, 409–418. doi: 10.1556/036.102.2015.4.8

Ramos-Campo, D. J., Scott, B. R., Alcaraz, P. E., and Rubio-Arias, J. A. (2018). The efficacy of resistance training in hypoxia to enhance strength and muscle growth: a systematic review and meta-analysis. *Eur. J. Sport Sci.* 18, 92–103. doi: 10.1080/17461391.2017.1388850

Rathat, C., Richalet, J. P., Herry, J. P., and Larmignat, P. (1992). Detection of high-risk subjects for high altitude diseases. *Int. J. Sports Med.* 13 (Suppl. 1), S76–S78. doi: 10.1055/s-2007-1024602

Rey, S., and Semenza, G. L. (2010). Hypoxia-inducible factor-1-dependent mechanisms of vascularization and vascular remodelling. *Cardiovasc. Res.* 86, 236–242. doi: 10.1093/cvr/cvq045

Reynafarje, B. D., and Marticorena, E. (2002). Bioenergetics of the heart at high altitude: environmental hypoxia imposes profound transformations on the myocardial process of ATP synthesis. *J. Bioenerg. Biomembr.* 34, 407–412. doi: 10.1023/A:1022597523483

Ricart, A., Casas, H., Casas, M., Pagés, T., Palacios, L., Rama, R., et al. (2000). Acclimatization near home? Early respiratory changes after short-term intermittent exposure to simulated altitude. *Wilderness Environ. Med.* 11, 84–88. doi: 10.1580/1080-6032(2000)011[0084:ANHERC]2.3.CO;2

Richalet, J. P., Bittel, J., Herry, J. P., Savourey, G., Le Trong, J. L., Auvert, J. F., et al. (1992). Use of a hypobaric chamber for pre-acclimatization before climbing Mount Everest. *Int. J. Sports Med.* 13 (Suppl. 1), S216–S220. doi: 10.1055/s-2007-1024644

Richalet, J. P., Souberbielle, J. C., Antezana, A. M., Déchaux, M., Le Trong, J. L., Bienvenu, A., et al. (1994). Control of erythropoiesis in humans during prolonged exposure to the altitude of 6,542 m. *Am. J. Physiol.* 266, R756–R764. doi: 10.1152/ajpregu.1994.266.3.R756

Richalet, J.-P., and Gore, C. J. (2008). Live and/or sleep high:train low, using normobaric hypoxia. *Scand. J. Med. Sci. Sports* 18 (Suppl. 1), 29–37. doi: 10.1111/j.1600-0838.2008.00830.x

Richalet, J.-P., and Lhuissier, F. J. (2015). Aging, tolerance to high altitude, and cardiorespiratory response to hypoxia. *High Alt. Med. Biol.* 16:117–124. doi: 10.1089/ham.2015.0030

Rizo-Roca, D., Bonet, J. B., Inal, B., Ríos-Kristjánsson, J. G., and Pagès, T., Viscor, G., et al. (2018). Contractile activity is necessary to trigger intermittent hypobaric hypoxia-induced fibre size and vascular adaptations in skeletal muscle. *Front. Physiol.* 9:481. doi: 10.3389/FPHYS.2018.00481

Rizo-Roca, D., Ríos-Kristjánsson, J. G., Núñez-Espinosa, C., Santos-Alves, E., Gonçalves, I. O., Magalhães, J., et al. (2017a). Intermittent hypobaric hypoxia combined with aerobic exercise improves muscle morphofunctional recovery after eccentric exercise to exhaustion in trained rats. *J. Appl. Physiol.* 122, 580–592. doi: 10.1152/japplphysiol.00501.2016

Rizo-Roca, D., Ríos-Kristjánsson, J. G., Núñez-Espinosa, C., Santos-Alves, E., Magalhães, J., Ascensão, A., et al. (2017b). Modulation of mitochondrial biomarkers by intermittent hypobaric hypoxia and aerobic exercise after eccentric exercise in trained rats. *Appl. Physiol. Nutr. Metab.* 42, 683–693. doi: 10.1139/apnm-2016-0526

Rodríguez, F. A., Casas, H., Casas, M., Pagés, T., Rama, R., Ricart, A., et al. (1999). Intermittent hypobaric hypoxia stimulates erythropoiesis and improves aerobic capacity. *Med. Sci. Sports Exerc.* 31, 264–268. doi: 10.1097/00005768-199902000-00010

Rodríguez, F. A., Iglesias, X., Feriche, B., Calderón-Soto, C., Chaverri, D., Wachsmuth, N. B., et al. (2015). Altitude Training in Elite Swimmers for Sea Level Performance (Altitude Project). *Med. Sci. Sports Exerc.* 47, 1965–1978. doi: 10.1249/MSS.0000000000000626

Rodríguez, F. A., Truijens, M. J., Townsend, N. E., Gore, C. J., Levine, B. D., Truijens, M. J., et al. (2007). Performance of runners and swimmers after four weeks of intermittent hypobaric hypoxic exposure plus sea level training. *J. Appl. Physiol.* 103, 1523–1535. doi: 10.1152/japplphysiol.01320.2006

Rodríguez, F. A., Ventura, J. L., Casas, M., Casas, H., Pagés, T., Rama, R., et al. (2000). Erythropoietin acute reaction and haematological adaptations to short, intermittent hypobaric hypoxia. *Eur. J. Appl. Physiol.* 82, 170–177. doi: 10.1007/s004210050669

Ross, H. H., Sandhu, M. S., Cheung, T. F., Fitzpatrick, G. M., Sher, W. J., Tiemeier, A. J., et al. (2012). *In vivo* intermittent hypoxia elicits enhanced expansion and neuronal differentiation in cultured neural progenitors. *Exp. Neurol.* 235, 238–245. doi: 10.1016/j.expneurol.2012.01.027

Salpeter, S. R., Buckley, N. S., Ormiston, T. M., and Salpeter, E. E. (2006). Meta-analysis: effect of long-acting beta-agonists on severe asthma exacerbations and asthma-related deaths. *Ann. Intern. Med.* 144, 904–912. doi: 10.7326/0003-4819-144-12-200606200-00126

Sanchez, A. M. J., and Borrani, F. (2018). Effects of intermittent hypoxic training performed at high hypoxia level on exercise performance in highly trained runners. *J. Sports Sci.* 36, 2045–2052. doi: 10.1080/02640414.2018.1434747

Saugy, J. J., Schmitt, L., Hauser, A., Constantin, G., Cejuela, R., Faiss, R., et al. (2016). Same Performance Changes after Live High-Train Low in Normobaric vs. *Hypobaric Hypoxia. Front. Physiol.* 7:138. doi: 10.3389/fphys.2016.00138

Savourey, G., Launay, J.-C., Besnard, Y., Guinet, A., and Travers, S. (2003). Normo- and hypobaric hypoxia: are there any physiological differences? *Eur. J. Appl. Physiol.* 89, 122–126. doi: 10.1007/s00421-002-0789-8

Schommer, K., Wiesegart, N., Menold, E., Haas, U., Lahr, K., Buhl, H., et al. (2010). Training in normobaric hypoxia and its effects on acute mountain sickness after rapid ascent to 4559 m. *High Alt. Med. Biol.* 11, 19–25. doi: 10.1089/ham.2009.1019

Schultze-Werninghaus, G. (2006). Should asthma management include sojourns at high altitude? *Chem. Immunol. Allergy* 91, 16–29. doi: 10.1159/000090227

Schultze-Werninghaus, G. (2008). [Effects of high altitude on bronchial asthma]. *Pneumologie* 62, 170–176. doi: 10.1055/s-2007-1016442

Serebrovska, T. V., Portnychenko, A. G., Drevytska, T. I., Portnichenko, V. I., Xi, L., Egorov, E., et al. (2017). Intermittent hypoxia training in prediabetes patients: Beneficial effects on glucose homeostasis, hypoxia tolerance and gene expression. *Exp. Biol. Med. (Maywood).* 242, 1542–1552. doi: 10.1177/1535370217723578

Serebrovska, T. V., Serebrovska, Z. O., and Egorov, E. (2016). Fitness and therapeutic potential of intermittent hypoxia training: a matter of dose. *Fiziol. Zh.* 62, 78–91. Available online at: https://fz.kiev.ua/journals/2016_V.62/2016_3/2016_3-78-91.pdf

Serebrovskaya, T. V., Manukhina, E. B., Smith, M. L., Downey, H. F., and Mallet, R. T. (2008). Intermittent hypoxia: cause of or therapy for systemic hypertension? *Exp. Biol. Med. (Maywood).* 233, 627–650. doi: 10.3181/0710-MR-267

Serebrovskaya, T. V., Swanson, R. J., and Kolesnikova, E. E. (2003). Intermittent hypoxia: mechanisms of action and some applications to bronchial asthma treatment. *J. Physiol. Pharmacol.* 54 (Suppl. 1), 35–41. doi: 10.318/0710-MR-

Serebrovskaya, T., V (2002). Intermittent hypoxia research in the former Soviet Union and the Commonwealth of Independent States: history and review of the concept and selected applications. *High Alt. Med. Biol.* 3, 205–221. doi: 10.1089/15270290260131939

Simon, H. U., Grotzer, M., Nikolaizik, W. H., Blaser, K., and Schöni, M. H. (1994). High altitude climate therapy reduces peripheral blood T lymphocyte activation, eosinophilia, and bronchial obstruction in children with house-dust mite allergic asthma. *Pediatr. Pulmonol.* 17, 304–311. doi: 10.1002/ppul.1950170507

Singh, I., Chohan, I. S., Lal, M., Khanna, P. K., Srivastava, M. C., Nanda, R. B., et al. (1977). Effects of high altitude stay on the incidence of common diseases in man. *Int. J. Biometeorol.* 21, 93–122. doi: 10.1007/BF01553705

Steiner, C. (2009). [Atopic dermatitis and psoriasis: what is the benefit of in-patient high altitude climate therapy?]. *Praxis (Bern. 1994).* 98, 1373–1376. doi: 10.1024/1661-8157.98.23.1373

Stray-Gundersen, J., and Levine, B. D. (1999). "Living high and training low" can improve sea level performance in endurance *athletes.* 33, 150–151. doi: 10.1136/bjsm.33.3.150

Stray-Gundersen, J., Chapman, R. F., and Levine, B. D. (2001). "Living high-training low" altitude training improves sea level performance in male and female elite runners. *J. Appl. Physiol.* 91, 1113–1120. doi: 10.1152/jappl.2001.91.3.1113

Streeter, K. A., Sunshine, M. D., Patel, S., Gonzalez-Rothi, E. J., Reier, P. J., Baekey, D. M., et al. (2017). Intermittent hypoxia enhances functional connectivity of midcervical spinal interneurons. *J. Neurosci.* 37, 8349–8362. doi: 10.1523/JNEUROSCI.0992-17.2017

Sy, D. Q., Thanh Binh, M. H., Quoc, N. T., Hung, N. V., Quynh Nhu, D. T., Bao, N. Q., et al. (2007). Prevalence of asthma and asthma-like symptoms in Dalat Highlands, Vietnam. *Singapore Med. J.* 48, 294–303. Available online at: http://smj.sma.org.sg/4804/4804a4.pdf

Thanigaimani, S., McLennan, E., Linz, D., Mahajan, R., Agbaedeng, T. A., Lee, G., et al. (2017). Progression and reversibility of stretch induced atrial remodeling: characterization and clinical implications. *Prog. Biophys. Mol. Biol.* 130, 376–386. doi: 10.1016/j.pbiomolbio.2017.07.010

Tin'kov, A. N., and Aksenov, V. A. (2002). Effects of intermittent hypobaric hypoxia on blood lipid concentrations in male coronary heart disease patients. *High Alt. Med. Biol.* 3, 277–282. doi: 10.1089/152702902320604250

Truijens, M. J., Rodríguez, F. A., Townsend, N. E., Stray-Gundersen, J., Gore, C. J., and Levine, B. D. (2008). The effect of intermittent hypobaric hypoxic exposure and sea level training on submaximal economy in well-trained swimmers and runners. *J. Appl. Physiol.* 104, 328–337. doi: 10.1152/japplphysiol.01324.2006

Trumbower, R. D., Hayes, H. B., Mitchell, G. S., Wolf, S. L., and Stahl, V. A. (2017). Effects of acute intermittent hypoxia on hand use after spinal cord trauma: a preliminary study. *Neurology* 89, 1904–1907. doi: 10.1212/WNL.0000000000004596

Tsai, Y.-W., Yang, Y.-R., Sun, S. H., Liang, K.-C., and Wang, R.-Y. (2013). Post ischemia intermittent hypoxia induces hippocampal neurogenesis and synaptic alterations and alleviates long-term memory impairment. *J. Cereb. Blood Flow Metab.* 33, 764–773. doi: 10.1038/jcbfm.2013.15

Turban, K., and Spengler, L. (1906). Resultate der Asthmabehandlung im Hochgebirge. *Jahresbericht der Schweiz Balneol. Gesellschaft* 2:72.

Valle, M., del, P., García-Godos, F., Woolcott, O. O., Marticorena, J. M., Rodríguez, V., et al. (2006). Improvement of myocardial perfusion in coronary patients after intermittent hypobaric hypoxia. *J. Nucl. Cardiol.* 13, 69–74. doi: 10.1016/j.nuclcard.2005.11.008

van der Woude, H. J., Winter, T. H., and Aalbers, R. (2001). Decreased bronchodilating effect of salbutamol in relieving methacholine induced moderate to severe bronchoconstriction during high dose treatment with long acting beta2 agonists. *Thorax* 56, 529–535. doi: 10.1136/thorax.56.7.529

van Velzen, E., van den Bos, J. W., Benckhuijsen, J. A., van Essel, T., de Bruijn, R., and Aalbers, R. (1996). Effect of allergen avoidance at high altitude on direct and indirect bronchial hyperresponsiveness and markers of inflammation in children with allergic asthma. *Thorax* 51, 582–584. doi: 10.1136/thx.51.6.582

Virués-Ortega, J., Garrido, E., Javierre, C., and Kloezeman, K. C. (2006). Human behaviour and development under high-altitude conditions. *Dev. Sci.* 9, 400–410. doi: 10.1111/j.1467-7687.2006.00505.x

Viscor, G., Javierre, C., Pagès, T., Ventura, J.-L., Ricart, A., Martin-Henao, G., et al. (2009). Combined intermittent hypoxia and surface muscle electrostimulation as a method to increase peripheral blood progenitor cell concentration. *J. Transl. Med.* 7:91. doi: 10.1186/1479-5876-7-91

Viscor, G., Ricart, A., Pagès, T., Corral, L., Javierre, C. F., and Ventura, J. L. (2014). Intermittent hypoxia for obstructive sleep apnea? *High Alt. Med. Biol.* 15, 520–521. doi: 10.1089/ham.2014.1060

Vocks, E., Schuh, A., Liebich, C., Topperzer, U., and Ring, J. (1999). High altitude stay and plasma cortisol level in psoriasis. *Phys. Medizin Rehabil. Kurortmedizin* 9, 197–201. doi: 10.1055/s-2008-1061805

Wang, G. L., and Semenza, G. L. (1993). General involvement of hypoxia-inducible factor 1 in transcriptional response to hypoxia. *Proc. Natl. Acad. Sci.U.S.A.* 90, 4304–4308. doi: 10.1073/pnas.90.9.4304

Ward, M. (1954). High altitude deterioration. *Proc. R. Soc. London. Ser. B Biol. Sci.* 143, 40–42. doi: 10.2307/83018

West, J. B., Schoene, R. B., Luks, A. M., and Milledge, J. S. (2013). *High Altitude Medicine and Physiology. 5th Edn.* Boca Raton, FL: CRC Press/Taylor & Francis Group

Wiesner, S., Haufe, S., Engeli, S., Mutschler, H., Haas, U., Luft, F. C., et al. (2010). Influences of normobaric hypoxia training on physical fitness and metabolic risk markers in overweight to obese subjects. *Obesity* 18, 116–120. doi: 10.1038/oby.2009.193

Wilber, R. L. (2004). *Altitude training and Athletic Performance.* Champaign, IL: Human Kinetics.

Wilber, R. L., Stray-Gundersen, J., and Levine, B. D. (2007). Effect of hypoxic "dose" on physiological responses and sea-level performance. *Med. Sci. Sports Exerc.* 39, 1590–1599. doi: 10.1249/mss.0b013e3180de49bd

Wille, M., Gatterer, H., Mairer, K., Philippe, M., Schwarzenbacher, H., Faulhaber, M., et al. (2012). Short-term intermittent hypoxia reduces the severity of acute mountain sickness. *Scand. J. Med. Sci. Sport.* 22, 79–85. doi: 10.1111/j.1600-0838.2012.01499.x

Wu, Q., Yu, K. X., Ma, Q. S., and Liu, Y. N. (2015). Effects of intermittent hypobaric hypoxia preconditioning on the expression of neuroglobin and Bcl-2 in the rat hippocampal CA1 area following ischemia-reperfusion. *Genet. Mol. Res.* 14, 10799–10807. doi: 10.4238/2015.September.9.18

Xi, L., and Serebrovskaya, T. V. (eds) (2012). *Intermittent Hypoxia and Human Diseases.* London: Springer.

Xing, B., Chen, H., Zhang, M., Zhao, D., Jiang, R., Liu, X., et al. (2008). Ischemic postconditioning inhibits apoptosis after focal cerebral ischemia/reperfusion injury in the rat. *Stroke* 39, 2362–2369. doi: 10.1161/STROKEAHA.107.507939

Xu, Q., Wang, S., Jiang, X., Zhao, Y., Gao, M., Zhang, Y., et al. (2007). Hypoxia-induced astrocytes promote the migration of neural progenitor cells via vascular endothelial factor, stem cell factor, stromal-derived factor-1alpha and monocyte chemoattractant protein-1 upregulation *in vitro. Clin. Exp. Pharmacol. Physiol.* 34, 624–631. doi: 10.1111/j.1440-1681.2007.04619.x

Yangzong, Nafstad, P., Madsen, C., and Bjertness, E. (2006). Childhood asthma under the north face of Mount Everest. *J. Asthma* 43, 393–398. doi: 10.1080/02770900600710326

Zhang, H., Li, Q., Li, Z., Mei, Y., and Guo, Y. (2008). The protection of Bcl-2 overexpression on rat cortical neuronal injury caused by analogous ischemia/reperfusion *in vitro. Neurosci. Res.* 62, 140–146. doi: 10.1016/j.neures.2008.07.002

Zhang, K., Zhao, T., Huang, X., Wu, L., Wu, K., Zhu, L., et al. (2014a). Notch1 mediates postnatal neurogenesis in hippocampus enhanced by intermittent hypoxia. *Neurobiol. Dis.* 64, 66–78. doi: 10.1016/j.nbd.2013.12.010

Zhang, S., Guo, Z., Yang, S., Ma, H., Fu, C., Wang, S., et al. (2016a). Chronic intermittent hybobaric hypoxia protects against cerebral ischemia via modulation of mitoKATP. *Neurosci. Lett.* 635, 8–16. doi: 10.1016/j.neulet.2016.10.025

Zhang, Y., Wang, L., Dey, S., Alnaeeli, M., Suresh, S., Rogers, H., et al. (2014b). Erythropoietin action in stress response, tissue maintenance and metabolism. *Int. J. Mol. Sci.* 15, 10296–10333. doi: 10.3390/ijms150610296

Zhang, Z., Yan, J., and Shi, H. (2016b). Role of hypoxia Inducible Factor 1 in hyperglycemia-exacerbated blood-brain barrier disruption in ischemic stroke. *Neurobiol. Dis.* 95, 82–92. doi: 10.1016/j.nbd.2016.07.012

Zhou, S., Yi, T., Liu, R., Bian, C., Qi, X., He, X., et al. (2012). Proteomics identification of annexin A2 as a key mediator in the metastasis and proangiogenesis of endometrial cells in human adenomyosis. *Mol. Cell. Proteomics* 11:M112.017988. doi: 10.1074/mcp.M112.017988

Zhu, L., Zhao, T., Li, H., Zhao, H., Wu, L.-Y., Ding, A., et al. (2005). Neurogenesis in the adult rat brain after intermittent hypoxia. *Brain Res.* 1055, 1–6. doi: 10.1016/j.brainres.2005.04.075

Zimna, A., and Kurpisz, M. (2015). Hypoxia-inducible factor-1 in physiological and pathophysiological angiogenesis: applications and therapies. *Biomed Res. Int.* 2015:549412. doi: 10.1155/2015/549412

10

Chronic Intermittent Hypoxia-Induced Vascular Dysfunction in Rats is Reverted by *N*-Acetylcysteine Supplementation and Arginase Inhibition

Bernardo J. Krause[1*†], Paola Casanello[1,2], Ana C. Dias[3], Paulina Arias[3], Victoria Velarde[3], German A. Arenas[3], Marcelo D. Preite[4] and Rodrigo Iturriaga[3†]

[1] Division of Pediatrics, Faculty of Medicine, Pontificia Universidad Católica de Chile, Santiago, Chile, [2] Division of Obstetrics & Gynecology, Faculty of Medicine, Pontificia Universidad Católica de Chile, Santiago, Chile, [3] Laboratorio de Neurobiología, Facultad de Ciencias Biológicas, Pontificia Universidad Católica de Chile, Santiago, Chile, [4] Departamento de Química Orgánica, Facultad de Química, Pontificia Universidad Católica de Chile, Santiago, Chile

***Correspondence:**
Bernardo J. Krause
bjkrause@uc.cl

† These authors have contributed equally to this work.

Chronic intermittent hypoxia (CIH), the main attribute of obstructive sleep apnea (OSA), produces oxidative stress, endothelial dysfunction, and hypertension. Nitric oxide (NO) plays a critical role in controlling the vasomotor tone. The NO level depends on the L-arginine level, which can be reduced by arginase enzymatic activity, and its reaction with the superoxide radical to produce peroxynitrite. Accordingly, we hypothesized whether a combination of an arginase inhibitor and an antioxidant may restore the endothelial function and reduced arterial blood pressure (BP) in CIH-induced hypertensive rats. Male Sprague-Dawley rats 200 g were exposed either to CIH (5% O_2, 12 times/h 8 h/day) or sham condition for 35 days. BP was continuously measured by radio-telemetry in conscious animals. After 14 days, rats were treated with 2(*S*)-amino-6-boronohexanoic acid (ABH 400 μg/kg day, osmotic pump), *N*-acetylcysteine (NAC 100 mg/kg day, drinking water), or the combination of both drugs until day 35. At the end of the experiments, external carotid and femoral arteries were isolated to determine vasoactive contractile responses induced by KCL and acetylcholine (ACh) with wire-myography. CIH-induced hypertension (~8 mmHg) was reverted by ABH, NAC, and ABH/NAC administration. Carotid arteries from CIH-treated rats showed higher contraction induced by KCl (3.4 ± 0.4 vs. 2.4 ± 0.2 N/m^2) and diminished vasorelaxation elicits by ACh compared to sham rats (12.8 ± 1.5 vs. 30.5 ± 4.6%). ABH reverted the increased contraction (2.5 ± 0.2 N/m^2) and the reduced vasorelaxation induced by ACh in carotid arteries from CIH-rats (38.1 ± 4.9%). However, NAC failed to revert the enhanced vasocontraction (3.9 ± 0.6 N/m^2) induced by KCl and the diminished ACh-induced vasorelaxation in carotid arteries (10.7 ± 0.8%). Femoral arteries from CIH rats showed an increased contractile response, an effect partially reverted by ABH, but completely reverted by NAC and ABH/NAC. The impaired endothelial-dependent relaxation in femoral arteries from CIH rats was reverted by ABH and ABH/NAC. In addition, ABH/NAC at high doses had no effect on liver and kidney gross morphology and biochemical parameters. Thus, although ABH, and NAC alone and the combination of ABH/NAC were able to normalize the elevated BP, only the combined treatment of ABH/NAC normalized the vascular reactivity and the systemic oxidative stress in CIH-treated rats.

Keywords: arginase, chronic intermittent hypoxia, endothelial dysfunction, nitric oxide, oxidative stress, vascular reactivity

INTRODUCTION

Obstructive sleep apnea (OSA), a growing breathing disorder featured by cyclic episodes of partial or total airflow occlusions during sleep, is considered an independent risk factor for develop systemic hypertension and is linked with stroke, coronary artery disease, and pulmonary hypertension (McNicholas et al., 2007; Dempsey et al., 2010). The airflow occlusion produces hypoxia and hypercapnia, which in turn stimulates the carotid body (CB) causing sympathetic, hypertensive, and ventilatory responses. Among these alterations, chronic intermittent hypoxia (CIH) is considered the main factor to develop systemic hypertension (Lavie, 2003; Kheirandish-Gozal and Gozal, 2008; Dempsey et al., 2010). Pre-clinical models of rodents exposed to CIH, which mimics most of the pathologic features of OSA including hypoxemia and hypertension, are used to study the mechanisms involved in cardiovascular and autonomic alterations induced by OSA (Fletcher, 2000; Del Rio et al., 2010; Prabhakar and Kumar, 2010; Iturriaga et al., 2017). Although the link between OSA and hypertension is well established, the mechanisms underlying the onset and progression of the arterial blood pressure (BP) elevation are not well-known. It has been proposed that CIH produces oxidative stress, inflammation, and sympathetic overflow, endothelial dysfunction, and hypertension (Lévy et al., 2008; Garvey et al., 2009; Iturriaga et al., 2009). In addition, new evidences suggest that the CB is involved in generation of autonomic and cardiovascular and ventilatory alterations elicited by CIH (Iturriaga et al., 2014, 2017; Prabhakar et al., 2015). The cycles of hypoxia-reoxygenation produce oxidative stress in the CB and enhance its chemosensory responsiveness to hypoxia. The enhanced CB chemosensory drive leads to sympathetic hyperactivation of the sympatho-adrenal axis and the renin-angiotensin system (Fletcher, 2000; Iturriaga et al., 2009; Prabhakar et al., 2012).

OSA patients show endothelial dysfunction with reduced vasodilatation to ACh, and vascular remodeling characterized by increased intima-media thickness (Ip et al., 2004; Patt et al., 2010) Similarly, CIH diminish the vasodilatation induced by ACh in rats (Tahawi et al., 2001; Dopp et al., 2011). CIH produces structural changes in the rat skeletal muscle resistance arteries in the first 14 days of CIH (Philippi et al., 2010). We previously found evidence that endothelial dysfunction in CIH-induced hypertension, may result from an imbalance in the ratio of arginase-1 to eNOS expression, vascular remodeling and increased contractile capacity (Krause et al., 2015). Indeed, we found that *ex vivo* acute arginase inhibition in carotid arteries of CIH-treated rats reverted the impaired ACh-induced relaxation, an effect completely blocked by the NO-synthase inhibitors NG-nitro-L-arginine (L-NA). In addition, we found that arginase-1 protein level was increased, whereas eNOS levels decreased in CIH-derived arteries (Krause et al., 2015). Thus, it is plausible that the reduction of the oxidative stress and inhibition of the arginase enzymatic activity and may revert the vascular dysfunction and hypertension associated with CIH. It is well-known that NO levels play a critical role in vasomotor regulation, depending on L-arginine availability, which can be reduced in conditions where high arginase expression and activity have been evidenced (Demougeot et al., 2005; Bagnost et al., 2010; Krause et al., 2012; Cowburn et al., 2016). In addition, NO may react with the superoxide radical to produce peroxynitrite ($ONOO^-$). Accordingly, we hypothesized whether the administration of an arginase inhibitor and a precursor of the potent antioxidant glutathione, *N*-acetylcysteine (NAC) (Rushworth and Megson, 2014; Lasram et al., 2015; Schmitt et al., 2015), may reduce the endothelial dysfunction and hypertension induced by CIH. Thus, we assessed the effects of the arginase inhibitor 2(S)-amino-6-boronohexanoic (ABH) and the antioxidant NAC on the elevated BP and endothelial dysfunction in carotid and femoral arteries, from CIH-induced hypertensive rats. Furthermore, since arginase inhibition could interfere with the urea pathway, the effects of high doses of ABH-NAC on renal and hepatic function on rats were assessed. In a separate series, we studied the effect of a large dose of ABH of 400 μg/kg day and NAC 400 mg /kg day on renal and hepatic function and histology in rats. Proteins, creatinine, and urea were determined in urine and creatinine, urea, glutamic-oxalacetic transaminase (GOT), glutamic-pyruvic transaminase (GPT), and lactate dehydrogenase (LDH) were measured in plasma.

MATERIALS AND METHODS

Animal Care and Ethics Approval

This study was carried out in accordance with the recommendation of the Guide for the Care and Use of Laboratory Animals of the Bioethics Committee, CONICYT Chile. The experimental protocol for the animal was approved by the Bioethics Committee of the Faculty of Biological Sciences of the Pontificia Universidad Católica de Chile. For human samples the research was conducted in accordance with the Declaration of Helsinki and was approved by the Ethics Committee from the Faculty of Medicine of the Pontificia Universidad Católica de Chile (Protocol #11-247) as well as patient informed consent was obtained. Placentae were collected immediately after delivery from full-term normal normotensive, non-alcohol non-smoking, or drug consuming mothers, without any other obstetrical or medical problem.

Animals and Exposure to Chronic Intermittent Hypoxia

Experiments were done on male Sprague-Dawley rats, weighing initially ~200 g. Rats were fed with standard rat chow diet *ad libitum*, and kept on a 12-h light/dark schedule (8:00 a.m.–8:00 p.m.). Rats were exposed to CIH for 35 days, as previously described (Iturriaga et al., 2010; Del Rio et al., 2016). Briefly, unrestrained, freely moving rats were housed in individual chambers. The CIH protocol consisted of hypoxic cycles of 5–6% inspired O_2 for 20 s, followed by room air for 280 s, applied 12 times/h, 8 h/day. The chambers had a rear N_2 inlet and a front air extractor, which enables the recovery to normoxia. A computerized system controlled the valve inlets and the alternating cycles of the extractors. During hypoxia, the extractors stopped for 30 s, and the rear solenoid valves allowed 100% N_2 flow into the chambers. The O_2 level in the chambers was continuously monitored with an oxygen analyzer (Teledyne AX 380, USA). The CO_2 in the chamber was maintained low by continuous air extraction. In the Sham condition, rats were exposed to compressed air flow into chambers.

Arterial Blood Pressure Recordings

Arterial blood pressure (BP) was measured in conscious rats using radio-telemetry. Seven days before the beginning of the experiments, rats were anesthetized with 5% isoflurane and maintained with 2% isoflurane in 100% O_2 during the surgical procedure. The tip of a cannula-coupled telemetry device (PC40A-40, Data Science International, USA) was introduced into the femoral artery (Del Rio et al., 2016). After surgery rats received a subcutaneous injection of ketoprofen (1%) and enrofloxacin (1%). The BP recording was started after 5 days of recovery. The raw data from each rat was continuously collected at a sample rate of 1 KHz, and average every 24 h with the ART Dataquest Platform (Data Science International, USA).

Synthesis and Functional Studies of ABH

The 2(*S*)-amino-6-boronohexanoic acid (ABH) was synthesized by an optimization of a method previously reported by Vadon-Legoff et al. (2005), which was itself based in the previous work of Collet et al. (2000). The synthesis of ABH consisted of the preparation of the Gly-Ni-BPB complex, which was obtained by reaction of glycine (Gly), nickel(II) chloride, and 2[N-(N′-benzylprolyl)amino]benzophenone (BPB) in the presence of excess KOH in methanol. The Gly-Ni-BPB complex was treated with a base at low temperature and enantioselectively alkylated with the corresponding catechol-protected boronated bromide. The alkylated complex was then hydrolyzed with aqueous acid and purified by ion-exchange chromatography. The effectiveness of synthesized ABH was determined by measuring its ability to inhibit arginase activity, as described previously for endothelial cells (Krause et al., 2012). Briefly, basal arginase activity was determined in the presence of the synthesized inhibitor ABH and, compared with the effect of the commercial inhibitor of arginase, S-(2-boronoethyl)-L-cysteine (BEC. Sigma, USA) in protein extracts obtained from total human placental homogenates (i.e., vascular, syncytium and connective tissue) obtained with lysis buffer [1 mmol/l pepstatine A, 1 mmol/l leupeptine, 200 mmol/l phenylmethylsulfonyl fluoride (PMSF), 50 mmol/l Tris-HCl (pH 7.5), 0.2% Triton X-100] sonicated (20 pulses, 150 W, 3 min). The production of urea was measured using 70 μg of placental homogenate protein in 100 μl of reaction incubated at 37°C for 1 h in the presence of L-arginine (50 mM) and the cofactor Mn2+ (5 Mm), and the presence or absence of BEC (100 μM) or, increasing concentrations of synthesized ABH (10–1,000 μM). The catalysis was stopped by adding 4 volumes of acid solution (H2SO4: H3PO4: H2O = 1: 3: 7), and the urea formed was determined by adding 25 μl of α-isonitrosopropiophenone (9% ISPF in absolute ethanol) to the assay and heating the mixture (100°C for 45 min). The concentration of urea was measured by spectrophotometry (OD 450 nm) in an automatic plate reader based on results obtained from a urea calibration curve. We found that synthesized ABH produced a concentration-dependent inhibition of the arginase activity and that it reached levels comparable to those observed in the presence of the commercial inhibitor BEC. The Ki for ABH was 4.78 ± 1.76 μM and the solubility in water 125 g/L or 0.7 mol/L.

Experimental Procedure and Drug Administration

The antioxidant *N*-acetylcysteine (NAC, Sigma USA) was administered through drinking tap water (400 mg/kg day) from the day 14 of CIH exposure until the end of the experimental protocol. The NAC solution was prepared daily and preserved in dark condition to avoid oxidation. ABH was administrated with osmotic pumps (2ML4, Alzet Scientific Products, USA). Rats were anesthetized with isoflurane in O_2, and the osmotic pumps were implanted subcutaneously on the back. Pumps deliver ABH in saline solution at a rate of 400 μg/kg/ day. Animals were implanted with the same osmotic pumps (Alzet Scientific Products, USA) filled with saline solution. Rats were out of the hypoxic chambers for 2–3 h for the surgical implant of the osmotic pumps. After surgical procedures, rats were treated with enrofloxacin and ketoprofen as mentioned before.

Wire Myography

At the end of the experiments, external carotid and femoral arteries were surgically removed from rats anesthetized with sodium pentobarbitone (50 mg/kg ip) and placed in ice-cold PBS. Vessel segments (~2 mm) of external carotid arteries and second/third-order femoral arteries were mounted on a wire-myograph (model 610A; Danish Myo Technology A/S, Denmark) and contractile responses were studied as previously described (Krause et al., 2015). Animals were euthanized with a higher dose of sodium pentobarbitone (200 mg/kg ip). The internal diameter of vessels was defined by determining the stretch condition at which the maximal contractile response to KCl was obtained (Delaey et al., 2002). Indeed, the internal diameter of the vessels for wire myography was established by determining the opening length (or stretching condition) at which the vessel presents its maximal contractile response (Mulvany and Aalkjaer, 1990). This *ex vivo* method has been shown to accurately represent the *in vivo* internal arterial perimeter in different models (Mulvany and Aalkjaer, 1990; Delaey et al., 2002). Likewise, through this methodology, a direct correlation of the *ex vivo* contractile response with the biomechanical and structural properties of different blood vessels has been observed (Cañas et al., 2017). Isometric force in response to cumulative concentrations of KCl (16–125 mM) was assayed to determine the maximal contractile force. Similarly, isometric force in response to acetylcholine (ACh, 10^{-8}-10^{-5} mol/L) in pre-constricted vessels with 37.5 mmol/L KCl were determined. Responses were expressed as percentage of the maximal contractile effect induced by KCl at 40.8 mmol/L (%Kmax). Concentration-response curves were fit with the GraphPad Prism version 5.00 (CA, USA) to obtain the maximal effect and potency ($pD_2 = -\log EC_{50}$).

Measurement of Systemic Oxidative Stress

Plasmatic oxidative stress was measured with the TBARS assay (Cat N° 10009055, Cayman, USA) according to the protocol provided by the supplier. The concentration of thiobarbituric acid-reactive species were expressed as malondialdehyde (MDA) μmol/L. Blood samples were collected from the common carotid artery and placed in heparinized ice-cold microcentrifuge tubes after 1–2 h of the last intermittent hypoxic cycle. Plasma was separated by centrifugation and stored at −80°C.

Biosafety of NAC and ABH

Since arginase inhibition may affect the urea pathway, we evaluated whether high doses of ABH and NAC could have a hepatotoxic or nephrotoxic effect. In a separate series, two independent groups were used: one group without treatment (n = 4) and one treated with the combination of ABH and NAC (n = 8). Under isoflurane anesthesia, osmotic pumps were implanted subcutaneously (2ML4, Alzet Scientific Products USA). In the untreated animals, pumps were filled with saline solution. In the rats treated with ABH/NAC, the same osmotic pumps with ABH dissolved in saline solution were installed. Each rat received a dose of ABH of 400 μg/kg day and NAC 400 mg /kg day. Rats were kept for 28 days, and placed in metabolic cages to collect urine. Blood was collected from the ocular orbital sinus under isoflurane 5% in O_2 anesthesia. Proteins, creatinine, and urea were determined in urine and creatinine, urea, lactate dehydrogenase (LDH), glutamic-pyruvic transaminase (GPT), and glutamic-oxalacetic transaminase (GOT) were measured in plasma.

In a separate experimental series of rats (n = 6) without treatment and a group of 6 rats treated with the combination ABH/NAC, creatinine clearance was measured. The collected urine was measured to determine the 24 h volume and then centrifuged at 3,000 rpm for 10 min at 4°C to discard any precipitate. Under anesthesia with isoflurane, blood was obtained from the left ventricle. Blood was collected in heparinized tubes, centrifuged at 3,000 rpm to obtain plasma. Creatinine was measured in both plasma and urine using the Creatinine Liquicolor kit from human (Wiesbaden, Germany), which evaluates the kinetics of the reaction. Briefly, plasma and urine samples (diluted 1:50) were mixed with a solution of picric acid and alkaline buffer (NaOH/bicarbonate). Immediately the samples were transferred to a reading cell and their absorbance was measured at 492 nm at 30 s and at 2 min after the start of the reaction. With these values and using a creatinine standard, the concentration of creatinine present in each sample was determined.

Histological Staining and Examination

Anesthetized rats were perfused intracardially with phosphate buffer saline (PBS; pH 7.4) for 10 min, followed by buffered paraformaldehyde (PFA 4%, Sigma, St Louis, USA) for 10 min. The saline and PFA solutions were perfused at constant pressure of 95 mmHg. Pieces of the carotid external artery (3–4 mm length) were collected 2 mm rostral from the carotid sinus and post-fixed by immersion in buffered-PFA 4% for 12 h at 4°C. Carotid arteries were dehydrated in graded ethanol solutions followed by xylol, included in paraffin, sectioned at 5 μm and mounted on silanized slides. The vessels were stained with hematoxylin and eosin and photomicrographs were taken with an Olympus CX 31 microscope with a CCD camera (Olympus Corp, Japan). The internal diameter (ID) was measured from fixed tissues with the ImageJ software (NIH, USA).

Liver and kidney samples obtained from euthanized rats were fixed with 4% paraformaldehyde (Sigma, St Louis, USA), dehydrated and paraffin-embedded. Transverse sections (5 μM) were stained with Harris hematoxylin (5 min) and eosin (30 s) and mounted with Entellan (Merck, Whitehouse Station, NJ, USA). Microphotographs were obtained at 40x and 100x with and Olympus CX31 microscope (Olympus Corporation, Tokyo, Japan).

Statistical Data Analysis

Data were expressed as mean ± SEM. For BP recordings, the average daily MABP for each animal were grouped and compared through one-way ANOVA followed by Dunnet' multiple comparison test among the treatment groups. Comparisons between two groups were performed with the U Mann-Whitney test, and differences between more groups were assessed with one or two-way ANOVA tests, followed by Dunnet *post-hoc* comparisons. Significance was accepted to $p < 0.05$.

RESULTS

Effects of ABH and NAC on the Arterial Blood Pressure in CIH-Treated Rats

Rats submitted to CIH showed a sustained increase in mean arterial blood pressure (MABP) of ~8 mmHg after 3–4 days of exposure (**Figure 1** and **Table 1**). To demonstrate the role of arginase activity and oxidative stress in this increased arterial BP, rats exposed to CIH were treated with the arginase inhibitor ABH and/or NAC from day 14 of CIH. ABH and NAC treatment progressively reduced MABP in CIH-rats reaching basal values (**Figures 1B,C**). Similarly, simultaneous administration of ABH and NAC restored the normal MABP levels in CIH-treated rats (**Figure 1D**).

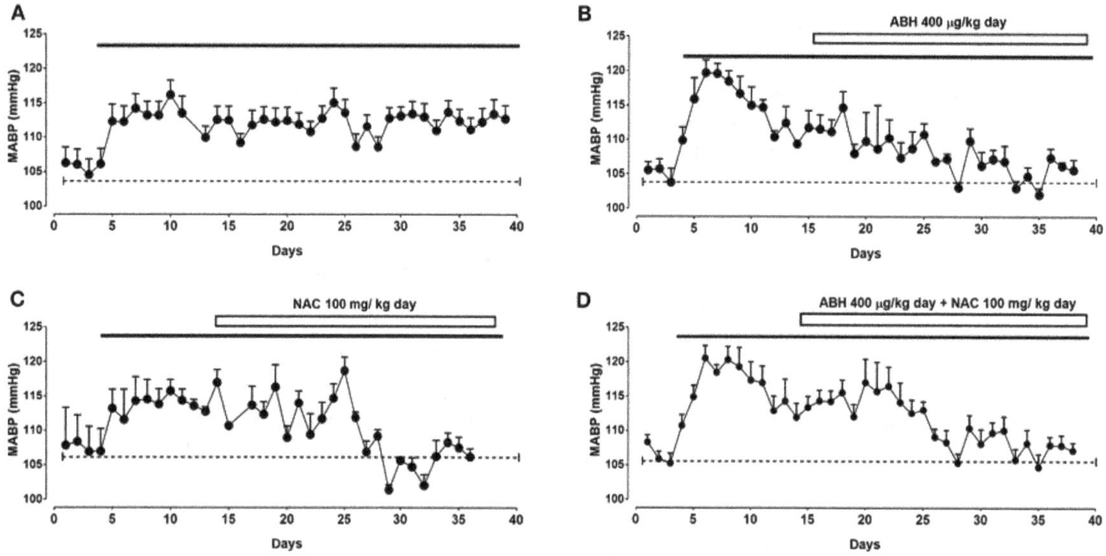

FIGURE 1 | Effects of ABH and NAC on CIH-induced hypertension. Mean arterial blood pressure (MABP) determined by telemetry in rats submitted to CIH. After 14 days rats were maintained in CIH without treatment (**A**, $n = 8$) or receiving the arginase inhibitor ABH (**B**, $n = 8$), the glutathione precursor NAC (**C**, $n = 6$), or the combination of both ABH/NAC (**D**, $n = 8$).

TABLE 1 | Effects of ABH, NAC, and ABH/NAC on arterial blood pressure.

	MABP baseline (mm Hg)	MABP 7–14 days (mm Hg)	MABP 28–35 days (mm Hg)
SHAM	106.0 ± 1.4	107.4 ± 1.5	107.1 ± 1.1
CIH	105.8 ± 0.4	112.4 ± 0.1*	112.6 ± 0.4*
CIH+ABH	105.0 ± 0.6	112.9 ± 0.6*	105.1 ± 0.7
CIH+NAC	107.5 ± 0.4	114.0 ± 0.3*	105.9 ± 0.9
CIH+ABH/NAC	106.5 ± 1.4	116.7 ± 1.4*	107.1 ± 0.8

*Mean ± SEM. *$P < 0.05$ vs. baseline. One-way ANOVA followed by Dunnet ($n = 6$–8 rats per group).*

Effect of ABH and NAC on the Contractile Responses in Arteries From CIH-Treated Rats

To determine the effects of ABH and NAC on vascular reactivity in CIH-rats, the vasoactive response to KCl of carotid and femoral artery segments were assayed using wire myography. Carotid arteries from CIH-rats showed a significant decreased internal diameter measured in histological sections of fixed tissues, whilst the treatment with ABH, NAC and their combination ABH/NAC prevented the reduction in internal diameter (**Figure 2A**). Compared with sham, maximal KCl-induced constriction was increased in CIH and CIH NAC groups, while this effect was reverted by ABH, as well as the combination of ABH/NAC (**Figure 2B**). There were no significant changes in the internal diameter of femoral arteries in the groups studied compared with sham rats (**Figure 2C**). However, maximal KCl-induced constriction was increased in CIH. The latter effect was partially reverted by ABH treatment and completely prevented by NAC, as well as ABH/NAC (**Figure 2D**).

Effect of ABH and NAC on the NOS-Dependent Relaxation in Arteries From CIH-Treated Rats

Carotid arteries from rats exposed to CIH showed a decrease in the concentration-dependent relaxation (**Figure 3A**) and maximal response (**Figure 3B**) to ACh compared to the sham group, and this effect was reverted by the combination of ABH/NAC. Similarly, treatment with NAC did not improve the response to ACh in CIH-rats, whilst ABH treated rats showed a significant increase in the maximal response compared to sham. Sensitivity (pD_2) to ACh was comparable between sham, CIH and CIH- NAC groups, but substantially increased (>1 Log unit) in CIH rats treated with ABH and ABH in combination with NAC (**Figure 3C**). Femoral arteries from rats exposed to CIH showed a decrease in the concentration-dependent relaxation (**Figure 4A**) and maximal response (**Figure 4B**) to ACh related to sham, effect reverted by NAC and ABH/NAC. CIH-ABH-treated rats showed a ~2-fold increase in the maximal response to ACh relative to the sham. Conversely, sensitivity to ACh was comparable between sham, CIH,

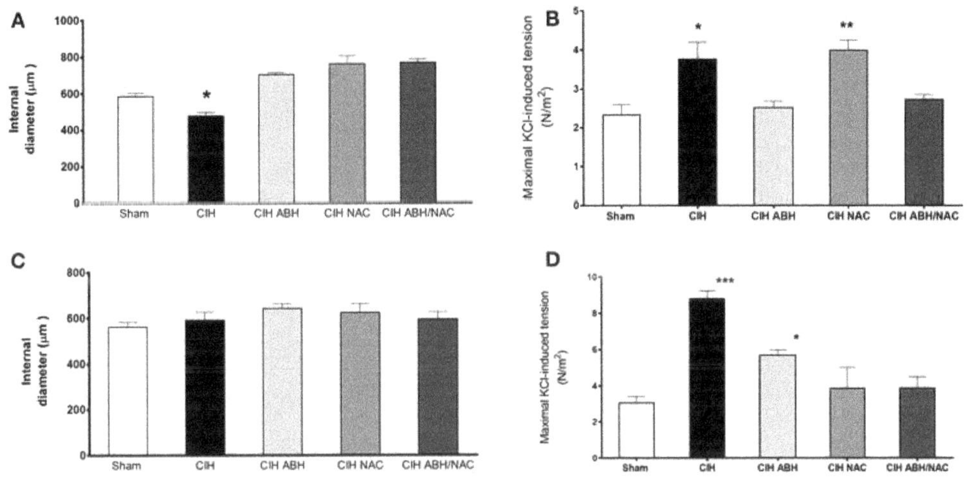

FIGURE 2 | Effects of ABH and NAC on the CIH-induced vascular remodeling. Internal diameter measured by histology in fixed tissues **(A,C)** and maximal contractile response to KCl **(B,D)** of carotid **(A,B)** and femoral **(C,D)** arteries from sham (open bars, $n = 10$), CIH (solid bars, $n = 10$), CIH treated with ABH (light gray bars, $n = 5$), CIH treated with NAC (gray bars, $n = 5$), and CIH treated with ABH, and NAC (dark gray bars, $n = 5$) rats. Values expressed as mean ± SEM, $^{*}p < 0.05$, $^{**}p < 0.01$, $^{***}p < 0.001$ vs. sham, ANOVA.

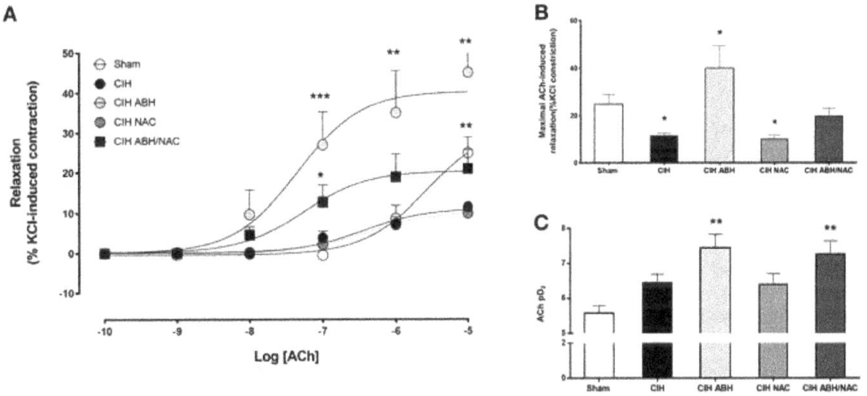

FIGURE 3 | Endothelial-dependent relaxation in carotid arteries from CIH-rats. **(A)** Concentration-dependent relaxation curves in response to acetylcholine of carotid arteries from sham (open circles, $n = 6$), CIH (solid circles, $n = 6$), CIH treated with ABH (light gray circles, $n = 6$), CIH treated with NAC (gray circles, $n = 6$) and CIH treated with ABH, and NAC (dark gray square, $n = 6$) rats. Maximal acetylcholine-induced response **(B)** and pharmacological potency (pD_2, i.e., sensitivity) **(C)** from sham (open bars), CIH (solid bars), CIH treated with ABH (light gray bars), CIH treated with NAC (gray bars), and CIH treated with ABH, and NAC (dark gray bars) rats were derived from **(A)**. Values expressed as mean ± SEM, $^{*}p < 0.05$, $^{**}p < 0.01$, $^{***}p < 0.001$ vs. sham, ANOVA.

CIH-ABH, and CIH-NAC groups, but substantially increased in CIH-rats treated with ABH in combination with NAC (**Figure 4C**).

Effects of ABH and NAC on Systemic Oxidative Stress in CIH-Rats

Systemic oxidative stress in CIH-treated rats was evaluated by determining plasma levels of MDA as an index of lipids peroxidation after 35 days of CIH or sham condition. CIH-treated rats showed a substantial increase (~2-fold) in MDA levels compared with the sham group, an effect also observed in CIH-rats treated with ABH (**Figure 5**). On the contrary, CIH-rats treated with NAC, as well as with ABH/NAC, showed plasma levels of TBARS comparable to sham rats (**Figure 5**).

Biosafety Testing of ABH-NAC Combination

Considering the effect of ABH/NAC combination on normalizing the BP and vascular reactivity in CIH rats, liver and kidney morphology as well as the renal function was evaluated in sham rats treated for 14 days with high doses of ABH (400 µg/kg day) and NAC (400 mg/kg day). Kidney (**Figure 6A**) and liver (**Figure 6B**) morphology were not altered by the treatment. Similarly, we did not found changes in plasma urea concentration and creatinine clearance

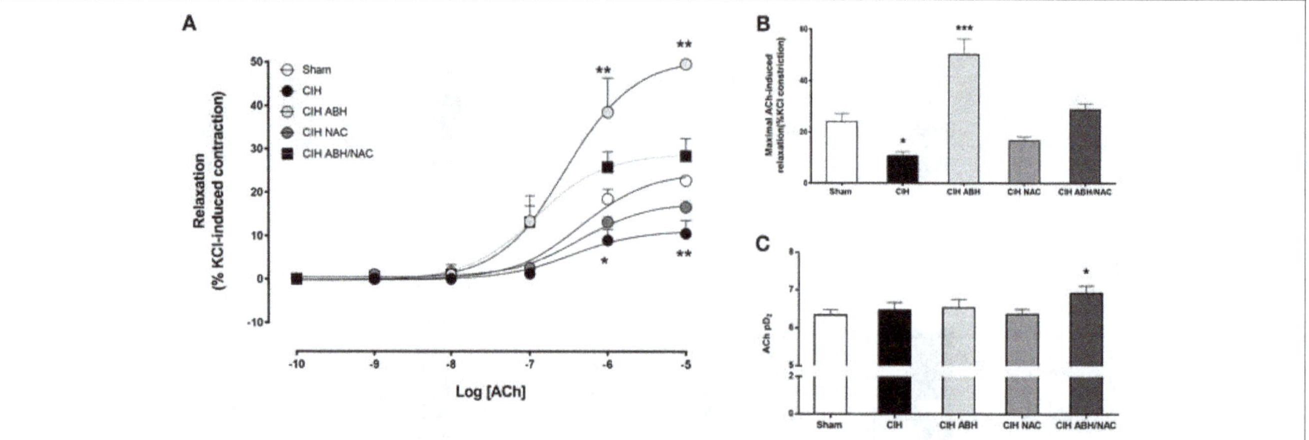

FIGURE 4 | Endothelial-dependent relaxation in femoral arteries from CIH-rats. **(A)** Concentration-dependent relaxation curves in response to acetylcholine of femoral arteries from sham (open circles, $n = 6$), CIH (solid circles, $n = 6$), CIH treated with ABH (light gray circles, $n = 6$), CIH treated with NAC (gray circles, $n = 6$) and CIH treated with ABH, and NAC (dark gray square, $n = 6$) rats. Maximal acetylcholine-induced response **(B)** and pharmacological potency (pD_2, i.e., sensitivity) **(C)** from sham (open bars), CIH (solid bars), CIH treated with ABH (light gray bars), CIH treated with NAC (gray bars), and CIH treated with ABH, and NAC (dark gray bars) rats were derived from **(A)**. Values expressed as mean ± SEM, $^{*}p < 0.05$, $^{**}p < 0.01$, $^{***}p < 0.001$ vs. sham, ANOVA.

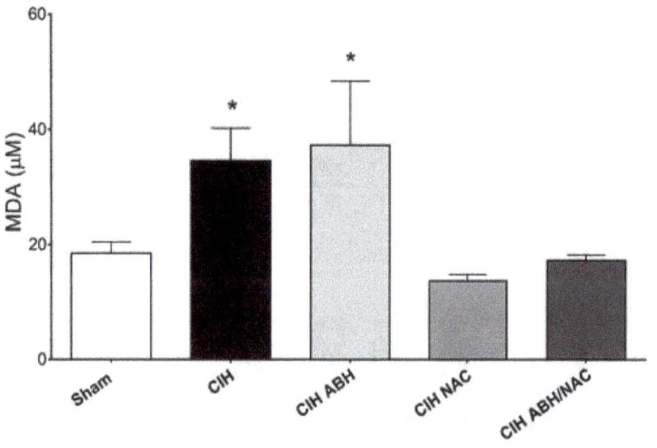

FIGURE 5 | Circulating levels of oxidized lipids in CIH-rats. Plasma levels of the oxidative stress marker MDA in sham (open bars, $n = 16$), CIH (solid bars, $n = 13$), CIH treated with ABH (light gray bars, $n = 7$), CIH treated with NAC (gray bars, $n = 5$), and CIH treated with ABH, and NAC (dark gray bars, $n = 10$) rats. Values expressed as mean ± SEM, $^{*}p < 0.05$ vs. sham, ANOVA.

between the rats with or without ABH/NAC treatment (**Table 2**).

DISCUSSION

This study aimed to determine whether the administration of the arginase inhibitor ABH and the glutathione precursor NAC may revert the hypertension and endothelial dysfunction in rats exposed to CIH. The results showed that ABH and NAC, as well as the combination of both drugs, reverted the increase in BP induced by CIH. However, only the combination of ABH and NAC leads to a normalization of BP and endothelial function along with a reversion of vascular remodeling markers, as suggests the changes in contractile force and internal diameter. In addition, the combination of ABH and NAC at high doses had no

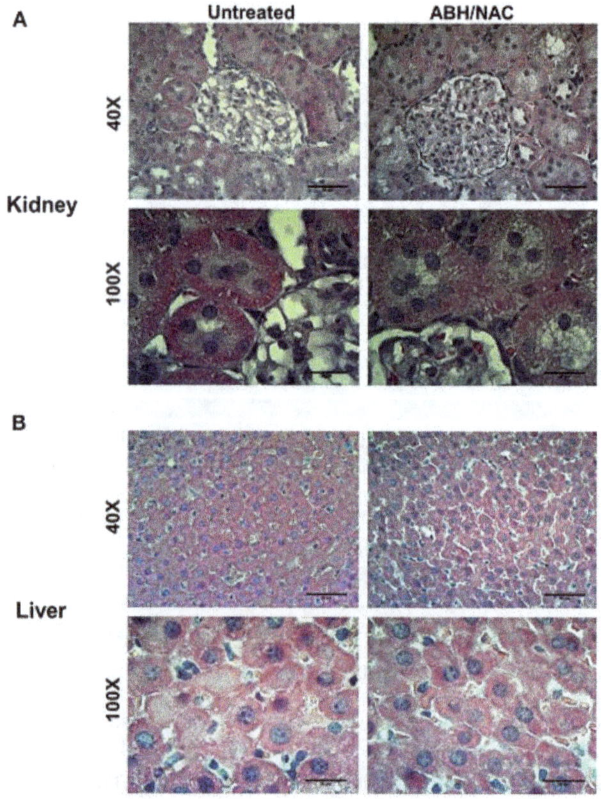

FIGURE 6 | Effects of ABH/NAC treatment on kidney and liver morphology. Micrograph of transverse sections of kidney **(A)** and liver **(B)** samples stained with Harris hematoxylin and eosin from untreated and ABH/NAC treated rats.

TABLE 2 | Effect of ABH/NAC on rats renal and hepatic variables.

	Untreated	ABH/NAC
Initial body weight (g)	199.8 ± 3.7	197.3 ± 1.9
Body weight at 28 days (g)	330.3 ± 4.2	298.3 ± 7.0*
Body weight as % initial (%)	165.3 ± 2.2	146.6 ± 3.6*
Plasma urea (mg/dL)	41.9 ± 3.4	48.0 ± 4.8
Urine urea (mg/24 h)	6.5 ± 0.4	5.4 ± 0.5
Proteins (mg/24 h)	10.7 ± 1.2	12.5 ± 1.3
Plasma creatinine (mg/dL)	0.56 ± 0.2	0.57 ± 0.3
Urine creatinine (mg/24 h)	972.0 ± 87.5	941.5 ± 57.1
Creatinine clearance (ml/min)	1.78 ± 0.3	1.76 ± 0.2
Lactate dehydrogenase LDH (U/L)	1111.0 ± 435.3	768.6 ± 188.9
Glutamic-oxalacetic transaminase GOT (U/L)	60.0 ± 4.5	61.0 ± 11.4
Glutamic-pyruvic transaminase GTP (U/L)	21.7 ± 1.1	16.5 ± 2.9

$^*P < 0.05$ U-Mann-Whitney treated vs. non-treated rats (Untreated Rats n = 4 and ABH-NAC rats = 8).

effect on liver and kidney morphology and biochemical function.

Compelling evidence shows that, in humans, oxidative stress has a prominent role in the cardiovascular dysfunction induced by OSA, a fact that is present also in preclinical models. In this study, similar to previous reports antioxidant treatment reverted the increase in BP in CIH rats. Indeed, Moya et al. (2016) found that rats treated with the antioxidant ebselen and exposed to CIH displayed a significant decreased of the elevated BP, suggesting that CIH-induced hypertension is critically dependent on oxidative stress. In this study, to understand the cardiovascular effects of antioxidants in CIH, we assayed the *ex vivo* vascular function in two representative arteries (i.e., carotid and femoral). It is well established that NAC antioxidant effect occurs mainly by restoring the potent intracellular reducing agent glutathione, under oxidative stress conditions (Rushworth and Megson, 2014). Notably, *in vivo* NAC treatment had limited effects on the *ex vivo* impaired endothelial dependent-relaxation and increased contractile reactivity in carotid arteries, as well as partially reverted the endothelial dysfunction in femoral arteries from animals exposed to CIH. These data suggest that the antihypertensive effect of NAC and other antioxidants occurs partially by improving vascular reactivity and, in a higher degree, by preventing the overactivation of the CB in CIH. Indeed, previous reports have shown that oxidative stress in the CB drives the chemosensory potentiation and hypertensive effects of CIH (Del Rio et al., 2016; Iturriaga et al., 2017). However, considering that our studies on endothelial-dependent relaxation were carried-out after pre-constriction with KCl, a potential effect of NAC enhancing the role of endothelium-derived hyperpolarizing factor (EDHF) (Krummen et al., 2006) or alternative glutathione-dependent vasodilator pathways (Yang and Wang, 2015) cannot be ruled out.

Conversely, endothelial dysfunction has been proposed to play a key role in the cardiovascular risk associated with OSA and CIH. Indeed, OSA patients show a reduced flow-mediated dilation (Ip et al., 2004), and endothelial dysfunction has been directly demonstrated in middle cerebral (Phillips et al., 2004) and carotid arteries from rats exposed to CIH (Krause et al., 2015). In the present study, we add new evidence that vascular dysfunction in CIH is associated with an increased contractile response and impaired NOS-dependent relaxation in femoral arteries. This new data shows the effects of CIH on the vascular function on carotid and femoral arteries. In this context, we previously reported that the reduced relaxation in response to ACh in carotid arteries from CIH-treated rats can be prevented by the *ex vivo* inhibition of arginase activity, and this effect could be explained by an unbalanced endothelial expression of eNOS and arginase-1 (Krause et al., 2015). Increased arginase expression and its effect on NOS-dependent relaxation have been extensively reported in hypertension and cardiovascular diseases (Caldwell et al., 2015). For instance, a study in humans shows that plasma levels of arginase are increased in subjects with OSA that present a normal cardiovascular function compared with health controls, and these levels are further increased when OSA is associated to vascular dysfunction (Yüksel et al., 2014). In that regard, a higher arginase expression and activity has been reported in diverse models of hypoxia (i.e., intermittent and sustained) in which an increased expression of arginases 1 or 2 occurs in the endothelium leading to a decreased NO synthesis (Krotova et al., 2010; Krause et al., 2013, 2015; Singh et al., 2014; Cowburn et al., 2016). Here we found that chronic *in vivo* arginase inhibition with ABH reverted the increase in BP induced by CIH, with no effects on circulating markers of oxidative stress. Furthermore, the treatment with ABH potentiated the vasorelaxation response to ACh in carotid and femoral arteries, as well as partially reverted the increased contractile response to KCl. The later effect of ABH treatment on the contractile response could result from the inhibition of the proliferative stimulus by arginases-derived polyamines on vascular smooth muscle cells (Ignarro et al., 2001; Wei et al., 2001; Chen et al., 2009). Similar to our results, previous studies in spontaneously hypertensive rats have demonstrated the potential therapeutic role of arginase inhibitors decreasing arterial blood pressure and restoring endothelial function (Demougeot et al., 2005; Bagnost et al., 2008, 2010). Altogether, the available information reinforces the idea that arginase-mediated impaired endothelial NO synthesis plays a key role in the vascular dysfunction associated with CIH and OSA.

It is worth to note that neither NAC nor ABH treatments separately led to a complete normalization of *ex vivo* vascular responses in carotid or femoral arteries from CIH rats, despite that they had a clear effect decreasing BP, but a heterogeneous outcome on systemic oxidative stress levels. This confirms the notion that CIH-induced increase in BP (Del Rio et al., 2016; Iturriaga et al., 2017), similarly to other hypertensive models (Godo and Shimokawa, 2017; Handy and Loscalzo, 2017; Mancia et al., 2017), is a multifactorial process in which a CB chemosensory and sympathetic overactivity, oxidative stress and endothelial dysfunction are the cornerstones. Considering this idea, we aimed to determine whether the combined treatment with ABH and NAC could normalize the vascular function in CIH rats. Clearly, the combination of both drugs normalized

BP and oxidative stress markers; effects accompanied by the restoration of normal *ex vivo* contractile and relaxing responses. Compared with ABH treatment, the NAC/ABH combination led to a lower, but normal, maximal NOS-dependent relaxation in carotid and femoral arteries. This counterintuitive finding could result from the buffering effect of NAC, as well as glutathione, on NO levels (Hu et al., 2006; Keszler et al., 2010; Kolesnik et al., 2013), that would be limiting the enhanced levels of NO as a consequence of arginase inhibition. Conversely, ABH/NAC combination reverted the increase in the KCl contractile response induced by CIH. Notably, in a recent study we found that an increased KCl-induced contractile response is directly associated with biomechanical and histological markers of vascular remodeling (Cañas et al., 2017). Altogether, this data strongly suggests that ABH/NAC combination reverted the vascular remodeling observed in rats exposed to CIH (Krause et al., 2015). The mechanisms involved in the combined effect of ABH-NAC, as well as, the heterogeneous changes induced in femoral and carotid arteries need further studies that would include the analysis of alternative vasodilator pathways involving the cysteine and glutathione metabolism (Yang and Wang, 2015). Nonetheless, considering the changes in ACh potency (i.e., sensitivity) and markers of vascular remodeling, this combined effect could result from an increased vascular bioavailability of NO.

Present results show that CIH increased BP in 3–5 days. This fast increase in BP is probably triggered by a potentiated sympathetic vasoconstrictor tone on the arterial blood vessels, that would result from the cyclic hypoxic excitation of the CB (Iturriaga et al., 2017). In agreement to this explanation, we found that external carotid arteries from rats submitted to CIH for 21 days showed moderate enhanced contractile responses to KCl and a diminished vasorelaxation to ACh (Krause et al., 2015). Recently, Del Rio et al. (2016) found that the ablation of both CBs completely reverts the increased BP and sympathetic overflow in hypertensive rats exposed to CIH for 21 days, indicating that the CIH-enhanced CB chemosensory drive mediates the onset and maintenance of neurogenic hypertension. It is known that CIH reduced the ACh-mediated vasodilation (Tahawi et al., 2001; Dopp et al., 2011; Krause et al., 2015). However, there are some reports showing normal endothelial function in hypertensive rats exposed to CIH (Julien et al., 2003; Lefebvre et al., 2006). Indeed, Lefebvre et al. (2006) found that the ACh-induced vasodilation in carotid, aortic and mesenteric vascular beds, as well as the contractile responses to noradrenaline and angiotensin II (Ang II), are similar between CIH-treated and sham rats, while the contraction induced by exogenous application of ET-1 is augmented in CIH-treated rats. Oxidative stress is associated with the endothelial dysfunction in CIH-treated rats. Indeed, treatment of CIH-exposed rats with allopurinol improves the reduced vasodilatation induced by ACh in gracillis arteries, although neither allopurinol nor CIH affect the vessel morphometry and systemic markers of oxidative stress in rats exposed to CIH for 14 days (Dopp et al., 2011). Similarly, Philippi et al. (2010) report that CIH elicited systemic oxidative stress, although they found that CIH has an inconsistent effect on the oxidative stress marker 3-nitrotyrosine in the vascular wall. Therefore, it is plausible that NAC and ABH may affect CIH-induced hypertension acting at different levels. It is likely that NAC may reduce the enhanced CB chemosensory discharge as all tested antioxidants do (Peng et al., 2003; Del Rio et al., 2010; Moya et al., 2016), while ABH may act at the level of the arteries. In addition, it is plausible that NAC may affect the arginase activity in the blood vessels or ABH may affect the oxidative stress in the blood vessels. If these aspects are different, it may explain the heterogeneous effect of the drugs in the femoral and carotid arteries.

PERSPECTIVES

Present results support a potential therapeutic application of a combined antihypertensive treatment with an antioxidant and an arginase inhibitor, which not only decrease BP but also normalize endothelial vascular reactivity and revert vascular remodeling, without compromising kidney and liver functions. Further studies are required to demonstrate whether this increased antihypertensive effect is limited to the drugs tested in the present study or can be applied to other combination of antioxidant and antihypertensive agents.

AUTHOR CONTRIBUTIONS

BK, PC, and RI conceived and designed the experiments. MP synthetized ABH. BK, ACD, PA, RI, VV, and GA performed the experiments. BK, RI, GA, VV, and ACD analyzed the data. RI and BK wrote the draft paper and all authors contributed to the manuscript and approved the final version.

FUNDING

This work was supported by FONDEF D11I1098 and FONDECYT 1150040.

REFERENCES

Bagnost, T., Berthelot, A., Bouhaddi, M., Laurant, P., Andre, C., Guillaume, Y., et al. (2008). Treatment with the arginase inhibitor N(omega)-hydroxy-nor-L-arginine improves vascular function and lowers blood pressure in adult spontaneously hypertensive rat. *J. Hypertens.* 26, 1110–1118. doi: 10.1097/HJH.0b013e3282fcc357

Bagnost, T., Ma, L., Da Silva, R. F., Rezakhaniha, R., Houdayer, C., Stergiopulos, N., et al. (2010). Cardiovascular effects of arginase inhibition in spontaneously hypertensive rats with fully developed hypertension. *Cardiovasc. Res.* 87, 569–577. doi: 10.1093/cvr/cvq081

Caldwell, R. B., Toque, H. A., Narayanan, S. P., and Caldwell, R. W. (2015). Arginase: an old enzyme with new tricks. *Trends Pharmacol. Sci.* 36, 395–405. doi: 10.1016/j.tips.2015.03.006

Cañas D., Herrera, E. A., García-Herrera, C., Celentano, D., and Krause, B. J. (2017). Fetal growth restriction induces heterogeneous effects on vascular biomechanical and functional properties in guinea pigs (*Cavia porcellus*). *Front. Physiol.* 8, 144. doi: 10.3389/fphys.2017.00144

Chen, B., Calvert, A. E., Cui, H., and Nelin, L. D. (2009). Hypoxia promotes human pulmonary artery smooth muscle cell proliferation through induction of arginase. *Am. J. Physiol. Lung Cell. Mol. Physiol.* 297, L1151–L1159. doi: 10.1152/ajplung.00183.2009

Collet, S., Carreaux, F., Boucher, J.-L., Pethe, S., Lepoivre, M., Danion-Bougot, R., et al. (2000). Synthesis and evaluation of [ω]-borono-[α]-amino acids as active-site probes of arginase and nitric oxide synthases. *J. Chem. Soc. Perkin Trans.* 1, 177–182. doi: 10.1039/a908140b

Cowburn, A. S., Crosby, A., Macias, D., Branco, C., Colaco, R. D., Southwood, M., et al. (2016). HIF2alpha-arginase axis is essential for the development of pulmonary hypertension. *Proc. Natl. Acad. Sci. U.S.A.* 113, 8801–8806. doi: 10.1073/pnas.1602978113

Delaey, C., Boussery, K., and Van De Voorde, J. (2002). Contractility studies on isolated bovine choroidal small arteries: determination of the active and passive wall tension-internal circumference relation. *Exp. Eye Res.* 75, 243–248. doi: 10.1006/exer.2002.2028

Del Rio, R., Moya, E. A., and Iturriaga, R. (2010). Carotid body and cardiorespiratory alterations in intermittent hypoxia: the oxidative link. *Eur. Respir. J.* 36, 143–150. doi: 10.1183/09031936.00158109

Del Rio, R., Andrade, D. C., Lucero, C., Arias, P., and Iturriaga, R. (2016). Carotid body ablation abrogates hypertension and autonomic alterations induced by intermittent hypoxia in rats. *Hypertension* 68, 436–445. doi: 10.1161/HYPERTENSIONAHA.116.07255

Demougeot, C., Prigent-Tessier, A., Marie, C., and Berthelot, A. (2005). Arginase inhibition reduces endothelial dysfunction and blood pressure rising in spontaneously hypertensive rats. *J. Hypertens.* 23, 971–978. doi: 10.1097/01.hjh.0000166837.78559.93

Dempsey, J. A., Veasey, S. C., Morgan, B. J., and O'donnell, C. P. (2010). Pathophysiology of sleep apnea. *Physiol. Rev.* 90, 47–112. doi: 10.1152/physrev.00043.2008

Dopp, J. M., Philippi, N. R., Marcus, N. J., Olson, E. B., Bird, C. E., Moran, J. J., et al. (2011). Xanthine oxidase inhibition attenuates endothelial dysfunction caused by chronic intermittent hypoxia in rats. *Respiration* 82, 458–467. doi: 10.1159/000329341

Fletcher, E. C. (2000). Effect of episodic hypoxia on sympathetic activity and blood pressure. *Respir. Physiol.* 119, 189–197. doi: 10.1016/S0034-5687(99)00114-0

Garvey, J. F., Taylor, C. T., and McNicholas, W. T. (2009). Cardiovascular disease in obstructive sleep apnoea syndrome: the role of intermittent hypoxia and inflammation. *Eur. Respir. J.* 33, 1195–1205. doi: 10.1183/09031936.001 11208

Godo, S., and Shimokawa, H. (2017). Divergent roles of endothelial nitric oxide synthases system in maintaining cardiovascular homeostasis. *Free Radic. Biol. Med.* 109, 4–10. doi: 10.1016/j.freeradbiomed.2016.12.019

Handy, D. E., and Loscalzo, J. (2017). Responses to reductive stress in the cardiovascular system. *Free Radic. Biol. Med.* 109, 114–124. doi: 10.1016/j.freeradbiomed.2016.12.006

Hu, T. M., Hayton, W. L., and Mallery, S. R. (2006). Kinetic modeling of nitric-oxide-associated reaction network. *Pharm. Res.* 23, 1702–1711. doi: 10.1007/s11095-006-9031-4

Ignarro, L. J., Buga, G. M., Wei, L. H., Bauer, P. M., Wu, G., and Del Soldato, P. (2001). Role of the arginine-nitric oxide pathway in the regulation of vascular smooth muscle cell proliferation. *Proc. Natl. Acad. Sci. U.S.A.* 98, 4202–4208. doi: 10.1073/pnas.071054698

Ip, M. S., Tse, H. F., Lam, B., Tsang, K. W., and Lam, W. K. (2004). Endothelial function in obstructive sleep apnea and response to treatment. *Am. J. Respir. Crit. Care Med.* 169, 348–353. doi: 10.1164/rccm.200306-767OC

Iturriaga, R., Andrade, D. C., and Del Rio, R. (2014). Enhanced carotid body chemosensory activity and the cardiovascular alterations induced by intermittent hypoxia. *Front. Physiol.* 5:468. doi: 10.3389/fphys.2014.00468

Iturriaga, R., Moya, E. A., and Del Rio, R. (2009). Carotid body potentiation induced by intermittent hypoxia: implications for cardiorespiratory changes induced by sleep apnoea. *Clin. Exp. Pharmacol. Physiol.* 36, 1197–1204. doi: 10.1111/j.1440-1681.2009.05213.x

Iturriaga, R., Moya, E. A., and Del Rio, R. (2010). Cardiorespiratory alterations induced by intermittent hypoxia in a rat model of sleep apnea. *Adv. Exp. Med. Biol.* 669, 271–274. doi: 10.1007/978-1-4419-5692-7_55

Iturriaga, R., Oyarce, M. P., and Dias, A. C. R. (2017). Role of carotid body in intermittent hypoxia-related hypertension. *Curr. Hypertens. Rep.* 19, 38. doi: 10.1007/s11906-017-0735-0

Julien, C., Bayat, S., and Levy, P. (2003). Vascular reactivity to norepinephrine and acetylcholine after chronic intermittent hypoxia in mice. *Respir. Physiol. Neurobiol.* 139, 21–32. doi: 10.1016/j.resp.2003.09.005

Keszler, A., Zhang, Y., and Hogg, N. (2010). Reaction between nitric oxide, glutathione, and oxygen in the presence and absence of protein: how are S-nitrosothiols formed? *Free Radic. Biol. Med.* 48, 55–64. doi: 10.1016/j.freeradbiomed.2009.10.026

Kheirandish-Gozal, L., and Gozal, D. (2008). The multiple challenges of obstructive sleep apnea in children: diagnosis. *Curr. Opin. Pediatr.* 20, 650–653. doi: 10.1097/MOP.0b013e328316bdb2

Kolesnik, B., Palten, K., Schrammel, A., Stessel, H., Schmidt, K., Mayer, B., et al. (2013). Efficient nitrosation of glutathione by nitric oxide. *Free Radic. Biol. Med.* 63, 51–64. doi: 10.1016/j.freeradbiomed.2013.04.034

Krause, B. J., Carrasco-Wong, I., Caniuguir, A., Carvajal, J., Farias, M., and Casanello, P. (2013). Endothelial eNOS/arginase imbalance contributes to vascular dysfunction in IUGR umbilical and placental vessels. *Placenta* 34, 20–28. doi: 10.1016/j.placenta.2012.09.015

Krause, B. J., Del Rio, R., Moya, E. A., Marquez-Gutierrez, M., Casanello, P., and Iturriaga, R. (2015). Arginase-endothelial nitric oxide synthase imbalance contributes to endothelial dysfunction during chronic intermittent hypoxia. *J. Hypertens.* 33, 515–524. doi: 10.1097/HJH.0000000000000453

Krause, B. J., Prieto, C. P., Munoz-Urrutia, E., San Martin, S., Sobrevia, L., and Casanello, P. (2012). Role of arginase-2 and eNOS in the differential vascular reactivity and hypoxia-induced endothelial response in umbilical arteries and veins. *Placenta* 33, 360–366. doi: 10.1016/j.placenta.2012.02.006

Krotova, K., Patel, J. M., Block, E. R., and Zharikov, S. (2010). Hypoxic upregulation of arginase II in human lung endothelial cells. *Am. J. Physiol. Cell Physiol.* 299, C1541–C1548. doi: 10.1152/ajpcell.00068.2010

Krummen, S., Drouin, A., Gendron, M. E., Falck, J. R., and Thorin, E. (2006). ROS-sensitive cytochrome P450 activity maintains endothelial dilatation in ageing but is transitory in dyslipidaemic mice. *Br. J. Pharmacol.* 147, 897–904. doi: 10.1038/sj.bjp.0706679

Lasram, M. M., Dhouib, I. B., Annabi, A., El Fazaa, S., and Gharbi, N. (2015). A review on the possible molecular mechanism of action of N-acetylcysteine against insulin resistance and type-2 diabetes development. *Clin. Biochem.* 48, 1200–1208. doi: 10.1016/j.clinbiochem.2015.04.017

Lavie, L. (2003). Obstructive sleep apnoea syndrome–an oxidative stress disorder. *Sleep Med. Rev.* 7, 35–51. doi: 10.1053/smrv.2002.0261

Lefebvre, B., Godin-Ribuot, D., Joyeux-Faure, M., Caron, F., Bessard, G., Levy, P., et al. (2006). Functional assessment of vascular reactivity after chronic intermittent hypoxia in the rat. *Respir. Physiol. Neurobiol.* 150, 278–286. doi: 10.1016/j.resp.2005.05.020

Lévy, P., Pépin, J. L., Arnaud, C., Tamisier, R., Borel, J. C., Dematteis, M., et al. (2008). Intermittent hypoxia and sleep-disordered breathing: current concepts and perspectives. *Eur. Respir. J.* 32, 1082–1095. doi: 10.1183/09031936.00013308

Mancia, G., Rea, F., Cuspidi, C., Grassi, G., and Corrao, G. (2017). Blood pressure control in hypertension. Pros and cons of available treatment strategies. *J. Hypertens.* 35, 225–233. doi: 10.1097/HJH.0000000000001181

McNicholas, W. T., Bonsigore, M. R., and Management Committee of EU COST ACTION B26. (2007). Sleep apnoea as an independent risk factor for cardiovascular disease: current evidence, basic mechanisms and research priorities. *Eur. Respir. J.* 29, 156–178. doi: 10.1183/09031936.00027406

Moya, E. A., Arias, P., Varela, C., Oyarce, M. P., Del Rio, R., and Iturriaga, R. (2016). Intermittent hypoxia-induced carotid body chemosensory potentiation and hypertension are critically dependent on peroxynitrite formation. *Oxid. Med. Cell Longev.* 2016:9802136. doi: 10.1155/2016/9802136

Mulvany, M. J., and Aalkjaer, C. (1990). Structure and function of small arteries. *Physiol. Rev.* 70, 921–961. doi: 10.1152/physrev.1990.70.4.921

Patt, B. T., Jarjoura, D., Haddad, D. N., Sen, C. K., Roy, S., Flavahan, N. A., et al. (2010). Endothelial dysfunction in the microcirculation of patients with obstructive sleep apnea. *Am. J. Respir. Crit. Care Med.* 182, 1540–1545. doi: 10.1164/rccm.201002-0162OC

Peng, Y., Yuan, G., Overholt, J. L., Kumar, G. K., and Prabhakar, N. R. (2003). Systemic and cellular responses to intermittent hypoxia: evidence for oxidative stress and mitochondrial dysfunction. *Adv. Exp. Med. Biol.* 536, 559–564. doi: 10.1007/978-1-4419-9280-2_71

Philippi, N. R., Bird, C. E., Marcus, N. J., Olson, E. B., Chesler, N. C., and Morgan, B. J. (2010). Time course of intermittent hypoxia-induced impairments in resistance artery structure and function. *Respir. Physiol. Neurobiol.* 170, 157–163. doi: 10.1016/j.resp.2009.12.003

Phillips, S. A., Olson, E. B., Morgan, B. J., and Lombard, J. H. (2004). Chronic intermittent hypoxia impairs endothelium-dependent dilation in rat cerebral and skeletal muscle resistance arteries. *Am. J. Physiol. Heart Circ. Physiol.* 286, H388–H393. doi: 10.1152/ajpheart.00683.2003

Prabhakar, N. R., and Kumar, G. K. (2010). Mechanisms of sympathetic activation and blood pressure elevation by intermittent hypoxia. *Respir. Physiol. Neurobiol.* 174, 156–161. doi: 10.1016/j.resp.2010.08.021

Prabhakar, N. R., Kumar, G. K., and Peng, Y. J. (2012). Sympatho-adrenal activation by chronic intermittent hypoxia. *J. Appl. Physiol.* 113, 1304–1310. doi: 10.1152/japplphysiol.00444.2012

Prabhakar, N. R., Peng, Y. J., Kumar, G. K., and Nanduri, J. (2015). Peripheral chemoreception and arterial pressure responses to intermittent hypoxia. *Compr. Physiol.* 5, 561–577. doi: 10.1002/cphy.c140039

Rushworth, G. F., and Megson, I. L. (2014). Existing and potential therapeutic uses for N-acetylcysteine: the need for conversion to intracellular glutathione for antioxidant benefits. *Pharmacol. Ther.* 141, 150–159. doi: 10.1016/j.pharmthera.2013.09.006

Schmitt, B., Vicenzi, M., Garrel, C., and Denis, F. M. (2015). Effects of N-acetylcysteine, oral glutathione (GSH) and a novel sublingual form of GSH on oxidative stress markers: a comparative crossover study. *Redox Biol.* 6, 198–205. doi: 10.1016/j.redox.2015.07.012

Singh, M., Padhy, G., Vats, P., Bhargava, K., and Sethy, N. K. (2014). Hypobaric hypoxia induced arginase expression limits nitric oxide availability and signaling in rodent heart. *Biochim. Biophys. Acta* 1840, 1817–1824. doi: 10.1016/j.bbagen.2014.01.015

Tahawi, Z., Orolinova, N., Joshua, I. G., Bader, M., and Fletcher, E. C. (2001). Altered vascular reactivity in arterioles of chronic intermittent hypoxic rats. *J. Appl. Physiol.* 90, 2007–2013. doi: 10.1152/jappl.2001.90.5.2007

Vadon-Legoff, S., Dijols, S., Mansuy, D., and Boucher, J.-L. (2005). Improved and high yield synthesis of the potent arginase inhibitor: 2(S)-amino-6-boronohexanoic acid. *Organ. Process Res. Dev.* 9, 677–679. doi: 10.1021/op050096n

Wei, L. H., Wu, G., Morris, S. M. Jr., and Ignarro, L. J. (2001). Elevated arginase I expression in rat aortic smooth muscle cells increases cell proliferation. *Proc. Natl. Acad. Sci. U.S.A.* 98, 9260–9264. doi: 10.1073/pnas.161294898

Yang, G., and Wang, R. (2015). H2S and blood vessels: an overview. *Handb. Exp. Pharmacol.* 230, 85–110. doi: 10.1007/978-3-319-18144-8_4

Yüksel, M., Okur, H. K., Pelin, Z., Ögünç, A. V., and Öztürk, L. (2014). Arginase activity and nitric oxide levels in patients with obstructive sleep apnea syndrome. *Clinics* 69, 247–252. doi: 10.6061/clinics/2014(04)05

11

Carotid Body Type-I Cells Under Chronic Sustained Hypoxia: Focus on Metabolism and Membrane Excitability

Raúl Pulgar-Sepúlveda[1], Rodrigo Varas[1,2], Rodrigo Iturriaga[3], Rodrigo Del Rio[4,5,6] and Fernando C. Ortiz[1]**

[1] Instituto de Ciencias Biomédicas, Facultad de Ciencias de la Salud, Universidad Autónoma de Chile, Santiago, Chile, [2] Facultad de Ciencias de la Salud, Universidad Autónoma de Chile, Talca, Chile, [3] Laboratorio de Neurobiología, Facultad de Ciencias Biológicas, Pontificia Universidad Católica de Chile, Santiago, Chile, [4] Laboratory of Cardiorespiratory Control, Department of Physiology, Pontificia Universidad Católica de Chile, Santiago, Chile, [5] Centro de Envejecimiento y Regeneración, Pontificia Universidad Católica de Chile, Santiago, Chile, [6] Centro de Excelencia en Biomedicina de Magallanes, Universidad de Magallanes, Punta Arenas, Chile

***Correspondence:**
Rodrigo Del Rio
rdelrio@bio.puc.cl
Fernando C. Ortiz
fernando.ortiz@uautonoma.cl

Chronic sustained hypoxia (CSH) evokes ventilatory acclimatization characterized by a progressive hyperventilation due to a potentiation of the carotid body (CB) chemosensory response to hypoxia. The transduction of the hypoxic stimulus in the CB begins with the inhibition of K+ currents in the chemosensory (type-I) cells, which in turn leads to membrane depolarization, Ca^{2+} entry and the subsequent release of one- or more-excitatory neurotransmitters. Several studies have shown that CSH modifies both the level of transmitters and chemoreceptor cell metabolism within the CB. Most of these studies have been focused on the role played by such putative transmitters and modulators of CB chemoreception, but less is known about the effect of CSH on metabolism and membrane excitability of type-I cells. In this mini-review, we will examine the effects of CSH on the ion channels activity and excitability of type-I cell, with a particular focus on the effects of CSH on the TASK-like background K+ channel. We propose that changes on TASK-like channel activity induced by CSH may contribute to explain the potentiation of CB chemosensory activity.

Keywords: carotid body, chronic hypoxia, membrane depolarization, ion channels, TASK-like channel

INTRODUCTION

The carotid body (CB) is the main peripheral chemoreceptor in mammals. Natural stimuli such as hypoxemia, hypercapnia, and/or acidosis increase the firing rate of the petrosal ganglion (PG) sensory afferent neurons projecting to the cardiovascular and respiratory regions in the brain stem (Gonzalez et al., 1994).

The current model for hypoxic chemoreception states that hypoxia evokes a depolarization of CB type-I (glomus) cells, leading to an increment of intracellular Ca^{2+} and the subsequent release of one- or more-excitatory neurotransmitters to the nerve terminals of the PG neurons (Gonzalez et al., 1994; Iturriaga and Alcayaga, 2004; Nurse, 2005). It is well established that a key event in triggering the hypoxic response is the depolarization of the type-I cells (Buckler and Vaughan-Jones, 1994). In type-I cells from several species it has been found that hypoxia produces a fast and reversible inhibition of K^+ currents (López-Barneo et al., 1988; López-López and González, 1992; Wyatt and Peers, 1995; Buckler, 1997) leading to a depolarization of type-I cells membrane and the consequence Ca^{2+}entry, mainly throughout L-type Ca^{2+} channels (Fieber and McCleskey, 1993; Wyatt et al., 1994). Among several molecules present in type-I cells, acetylcholine (ACh) and adenosine triphosphate (ATP) meets most of the criteria to be consider excitatory transmitters in the pathway (Varas et al., 2003; Iturriaga and Alcayaga, 2004), while dopamine (DA), nitric oxide (NO), and endothelin-1 (ET-1) modulate the chemosensory process (Iturriaga and Alcayaga, 2004).

Mammals exposed to sustained hypoxia (i.e., high altitude) develop ventilatory acclimatization featured by a progressively hyperventilation, due to an augmented CB responsiveness to hypoxia (Bisgard, 2000). In addition to the enhanced CB chemosensory responses, chronic sustained hypoxia (CSH) for weeks or months induces angiogenesis in the CB along with type-I cell hypertrophy and hyperplasia (Heath et al., 1985). Most of the studies on CB hypoxia acclimatization have been focused on putative changes in transmitters or modulators of CB chemoreception. Interestingly, DA, NO, and ET-1 are up-regulated in the CB during the first week of chronic hypoxia (Bisgard, 2000). In addition, some reports indicate that CSH increases type-I cell excitability due to changes in K^+ and Na^+ channels expression. In spite of the efforts, the mechanisms by which CSH enhances CB chemosensory responses to hypoxia remains to be established. In this review, we will examine the effects of sustained hypoxia on CB metabolism and ion channels function, focusing on the type-I cell excitability.

ELECTRICAL PROPERTIES OF TYPE-I CELLS

Type-I cells are small round-shaped cells (diameter $\sim$10 μm in the rat), with high input resistance of 5–6 GΩ (Duchen et al., 1988; Xu et al., 2005), and resting membrane potential ranging from −50 to −70 mV (Gonzalez et al., 1994). Regarding to the inward currents expressed by type-I cells, in the adult rabbit it has been reported a tetrodotoxin-sensitive, voltage-gated Na^+ current with fast activation and inactivation kinetics (Duchen et al., 1988). However, in both adult and neonatal rat type-I cells, there are contradictory results regarding the expression of functional voltage gated Na^+ channels (Fieber and McCleskey, 1993; Hempleman, 1995; Stea et al., 1995; Cáceres et al., 2007). Voltage-gated Ca^{2+} channels have been found in both rat and rabbit type-I cells (Fieber and McCleskey, 1993; Buckler and Vaughan-Jones, 1994; Wyatt et al., 1994). Most of the studies agree that L-type Ca^{2+} channel is the most abundant subtype of Ca^{2+} channel in type-I cells, however, in rabbit CB type-I cells, pharmacological evidences suggest the additional presence of N-, P/Q-type Ca^{2+} channels and a ω-conotoxin-resistent Ca^{2+} current (Overholt and Prabhakar, 1997, 1999). In addition, rat type-I cells express anionic currents (mainly Cl^-) which are involved in the chemosensory transduction of acidic and hypercapnic stimuli (Carpenter and Peers, 1997; Iturriaga et al., 1998).

Type-I cells express a wide variety of K^+ channels. Rabbit type-I cells express at least two voltage-gated, TEA-sensitive Ca^{2+} - independent K^+ currents. One of these conductances correspond to an oxygen-sensitive voltage-gated K^+ channel with a unitary conductance of $\sim$40 pS and an activation threshold around −40 to −30 mV (hereafter KO_2; López-Barneo et al., 1988). The opening of this K^+ channel is reversibly inhibited by hypoxia with an IP_{50} (PO_2 at which 50% of maximal inhibition is reached) near to 5–10 mmHg. This inhibition by hypoxia depends on membrane potential: maximal inhibition (40% of control activity) is reached at 0 mV (López-Barneo et al., 1988). The KO_2 channel has at least four closed states (C0–C4), one open state (O) and two inactivated states (I1–I2). Hypoxia induces both, stabilization of the "C0" state and promoting the channel from "O" state to inactivation state "I1" (Ganfornina and Lopez-Barneo, 1992).

Neonatal rat type-I cells express a maxi-K (BK) channel, whose opening depends on the PO_2. This maxi-K channel has a large unitary conductance of $\sim$200 pS, it is blocked by charybdotoxin and activated by both membrane depolarization (threshold ranging from −40 to −20 mV) and by a rise in intracellular $[Ca^{2+}]$ above 100 nM (Peers, 1990; Wyatt and Peers, 1995). Wyatt and Peers (1995) found that hypoxia (PO_2 = 5–10 mmHg) causes a reversible inhibition of this maxi-K current in cell-attached patch-clamp recordings. Later, Williams et al. (2004) proposed that the oxygen-sensitivity of the rat type-I cells is mediated by a heme oxygenase-2 (HO-2) associated with the maxi-K channel complex. However, this proposition was challenged by Ortega-Sáenz et al. (2006), when they found that hypoxic response of type-I cells remains intact in HO-2 null mice.

Interestingly, Buckler (1997) found that voltage gated K^+ channel blockers (10 mM TEA plus 5 mM 4-aminopyridine and 20 nM charybdotoxin) failed to depolarize type-I cells and to modify intracellular $[Ca^{2+}]$. However, in the presence of these K^+ channel blockers, a hypoxic stimulus was able to evoke cell depolarization and a rise in intracellular Ca^{2+} levels. This background K^+ current was inhibited by hypoxia with an IP_{50} $\sim$10 mmHg, reaching a maximal $\sim$70% inhibition during anoxia. Hypoxia stabilized the background K^+ channel in its close state, but did not affect the opening/closing kinetics, or the open state duration (Williams and Buckler, 2004). This background K^+ channel correspond to a TWIK-related acid-sensitive K^+ channel (TASK), member of the two-pore domain K^+ channel superfamily (Buckler et al., 2000). Additional evidences suggest the presence of TASK-1, TASK-2, TASK-3, TRAAK, and TREK (Buckler, 1997; Buckler et al., 2000; Yamamoto et al., 2002; Yamamoto and Taniguchi, 2006).

The discovery of oxygen-dependent voltage-gated K^+ channels promptly leads to the suggestion that hypoxia inhibits K^+ channels, which in turn produces type-I cells depolarization. Nevertheless, the resting membrane potential of type-I cells is quite stable at least 10 mV below the threshold activation of both maxi-K and KO_2 channels. Therefore, it was hard to conciliate a possible role of these K^+ channels in initiating the depolarization in response to hypoxia in type-I cells. Since background K^+ channels (Buckler, 1997; Buckler et al., 2000)

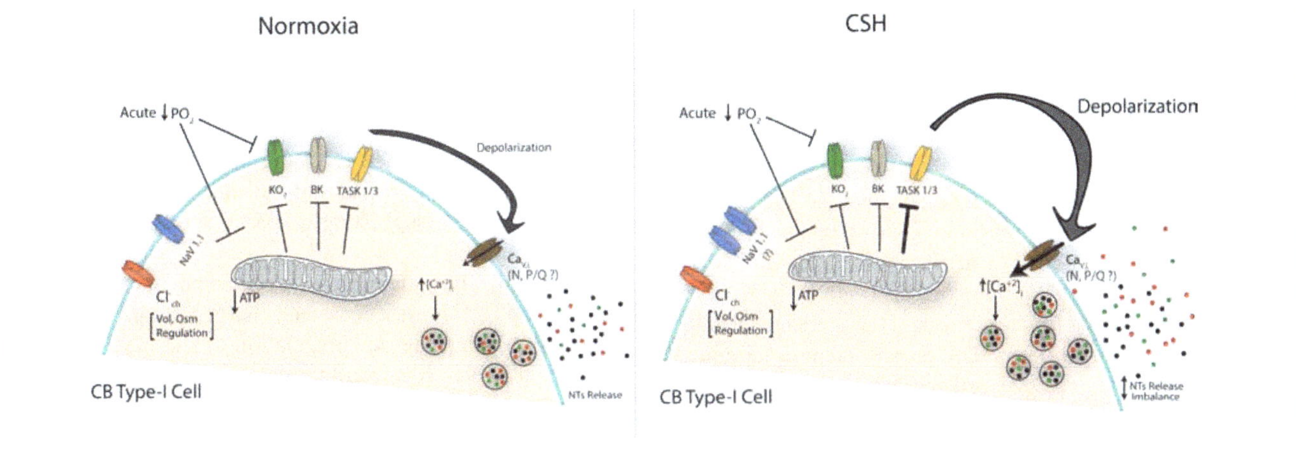

FIGURE 1 | Proposed mechanisms of CB type-I cell hyperexcitability under chronic sustained hypoxia (CSH). The scheme depicts the main ion channels described in CB type-I cells. Acute fall in the PO_2 inhibits K^+ conductance(s) either directly on membrane components (i.e., KO_2) or indirectly by reducing mitochondrial ATP production ('metabolic hypothesis') triggering a membrane depolarization that leads to the calcium-dependent neurotransmitters (NTs) release, initiating the chemosensory response to hypoxia. Under CSH an increased Na-current has been suggested [Nav1.1 subunit increased expression (Cáceres et al., 2007)] while a potentiated inhibition of a TASK-like K^+–channel activity which induced a larger depolarization has been described (Ortiz et al., 2007, 2013). A major voltage-dependent calcium entry (mainly through L-type Ca-channels) is expected, which could explain the CB neurotransmitter release imbalance under CSH. Chloride channel(s) have been related with volume (Vol) and osmolarity (Osm) regulation but they would not participate in CSH mechanisms.

are active at resting conditions, the closure of these channels may explain the initiation of the depolarization evoked by hypoxia. The precise mechanism by which acute hypoxia is sensed remains controversial, but is clear that TASK, maxi-K, and KO_2 channels plays a key role in the depolarization required for the neurotransmitters release from type-I cells in response to hypoxia (**Figure 1**).

CHRONIC SUSTAINED HYPOXIA (CSH)

Hypoxic-hypoxia (a PO_2 fall), could be classified as acute (seconds to minutes) or chronic (days to years). Acute hypoxia produced CB chemosensory excitation that evokes a reflex hyperventilation. CB increases its size in response to chronic sustained hypoxia (CSH) – to differentiate it from the *intermittent* paradigm – due to both increased number of cells and enhanced cell bodies diameter (Pequignot et al., 1984; Mills and Nurse, 1993). In this line, Pardal et al. (2007) have reported that in mice exposed to 10% O_2 for 7 days, a subpopulation of type-II cells acts like stem-cells, differentiating into new type-I cells. This mechanism may explain why CB hyperplasia is induced by CSH (Pardal et al., 2007). Likewise, several evidences suggest an important role of type-II cells in CB adaptation to different paradigms of chronic hypoxia (see Leonard et al., 2018 for a recent revision on this subject). The progressively increases in ventilation elicited by CSH, it is known as ventilatory acclimatization (Bisgard, 2000). Ventilatory acclimatization induced by CSH depends on the potentiation of the CB chemosensory response to hypoxia in several species (Bouverot et al., 1973; Olson and Dempsey, 1978; Smith et al., 1986; Vizek et al., 1987; Di Giulio et al., 2003). In this section we summarized some evidences concerning possible mechanisms behind this phenomenon.

Increased Levels of NO and ET-1 in the CB

Chronic sustained hypoxia increases the levels of NO in the CB (Ye et al., 2002) due to an augmented expression of endothelial and inducible nitric oxide synthase (Ye et al., 2002). An increased NO levels evoked by CSH may change the oxidative state and/or produce protein nitrosylation in type-I cells (Monteiro et al., 2005). It is possible that increased levels of NO induced by CSH may contribute to enhances the oxygen sensitivity in the CB. Iturriaga et al. (2000) reported that during steady chemosensory excitation induced by hypoxia, bolus injections of a NO donor transiently reduced chemosensory discharges. However, during normoxia the same concentration of NO increased chemosensory discharge, suggesting a dual role of NO (see also Iturriaga, 2001). Endothelin-1 (ET-1) is also present in the CB. Chronic hypoxia for 2 weeks increases the ET-1 levels and the expression of the ETA receptor in rat type-I cells (Chen Y. et al., 2002). ET peptides have a proliferative effect in the CB stimulating cellular proliferation in CB primary cultures trough the ETA receptor activation (Paciga et al., 1999). In the rabbit CB superfused *in vitro*, Chen et al. (2000) found that ET-1 did not modify basal CB chemosensory discharge, but potentiates the response induced by hypoxia. In addition, Chen Y. et al. (2002) found that ET-1 increases Ca^{2+} acting on L-type Ca^{2+} channels in rabbit type-I cells. Although, ET may enhance the CB response to hypoxia in a CB preparation devoid of vascular effects, the excitatory effect of ET-1 on CB chemoreception is most likely mediated by its vasoconstrictor effect (Rey and Iturriaga, 2004). Chen et al. (2007) found that the enhanced basal and hypoxic evoked chemosensory activity following CSH was significantly reduced by concurrent treatment with the ETA receptors blocker bosentan. Thus, it is plausible that CSH-induced CB acclimatization would be partially mediated by ETA receptors.

Changes in Levels and Secretion of DA, ACh, ATP, or Their Receptors

Carotid body type-I cells contains high levels of dopamine (DA), thus tyrosine hydroxylase (TH) is a conventional marker for the identification of type-I cells (Chou et al., 1998). CSH enhances both, the expression and activity of TH in CBs (Hanbauer, 1977; Czyzyk-Krzeska et al., 1992); as a consequence, there is an increased DA content. It is worth to mention that even though DA is released in response to acute hypoxia, its role in CB neurotransmission remains controversial (Fidone et al., 1990; Alcayaga et al., 2006). In most species, the evidence strongly suggests an inhibitory role for DA on CB chemoreception. It has been proposed that DA is involved in an auto-regulatory mechanism mediated by D2 dopaminergic receptors expressed in type-I cells (Fidone et al., 1990). Some evidences suggesting that the inhibitory role of DA could be attenuated in CBs exposed to CSH, leading to the increased chemoreactivity (Tatsumi et al., 1995). However, this is in sharp contrast with the increased TH activity during chronic hypoxia. Zhang et al. (2017) proposed that adenosine and DA control CB chemosensory discharge acting on petrosal neurons via their opposing actions on the hyperpolarization-activated, cyclic nucleotide-gated (HCN) cation current (Ih). By using a functional *in vitro* preparation of rat type-I cells/petrosal neurons co-cultures, they found that adenosine enhanced Ih in petrosal neurons acting on A2a receptors, while DA had the opposite effect via D2 receptors. Indeed, adenosine modified the Ih activation curve and increased firing frequency, while DA caused a hyperpolarizing shift in the curve and decreased the firing frequency (Zhang et al., 2017).

Acetylcholine and ATP have been proposed as excitatory transmitters in the CB, acting on nicotinic and P2X receptors, respectively (Zhang et al., 2000; Varas et al., 2003; Meza et al., 2012). In response to CSH, an increase of nicotinic acetylcholine receptor (nAChR) expression in chemosensory afferents has been reported (He et al., 2005). Paradoxically, nAChRs blockers does not revert the CB hyperreactivity evoked by chronic hypoxia (Bisgard, 2000). Regarding to the role played by ATP, it seems that CSH has no effect on P2X receptors expression in both, type-I cells and postsynaptic terminals of petrosal neurons. However, administration of P2X receptor blockers reduced the enhanced chemosensory response to acute hypoxia induced by CSH (He et al., 2006). Therefore, reports suggest that ACh and ATP may play a role in the hyperreactivity of the CB induced by CSH. Hence, it seems that chronic hypoxia enhances both the excitatory (purinergic and cholinergic) and inhibitory (dopaminergic) chemoreception pathways, in agreement with the proposal stating that the balance between excitatory and inhibitory transmitters is more relevant during chronically hypoxic conditions rather than normoxia (Prabhakar, 2006).

Increase in the Proportion of Na^+ Currents and a Decrease in K^+ Currents

In type-I cells of neonatal rats subjected to long-lasting chronic hypoxia there is an increase in the proportion of Na^+ currents and a decrease in oxygen-sensitive K^+ current density (Hempleman, 1995). Likewise, Cáceres et al. (2007) found that rat CB hyperreactivity induced by CSH correlated with an increased expression of voltage-gated Na^+ channel Nav1.1 subunit. Carpenter et al. (1998) found that exposing adult rats to 10% O_2 for 3 weeks significantly reduced K^+ current density with no change in voltage-gated K^+ current amplitudes. However, rabbit CBs cultured in 5% O_2 for 2 days shows a decrease in expression of the Kv3.4 subunit of the voltage-gated K^+ channel (Kääb et al., 2005), suggesting a species-specific effect on Kv-conductance.

Additionally, neonatal rat type-I cells exposed to hypoxia (9–14 days, 10% O_2) shows a decreased charybdotoxin-sensitive K^+ current, suggesting the downregulation of the maxi-K channel (Wyatt et al., 1995). It is worth to mention that in this paradigm, the rats have "blunted" rather hyperreactive responses to acute hypoxia (Wyatt et al., 1995). In culture, human maxi-K channels show an increased calcium sensitivity after 72 h of hypoxia. This is probably due to the reported threefold increase in maxi-K β-regulatory subunit expression induced by CSH (Hartness et al., 2003). However, cultured type-I cells from neonatal rat subjected to CSH, express normal levels of maxi-K and TASK-1 channels (Nurse and Fearon, 2002). Additionally, cultured CBs cells exposed to chronic hypoxia for 2 weeks showed an increase in Na^+ currents, but no changes in Ca^{2+} currents were reported (Stea et al., 1995), findings confirmed later in a paradigm of adult rats exposed to CSH (Peers et al., 1996).

We found an enhanced inhibition of the TASK-like current in neonatal rat type-I cells in cultured exposed to hypoxia for 2 days (Ortiz et al., 2007). While acute hypoxia (1% O_2) evokes a ~70% inhibition of the TASK-like current in control conditions, after 48 h of hypoxia current inhibition reaches ~90%. Importantly, these results were later reproduced (Ortiz et al., 2013) in an animal model for chronic *intermittent* hypoxia suggesting a common preserved mechanism of CB adaptation to hypoxic environments.

The evidence suggests that regulation of the expression and/or function of ionic currents are important adaptive mechanisms for the CB subjected to chronic hypoxia. Nevertheless, with the exception of the work of Cáceres et al. (2007), there is no physiological evidence that the CSH protocols used in above mentioned studies (Hempleman, 1995; Stea et al., 1995; Carpenter et al., 1998) really potentiated the CB chemosensory responses to acute hypoxia. On the contrary, most of them used long-term CSH exposition (>2 weeks) which is associated with an attenuation rather than a potentiation of CB chemosensory responses to acute hypoxia (Tatsumi et al., 1991). Hence, no convincing conclusion can be draw.

Increased Activity of AMP-Dependent Kinase and Protein Kinase C (PKC)

The activities of maxi-K and TASK channels are modulated by cell metabolism. Wyatt et al. (2007) found that AMP-dependent kinase (AMPK) is colocalized with both maxi-K and TASK channels in rat type-I cells. They found that AMPK activation inhibits those K^+ currents triggering membrane depolarization, whereas AMPK-antagonist application prevents the depolarization induced by hypoxia (Wyatt et al., 2007).

TASK channel current is activated by intracellular nucleotides, such as ATP (Varas et al., 2007). At physiological concentrations (1–3 mM) ATP strongly promotes channel opening. Accordingly, in absence of ATP, TASK channel activity decreases in ~50 % in inside-out patches (Williams and Buckler, 2004; Varas et al., 2007). Thus, ATP production seems to be central in regulating the activity of TASK-like and other potassium channels such as maxi-K (Williams and Buckler, 2004; Varas et al., 2007; Holmes et al., 2018). Even though some reports postulate a null or small effect of ATP on these conductances (Xu et al., 2005) one of the earliest proposition, the "metabolic hypothesis", states that CB oxygen sensing is mediated by oxidative phosphorylation, supported by the fact that virtually all metabolic poisons or oxidative phosphorylation inhibitors induce CB type-I cell excitation (Mulligan and Lahiri, 1982; Buerk et al., 1994; Wilson et al., 1994; Buckler and Turner, 2013). This response is normally triggered by potassium conductance(s) inhibition leading to the depolarization of the type-I cell membrane, reinforcing the notion that low PO_2 trigger potassium current blockage (**Figure 1**, see also Holmes et al., 2018). In this regard, it has been postulated that CB-mitochondria express a particular subtype of *cytochrome a3* – the functional core of mitochondrion complex IV – which is at least seven times more sensitive to a drop in the PO_2, further supporting a pivotal role of mitochondrial metabolism on CB-type-I cell excitation (for a full revision on this matter see Holmes et al., 2018 in this same research topic).

Therefore, in addition to changes in the expression and intrinsic function of ion channels, the fact that cellular metabolism is modified by CSH provides a potential link between CSH and the type-I cell membrane excitability. It is known that CSH increases the cytosolic AMP/ATP ratio in type-I cells. Thus, several enzymatic systems can be activated, including AMPK (Laderoute et al., 2006). Likewise, CSH induces an increase in cAMP levels in CB cells (Nurse et al., 1994). Protein kinase C (PKC) activity is enhanced by chronic hypoxia in several tissues (Zhang et al., 2004; Neckar et al., 2005), whereas the protein kinase A (PKA) activity decreases (Kobayashi et al., 1998). Increased PKC activity in response to acute hypoxia (Summers et al., 2000) was associated to the regulation of L-type Ca^{2+}, maxi-K channels and background K^+ channels in type-I cells (Peers and Carpenter, 1998; Summers et al., 2000; Zhang et al., 2003). Since PKC inhibits TASK channel activity, whereas PKA enhanced it (Zilberberg et al., 2000; Besana et al., 2004) these pathways are well-suited as potential effectors of CSH induced-changes.

Activation of Hypoxia-Inducible Transcription Factors (HIFs)

The cellular long-term response to hypoxia is driven by changes in the expression of several genes to cope with the new hypoxic environment. These cellular transcriptional responses are largely dependent on the activation of the so-called hypoxia-inducible transcription factors (Shimoda and Semenza, 2011). HIFs are composed by a HIFα subunit (mainly 1α and 2α), regulated by hypoxia and a constitutive β subunit (HIF-1β). Under normoxic conditions, HIFα is continuously degraded through hydroxylation modification catalyzed by a set of oxygen sensitive prolyl-hydroxylases enzymes. During hypoxia, the activity of prolyl-hydroxylases are dramatically reduced, allowing the translocation of HIFα to the cell nuclei where it forms an heterodimer with HIF-1β. Following translocation and dimerization, the HIF-1α/HIF-1β complex bind to hypoxia response elements (HRE) present in the DNA to regulate gene expression (Shimoda and Semenza, 2011). In the CB, the contribution of HIF-1α and HIF-2α has been largely studied in the setting of intermittent hypoxia; much less it is known in the context of CSH. Nevertheless, it has been shown that activation of the HIF-1α pathway promotes the up-regulation of pro-oxidant enzymes (i.e., NADPH) in the CB. On the contrary, intermittent hypoxia reduced the expression of HIF-2α within the CB, resulting in a significant down-regulation of antioxidant enzymes (i.e., SOD) levels being the outcome an increase ROS formation within CB glomus cells, increasing both intracellular Ca^{2+} and neurotransmitter release (Prabhakar and Semenza, 2016). The specific contribution of HIF-1α and HIF-2α pathways on the sensitization of the CB to hypoxia under CSH remains to be fully determined. Nevertheless, it is possible to speculate that activation of HIF-1α and inhibition of HIF-2α pathways may occur in the CBs of animals exposed to sustained hypoxia.

We have here discussed some of the mechanisms explaining CB chemosensory hyperreactivity under CSH. This exacerbated activity has systemic consequences inducing the adaptation to CSH. In this regard, a central aspect is the CB-mediated autonomic function and even though the neural mechanism associated to autonomic responses to CSH are not completely elucidated, it has been described that CB type-I cells could be involved. During acute hypoxic exposure, excitatory inputs from the CB activate neural pathways in the brainstem increasing minute ventilation and sympathetic outflow (Barros et al., 2002; Braga et al., 2007). However, during CSH the baseline minute ventilation increases in a time-dependent manner (ventilatory acclimatization to hypoxia), probably related to the changes in oxygen sensitivity of the CB as well as the neural network in the brainstem related to sympathetic response to hypoxia (Powell et al., 2000; Powell, 2007). It has been proposed that hypoxia-mediated sympathetic activation act as a compensatory mechanism to increase oxygen supply to critical organs through regulating cardiac output and vascular conductance (Leuenberger et al., 1991; Calbet, 2003). Indeed, exposure of healthy humans to CSH produces a significant increase in circulating norepinephrine levels reflecting increases in sympathetic outflow during hypoxic exposure (Calbet, 2003; Hansen and Sander, 2003). In addition, it has been shown that rats subjected to 24 h of FiO_2 10% displayed an increase of pre-sympathetic neurons activation located in the rostral aspect of the ventral medullary surface (RVLM). Furthermore, these set of neurons showed a further increase activation during the late expiratory phase during hypoxia stimulation suggesting a potential role on regulating the neural circuitry related to the respiratory-sympathetic coupling observed during CSH (Moraes et al., 2014). Interestingly, previous studies from our group showed that chronic activation of the CB afferent input to the brainstem using episodic hypoxic stimulation induces the activation of RVLM neurons (Del Rio et al., 2016). Therefore, it is plausible to hypothesize that during CSH, activation of the CB may contribute to the regulation of sympathetic drive. This hypothesis remains to be determined.

CONCLUSION

Potentiation of CB chemosensory responses is an absolute requirement for ventilatory acclimatization. How the increased response to acute hypoxia in chronically hypoxic CBs is achieved? There are probably multiple mechanisms underlying such phenomena. In the present review we focused on evidences suggesting that type-I cells excitability and metabolism undergoes substantial changes when exposed to CSH. Interestingly, ion channels, including some involved in the generation of the chemosensory response to acute hypoxia (i.e., maxi-K and TASK channels) are tightly regulated by PKC, PKA, AMPK, and ATP. Therefore, it is possible that throughout changes in cell metabolism, in addition to modifications on ion channels expression, CSH generates changes in type-I cells excitability, ultimate leading to increased depolarization during acute hypoxia. Importantly, increased inhibition of TASK-like currents under chronic - sustained and intermittent - hypoxia provide a novel potential mechanism to explain the CB hyperreactivity (Ortiz et al., 2007, 2013). It seems clear that there is no a single mechanism as full explanation for CB hyperreactivity during CSH. Combined studies covering from cellular/molecular studies to functional approaches will help to understand the physiology of ventilatory acclimatization during chronic sustained hypoxia.

AUTHOR CONTRIBUTIONS

All authors contributed to writing the article. RV, RI, RDR, and FO designed and edited the paper.

FUNDING

This work was supported by grants FONDECYT 11160616 to FO, FONDECYT 1180172 to RDR, and FONDECYT 1150040 to RI.

REFERENCES

Alcayaga, J., Soto, C. R., Vargas, R. V., Ortiz, F. C., Arroyo, J., and Iturriaga, R. (2006). Carotid body transmitters actions on rabbit petrosal ganglion in vitro. *Adv. Exp. Med. Biol.* 580, 331–337. doi: 10.1007/0-387-31311-7_51

Barros, R. C., Bonagamba, L. G., Okamoto-Canesin, R., de Oliveira, M., Branco, L. G., and Machado, B. H. (2002). Cardiovascular responses to chemoreflex activation with potassium cyanide or hypoxic hypoxia in awake rats. *Auton. Neurosci.* 97, 110–115. doi: 10.1016/S1566-0702(02)00050-4

Besana, A., Barbuti, A., Tateyama, M. A., Symes, A. J., Robinson, R. B., and Feinmark, S. J. (2004). Activation of protein kinase C epsilon inhibits the two-pore domain K^+ channel, TASK-1, inducing repolarization abnormalities in cardiac ventricular myocytes. *J. Biol. Chem.* 279, 33154–33160. doi: 10.1074/jbc.M403525200

Bisgard, G. E. (2000). Carotid body mechanisms in acclimatization to hypoxia. *Respir. Physiol.* 121, 237–246. doi: 10.1016/S0034-5687(00)00131-6

Bouverot, P., Candas, V., and Libert, J. P. (1973). Role of the arterial chemoreceptors in ventilatory adaptation to hypoxia of awake dogs and rabbits. *Respir. Physiol.* 17, 209–219. doi: 10.1016/0034-5687(73)90062-5

Braga, V. A., Soriano, R. N., Braccialli, A. L., de Paula, P. M., Bonagamba, L. G., Paton, J. F., et al. (2007). Involvement of L-glutamate and ATP in the neurotransmission of the sympathoexcitatory component of the chemoreflex in the commissural nucleus tractus solitarii of awake rats and in the working heart-brainstem preparation. *J. Physiol.* 581, 1129–1145. doi: 10.1113/jphysiol.2007.129031

Buckler, K. (1997). A novel oxygen-sensitive potassium current in rat carotid body type I cells. *J. Physiol.* 498, 649–662. doi: 10.1113/jphysiol.1997.sp021890

Buckler, K., Williams, B., and Honoré, E. (2000). An oxygen, acid and anaesthetic sensitive TASK-like background potassium channel in rat arterial chemoreceptor cells. *J. Physiol.* 525, 135–142. doi: 10.1111/j.1469-7793.2000.00135.x

Buckler, K. J., and Turner, P. J. (2013). Oxygen sensitivity of mitochondrial function in rat arterial chemoreceptor cells. *J. Physiol.* 591, 3549–3563. doi: 10.1113/jphysiol.2013.257741

Buckler, K. J., and Vaughan-Jones, R. D. (1994). Effects of hypoxia on membrane potential and intracellular calcium in rat neonatal carotid body type I cells. *J. Physiol.* 476, 423–428. doi: 10.1113/jphysiol.1994.sp020143

Buerk, D. G., Iturriaga, R., and Lahiri, S. (1994). Testing the metabolic hypothesis of O2 chemoreception in the cat carotid body in vitro. *J. Appl. Physiol.* 76, 1317–1323. doi: 10.1152/jappl.1994.76.3.1317

Cáceres, A. I., Obeso, A., Gonzalez, C., and Rocher, A. (2007). Molecular identification and functional role of voltage-gated sodium channels in rat carotid body chemoreceptor cells.n Regulation of expression by chronic hypoxia in vivo. *J. Neurochem.* 102, 231–245. doi: 10.1111/j.1471-4159.2007.04465.x

Calbet, J. A. L. (2003). Chronic hypoxia increases blood pressure and noradrenaline spillover in healthy humans. *J. Physiol.* 551, 379–386. doi: 10.1113/jphysiol.2003.045112

Carpenter, E., Bee, D., and Peers, C. (1998). Ionic currents in carotid body type I cells isolated from normoxic and chronically hypoxic adult rats. *Brain Res.* 811, 79–87. doi: 10.1016/S0006-8993(98)00962-7

Carpenter, E., and Peers, C. (1997). Swelling- and cAMP-activated Cl- currents in isolated rat carotid body type I cells. *J. Physiol.* 503, 497–511. doi: 10.1111/j.1469-7793.1997.497bg.x

Chen, J., He, L., Dinger, B., and Fidone, S. (2000). Pharmacological effects of endothelin in rat carotid body. Activation of second messenger pathways and potentiation of chemoreceptor activity. *Adv. Exp. Med. Biol.* 475, 517–525.

Chen, Y., Tipoe, G. L., Liong, E., Leung, S., Lam, S. Y., Iwase, R., et al. (2002). Chronic hypoxia enhances endothelin-1-induced intracellular calcium elevation in rat carotid body chemoreceptors and up-regulates ETA receptor expression. *Pflugers Arch.* 443, 565–573. doi: 10.1007/s00424-001-0728-2

Chen, J., He, L., Liu, X., Dinger, B., Stensaas, L., and Fidone, S. (2007). Effect of the endothelin receptor antagonist bosentan on chronic hypoxia-induced morphological and physiological changes in rat carotid body. *Am. J. Physiol. Lung. Cell. Mol. Physiol.* 292, L1257–L1262. doi: 10.1152/ajplung.00419.2006

Chou, C. L., Sham, J. S., Schofield, B., and Shirahata, M. (1998). Electrophysiological and immunocytological demonstration of cell-type specific responses to hypoxia in the adult cat carotid body. *Brain Res.* 789, 229–238. doi: 10.1016/S0006-8993(97)01472-8

Czyzyk-Krzeska, M. F., Bayliss, D. A., Lawson, E. E., and Millhorn, D. E. (1992). Regulation of tyrosine hydroxylase gene expression in the rat carotid body by hypoxia. *J. Neurochem.* 58, 1538–1546. doi: 10.1111/j.1471-4159.1992.tb11376.x

Del Rio, R., Andrade, D. C., Lucero, C., Arias, P., and Iturriaga, R. (2016). Carotid body ablation abrogates hypertension and autonomic alterations induced by intermittent hypoxia in rats. *Hypertension* 68, 436–445. doi: 10.1161/HYPERTENSIONAHA.116.07255

Di Giulio, C., Huang, W. X., Mokashi, A., Roy, A., Cacchio, M., Macrí, M. A., et al. (2003). Sustained hypoxia promotes hyperactive response of carotid body in the cat. *Respir. Physiol. Neurobiol.* 134, 69–74. doi: 10.1016/S1569-9048(02)00203-3

Duchen, M. R., Caddy, K. W., Kirby, G. C., Patterson, D. L., Ponte, J., and Biscoe, T. J. (1988). Biophysical studies of the cellular elements of the rabbit carotid body. *Neuroscience* 26, 291–313. doi: 10.1016/0306-4522(88)90146-7

Fidone, S. J., Gonzalez, C., Obeso, A., Gomez-Nino, A., and Dinger, B. (1990). "Biogenic amine and neuropeptide transmitters in carotid body chemotransmission: experimental findings and perspectives," in *Hypoxia: the Adaptations*, ed. J. E. Remmers (Toronto: B.C. Decker Inc), 116–126.

Fieber, L. A., and McCleskey, E. W. (1993). L-type calcium channels in type I cells of the rat carotid body. *J. Neurophysiol.* 70, 1378–1384. doi: 10.1152/jn.1993.70.4.1378

Ganfornina, M. D., and Lopez-Barneo, J. (1992). Gating of O2-sensitive K^+ channels of arterial chemoreceptor cells and kinetic modifications induced by low PO2. *J. Gen. Physiol.* 100, 427–455. doi: 10.1085/jgp.100.3.427

Gonzalez, C., Almaraz, L., Obeso, A., and Rigual, R. (1994). Carotid body chemoreceptors: from natural stimuli to sensory discharges. *Physiol. Rev.* 74, 829–898. doi: 10.1152/physrev.1994.74.4.829

Hanbauer, I. (1977). Regulation of tyrosine hydroxylase in carotid body. *Adv. Biochem. Psychopharmacol.* 16, 275–280.

Hansen, J., and Sander, M. (2003). Sympathetic neural overactivity in healthy humans after prolonged exposure to hypobaric hypoxia. *J. Physiol.* 546, 921–929. doi: 10.1113/jphysiol.2002.031765

Hartness, M. E., Brazier, S. P., Peers, C., Bateson, A. N., Ashford, M. L., and Kemp, P. J. (2003). Post-transcriptional control of human maxiK potassium channel activity and acute oxygen sensitivity by chronic hypoxia. *J. Biol. Chem.* 278, 51422–51432. doi: 10.1074/jbc.M309463200

He, L., Chen, J., Dinger, B., Stensaas, L., and Fidone, S. (2006). Effect of chronic hypoxia on purinergic synaptic transmission in rat carotid body. *J. Appl. Physiol.* 100, 157–162. doi: 10.1152/japplphysiol.00859.2005

He, L., Dinger, B., and Fidone, S. (2005). Effect of chronic hypoxia on cholinergic chemotransmission in rat carotid body. *J. Appl. Physiol.* 98, 614–619. doi: 10.1152/japplphysiol.00714.2004

Heath, D., Smith, P., and Fitch, R. (1985). Comparative pathology of the enlarged carotid body. *J. Comp. Pathol.* 95, 259–271. doi: 10.1016/0021-9975(85)90012-X

Hempleman, S. C. (1995). Sodium and potassium current in neonatal rat carotid body cells following chronic in vivo hypoxia. *Brain Res.* 699, 42–50. doi: 10.1016/0006-8993(95)00850-P

Holmes, A. P., Ray, C. J., Coney, A. M., and Kumar, P. (2018). Is carotid body physiological o2 sensitivity determined by a unique mitochondrial phenotype? *Front. Physiol.* 9:562. doi: 10.3389/fphys.2018.00562

Iturriaga, R. (2001). Nitric oxide and carotid chemoreception. *Biol. Res.* 34, 135–139. doi: 10.4067/S0716-97602001000200019

Iturriaga, R., and Alcayaga, J. (2004). Neurotransmission in the carotid body: transmitters and modulators between glomus cells and petrosal ganglion nerve terminals. *Brain Res. Rev.* 47, 46–53. doi: 10.1016/j.brainresrev.2004.05.007

Iturriaga, R., Mokashi, A., and Lahiri, S. (1998). Anion exchanger and chloride channel in cat carotid body chemotransduction. *J. Auton. Nerv. Syst.* 70, 23–31. doi: 10.1016/S0165-1838(98)00019-8

Iturriaga, R., Villanueva, S., and Mosqueira, M. (2000). Dual effects of nitric oxide on cat carotid body chemoreception. *J. Appl. Physiol.* 89, 1005–1012. doi: 10.1152/jappl.2000.89.3.1005

Kääb, S., Miguel-Velado, E., López-López, J. R., and Pérez-García, M. T. (2005). Down regulation of kv3.4 channels by chronic hypoxia increases acute oxygen sensitivity in rabbit carotid body. *J. Physiol.* 566(Pt 2), 395–408. doi: 10.1113/jphysiol.2005.085837

Kobayashi, S., Beitner-Johnson, D., Conforti, L., and Millhorn, D. E. (1998). Chronic hypoxia reduces adenosine A2A receptor-mediated inhibition of calcium current in rat PC12 cells via downregulation of protein kinase A. *J. Physiol.* 512, 351–363. doi: 10.1111/j.1469-7793.1998.351be.x

Laderoute, K. R., Amin, K., Calaoagan, J. M., Knapp, M., Le, T., Orduna, J., et al. (2006). 5'-AMP-activated protein kinase (AMPK) is induced by low-oxygen and glucose deprivation conditions found in solid-tumor microenvironments. *Mol. Cell. Biol.* 26, 5336–5347. doi: 10.1128/MCB.00166-06

Leonard, E. M., Salman, S., and Nurse, C. A. (2018). Sensory processing and integration at the carotid body tripartite synapse: neurotransmitter functions and effects of chronic hypoxia. *Front. Physiol.* 9:225. doi: 10.3389/fphys.2018.00225

Leuenberger, U., Gleeson, K., Wroblewski, K., Prophet, S., Zelis, R., Zwillich, C., et al. (1991). Norepinephrine clearance is increased during acute hypoxemia in humans. *Am. J. Physiol.* 261, H1659–H1664.

López-Barneo, J., López-López, J. R., Ureña, J., and González, C. (1988). Chemotransduction in the carotid body: current modulated by PO2 in type I chemoreceptor cells. *Science* 241, 580–582. doi: 10.1126/science.2456613

López-López, J. R., and González, C. (1992). Time course of K+ current inhibition by low oxygen in chemoreceptor cells of adult rabbit carotid body. Effects of carbon monoxide. *FEBS Lett.* 299, 251–254. doi: 10.1016/0014-5793(92)80126-2

Meza, R. C., Ortiz, F. C., Bravo, E., Iturriaga-Vásquez, P., Eugenín, J. L., and Varas, R. (2012). Functional expression of the $\alpha 7$ and $\alpha 4$-containing nicotinic acetylcholine receptors on the neonatal rat carotid body. *Neurochem. Int.* 60, 115–124. doi: 10.1016/j.neuint.2011.11.011

Mills, L., and Nurse, C. (1993). Chronic hypoxia in vitro increases volume of dissociated carotid body chemoreceptors. *Neuroreport* 4, 619–622. doi: 10.1097/00001756-199306000-00004

Monteiro, H. P., Rocha Oliveira, C. J., Curcio, M. F., Moraes, M. S., and Arai, R. J. (2005). Tyrosine phosphorylation in nitric oxide-mediated signaling events. *Methods Enzymol.* 396, 350–358. doi: 10.1016/S0076-6879(05)96029-1

Moraes, D. J. A., Bonagamba, L. G. H., Costa, K. M., Costa-Silva, J. H., Zoccal, D. B., and Machado, B. H. (2014). Short-term sustained hypoxia induces changes in the coupling of sympathetic and respiratory activities in rats. *J. Physiol.* 592, 2013–2033. doi: 10.1113/jphysiol.2013.262212

Mulligan, E., and Lahiri, S. (1982). Separation of carotid body chemoreceptor responses to O2 and CO2 by oligomycin and by antimycin A. *Am. J. Physiol.* 242, C200–C206. doi: 10.1152/ajpcell.1982.242.3.C200

Neckar, J., Markova, I., Novak, F., Novakova, O., Szarszoi, O., Ost'adal, B., et al. (2005). Increased expression and altered subcellular distribution of PKC-δ in chronically hypoxic rat myocardium: involvement in cardioprotection. *Am. J. Physiol. Heart Circ. Physiol.* 288, H1566–H1572.

Nurse, C. A. (2005). Neurotransmission and neuromodulation in the chemosensory carotid body. *Auton. Neurosci.* 120, 1–9. doi: 10.1016/j.autneu.2005.04.008

Nurse, C. A., and Fearon, I. M. (2002). Carotid body chemoreceptors in dissociated cell culture. *Microsc. Res. Tech.* 59, 249–255. doi: 10.1002/jemt.10199

Nurse, C. A., Jackson, A., and Stea, A. (1994). Plasticity in cultured arterial chemoreceptors: effects of chronic hypoxia and cyclic AMP analogs. *Adv. Exp. Med. Biol.* 360, 167–170. doi: 10.1007/978-1-4615-2572-1_20

Olson, E. B. J. R., and Dempsey, J. A. (1978). Rat as a model for human like ventilatory adaptation to chronic hypoxia. *J. Appl. Physiol.* 44, 763–769. doi: 10.1152/jappl.1978.44.5.763

Ortega-Sáenz, P., Pascual, A., Gómez-Díaz, R., and López-Barneo, J. (2006). Acute oxygen sensing in heme oxygenase-2 null mice. *J. Gen. Physiol.* 128, 405–411. doi: 10.1085/jgp.200609591

Ortiz, F., Varas, R., and Iturriaga, R. (2007). Chronic hypoxia enhanced the TASK-like current inhibition evoked by acute hypoxia. *Biol. Res.* 40:135.

Ortiz, F. C., Del Rio, R., Ebensperger, G., Reyes, V. R., Alcayaga, J., Varas, R., et al. (2013). Inhibition of rat carotid body glomus cells TASK-like channels by acute hypoxia is enhanced by chronic intermittent hypoxia. *Respir. Physiol. Neurobiol.* 185, 600–607. doi: 10.1016/j.resp.2012.11.015

Overholt, J. L., and Prabhakar, N. R. (1997). Ca^{2+} current in rabbit carotid body glomus cells is conducted by multiple types of high-voltage-activated Ca^{2+} channels. *J. Neurophysiol.* 78, 2467–2474. doi: 10.1152/jn.1997.78.5.2467

Overholt, J. L., and Prabhakar, N. R. (1999). Norepinephrine inhibits a toxin resistant Ca^{2+} current in carotid body glomus cells: evidence for a direct G protein mechanism. *J. Neurophysiol.* 81, 225–233. doi: 10.1152/jn.1999.81.1.225

Paciga, M., Vollmer, C., and Nurse, C. (1999). Role of ET-1 in hypoxia-induced mitosis of cultured rat carotid body chemoreceptors. *Neuroreport* 10, 3739–3744. doi: 10.1097/00001756-199912160-00003

Pardal, R., Ortega-sáenz, P., Durán, R., and López-barneo, J. (2007). Glia-like stem cells sustain physiologic neurogenesis in the adult mammalian carotid body. *Cell* 131, 234–236. doi: 10.1016/j.cell.2007.07.043

Peers, C. (1990). Hypoxic suppression of K^+ currents in type I carotid body cells: selective effect on the Ca^{2+}-activated K^+ current. *Neurosci. Lett.* 119, 253–256. doi: 10.1016/0304-3940(90)90846-2

Peers, C., and Carpenter, E. (1998). Inhibition of Ca^{2+}-dependent K^+ channels in rat carotid body type I cells by protein kinase C. *J. Physiol.* 512, 743–750. doi: 10.1111/j.1469-7793.1998.743bd.x

Peers, C., Carpenter, E., Hatton, C. J., Wyatt, C. N., and Bee, D. (1996). Ca^{2+} channeln currents in type I carotid body cells of normoxic and chronically hypoxic neonatal rats. *Brain Res.* 739, 251–257. doi: 10.1016/S0006-8993(96)00832-3

Pequignot, J. M., Hellstrom, S., and Johannsson, H. (1984). Intact and sympathectomized carotid bodies of long-term hypoxic rats: a morphometric ultrastructural study. *J. Neurocytol.* 13, 481–493. doi: 10.1007/BF01148336

Powell, F. L. (2007). The influence of chronic hypoxia upon chemoreception. *Respir. Physiol. Neurobiol.* 157, 154–161. doi: 10.1016/j.resp.2007.01.009

Powell, F. L., Huey, K. A., and Dwinell, M. R. (2000). Central nervous system mechanisms of ventilatory acclimatization to hypoxia. *Respir. Physiol.* 121, 223–236. doi: 10.1016/S0034-5687(00)00130-4

Prabhakar, N. R. (2006). O2 sensing at the mammalian carotid body: why multiple O2 sensors and multiple transmitters? *Exp. Physiol.* 91, 17–23.

Prabhakar, N. R., and Semenza, G. L. (2016). Regulation of carotid body oxygen sensing by hypoxia-inducible factors. *Pflugers Arch.* 468, 71–75. doi: 10.1007/s00424-015-1719-z

Rey, S., and Iturriaga, R. (2004). Endothelins and nitric oxide: vasoactive modulators of carotid body chemoreception. *Curr. Neurovasc. Res.* 1, 465–473. doi: 10.2174/1567202043361857

Shimoda, L. A., and Semenza, G. L. (2011). HIF and the lung: role of hypoxia-inducible factors in pulmonary development and disease. *Am. J. Respir. Crit. Care Med.* 183, 152–156. doi: 10.1164/rccm.201009-1393PP

Smith, C. A., Bisgard, G. E., Nielsen, A. M., Daristotle, L., Kressin, N. A., Forster, H. V., et al. (1986). Carotid bodies are required for ventilatory acclimatization to chronic hypoxia. *J. Appl. Physiol.* 60, 1003–1010. doi: 10.1152/jappl.1986.60.3.1003

Summers, B. A., Overholt, J. L., and Prabhakar, N. R. (2000). Augmentation of calcium current by hypoxia in carotid body glomus cells. *Adv. Exp. Med. Biol.* 475, 589–599. doi: 10.1007/0-306-46825-5_57

Stea, A., Jackson, A., Macintyre, L., and Nurse, C. A. (1995). Long-term modulation of inward currents in O2 chemoreceptors by chronic hypoxia and cyclic AMP in vitro. *J. Neurosci.* 15, 2192–2202. doi: 10.1523/JNEUROSCI.15-03-02192.1995

Tatsumi, K., Pickett, C. K., and Weil, J. V. (1991). Attenuated carotid body hypoxic sensitivity after prolonged hypoxic exposure. *J. Appl. Physiol.* 70, 748–755. doi: 10.1152/jappl.1991.70.2.748

Tatsumi, K., Pickett, C. K., and Weil, J. V. (1995). Possible role of dopamine in ventilatory acclimatization to high altitude. *Respir. Physiol.* 99, 63–73. doi: 10.1016/0034-5687(94)00084-D

Varas, R., Alcayaga, J., and Iturriaga, R. (2003). ACh and ATP mediate excitatory transmission in cat carotid identified chemoreceptor units in vitro. *Brain Res.* 988, 154–163. doi: 10.1016/S0006-8993(03)03366-3

Varas, R., Wyatt, C. N., and Buckler, K. J. (2007). Modulation of TASK-like backgroundn potassium channels in rat arterial chemoreceptor cells by intracellular ATP and other nucleotides. *J. Physiol.* 583, 521–536. doi: 10.1113/jphysiol.2007.135657

Vizek, M., Pickett, C. K., and Weil, J. V. (1987). Increased carotid body hypoxic sensitivity during acclimatization to hypobaric hypoxia. *J. Appl. Physiol.* 63, 2403–2410. doi: 10.1152/jappl.1987.63.6.2403

Williams, B. A., and Buckler, K. J. (2004). Biophysical properties and metabolic regulation of a TASK-like potassium channel in rat carotid body type 1 cells. *Am. J. Physiol. Lung Cell. Mol. Physiol.* 286, L221–L230. doi: 10.1152/ajplung.00010.2003

Williams, S. E., Wootton, P., Mason, H. S., Bould, J., Iles, D. E., Riccardi, D., et al. (2004). Hemoxygenase-2 is an oxygen sensor for a calcium-sensitive potassium channel. *Science* 306, 2093–2097. doi: 10.1126/science.1105010

Wilson, D. F., Mokashi, A., Chugh, D., Vinogradov, S., Osanai, S., and Lahiri, S. (1994). The primary oxygen sensor of the cat carotid body is cytochromea3 of the mitochondrial respiratory chain. *FEBS Lett.* 351, 370–374. doi: 10.1016/0014-5793(94)00887-6

Wyatt, C. N., Mustard, K. J., Pearson, S. A., Dallas, M. L., Atkinson, L., Kumar, P., et al. (2007). AMP-activated protein kinase mediates carotid body excitation by hypoxia. *J. Biol. Chem.* 282, 8092–8098. doi: 10.1074/jbc.M608742200

Wyatt, C. N., and Peers, C. (1995). Ca^{2+}-activated K^+ channels in isolated type I cells of the neonatal rat carotid body. *J. Physiol.* 483, 559–565. doi: 10.1113/jphysiol.1995.sp020606

Wyatt, C. N., Weir, E. K., and Peers, C. (1994). Diphenylene iodonium blocks K^+ and Ca^{2+} currents in type I cells isolated from the neonatal rat carotid body. *Neurosci. Lett.* 172, 63–66. doi: 10.1016/0304-3940(94)90663-7

Wyatt, C. N., Wright, C., Bee, D., and Peers, C. (1995). O2-sensitive K^+ currents in carotid body chemoreceptor cells from normoxic and chronically hypoxic rats and their roles in hypoxic chemotransduction. *Proc. Natl. Acad. Sci. U.S.A.* 92, 295–299. doi: 10.1073/pnas.92.1.295

Xu, J., Xu, F., Tse, F., and Tse, A. (2005). ATP inhibits the hypoxia response in type I cells of rat carotid bodies. *J. Neurochem.* 92, 1419–1430. doi: 10.1111/j.1471-4159.2004.02978.x

Yamamoto, Y., Kummer, W., Atoji, Y., and Suzuki, Y. (2002). TASK-1, TASK-2, TASK-3 and TRAAK immunoreactivities in the rat carotid body. *Brain Res.* 950, 304–307. doi: 10.1016/S0006-8993(02)03181-5

Yamamoto, Y., and Taniguchi, K. (2006). Expression of tandem P domain K^+ channel, TREK-1, in the rat carotid body. *J. Histochem. Cytochem.* 54, 467–472. doi: 10.1369/jhc.5A6755.2005

Ye, J. S., Tipoe, G. L., Fung, P. C., and Fung, M. L. (2002). Augmentation of hypoxia-induced nitric oxide generation in the rat carotid body adapted to chronic hypoxia: an involvement of constitutive and inducible nitric oxide synthases. *Pflugers Arch.* 444, 178–185. doi: 10.1007/s00424-002-0785-1

Zhang, M., Fearon, I. M., Zhong, H., and Nurse, C. A. (2003). Presynaptic modulation of rat arterial chemoreceptor function by 5-HT: role of K^+ channel inhibition via protein kinase C. *J. Physiol.* 551, 825–842. doi: 10.1113/jphysiol.2002.038489

Zhang, M., Vollmer, C., and Nurse, C. A. (2017). Adenosine and dopamine oppositely modulate a hyperpolarization-activated current Ih in chemosensory neurons of the rat carotid body in co-culture. *J. Physiol.* doi: 10.1113/JP274743 [Epub ahead of print].

Zhang, M., Zhong, H., Vollmer, C., and Nurse, C. A. (2000). Co-release of ATP and ACh mediates hypoxic signaling at rat carotid body chemoreceptors. *J. Physiol.* 1, 143–158. doi: 10.1111/j.1469-7793.2000.t01-1-00143.x

Zhang, Y. C., Ni, W., Zhang, Z. K., and Xu, Y. J. (2004). The effect of protein kinase C on voltagegated potassium channel in pulmonary artery smooth muscle cells from rats exposed to chronic hypoxia. *Chin. Med. J.* 117, 19–23.

Zilberberg, N., Ilan, N., Gonzalez-Colaso, R., and Goldstein, S. A. (2000). Opening and closing of KCNKO potassium leak channels is tightly regulated. *J. Gen. Physiol.* 116, 721–734. doi: 10.1085/jgp.116.5.721

12

Intrapartum Fetal Heart Rate: A Possible Predictor of Neonatal Acidemia and APGAR Score

Thâmila Kamila de Souza Medeiros[1,2], Mirela Dobre[3], Daniela Monteiro Baptista da Silva[1,2], Andrei Brateanu[4], Ovidiu Constantin Baltatu[1,2] and Luciana Aparecida Campos[1,2]**

[1] *Center of Innovation, Technology and Education at Anhembi Morumbi University – Laureate International Universities, São José dos Campos, Brazil,* [2] *School of Health Sciences at Anhembi Morumbi University – Laureate International Universities, São José dos Campos, Brazil,* [3] *Division of Nephrology and Hypertension, University Hospitals, Cleveland, OH, United States,* [4] *Medicine Institute, Cleveland Clinic, Cleveland, OH, United States*

Correspondence:
Ovidiu Constantin Baltatu
ocbaltatu@anhembi.br;
ocbaltatu@gmail.com
Luciana Aparecida Campos
labaltatu@anhembi.br;
camposbaltatu@gmail.com

Background: Predicting perinatal outcomes based on patterns of fetal heart rate (FHR) remains a challenge. The aim of this study was to evaluate intrapartum FHR variability as predictor for neonatal acidemia and APGAR score.

Methods: This was a retrospective observational study of 552 childbirths. Multivariable linear regression models were used to assess the association between FHR variability and each of the following outcomes: arterial cord blood pH and base deficit, Apgar 1, and 5 scores. Variables used for adjustment were maternal age, comorbidities (gestational diabetes, preeclampsia, maternal fever, and hypertension), parity, gravidity, uterine contractions, and newborn gestational age, and weight at birth.

Results: The following factors were associated with an increased risk of metabolic acidosis and low Apgar scores at birth: increased mean and coefficient of variation (CV) of the FHR, type of delivery and decreased parity. Each 10-beat/min increase in the FHR was associated with an increase of 0.43 mEq/L in the base deficit, and a decrease of 0.01 in the pH, 0.2 in the Apgar 1, and 0.14 in the Apgar 5 scores. Each 10% increase in the CV of the FHR was associated with an increase of 4.05 mEq/L in the base deficit and a decrease of 0.13 in the pH, 1.31 in the Apgar 1, and 0.86 in the Apgar 5 scores.

Conclusion: These data suggest the intrapartum FHR variability is physiologically relevant and can be used for predicting the acidemia and Apgar scores at birth of the newborn infants without severe cases of morbidity and from uncomplicated pregnancies.

Keywords: fetal monitoring, heart rate, perinatal outcome, noninvasive prenatal diagnosis, neonatal acidemia, APGAR

INTRODUCTION

Contemporary research aims to identify reliable and early markers for the neonatal acidemia and the physical condition of a newborn infant (Devane et al., 2012, 2017). Intrapartum cardiotocography monitors fetal heart rate (FHR) and uterine contractions and is commonly used for the early detection of fetal distress (Stout and Cahill, 2011).

It is theorized that intrapartum cardiotocography FHR could detect fetal hypoxia and/or acidosis allowing a timely intervention to reduce adverse neonatal outcomes such as postnatal cerebral palsy. This is based on the theory that intrapartum hypoxia may lead to alterations in the fetal central nervous system that directly affects the electrical activity of the fetal heart and could also induce neonatal cerebral palsy (Garabedian et al., 2017). Indeed, cardiotocography FHR parameters including baseline FHR and its variability appear to be independent predictors of fetal acidosis (Silberstein et al., 2017), were associated with a substantial decrease in early neonatal mortality and morbidity (Chen et al., 2011). At present, however, there is no consensus regarding sensitivity and specificity of cardiotocography classifications in predicting acidemia, with three guidelines for cardiotocography interpretation provided by the International Federation of Gynecology and Obstetrics (FIGO), American College of Obstetrics and Gynecology (ACOG), and National Institute for Health and Care Excellence (NICE) (Bhatia et al., 2017; Santo et al., 2017).

The improvement in the accuracy of FHR pattern interpretation through a continuous FHR centralization system is envisaged to be beneficial in reducing the incidence of neonatal acidemia (Michikata et al., 2016). To improve the predictive efficacy of cardiotocography FHR, diagnostic algorithms are currently being investigated to be used in real-time computerized systems for decision support (van Scheepen et al., 2016).

In this study, we aimed at investigating whether the intrapartum baseline and variability parameters of FHR are independently associated with neonatal acidemia and the APGAR scores of the newborn infants without severe cases of morbidity and from uncomplicated pregnancies.

MATERIALS AND METHODS

Study Design and Setting

A single-center retrospective observational study of 552 childbirths at the University Hospital Brno (UHB), Czechia (Chudacek et al., 2014). The hospital records were consecutively selected to pair both clinical and cardiotocography signal parameters.

Clinical Data

Clinical selection criteria (Chudacek et al., 2014) included maternal age (maternal age > 18 years), gravidity (only singleton, uncomplicated pregnancies), gestational week (weeks of gestation ≥ 37), delivery type (the majority of the database consists of vaginal deliveries), fetuses without known congenital defects or known intrauterine growth restriction (IUGR). Additional criteria considered were: sex of the fetus, parity, and risk factors including gestational diabetes, preeclampsia, maternal fever (>37.5°C), hypertension, and meconium stained fluid. The cohort included neonates without severe cases of neonatal morbidity, hypoxic ischemic encephalopathy, or seizures.

Cardiotocography Data

Cardiotocography recordings included contained time information and signal of FHR and uterine contractions sampled at 4 Hz were recorded starting 90 min preceding the delivery. Cardiotocography recordings selection criteria (Chudacek et al., 2014) were the signal length: 90 min preceding the delivery with 1st stage was limited to a maximum of 60 min and 2nd stage to 30 min in order to keep recordings easily comparable. Other criteria were: missing signal, noise and artifacts, and type of measurement device. The database is composed as a mixture of recordings acquired by ultrasound doppler probe, direct scalp measurement or combination of both, reflecting the clinical reality at the obstetrics ward. Cardiotocographies were recorded using STAN S21 and S31 (Neoventa Medical, Mölndal, Sweden) and Avalon FM40 and FM50 (Philips Healthcare, Andover, MA, United States) fetal monitors.

The cardiotocography recordings and clinical data were matched using anonymous unique identifiers generated by the hospital information system. A flowchart diagram describing the process of data selection for the final database is presented in the original publication (Chudacek et al., 2014).

The acid-base status (pH and base deficit) of umbilical cord arterial blood was measured at the moment of birth to evaluate the metabolic condition of neonates.

Apgar's scores (Apgar) at 1 and 5 min after birth evaluated the outcome of the delivery based on five categories: breathing effort, heart rate, muscle tone, reflexes, and skin color.

The CARDIOTOCOGRAPHY database is available at PhysioNet[1] ((Chudacek et al., 2014). All Physionet databases have been fully anonymized and may be used without further institutional review board approval.

Statistical Analysis

The FHR variability was determined using coefficient of variation (CV), which equals the standard deviation divided by the mean (Pereira et al., 2017). The characteristics of study participants were depicted using standard descriptive statistics, overall and stratified by quartiles of the mean of FHR. Chi-square (χ^2) test of independence for categorical (nominal) variables and Analysis of variance (ANOVA) test for continuous variables were used to analyze the covariates of interest.

Multivariable linear regression models were used to assess the association between FHRVand each of the following outcomes: pH, base deficit, Apgar 1, and 5 scores. Variables used for adjustment were maternal age, comorbidities, parity, gravidity,

[1] https://physionet.org/physiobank/database/ctu-uhb-ctgdb/

uterine contractions, and newborn gestational age, and weight at birth.

All statistical tests were two sided, and $P < 0.05$ was considered significant. IBM Corp (2016) SPSS Statistics for MAC, Version 24.0, was used for analyses.

RESULTS

Patient Characteristics

A total of 552 study participants were included in the study. The age of the mothers was 30 (27–33) median (IQR) years and gestational age was 40 (39–41) median (IQR) weeks. Characteristics of study participants distributed according to quartiles of the mean of FHR are summarized in **Table 1**. Patients in the lowest vs. highest quartile of the mean of FHR had a higher CV of the FHR (14.73 ± 3.56 vs. 11.24 ± 3.85). Mean of FHR was not associated with maternal age, history of diabetes mellitus or hypertension or preeclampsia, delivery type, gravidity, parity, gestational week, and mean of uterine contractions.

Association Between FHR and Metabolic Acidosis

The median pH values of the cohort were 7.25 (IQR: 7.17–7.3) [min to max: 6.85–7.47]. In multivariable adjusted models, the following factors were associated with an increased risk of metabolic acidosis at birth: increased mean and CV of the FHR, type of delivery (Caesarian section over vaginal), decreased parity (**Tables 2, 3**). The following parameters were not associated with risk of metabolic acidosis at birth: maternal age, history of diabetes mellitus, hypertension, preeclampsia, gravidity, gestational week, uterine contractions, newborn sex or weight.

Each 10-beat/min increase in the FHR was associated with a 0.01 decrease in the pH and a 0.43 mEq/L increase in the base deficit.

Each 10% increase in the CV of the FHR was associated with a 0.13 decrease in the pH and a 4.05 mEq/L increase in the base deficit.

Association Between FHR and Apgar Scores

In multivariable adjusted models, the following factors were associated with an increased risk of low Apgar scores at birth: increased mean and CV of the FHR, history of preeclampsia, type of delivery (Caesarian section over vaginal), decreased parity (**Tables 4, 5**). The following parameters were not associated with risk of low Apgar scores at birth: maternal age, history of diabetes mellitus, hypertension, gravidity, uterine contractions, newborn sex or weight.

TABLE 1 | Characteristics of study participants by quartile of mean fetal heart rate.

Characteristics		All participants	Quartiles of the mean fetal heart rate (FHR)				*P*-value
		N = 552 *N* (%) or Mean ± SD	*N* = 138 *N* (%) or Mean ± SD	*N* = 138 *N* (%) or Mean ± SD	*N* = 138 *N* (%) or Mean ± SD	*N* = 138 *N* (%) or Mean ± SD	
Maternal							
Age (years)		29.60 ± 4.72	30.22 ± 4.63	29.48 ± 4.47	29.15 ± 5.11	29.54 ± 4.64	0.29
History of diabetes	No	515 (93.3)	126 (91.3)	131 (94.9)	128 (92.8)	130 (94.2)	0.63
mellitus	Yes	37 (6.7)	12 (8.7)	7 (5.1)	10 (7.2)	8 (5.8)	
History of hypertension	No	508 (92)	125 (90.6)	127 (92)	127 (92)	129 (93.5)	0.85
	Yes	44 (8)	13 (9.4)	11 (8)	11 (8)	9 (6.5)	
History of Preeclampsia	No	535 (96.9)	131 (94.9)	134 (97.1)	134 (97.1)	136 (98.6)	0.38
	Yes	17 (3.1)	7 (5.1)	4 (2.9)	4 (2.9)	2 (1.4)	
Delivery type	1	506 (91.7)	127 (92)	132 (95.7)	127 (92)	120 (87)	0.07
	2	46 (8.3)	11 (8)	6 (4.3)	11 (8)	18 (13)	
Gravidity		1.41 ± 1.03	1.47 ± 1.08	1.36 ± 0.79	1.24 ± 0.79	1.55 ± 1.35	0.07
Parity		0.41 ± 0.72	038 ± 0.74	0.44 ± 0.65	0.38 ± 0.84	0.43 ± 0.66	0.83
Gestational week		39.94 ± 1.71	40.04 ± 1.11	39.81 ± 2.78	40.02 ± 1.20	39.88 ± 1.13	0.63
UC – mean (contractions/min)		24.82 ± 10.54	24.45 ± 11.48	24.16 ± 10.46	25.54 ± 10.12	25.14 ± 10.08	0.69
UC – CV		75.48 ± 25.70	74.90 ± 28.15	73.76 ± 27.29	80.70 ± 25.06	72.61 ± 21.29	0.04
Newborn							
FHR – mean (beats/min)		134,90 ± 11.73	120.85 ± 4.87	130.40 ± 2.33	138.02 ± 2.23	150.31 ± 7.19	<0.001
FHR – CV		12.86 ± 3.91	14.73 ± 3.56	12.88 ± 3.66	12.55 ± 3.77	11.24 ± 3.85	<0.001
Sex	Female	286 (51.8)	76 (55.1)	70 (50.7)	63 (45.7)	77 (55.8)	0.30
	Male	266 (48.2)	62 (44.9)	68 (49.3)	75 (54.3)	61 (44.2)	
Newborn weight (g)		3397.52 ± 459.58	3321.12 ± 442.09	3401.28 ± 472.53	3431.88 ± 447.37	3435.80 ± 471.34	0.13

UC, uterine contractions; FHR, fetal heart rate; CV, coefficient of variation.

Each 10-beat/min increase in the FHR was associated with a 0.2 and 0.14 decrease in the Apgar score at 1 and 5 min after birth, respectively.

Each 10% increase in the CV of the FHR was associated with a 1.31 and 0.86 decrease in the Apgar score at 1 and 5 min after birth, respectively.

TABLE 2 | Association between maternal and newborn parameters and pH.

	pH			
Parameters	**Unstandardized B Coefficients**	**95% Confidence interval**		***P*-value**
		Lower bound	**Upper bound**	
Maternal age	0.000	−0.003	0.002	0.70
History of diabetes mellitus	−0.009	−0.049	0.030	0.64
History of hypertension	−0.033	−0.069	0.004	0.08
History of preeclampsia	−0.005	−0.059	0.049	0.85
Delivery type	−0.042	−0.072	−0.013	0.005
Gravidity	−0.003	−0.015	0.010	0.67
Parity	0.036	0.019	0.053	< 0.001
Gestational week	0.006	−0.004	0.015	0.25
UC – mean (contractions/min)	−5.328*E* − 5	−0.001	0.001	0.91
UC – CV	0.000	−0.001	0.000	0.32
FHR – mean (beats/min)	−0.001	−0.002	−0.001	0.001
FHR – CV	−0.013	−0.015	−0.010	< 0.001
Newborn sex	−0.013	−0.033	0.007	0.19
Newborn weight (g)	−1.108*E* − 5	0.000	0.000	0.34

TABLE 3 | Association between maternal and newborn parameters and base deficit.

	Base deficit (mEq/L)			
Parameters	**Unstandardized B Coefficients**	**95% Confidence interval**		***P*-value**
		Lower bound	**Upper bound**	
Maternal age	0.052	−0.010	0.115	0.10
History of diabetes mellitus	0.709	−0.338	1.756	0.18
History of hypertension	0.185	−0.763	1.132	0.70
History of Preeclampsia	−0.244	−1.743	1.254	0.75
Delivery type	1.970	1.001	2.939	< 0.001
Gravidity	0.090	−0.210	0.391	0.55
Parity	−1.188	−1.635	−0.740	< 0.001
Gestational week	0.016	−0.139	0.171	0.84
UC – mean	−0.001	−0.026	0.025	0.96
UC – CV	−0.001	−0.011	0.010	0.90
FHR – mean	0.043	0.019	0.067	< 0.001
FHR – CV	0.405	0.334	0.476	< 0.001
Newborn sex	0.089	−0.439	0.617	0.74
Newborn weight (g)	0.000	0.000	0.001	0.54

TABLE 4 | Association between maternal and newborn parameters and Apgar 1 score (1 min after birth).

	Apgar 1 score			
Parameters	**Unstandardized B Coefficients**	**95% Confidence interval**		***P*-value**
		Lower bound	**Upper bound**	
Maternal age	−0.001	−0.031	0.029	0.94
History of diabetes mellitus	0.279	−0.247	0.805	0.30
History of hypertension	−0.279	−0.755	0.198	0.25
History of Preeclampsia	−0.767	−1.521	−0.014	0.05
Delivery type	−0.207	−0.678	0.264	0.39
Gravidity	−0.031	−0.181	0.120	0.69
Parity	0.367	0.144	0.589	0.001
Gestational week	0.165	0.087	0.242	< 0.001
UC – mean	0.000	−0.013	0.012	0.95
UC – CV	−0.002	−0.007	0.003	0.44
FHR – mean	−0.020	−0.031	−0.008	0.001
, FHR – CV	−0.131	−0.166	−0.095	< 0.001
Newborn sex	0.208	−0.056	0.471	0.12
Newborn weight (g)	−0.001	−0.001	0.000	< 0.001

TABLE 5 | Association between maternal and newborn parameters and Apgar 5 score (5 min after birth).

	Apgar 5 score			
Parameters	**Unstandardized B Coefficients**	**95% Confidence interval**		***P*-value**
		Lower bound	**Upper bound**	
Maternal age	−0.007	−0.028	0.015	0.54
History of diabetes mellitus	0.001	−0.374	0.376	0.99
History of hypertension	−0.126	−0.465	0.214	0.47
History of Preeclampsia	−0.938	−1.475	−0.400	0.001
Delivery type	−0.083	−0.419	0.253	0.63
Gravidity	−0.070	−0.177	0.038	0.20
Parity	0.234	0.076	0.393	0.004
Gestational week	0.053	−0.002	0.109	0.06
UC – mean	0.002	−0.007	0.011	0.63
UC – CV	0.000	−0.004	0.003	0.89
FHR – mean	−0.014	−0.023	−0.006	0.001
FHR – CV	−0.086	−0.111	−0.061	< 0.001
Newborn sex	0.060	−0.128	0.248	0.53
Newborn weight (g)	0.000	−0.001	0.000	0.003

DISCUSSION

The main findings of this study are that in a cohort of uncomplicated childbirths without severe cases of neonatal morbidity, hypoxic ischemic encephalopathy, or seizures: (1) increased mean and CV of the intrapartum FHR were associated with increased risk of metabolic acidosis and low Apgar scores at birth; (2) FHR was not associated with maternal age, history of diabetes mellitus or hypertension or preeclampsia, delivery type, gravidity, parity, gestational week, mean of uterine contractions. Besides the intrapartum cardiotocography FHR, delivery type, and decreased parity were also associated with neonatal acidemia and the physical condition of a newborn infant.

Intrapartum fetal hypoxia represents an important cause of postnatal cerebral palsy or other neurologic outcomes and in a significant proportion of cases there is evidence of suboptimal care related to fetal surveillance. Umbilical artery metabolic acidosis is commonly used to detect neurological injury (Ross and Gala, 2002).

A three-tiered FHR interpretation system for intrapartum cardiotocography FHR tracing interpretation was proposed (Macones et al., 2008; American College of Obestetricians and Gynecologists, 2009). As our study did not include complicated pregnancies, it supports using the normal cardiotocography FHR (category I), which has a predictive value of 99.7% of an Apgar score more than 7 (Macones et al., 2008; Crovetto et al., 2017; Raghuraman and Cahill, 2017).

Using multivariable models to control confounders, cardiotocography FHR was recently found to be an independent predictor of fetal acidosis (Silberstein et al., 2017), respiratory morbidity in term neonates (Liu et al., 2015), and indicator for preterm cesarean delivery for increased risk of neonatal and childhood morbidity (Mendez-Figueroa et al., 2015). In our multivariable model analysis, metabolic acidosis at birth had an independent relationship with the cardiotocography FHR mean and variability and also with the type of delivery (Caesarian section over vaginal) and parity. Our results are in agreement with the study of Heinonen et al. who also found that parity, but not maternal age, was an independent risk factor for neonatal acidosis (Heinonen and Saarikoski, 2001). Corroborating our results with another study of women with a singleton term pregnancy that found previous cesarean delivery and nulliparity as risk factors for neonatal metabolic acidosis (Westerhuis et al., 2012) may indicate that not only previous but also the current cesarean delivery may represent an actual challenge to the fetus. In two studies of poor neonatal adaptation at birth with severe neonatal acidosis (umbilical artery pH less than 7.10) independent risk factors included abnormal cardiotocography FHR, maternal age 35 years or older, parity, prior neonatal death or cesarean delivery (Maisonneuve et al., 2011; Crovetto et al., 2017). Our data extends a valuable role for cardiotocography FHR in predicting neonatal acidosis in deliveries with Apgar 5 ranging from fairly low to normal without neurological complications.

Heart rate variability (HRV) analysis with search for new algorithms is commonly employed to measure alterations in autonomic tone with predictive value in diseases (Campos et al., 2013). We have identified the CV of the heart rate as a sensitive measure of autonomic dysfunction (Miyabara et al., 2017) and independently associated with vascular atherosclerosis (Pereira et al., 2017). In this study, we found that CV of intrapartum cardiotocography FHR is an independent predictor of neonatal acidemia and Apgar scores.

Limitations and Strengths of the Study

There are important limitations associated with this study. First, since this was a retrospective study, we could only investigate factors that were available to us in the current dataset, mid-to-long term outcomes of the infants being not recorded in the database. Also, fetal sleep state was not considered in this study. Second, although robust statistical methods were used to account for differences between groups, the potential for residual confounding cannot be ruled out. This study, as with most retrospective studies, is susceptible to bias. Third, the results of the study cannot be generalizable to all patients, for instance to those with an APGAR score critically low or associated with neurological complications and did not include data from neonates with severe cases of neonatal morbidity, hypoxic ischemic encephalopathy, or seizures. Limitations notwithstanding there are key strengths to this paper. To our knowledge, this is the first study with a relatively large sample size providing sufficient statistical power to explore the relationship between intrapartum FHRV and neonatal acidemia or APGAR score. Also, we adjusted for several confounders including important comorbidities.

CONCLUSION

In conclusion, the present findings provide evidence that intrapartum cardiotocography FHR could be a predictor for neonatal acidemia and the physical condition of a newborn infant, as determined by arterial cord blood pH and base deficit, Apgar 1, and 5 scores. Further studies are warranted to examine the potential relationship between intrapartum FHR and neonatal pathologies including neurological complications.

AUTHOR CONTRIBUTIONS

OB, LC, AB, MD, TM, and DdS conceived and designed the study, and analyzed and interpreted the data. OB, LC, MD, and AB drafted the manuscript. TM, MD, DdS, AB, LC, and OB critically revised the manuscript. LC and OB are the guarantors of this work and, as such, had full access to all the data in the study and takes responsibility for the integrity of the data and the accuracy of the data analysis.

FUNDING

This research was supported by São Paulo Research Foundation to LC (FAPESP 17/11976-0).

ACKNOWLEDGMENTS

We gratefully acknowledge Prof. Dr. Václav Chudáèek and colleagues for making available the cardiotocography database to PhysioNet. No assistance in the preparation of this article is to be declared. We thank the reviewers for their thoughtful review of the manuscript. They raised important issues and their inputs were very helpful for improving the manuscript.

REFERENCES

American College of Obestetricians and Gynecologists (2009). ACOG Practice Bulletin No. 106: intrapartum fetal heart rate monitoring: nomenclature, interpretation, and general management principles. *Obstet. Gynecol.* 114, 192–202. doi: 10.1097/AOG.0b013e3181aef106

Bhatia, M., Mahtani, K. R., Nunan, D., and Reddy, A. (2017). A cross-sectional comparison of three guidelines for intrapartum cardiotocography. *Int. J. Gynaecol. Obstet.* 138, 89–93. doi: 10.1002/ijgo.12161

Campos, L. A., Pereira, V. L. Jr., Muralikrishna, A., Albarwani, S., Brás, S., and Gouveia, S. (2013). Mathematical biomarkers for the autonomic regulation of cardiovascular system. *Front. Physiol.* 4:279. doi: 10.3389/fphys.2013.00279

Chen, H. Y., Chauhan, S. P., Ananth, C. V., Vintzileos, A. M., and Abuhamad, A. Z. (2011). Electronic fetal heart rate monitoring and its relationship to neonatal and infant mortality in the United States. *Am. J. Obstet. Gynecol.* 204, 491.e1–491.e10. doi: 10.1016/j.ajog.2011.04.024

Chudacek, V., Spilka, J., Bursa, M., Janku, P., Hruban, L., Huptych, M., et al. (2014). Open access intrapartum CTG database. *BMC Pregnancy Childbirth* 14:16. doi: 10.1186/1471-2393-14-16

Crovetto, F., Fumagalli, M., De Carli, A., Baffero, G. M., Nozza, S., Dessimone, F., et al. (2017). Obstetric risk factors for poor neonatal adaptation at birth. *J. Matern. Fetal Neonatal Med.* 31, 2429–2435. doi: 10.1080/14767058.2017.1344635

Devane, D., Lalor, J. G., Daly, S., Mcguire, W., Cuthbert, A., and Smith, V. (2017). Cardiotocography versus intermittent auscultation of fetal heart on admission to labour ward for assessment of fetal wellbeing. *Cochrane Database Syst. Rev.* 1:CD005122. doi: 10.1002/14651858.CD005122.pub5

Devane, D., Lalor, J. G., Daly, S., Mcguire, W., and Smith, V. (2012). Cardiotocography versus intermittent auscultation of fetal heart on admission to labour ward for assessment of fetal wellbeing. *Cochrane Database Syst. Rev.* 2, 1–39.

Garabedian, C., De Jonckheere, J., Butruille, L., Deruelle, P., Storme, L., and Houfflin-Debarge, V. (2017). Understanding fetal physiology and second line monitoring during labor. *J. Gynecol. Obstet. Hum. Reprod.* 46, 113–117. doi: 10.1016/j.jogoh.2016.11.005

Heinonen, S., and Saarikoski, S. (2001). Reproductive risk factors of fetal asphyxia at delivery: a population based analysis. *J. Clin. Epidemiol.* 54, 407–410. doi: 10.1016/S0895-4356(00)00329-2

Liu, L., Tuuli, M. G., Roehl, K. A., Odibo, A. O., Macones, G. A., and Cahill, A. G. (2015). Electronic fetal monitoring patterns associated with respiratory morbidity in term neonates. *Am. J. Obstet. Gynecol.* 213, e681–e686. doi: 10.1016/j.ajog.2015.07.013

Macones, G. A., Hankins, G. D., Spong, C. Y., Hauth, J., and Moore, T. (2008). The 2008 National Institute of Child Health and Human Development workshop report on electronic fetal monitoring: update on definitions, interpretation, and research guidelines. *Obstet. Gynecol.* 112, 661–666. doi: 10.1097/AOG.0b013e3181841395

Maisonneuve, E., Audibert, F., Guilbaud, L., Lathelize, J., Jousse, M., Pierre, F., et al. (2011). Risk factors for severe neonatal acidosis. *Obstet. Gynecol.* 118, 818–823. doi: 10.1097/AOG.0b013e31822c9198

Mendez-Figueroa, H., Chauhan, S. P., Pedroza, C., Refuerzo, J. S., Dahlke, J. D., and Rouse, D. J. (2015). Preterm cesarean delivery for nonreassuring fetal heart rate: neonatal and neurologic morbidity. *Obstet. Gynecol.* 125, 636–642. doi: 10.1097/AOG.0000000000000673

Michikata, K., Sameshima, H., Urabe, H., Tokunaga, S., Kodama, Y., and Ikenoue, T. (2016). The regional centralization of electronic fetal heart rate monitoring and its impact on neonatal acidemia and the cesarean birth rate. *J. Pregnancy* 2016:3658527. doi: 10.1155/2016/3658527

Miyabara, R., Berg, K., Kraemer, J. F., Baltatu, O. C., Wessel, N., and Campos, L. A. (2017). Quantifying effects of pharmacological blockers of cardiac autonomous control using variability parameters. *Front. Physiol.* 8:10. doi: 10.3389/fphys.2017.00010

Pereira, V. L. Jr., Dobre, M., Dos Santos, S. G., Fuzatti, J. S., Oliveira, C. R., Campos, L. A., et al. (2017). Association between carotid intima media thickness and heart rate variability in adults at increased cardiovascular risk. *Front. Physiol.* 8:248. doi: 10.3389/fphys.2017.00248

Raghuraman, N., and Cahill, A. G. (2017). Update on fetal monitoring: overview of approaches and management of category II tracings. *Obstet. Gynecol. Clin. North Am.* 44, 615–624. doi: 10.1016/j.ogc.2017.08.007

Ross, M. G., and Gala, R. (2002). Use of umbilical artery base excess: algorithm for the timing of hypoxic injury. *Am. J. Obstet. Gynecol.* 187, 1–9. doi: 10.1067/mob.2002.123204

Santo, S., Ayres-De-Campos, D., Costa-Santos, C., Schnettler, W., Ugwumadu, A., Da Graca, L. M., et al. (2017). Agreement and accuracy using the FIGO, ACOG and NICE cardiotocography interpretation guidelines. *Acta Obstet. Gynecol. Scand.* 96, 166–175. doi: 10.1111/aogs.13064

Silberstein, T., Sheiner, E., Salem, S. Y., Hamou, B., Aricha, B., Baumfeld, Y., et al. (2017). Fetal heart rate monitoring category 3 during the 2nd stage of labor is an independent predictor of fetal acidosis. *J. Matern. Fetal Neonatal Med.* 30, 257–260. doi: 10.3109/14767058.2016.1172064

Stout, M. J., and Cahill, A. G. (2011). Electronic fetal monitoring: past, present, and future. *Clin. Perinatol.* 38, 127–142. doi: 10.1016/j.clp.2010.12.002

van Scheepen, J. A., Koster, M. P., Vasak, B., Redman, C., Franx, A., and Georgieva, A. (2016). Effect of signal acquisition method on the fetal heart rate analysis with phase rectified signal averaging. *Physiol. Meas.* 37, 2245–2259. doi: 10.1088/1361-6579/37/12/2245

Westerhuis, M. E., Schuit, E., Kwee, A., Zuithoff, N. P., Groenwold, R. H., Van Den Akker, E. S., et al. (2012). Prediction of neonatal metabolic acidosis in women with a singleton term pregnancy in cephalic presentation. *Am. J. Perinatol.* 29, 167–174. doi: 10.1055/s-0031-1284226

13

High Altitude Increases Alteration in Maximal Torque but not in Rapid Torque Development in Knee Extensors After Repeated Treadmill Sprinting

Olivier Girard[1,2], Franck Brocherie[1] and Grégoire P. Millet[1]*

[1] *ISSUL, Institute of Sport Sciences, Faculty of Biology and Medicine, University of Lausanne, Lausanne, Switzerland,* [2] *Athlete Health and Performance Research Centre, Orthopaedic and Sports Medicine Hospital, Aspetar, Doha, Qatar*

Correspondence:
Olivier Girard
oliv.girard@gmail.com

We assessed knee extensor neuromuscular adjustments following repeated treadmill sprints in different normobaric hypoxia conditions, with special reference to rapid muscle torque production capacity. Thirteen team- and racquet-sport athletes undertook 8 × 5-s "all-out" sprints (passive recovery = 25 s) on a non-motorized treadmill in normoxia (NM; FiO_2 = 20.9%), at low (LA; FiO_2 = 16.8%) and high (HA; FiO_2 = 13.3%) normobaric hypoxia (simulated altitudes of ∼1800 m and ∼3600 m, respectively). Explosive (∼1 s; "fast" instruction) and maximal (∼5 s; "hard" instruction) voluntary isometric contractions (MVC) of the knee extensors (KE), with concurrent electromyographic (EMG) activity recordings of the *vastus lateralis* (VL) and *rectus femoris* (RF) muscles, were performed before and 1-min post-exercise. Rate of torque development (RTD) and EMG (i.e., Root Mean Square or RMS) rise from 0 to 30, −50, −100, and −200 ms were recorded, and were also normalized to maximal torque and EMG values, respectively. Distance covered during the first 5-s sprint was similar ($P > 0.05$) in all conditions. A larger ($P < 0.05$) sprint decrement score and a shorter ($P < 0.05$) cumulated distance covered over the eight sprints occurred in HA (−8 ± 4% and 178 ± 11 m) but not in LA (−7 ± 3% and 181 ± 10 m) compared to NM (−5 ± 2% and 183 ± 9 m). Compared to NM (−9 ± 7%), a larger ($P < 0.05$) reduction in MVC torque occurred post-exercise in HA (−14 ± 9%) but not in LA (-12 ± 7%), with no difference between NM and LA ($P > 0.05$). Irrespectively of condition ($P > 0.05$), peak RTD (−6 ± 11%; $P < 0.05$), and normalized peak RMS activity for VL (−8 ± 11%; $P = 0.07$) and RF (−14 ± 11%; $P < 0.01$) muscles were reduced post-exercise, whereas reductions ($P < 0.05$) in absolute RTD occurred within the 0–100 (−8 ± 9%) and 0–200 ms (−10 ± 8%) epochs after contraction onset. After normalization to MVC torque, there was no difference in RTD values. Additionally, the EMG rise for VL muscle was similar ($P > 0.05$), whereas it increased ($P < 0.05$) for RF muscle during all epochs post-exercise, independently of the conditions. In summary, alteration in repeated-sprint ability and post-exercise MVC decrease were greater at high altitude than in normoxia or at low altitude. However, the post-exercise alterations in RTD were similar between normoxia and low-to-high hypoxia.

Keywords: repeated-sprint ability, hypoxia, rapid torque development, neural drive, voluntary force production

INTRODUCTION

Intense physical efforts performed at or near maximal speed and the ability to recover from it are important markers of successful in-game performance in high-intensity, intermittent sports (Spencer et al., 2005). Team- and racquet-sport players implement training methods, based on the repetition of maximal efforts in normoxia (e.g., repeated sprints, Bishop et al., 2011) or in hypoxia (e.g., repeated sprints in hypoxia; Brocherie et al., 2015a), for eliciting neuromuscular adaptations (e.g., enhanced muscle oxygenation and activation responses) and improving cardiovascular and metabolic function, in turn maximizing their physical performance. Although the physiological responses and potential metabolic limiting factors (i.e., limitations in energy supply, metabolite accumulation) associated with the completion of one repeated-sprint set have largely been described, there is comparatively less data on the neuromuscular consequences (Girard et al., 2011).

Neuromuscular fatigue is an exercise-induced reduction in the maximal isometric voluntary contraction (MVC) force/torque or power of a muscle group, which potentially involves alterations at any levels from the brain to skeletal muscles (Gandevia, 2001). Over the past decade, an increasing number of studies have quantified neuromuscular fatigue following repeated running (Perrey et al., 2010) or cycling (Racinais et al., 2007; Billaut et al., 2013; Girard et al., 2013; Hureau et al., 2014) sprints by comparing pre- to post-sprint values of force/torque, voluntary activation, electromyogram (EMG), and twitch responses. Recent studies assessed the neuromuscular function during the actual repeated-sprint sets (Goodall et al., 2015; Pearcey et al., 2015). With regard to MVC, however, it is important to note that maximal force/torque production capacity is most often obtained when exceeding 300 ms following contraction onset (Thorstensson et al., 1976). This is contrasting to the characteristics of muscular contraction occurring in several sporting events, where muscle force needs to be developed in less than 250 ms (e.g., sprints: Kuitunen et al., 2002; jumps: Luhtanen and Komi, 1979). Therefore, the ability to rapidly generate force/torque, i.e., the rate of force/torque development (RTD) within the initial (i.e., <250 ms) phase of an MVC which in turn correlates with sprint performance (Tillin et al., 2013), likely constitutes a more functional outcome measure (Girard and Millet, 2009). Therefore, RTD as a surrogate for explosive strength should be assessed for a better understanding of the acute neuromuscular adjustments to repeated sprinting.

Repeated-sprint ability is more altered at high (>3000–3500 m or FiO_2 below 13–14%) than lower altitudes, either normoxia or low-to-moderate (<3000 m or FiO_2 above 14%) altitude (Bowtell et al., 2014; Goods et al., 2014). Not only acute hypoxic exposure decreases convective O_2 transport (i.e., reduction in arterial O_2 saturation values or SpO_2), but also challenges multiple regulatory systems by increasing cardiorespiratory (i.e., higher heart rate, minute ventilation, O_2 debt), metabolic (i.e., slower muscle re-oxygenation responses) and/or neuromuscular (i.e., incomplete muscle activation) requirements during sprinting or subsequent recovery periods (Balsom et al., 1994; Billaut et al., 2013; Bowtell et al., 2014). Compared to normoxia, the completion of a repeated-sprint cycling protocol (15 × 5-s efforts, 25-s rest) in high hypoxia (FiO_2 = 14%) led to ~8% lower total mechanical work as a result of impaired muscle activation, which was also accompanied by ~6% lower post-exercise MVC (Billaut et al., 2013). However, these authors did not include any measure of explosive strength in their study.

To our knowledge, only one study has investigated the effect of repeated sprinting (i.e., 10 × 6-s "all out" cycling sprints, followed, after 6 min of passive rest, by 5 × 6-s sprints; recoveries = 30 s) performance on post-exercise alterations in rapid muscle torque production capacity of the knee extensors (KE) (Girard et al., 2013). MVC (−12%) and RTD (−15 to −26% from the 0–30 to 0–200 ms epochs after contraction onset) decreased during brief (i.e., 5 s) contractions after (i.e., 3 min) the repeated-sprint exercise. From this report, however, it is not entirely clear to which extent differences in RTD actually resulted from maximal voluntary strength adjustments, since RTD results were not normalized to MVC torque. Hence, whereas MVC torque losses following prolonged match-play tennis accounted for the dampened RTD values (Girard et al., 2014), fatigue induced by 10 sets of voluntary maximal explosive contractions exerted a more rapid and pronounced effect (particularly during the initial 50 ms of contraction) on explosive strength than MVC torque (Buckthorpe et al., 2014). Consequently, although repeated sprinting decreases RTD (Girard et al., 2013), the question of whether RTD at early and/or late intervals is more pronouncedly impaired than MVC has not been specifically addressed.

The analysis of EMG amplitude throughout the rising force-time curve can reveal how voluntary neural drive to skeletal muscle underlies the post-exercise decreased RTD. Hence, the rate of muscle activation is related to muscle shortening velocity (Nelson, 1996), a factor directly influencing RTD (Harridge et al., 1996). Furthermore, the determinants of explosive force production appear to change throughout the rising force-time curve (Folland et al., 2014) and fatigue may differentially affect the development of force throughout the time course of an explosive contraction. After repeated sprinting, non-significant reductions in *vastus lateralis* (VL) Root Mean Square (RMS) activities have been shown to accompany deteriorated RTD values (Girard et al., 2013). However, because the delay between exercise termination and post-exercise neuromuscular testing was 3 min in the aforementioned study, any meaningful changes in the central nervous performance may have already recovered. Furthermore, it has not been investigated if the early and later RTD time intervals (and associated rate of EMG activity rise) are in fact modified differently by performing repeated-sprint in various hypoxia severity levels. This question of the alteration in explosive strength post-hypoxic exposure/training is of high practical relevance in team- and racquet-sports but remains unclear: Hence, while countermovement jump performance increased to a similar extent after repeated-sprint training in normoxia vs. hypoxia (Brocherie et al., 2015a), movement velocity and power during the execution of a force-velocity in bench-press are improved when exposed to hypobaric vs. normobaric hypoxia in reference to normoxia (Feriche et al., 2014).

The aim of this study was therefore to assess the effects of repeated sprinting in different levels of normobaric hypoxia on the alterations in RTD and neuromuscular activity of KE. Given that there is "*extraordinarily little that changes with regard to maximal force-generating capacity with acute hypoxia*" (Perrey and Rupp, 2009), it was hypothesized that the already-known decrease in repeated sprint ability (i.e., lower fatigue resistance) under high hypoxic conditions would not be associated with more pronounced alterations in explosive force production (i.e., RTD) compared to normoxia or low hypoxia.

METHODS

Participants

Thirteen male recreational team- (i.e., football, rugby, basketball) and racket- (i.e., tennis, squash) sport athletes (Mean ± SD: 31.2 ± 4.8 years; 178.4 ± 6.6 cm; 74.3 ± 8.2 kg) participated in the study. All participants were born and raised at <1000 m and had not traveled to elevations >1000 m in the 3 months prior to investigation. They gave their informed, written consent preceding the commencement of the experiment. Experimental protocol was conducted according to the Declaration of Helsinki for use of Human Subjects and approved by the Ethics Committee of *Shafallah Medical Genetics Center.*

Study Design

Elements have previously been reported in Girard et al. (2015a). About a week prior to testing, participants undertook a complete preliminary session where they performed short (<5 s) treadmill sprints at increasing intensities wearing a facemask for habituation (i.e., with the hypoxic system turned off), with full recovery and until being comfortable with the running technique required (which generally necessitated 7–10 trials). Then they performed three maximal 5-s single sprints, separated by 2 min of passive recovery, and after 5 min of rest, the repeated-sprint exercise test in full. All of them satisfied the criteria of having a coefficient of variation < 2.2% for distance covered across three successive trials (Girard et al., 2015b). Strong verbal encouragement was given during all maximal efforts. Participants were also thoroughly familiarized with the neuromuscular function assessment protocol (see *Neuromuscular Function*) until they felt accustomed with the equipment (i.e., coefficient of variation in three successive KE trials for peak RFD and maximal torque with "fast" and "hard" instructions lower than 5 and 3%, respectively).

Participants reported to the laboratory (well-ventilated at a constant temperature of ~25°C and 40% relative humidity) on three different occasions (~1 h; counterbalanced randomized crossover design in double-blind fashion) at least 3–4 days apart to complete an experimental session. This involved performing a repeated-sprint running protocol on a sprint treadmill (ADAL3D-WR, Medical Development – HEF Tecmachine, Andrézieux-Bouthéon, France), allowing participants to produce realistic acceleration and high running velocities (Morin et al., 2010). Participants performed their trials at the same time of the day (± 1 h) and wore similar sports gear (running shoes, short, and T-shirt). They were instructed to maintain their normal diet (i.e., avoiding any nutritional supplements or alcohol consumption), sleeping (i.e., ≥7 h/night) and training (i.e., avoiding vigorous exercise 24 h before every trial) habits during the 1–2 weeks period of testing to prevent any possible interference on their sprinting abilities. Participants were instructed to drink 4–6 mL of water per kilogram of body mass every 2.5 h on the day before each experimental session to ensure euhydration at the start of exercise. They were permitted to drink *ad libitum* during the warm-up procedure.

Experimental Protocol

Upon arrival on testing days, participants were instrumented and pre-exercise (Pre-tests) neuromuscular function assessment (see *Neuromuscular Function*) was conducted in normoxia. Thereafter, they completed a running warm-up (i.e., on the sprint treadmill with participants breathing ambient air) consisting of 5 min of running at 10 km.h^{-1}, followed by 10 min of sprint-specific muscular warm-up exercises [i.e., 3 × (skipping, high knee, butt-kick, high heels for ~10 s with 30-s walking in between), followed by 3 × (3 steps accelerations at a subjective "sense of effort" of 7, 8, and 9 on a modified Borg 10 scale), then by 2 × (3-s sprints at a subjective "sense of effort" of 8 and 9)] (Christian et al., 2014). Afterwards, three maximal 5-s single sprints, separated by 2 min of passive recovery, were completed. After a facemask connected to a portable hypoxic generator (Altitrainer, SMTEC SA, Nyon, Switzerland) had been attached on participants, they were allowed 5-min of free cool-down prior to the repeated-sprint protocol. This exercise consisted of performing eight, 5-s "all-out" sprints interspersed with 25 s of passive rest and was randomly conducted in normoxia (NM; FiO_2 = 20.9%), in low and high simulated altitudes (normobaric hypoxia) of ~1800 m (LA; FiO_2 = 16.8%) and ~3600 m (HA; FiO_2 = 13.3%), respectively. Normobaric hypoxia was obtained by mixing nitrogen into ambient air under control of FiO_2. During recovery periods, participants stood quietly on the treadmill. Repeated-sprint ability was assessed from covered distance data using three scores: the largest (i.e., during the first sprint in all cases) distance ran, the cumulated distance covered over the eight sprints (i.e., sum of the eight sprints) and the sprint decrement score [i.e., ([cumulated distance/(largest distance × 8)]–1) × 100] (Girard et al., 2011). Finally, the neuromuscular function assessment was repeated (Post-tests) in normoxia (i.e., participants took off the facemask 25 s after completion of the last sprint) and was started exactly 1 min after the repeated-sprint exercise protocol ended.

Responses to Exercise

Heart rate and SpO_2 were monitored and estimated, respectively, via a Polar transmitter-receiver (Wearlink T-31, Polar Electro Oy, Kempele, Finland) and non-invasive pulse oximetry using a finger probe (Palmsat, 2500, NONIN Medical Inc., Plymouth, MI, USA). Together with heart rate and SpO_2, ratings of perceived exertion were recorded using the Borg 6–20 scale (i.e., 6 = no exertion at all, 20 = maximal exertion) exactly 10 s following each sprint (i.e., peak values likely to be obtained). Additionally, SpO_2 was recorded between before the warm-up and 4 min after the last sprint. These time points corresponded to the end of pre- and post-tests.

Neuromuscular Function

Neuromuscular test sessions began by the completion of three successful MVCs, all brief (~5 s) and separated by ≥30 s of rest, with a twitch delivered over the isometric plateau. Participants were instructed to increase torque production over a 1-s period, hold it for 3–4 s and then relax before completing the next contraction. Thereafter, participants were instructed to perform "explosive" MVCs (separated by ≥20 s). During all brief MVCs trials the participants were carefully instructed to contract "as fast as possible" for ~1 s from a fully relaxed state, in an attempt to achieve at least 90% of their MVC torque. Participants were asked to avoid any countermovement before torque onset; i.e., they were reminded not to flex the knee immediately prior to KE. They were strongly encouraged with verbal feedback and a visual display of the torque production. Contractions that had any discernable countermovement or pre-tension (i.e., change of baseline torque of >1.5 Nm during the 100 ms before contraction onset; Girard et al., 2014) were discarded and another attempt was made. To provide biofeedback on whether a countermovement had occurred, the resting torque level was displayed on a sensitive scale. The slope of the torque–time curve (10 ms time constant) was displayed throughout testing and the peak slope was used to provide visual performance feedback to participants after each contraction. Pre-tests assessment was preceded by a warm-up consisting of 10 isometric contractions of ~3–5 s in duration interspaced with ~10–20 s of recovery. Contraction intensity was progressively self-adjusted by the participant to attain maximal torque in the last three contractions.

Recordings

Torque Measurements

KE torque was measured with participants seated upright on a custom-built adjustable chair with the hips and knees flexed at 90°. Restraining straps placed across the chest and hips secured the participants in the chair to prevent extraneous movement, while the dynamometer (Captels, St Mathieu de Treviers, France) was attached 3–5 cm above the tip of the lateral malleoli. During all contractions the torque signals were amplified, sent through an A/D board and sampled at 2000 Hz by commercially available hardware and software (MP35 and BSL Pro Version 3.6.7, Biopac Systems Inc., Santa Barbara, USA).

Electromyography

The EMG activity of the VL and *rectus femoris* (RF) muscles was recorded via bipolar Ag/AgCl electrodes (Ambu Blue sensor T, Ambu A/S, Denmark; diameter = 9 mm; inter-distance electrode = 30 mm) fixed longitudinally over the muscle bellies. The reference electrode was attached to the right wrist. Low impedance between the two electrodes was obtained by abrading the skin with emery paper and cleaning with alcohol. The position of the electrodes was marked for consistent placement. EMG signals were amplified (gain = 1000), filtered (band-width frequency 30–500 Hz) and recorded (sampling frequency = 2000 Hz) by commercially available hardware (Biopac MP35, systems Inc., Santa Barbara, CA) and software (Acqknowledge 3.6.7, Biopac Systems Inc., Santa Barbara, CA).

Motor Nerve Stimulation

Femoral nerve stimulations (400 V, rectangular pulse of 0.2 ms) were delivered by a high-voltage stimulator (Digitimer DS7AH; Digitimer, Hertfordshire, UK) via a cathode electrode (diameter of 5 mm) placed in the inguinal crease and an anode (5 × 10 cm; Medicompex, SA, Ecublens, Switzerland) in the gluteal fold. The intensity of stimulation was determined during the familiarization test session using a passive isometric recruitment curve (Racinais et al., 2013). Briefly, the stimulation intensity was increased by 10-mA increments until a maximal peak twitch torque was achieved and then a further increased by 50% to ensure constant supramaximal stimulation throughout the protocol.

Data Analysis

All analyses were performed using Spike 2 Software (Cambridge Electronic Design, Cambridge, UK). The MVC torque was defined as the maximum value recorded for 1 s when the torque had reached a plateau (before the superimposed twitch), and the RMS of the EMG activity was computed during the same 1-s period (RMS_{MAX}). Similarly, the peak-to-peak amplitude of superimposed maximum compound action potential (M-wave) responses was measured for each agonist muscle, and RMS_{MAX} was divided by M-wave to give a ratio RMS_{MAX}/M-wave.

The contractile RTD (expressed as $Nm.s^{-1}$) was derived from the "explosive" MVC measurements, as the average slope of the initial time phase of the torque-time curve at 0–30, 0–50, 0–100, and 0–200 ms, relative to the onset of contraction (Aagaard et al., 2002; Suetta et al., 2004; Thorlund et al., 2009) using a custom written program (Spike 2 Software, Cambridge Electronic Design, Cambridge, UK). The onset of muscle contraction was defined as the time point at which the torque curve exceeded baseline by >4.5 Nm, corresponding to ~2.5% of MVC torque values (Andersen et al., 2010). The peak RTD was defined as the peak Δtorque/Δtime achieved during the initial 200 ms of the isometric contraction (de Oliveira et al., 2013; Girard et al., 2014). In addition, the rate of muscle activation (expressed as $mV.s^{-1}$) was measured as the raw RMS activity increase obtained at similar time intervals relative to onset integration (i.e., activity). The onset of EMG integration was shifted 50 ms before the onset of contraction to account for the presence of electromechanical delay (Aagaard et al., 2002; Girard et al., 2013). The RTD and EMG rise were also normalized relative to maximal MVC torque (%MVC) and maximal EMG activity (%RMS_{MAX}/M-wave). The mean over three trials was used for further analysis for each parameter.

Statistical Analysis

Values are expressed as means ± SD. Two-way repeated-measures ANOVAs [Time (Pre-tests vs. Post-tests) × Condition (NM, LA vs. HA)] were used to compare torque and muscle activation data for each time window (0–30, 0–50, 0–100, and 0–200 ms) independently for absolute and relative changes.

Outcome variables were tested using Mauchly's procedure for sphericity. Whenever the data violated the assumption of sphericity, *P*-values and adjusted degrees of freedom based on Greenhouse-Geisser correction were reported instead. Where significant effects were established, pairwise differences were identified using the Bonferroni *post-hoc* analysis procedure adjusted for multiple comparisons. For each ANOVA, partial eta-squared was calculated as measures of effect size. Values of 0.01, 0.06, and above 0.14 were considered as small, medium, and large, respectively. All statistical calculations were performed using SPSS statistical software V.21.0 (IBM Corp., Armonk, NY, USA). The significance level was set at $P < 0.05$.

RESULTS

Repeated-Sprint Ability and Responses to Exercise

Distance covered during the first 5-s sprint was similar (24.2 ± 1.4, 24.5 ± 1.5, and 24.4 ± 1.7 m for NM, LA, and HA, respectively; $P > 0.05$) across conditions (**Figure 1**). In reference to sprint 1, distance covered decreased from sprint 2 onwards ($P < 0.001$), independently of the condition ($P = 0.324$). The averaged values of distance covered for sprints 1–8 were lower in HA (22.3 ± 1.3 m) compared to NM (22.9 ± 1.2 m; $P = 0.044$) but not LA (22.7 ± 1.3 m; $P = 0.183$), with also no difference between NM and LA ($P = 0.710$). A larger sprint decrement score occurred in HA (−7.8 ± 3.6%) vs. NM (−5.3 ± 1.9%; $P = 0.015$) but not LA (−6.3 ± 3.5%; $P = 0.060$), with also no difference between NM and LA ($P = 0.237$). Compared to NM (183.2 ± 9.3 m), the cumulated distance covered over the eight sprints was shorter in HA (178.5 ± 10.7 m; $P = 0.014$) but not in LA (181.4 ± 10.3 m; $P = 0.056$), with also no difference between NM and LA ($P = 0.240$).

Whereas, it did not change in NM (96.8 ± 0.8 vs. 96.0 ± 1.6%; $P = 0.455$), SpO_2 values decreased from the first to the last sprint in LA (95.0 ± 2.0 vs. 89.7 ± 4.0%; $P = 0.050$) and HA (88.8 ± 2.5 vs. 81.8 ± 4.5%; $P = 0.001$) (**Table 1**). Compared to pre-tests (96.9 ± 0.4%), SpO_2 values were not different among conditions during post-tests after completion of the repeated-sprint ability protocol (96.2 ± 0.5%; all conditions pooled, $P > 0.05$). Heart rate (NM: 150 ± 15 vs. 176 ± 12 bpm; LA: 154 ± 9 vs. 176 ± 9 bpm; HA: 154 ± 12 vs. 174 ± 13 bpm, all $P < 0.001$) and ratings of perceived exertion (NM: 11.8 ± 1.4 vs. 18.5 ± 1.2 points; LA: 11.3 ± 1.4 vs. 18.1 ± 1.6 points; HA: 11.5 ± 1.8 vs. 19.1 ± 0.8 points, all $P < 0.001$) increased from sprint 1 to sprint 8, irrespective of the environmental condition ($P = 0.256$). Higher ratings of perceived exertion values were recorded for the average of eight sprints in HA (15.8 ± 0.3 points) vs. LA (15.2 ± 0.3 points; $P = 0.006$), but not NM (15.5 ± 0.3 points; $P = 0.452$).

Maximal Strength

Compared to NM (−9 ± 7%), a larger ($P < 0.05$) reduction in MVC torque occurred from pre- to post-exercise in HA (−14 ± 9%; $P = 0.021$) but not in LA (−12 ± 7%; $P = 0.270$), with

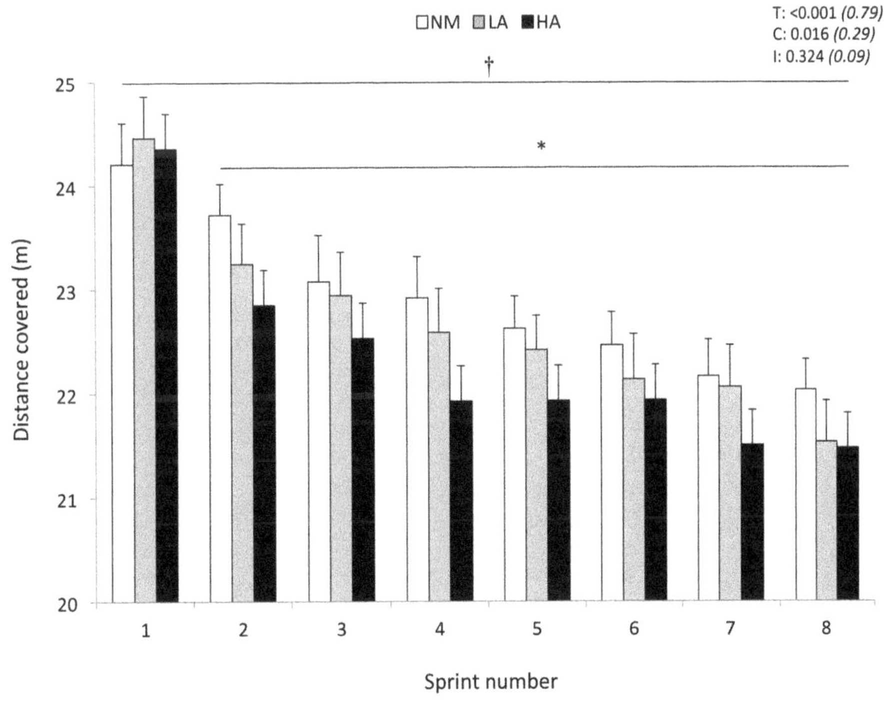

FIGURE 1 | Distance covered during the repeated-sprint ability test. Data are presented in normoxia (NM; $FiO_2 = 20.9\%$), at low (LA; $FiO_2 = 16.8\%$), and high (HA; $FiO_2 = 13.3\%$) normobaric hypoxia. Values are mean ± SD ($n = 13$). T, C, and I respectively refer to ANOVA main effects of time, condition, and interaction between these two factors with *P*-value and partial eta-squared in parentheses. *Significantly different from sprint 1 (all conditions pooled), $P < 0.05$. †NM different from HA (all sprints pooled), $P < 0.05$.

also no differences between LA and HA (P = 0.340) (**Table 2**). During MVCs, raw EMG signals of both VL and RF muscles were lower at post- relative to pre-, with no difference between conditions. Peak-to-peak M-wave amplitudes for both VL and RF muscles did not change. A global reduction of the RMS_{MAX}/M-wave ratio occurred from pre- to post-exercise for the RF (−14 ± 11%; $P = 0.002$), while failing to reach statistical significance for the VL (−8 ± 11%; $P = 0.075$).

Rapid Muscle Characteristics

Peak RTD (all conditions pooled: −6 ± 11%; $P = 0.031$) was significantly reduced from pre- to post-exercise (**Table 2**). Reduction in RTD (absolute values) occurred within the 0–100 (−8 ± 9%; $P = 0.011$) and 0–200 ms (−10 ± 8%; $P < 0.001$) epochs after contraction onset, independent of the condition ($P > 0.23$; **Figure 2**). No differences in RTD (relative values) were observed after normalization to MVC torque ($P > 0.197$; **Figure 3**). Furthermore, the relative rates of EMG rise for VL muscle for any epochs throughout the experimental protocol were not different between conditions ($P > 0.49$) and there were no interaction ($P > 0.42$) or time effects ($P > 0.12$) (**Figure 4**). The rate of EMG rise for RF muscle increased during the periods 0–30 (+22 ± 26%; $P = 0.006$), 0–50 (+25 ± 28%; $P = 0.002$), 0–100 (+27 ± 27%; $P < 0.001$), and 0–200 ms (+23 ± 2%; $P = 0.002$) post-exercise, independently of the condition ($P > 0.23$; **Figure 5**).

DISCUSSION

Repeated-Sprint Performance and Responses to Exercise

Distance ran during the first 5-s sprint was similar in all conditions, as an enhanced anaerobic energy release can compensate for the reduced aerobic ATP production during short maximal efforts in hypoxic conditions (Calbet et al., 2003). Compared to NM, a larger sprint decrement score and a shorter cumulated distance covered from sprint 1 to 8 occurred in HA, but not in LA, with also no difference between NM and LA. Consistent with previous repeated sprinting literature (Bowtell et al., 2014), our data therefore show that performance fatigability was significantly exacerbated relative to NM only under our severer hypoxic condition. The question of whether the same is true when completing identical repeated sprinting protocol at natural altitude (i.e., hypobaric hypoxia), known to induce severer physiological responses (Millet et al., 2012) and eventually larger neuromuscular alterations, has not been specifically addressed. Hence, the decrease in air density upon ascent to terrestrial altitude reduces air resistance, which is likely to decrease the energy cost of running at high velocities, and thereby improve single sprint performance (Levine et al., 2008). When sprints are repeated, however, hypobaric hypoxia would induce higher work of breathing responses and more detrimental neuromuscular consequences than exposure to gas mixtures lowering FiO_2. Despite lower SpO_2 values in the severer hypoxic condition, it is interesting to observe in this study that sensations that regulated the integrity of the performer (ratings of perceived exertion or perceived fatigability) and associated heart rate responses did not differ between SL and HA.

Neuromuscular Parameters during Maximal Contractions

Along with lower distance covered during the repeated-sprint test, post-exercise reduction in maximal KE torque, as measured from brief MVCs, was ∼5% larger in HA (−14%) compared to NM (−9%). This later result is in line with a previous study where the decrease in KE MVC torque under hypoxia (FiO_2 = 14%) was 6% larger in reference to normoxia after the completion

TABLE 1 | Changes in responses to exercise during the repeated-sprint ability test in normoxia (NM; FiO_2 = 20.9%), under low (LA; FiO_2 = 16.8%) and high (HA; FiO_2 = 13.3%) normobaric hypoxia.

Variables	Sprint number								ANOVA *(Partial eta-squared)*
	1	2	3	4	5	6	7	8	
SpO_2 (%)									
NM	96.8 ± 0.8	96.4 ± 1.9	96.3 ± 1.9	95.8 ± 2.0	96.2 ± 2.1	95.8 ± 2.0	95.8 ± 1.5	96.0 ± 1.6	T < 0.001 *(0.60)*
LA$^{\#}$	95.0 ± 2.0	94.3 ± 3.2	92.4 ± 3.4*	91.3 ± 2.9*	91.5 ± 3.0*	91.5 ± 3.0	89.6 ± 4.4*	89.7 ± 4.0*	C < 0.001 *(0.85)*
HA$^{\#,\dagger}$	88.8 ± 2.5	86.1 ± 4.5	84.5 ± 4.1*	84.0 ± 4.9*	83.6 ± 5.2*	83.2 ± 4.6*	82.5 ± 5.3*	81.8 ± 4.5*	I = 0.016 *(0.24)*
HR (bpm)									
NM	150 ± 15	164 ± 13*	169 ± 13*	171 ± 12*	174 ± 12*	175 ± 11*	175 ± 11*	176 ± 12*	T < 0.001 *(0.92)*
LA	154 ± 9	166 ± 11*	172 ± 9*	175 ± 10*	176 ± 10*	176 ± 11*	176 ± 10*	176 ± 9*	C = 0.427 *(0.07)*
HA	154 ± 12	166 ± 15*	171 ± 13*	174 ± 14*	174 ± 13*	175 ± 12*	174 ± 12*	174 ± 13*	I = 0.187 *(0.12)*
RPE (POINTS)									
NM	11.8 ± 1.4	13.0 ± 1.1*	14.3 ± 1.4*	15.5 ± 1.5*	16.4 ± 1.7*	17.1 ± 1.6*	17.7 ± 1.5*	18.5 ± 1.2*	T < 0.001 *(0.95)*
LA	11.3 ± 1.4	12.7 ± 1.1*	13.8 ± 1.2*	15.1 ± 1.1*	16.1 ± 1.2*	17.0 ± 1.5*	17.6 ± 1.4*	18.1 ± 1.6*	C = 0.034 *(0.25)*
HA†	11.5 ± 1.8	13.0 ± 1.6*	14.4 ± 1.6*	15.7 ± 1.6*	16.7 ± 1.4*	17.5 ± 1.3*	18.4 ± 1.1*	19.1 ± 0.8*	I = 0.256 *(0.10)*

Mean ± SD ($n = 13$).

SpO_2, arterial O_2 saturation; HR, heart rate; RPE, ratings of perceived exertion.

**Significantly different from sprint 1 ($P < 0.05$). $^{\#}$and †significantly different from NM and LA, respectively ($P < 0.05$).*

TABLE 2 | Neuromuscular parameters recorded during brief explosive maximal knee extension before (Pre-tests) and after (Post-tests) repeated sprinting in normoxia (NM; $FiO_2 = 20.9\%$), under low (LA; $FiO_2 = 16.8\%$) and high (HA; $FiO_2 = 13.3\%$) normobaric hypoxia.

Variables	Pre-tests			Post-tests			ANOVA (*Partial eta-squared*)		
	NM	LA	HA	NM	LA	HA	Time	Condition	Interaction
MVC torque (Nm)	271.0 ± 45.6	269.5 ± 41.9	270.1 ± 42.3	246.5 ± 35.4*	237.6 ± 39.0*	232.3 ± 40.8*#	<0.001 (*0.77*)	0.085 (*0.19*)	0.021 (*0.28*)
Peak RTD (Nm.s)	1018 ± 122	1074 ± 208	986 ± 195	965 ± 133*	948 ± 152*	942 ± 199*	0.031 (*0.33*)	0.024 (*0.11*)	0.040 (*0.24*)
RMS_{MAX}_VL (mV)	0.604 ± 0.112	0.599 ± 0.110	0.597 ± 0.111	0.568 ± 0.107	0.524 ± 0.093	0.553 ± 0.110	<0.001 (*0.59*)	0.159 (*0.14*)	0.117 (*0.16*)
RMS_{MAX}_RF (mV)	0.449 ± 0.173	0.451 ± 0.158	0.449 ± 0.160	0.403 ± 0.162	0.398 ± 0.147	0.395 ± 0.169	<0.001 (*0.65*)	0.927 (*0.06*)	0.777 (*0.13*)
M-wave_VL (mV)	11.4 ± 4.5	12.0 ± 4.5	11.4 ± 4.6	11.5 ± 4.5	11.3 ± 4.4	11.9 ± 4.9	0.903 (*0.01*)	0.905 (*0.08*)	0.176 (*0.15*)
M-wave_RF (mV)	12.4 ± 2.0	12.6 ± 3.2	12.4 ± 2.0	13.0 ± 2.1	12.5 ± 1.4	12.8 ± 1.7	0.436 (*0.051*)	0.914 (*0.07*)	0.570 (*0.05*)
RMS_{MAX}/M-wave_VL (mV)	0.054 ± 0.027	0.052 ± 0.025	0.056 ± 0.030	0.051 ± 0.025	0.049 ± 0.029	0.048 ± 0.022	0.075 (*0.24*)	0.643 (*0.04*)	0.395 (*0.07*)
RMS_{MAX}/M-wave_RF (mV)	0.038 ± 0.018	0.039 ± 0.020	0.037 ± 0.017	0.033 ± 0.016	0.033 ± 0.013	0.031 ± 0.015	0.002 (*0.57*)	0.053 (*0.05*)	0.813 (*0.02*)

Mean ± SD (n = 13).
MVC torque, maximal voluntary contraction torque; Peak RTD, peak rate of torque development; RMS_{MAX}, M-wave and RMS_{MAX}/M-wave represent the average of root mean square, maximal M-waves, and normalized electromyogram activity of vastus lateralis (VL) and rectus femoris (RF) muscles.
**Significantly different from Pre-tests (P < 0.05). #Significantly different from NM (P < 0.05).*

of 15 5-s cycling sprints interspersed with 25-s of rest (Billaut et al., 2013). Despite not supported by statistical analysis, our novel finding was that a graded effect of hypoxia was visible for strength losses post-repeated sprinting with progressively larger values (−9, −12, and −14%) with increasing severities of acute hypoxia. This extends similar findings following maximal intermittent dynamic leg extension where KE MVC torque losses increased (yet non-significantly) with hypoxia severity (−18, −19, and −27% in FiO_2 = 21, 14, and 10%, respectively) (Christian et al., 2014). Contrastingly, performing sets of intermittent, isometric, quadriceps contractions at 60% of MVC force to task failure in normoxia, mild hypoxia, moderate hypoxia and severe hypoxia (FiO_2 = 21, 16, 13, and 10%) resulted in ~30% declines in MVC force in all conditions, despite large differences in time-to-task failure (24.7 vs. 15.9 min in FiO_2 = 21 vs. 10%) (Goodall et al., 2010). Potentially, differences in exercise mode/duration/intensity and individuals' tolerance to hypoxic stress, in turn affecting the magnitude of reduction in convective O_2 transport, may explain aforementioned diverging results on MVC torque and further confirm that fatigue is task-dependent.

Also worth noticing, the effect of fatigue on M-wave changes during repeated sprinting is not clear-cut in literature, with reports of decreased (Perrey et al., 2010), unchanged (Girard et al., 2013), and increased (Racinais et al., 2007) amplitudes. Consequently, normalizing the raw EMG amplitude to a maximum compound action potential (M-wave) is a methodological requirement allowing control for any changes in neuromuscular junction and sarcolemma excitation, and hence, enhancing the sensitivity of EMG amplitude measurements. In this study, maximal normalized EMG activity (RMS_{MAX}/M-wave ratio) was dampened during MVCs in VL (−8%; albeit not significantly different) and RF (−14%) muscles. This suggests that the magnitude of the efferent motor outflow reaching the KE was adversely affected by the repetition of eight maximal sprints, confirming previous observations (Girard et al., 2015a; Brocherie et al., 2015b), while severity of hypoxic exposure had only minimal effect.

Rapid Muscle Force Characteristics

In addition to the post-exercise decrement in MVC torque, this study is unique as far as we are aware in reporting that the altitude severity (at least to 3600 m) did not modify the post-exercise RTD responses: the early phase RTD (30 and 50 ms) did not change, whereas the decline in peak RTD and absolute RTD values in the late phase (100 and 200 ms) of muscle contraction was similar between the normoxic and hypoxic conditions. In hot and cool conditions, a global (i.e., at all time intervals) downward-shift in the contractile RTD occurred after repeated cycling sprints (Girard et al., 2013). As it was unrelated to environmental conditions (i.e., modest hyperthermia), this was taken to reflect an overall fatigue-induced reduction in rapid muscle force characteristics. In the present study adopting a running mode, the difference between early (unchanged) and late (decreased) phases absolute RTDs may relate to the relative influence of passive stiffness in serial/lateral force transmission structures, myofiber cross-bridge kinetics and neural drive (Edman and Josephson, 2007).

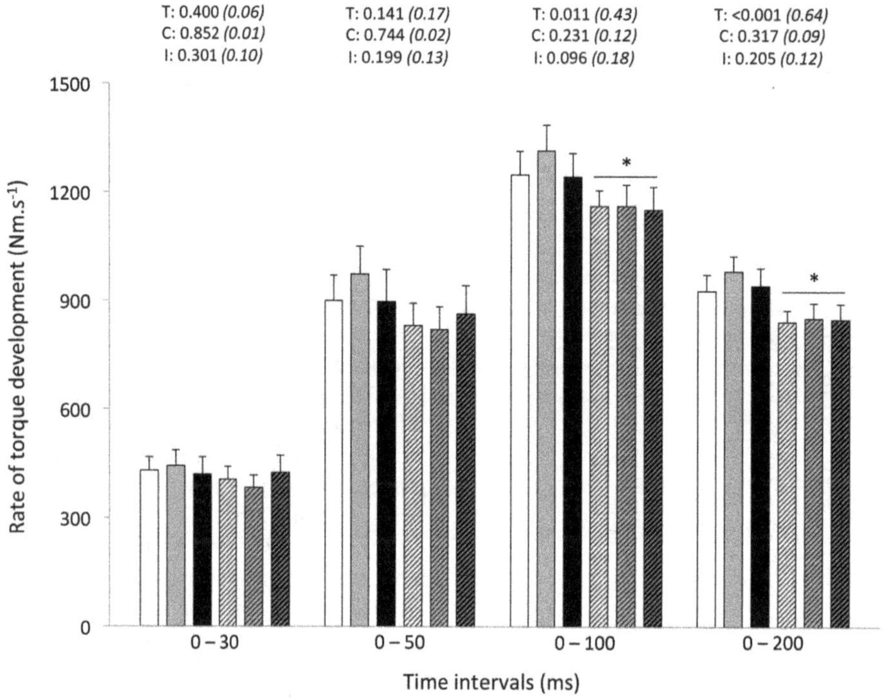

FIGURE 2 | Rate of torque development (absolute values) during explosive isometric knee extension obtained at 0–30, –50, –100, and –200 ms prior to (Pre-tests; full bars) and following (Post-tests; dashed bars) repeated sprinting in normoxia (NM; FiO_2 = 20.9%; white bars), at low (LA; FiO_2 = 16.8%; gray bars) and high (HA; FiO_2 = 13.3%; black bars) normobaric hypoxia. Values are mean ± SD (n = 13). T, C, and I respectively refer to ANOVA main effects of time, condition, and interaction between these two factors with P-value and partial eta-squared in parentheses. *Significantly different from Pre-tests, $P < 0.05$.

With late phase RTD more likely be affected by the fiber type composition (Penailillo et al., 2014), a more pronounced fatigue of faster fiber types after repeated running sprinting (Girard et al., 2015a), in turn associated with slower cross-bridge kinetics (Hamada et al., 2003), may dictate observed magnitude of post-exercise alterations in absolute RTD. Importantly, the exercise-related decline seen for the late-phase absolute RTD values occurred regardless of the environmental condition. In line with these findings, we have recently reported that heat stress does not exacerbate alterations in rapid muscle torque production capacity of KE neither after repeated cycling sprints (Girard et al., 2013) nor prolonged tennis playing (Girard et al., 2014).

In this study, when controlling for fatigue-induced reduction in maximal strength, we failed to demonstrate significant reductions in explosive strength post-exercise at any time interval. In fact, RTD is increasingly related to maximal muscle force, and reliance on muscle contractile properties decreases, as the time (mostly from 90 ms) from the onset of contraction increases (Andersen and Aagaard, 2006). The time interval in which RTD is determined influences the nature of the association between maximal muscle force and RTD and, in turn, the nature of fatigue-induced responses. By using different experimental designs (i.e., resistance training and verbal instructions during protocol), however, others have questioned the direct relationship between maximal force and RTD (Griffin and Cafarelli, 2005; Holtermann et al., 2007). Regardless, our data show the influence of maximal strength in maintaining normalized RFD values at all time intervals after repeated sprinting in differing hypoxic conditions.

Muscle Activation Rise

Whereas maximal VL muscle activation capacity (RMS_{MAX}/M-wave ratio) was impaired by sprints repetition, the ability to rapidly activate the VL muscle, as inferred from the rate of EMG amplitude rise, did not change in our study. Consistently, whole-body exercise studies, for instance following simulated team- (football: Thorlund et al., 2009; handball: Thorlund et al., 2008) and racket- (tennis: Girard et al., 2014) sport matches or a repeated cycling sprint protocol (Girard et al., 2013), show that reductions in RTDs are generally not associated with significant decreases in EMG values of quadriceps muscles. Opposite results have been reported by Morel et al. (2015) after the completion of 20 sets of 6-s isokinetic maximal KE at 240° s^{-1}, starting every 30 s. In their study, reductions of RTD were associated with a dampened activation capacity of the VL muscle in the early phase of muscle contraction, whereas participants were capable of producing similar maximal activation levels (Morel et al., 2015). Methodological differences (e.g., various time intervals, manual vs. automated methods to detect contraction onset; instructions to the participants during the contraction execution) preclude meaningful comparisons of EMG responses between studies.

In our study, the fact that RF muscle activation rise increased (at all time intervals) from pre- to post-exercise, despite

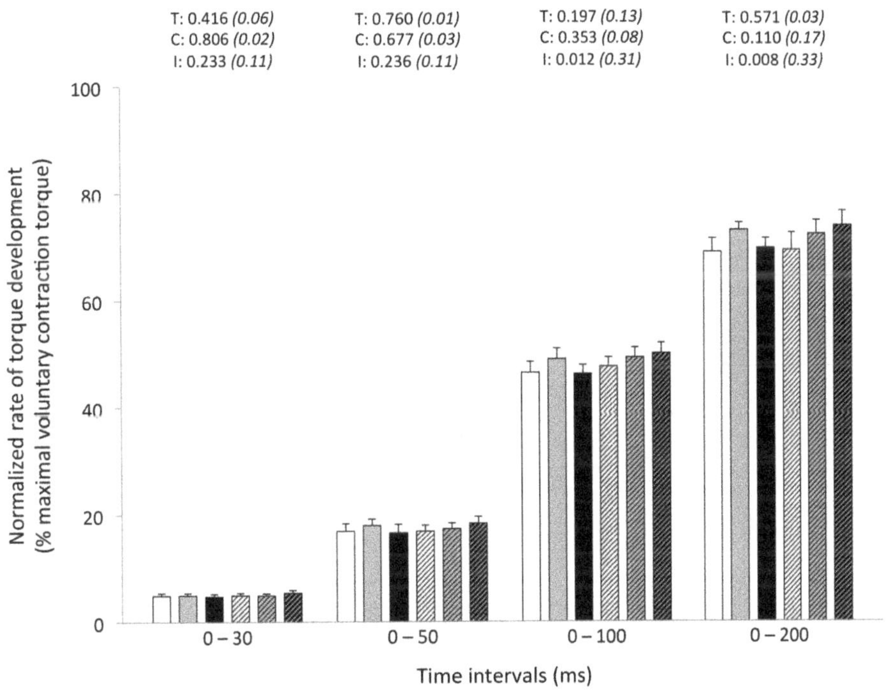

FIGURE 3 | Normalized rate of torque development (% maximal voluntary contraction torque) during explosive isometric knee extension obtained at 0–30, −50, −100, and −200 ms prior to (Pre-tests; full bars) and following (Post-tests; dashed bars) repeated sprinting in normoxia (NM; FiO_2 = 20.9%; white bars), at low (LA; FiO_2 = 16.8%; gray bars) and high (HA; FiO_2 = 13.3%; black bars) normobaric hypoxia. Values are mean ± SD (n = 13). T, C, and I respectively refer to ANOVA main effects of time, condition and interaction between these two factors with P-value and partial eta-squared in parentheses.

significant alteration of the ability to maximally activate this muscle, is an interesting observation. Considering the different activation sequences of this bi-articular muscle during sprinting (Morin et al., 2015) and the observation of reductions in RF RMS activity levels over sprints repetition (Brocherie et al., 2015b), it cannot be ruled out that this finding may partly depend on our non-specific testing position (i.e., marked hip extension while seating). Potentially, different results would occur when adopting another posture (i.e., when lying down) since knee position (RF muscle length) significantly affects quadriceps activation strategies (Krishnan et al., 2011). While this result was unexpected, larger activation in the *soleus* muscle has also been observed +24-h post-football game in hot vs. neutral environment (Girard et al., 2015c). Explosive force production depends on muscle fascicle shortening velocity and the tendon's elastic energy storage capacity, with tendon stiffness in turn affecting the time lag between muscle activation and muscle force production (i.e., electromechanical delay) (Proske and Morgan, 1987). In our study, a fixed electromechanical delay was used to determine EMG onset rise. As such, the role of tension-sensitive mechanoreceptors located in the muscle (e.g., Golgi tendon organs and muscle spindles) in influencing the tendon's stiffness, and thereby length change of the muscle fibers during explosive KE through proprioceptive feedback, probably did not change. A further result was to demonstrate that hypoxia severity had no effect on post-exercise adjustments in rapid muscle activation capacity. Potentially, longer sprints, shorter recoveries or combination of both (more intense exercise-to-rest ratios) and/or the use or severer hypoxic conditions might yield more unfavorable results with respect to RTD adjustments resulting directly to decreases in muscle activation rates if greater fatigue levels could be attained.

Additional Considerations

Importantly, a marked reduction in the intrinsic contractile capacity for explosive force production cannot be ruled out, as substantial peripheral locomotor muscle fatigue development (i.e., twitch torque decrease) usually occur as a result of repeated sprinting, independently of hypoxic severity (Billaut et al., 2013). Assessment of electrically evoked RTD can give insight into the intrinsic capacity of the muscle-tendon unit for explosive force production without the influence of voluntary control. This can be investigated by examining the response to a single or ideally high frequency contractions, such as an evoked octet (e.g., eight pulses at 300 Hz; Buckthorpe et al., 2012), to reliability evoke the maximum capacity for RTD.

In our study, all pre- and post-neuromuscular assessments were performed in normoxia with similar SpO_2 values of 96–97%. Reportedly, SpO_2 recovery response after an acute exposure to normobaric hypoxia (FiO_2 = 10%) decreasing SpO_2 to 85% is ~2 min (Krivoshchekov et al., 2014). With hypoxic simulation applied during the repeated sprint exercise through the use of a facemask, participants were switched

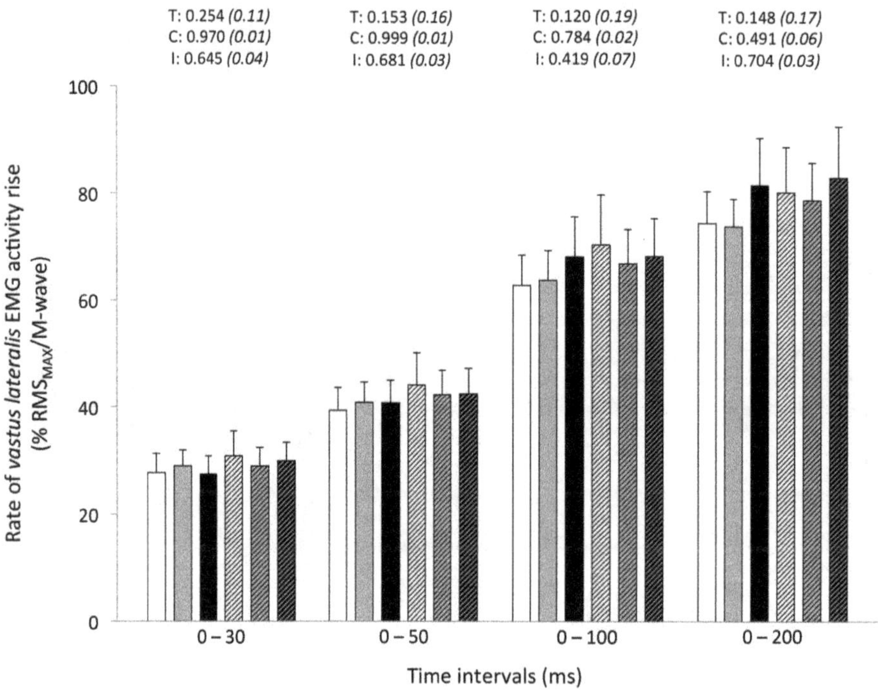

FIGURE 4 | Rate of *vastus lateralis* EMG activity rise (% RMS_{MAX}/M-wave) during explosive isometric knee extension obtained at 0–30, −50, −100, and −200 ms prior to (Pre-tests; full bars) and following (Post-tests; dashed bars) repeated sprinting in normoxia (NM; FiO_2 = 20.9%; white bars), at low (LA; FiO_2 = 16.8%; gray bars) and high (HA; FiO_2 = 13.3%; black bars) normobaric hypoxia. Values are mean ± SD (n = 13). T, C, and I respectively refer to ANOVA main effects of time, condition and interaction between these two factors with P-value and partial eta-squared in parentheses.

to normoxic breathing immediately (within seconds) after exercise cessation and seated on the chair, located near by the treadmill, for post-test assessment that started exactly 1 min after the last sprint completion. Whether this maneuver induced a faster recovery of neuromuscular function parameters, compared to situations where individuals continued breathing a hypoxic mixture (i.e., similar to exercise conditions), is unknown.

When evaluating RTD, most of the studies have used the same contraction, with a "hard and strong" instruction, to evaluate explosive and maximal voluntary strength capacities. The potential problem associated with this practice, however, is that only ballistic contractions (i.e., force production as fast as possible followed by muscle relaxation as soon the target force is reached) allow a careful evaluation of the maximal discharge rate of motor neurons (Duchateau and Baudry, 2014). Compared with a "hard-and-fast instruction," the steeper force development with a "fast" only instruction relates to a better activation of the agonist muscles at contraction onset (Sahaly et al., 2003). Although using this methodological precaution required a greater number of contractions (and potentially may have induced some recovery in neuromuscular function), we felt that it was a necessary prerequisite not to underestimate the true rate of muscle activation of our participants.

Because elite players are more accustomed to repeated-sprint activities, one can assume that, in comparison to recreational team-sport participants involved here, they may have been able to better resist fatigue. In a group of 17 healthy recreationally active individuals, those facing the greatest RTD reductions also experienced the largest fatigue rate during a Wingate cycle ergometer test and greater fatigue during an electrical stimulation protocol (Morris et al., 2010). Along the same line, only males were studied here, while females are generally less fatigable compared with men during repeated-sprint protocols (Billaut and Bishop, 2009). Whether performance level and/or gender differences exist regarding neuromuscular consequences (with special references to explosive strength), when completing repeated-sprint exercises at different altitudes, warrant further investigation.

CONCLUSION

In summary, alteration in repeated-sprint ability and post- KE MVC was greater under high altitude than in normoxia or at low altitude. In the KE, peak and late phase (>100 ms) contractile RTD decreased post-exercise to the same extent between conditions. However, contractile RTDs were not different after normalization to MVC torque, indicating that post-exercise strength losses accounted for the decrease in RTD. Additionally, we reported that repeated running sprints do not negatively influence the capacity of the central nervous

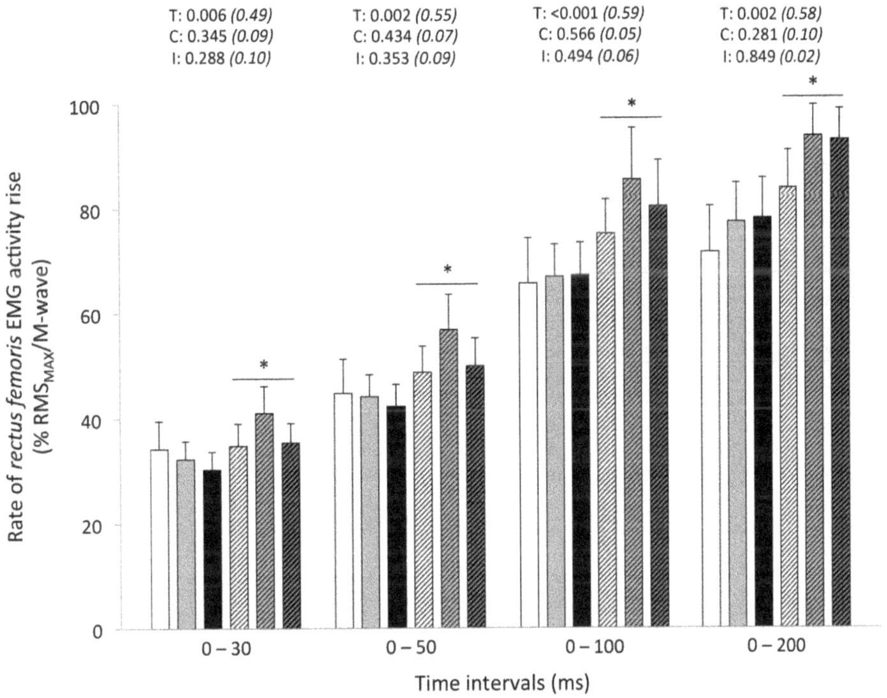

FIGURE 5 | Rate of *rectus femoris* EMG activity rise (% RMS_{MAX}/M-wave) during explosive isometric knee extension obtained at 0–30, −50, −100, and −200 ms prior to (Pre-tests; full bars) and following (Post-tests; dashed bars) repeated sprinting in normoxia (NM; FiO_2 = 20.9%; white bars), at low (LA; FiO_2 = 16.8%; gray bars) and high (HA; FiO_2 = 13.3%; black bars) normobaric hypoxia. Values are mean ± SD (n = 13). T, C, and I respectively refer to ANOVA main effects of time, condition and interaction between these two factors with P-value and partial eta-squared in parentheses. *Significantly different from Pre-tests, $P < 0.05$.

system to rapidly activate the VL (unchanged) and RF (improved) muscles during the first 200 ms, whereas maximal activation was dampened later during the contraction. Finally, normobaric hypoxia exposure had no additional influence on post-exercise alterations in rapid muscle torque production of the KE.

AUTHOR CONTRIBUTIONS

Conceived and designed the experiments: OG, FB, GM. Performed experiments: OG, FB. Analyzed data: OG. Interpreted results of research: OG. Drafted manuscript and prepared tables/figures: OG. Edited, critically revised paper, and approved final version of manuscript: OG, FB, GM.

FUNDING

This work is based on research funded by QNRF (NPRP 4–760–3–217).

ACKNOWLEDGMENTS

The authors thank the participants for their maximal efforts and cooperation.

REFERENCES

Aagaard, P., Simonsen, E. B., Andersen, J. L., Magnusson, P., and Dyhre-Poulsen, P. (2002). Increased rate of force development and neural drive of human skeletal muscle following resistance training. *J. Appl. Physiol.* 93, 1318–1326. doi: 10.1152/japplphysiol.00283.2002

Andersen, L. L., and Aagaard, P. (2006). Influence of maximal muscle strength and intrinsic muscle contractile properties on contractile rate of force development. *Eur. J. Appl. Physiol.* 96, 46–52. doi: 10.1007/s00421-005-0070-z

Andersen, L. L., Andersen, J. L., Zebis, M. K., and Aagaard, P. (2010). Early and late rate of force development: differential adaptive responses to resistance training? *Scand. J. Med. Sci. Sports* 20, 162–169. doi: 10.1111/j.1600-0838.2009.00933.x

Balsom, P. D., Gaitanos, G. C., Ekblom, B., and Sjödin, B. (1994). Reduced oxygen availability during high intensity intermittent exercise impairs performance. *Acta Physiol. Scand.* 152, 279–285. doi: 10.1111/j.1748-1716.1994.tb09807.x

Billaut, F., and Bishop, D. J. (2009). Muscle fatigue in males and females during multiple-sprint exercise. *Sports Med.* 39, 257–278. doi: 10.2165/00007256-200939040-00001

Billaut, F., Kerris, J. P., Rodriguez, R. F., Martin, D. T., Gore, C. J., and Bishop, D. J. (2013). Interactions of central and peripheral factors using repeated sprints at different levels of arterial O_2 saturation. *PLoS ONE* 8:e77297. doi: 10.1371/journal.pone.0077297

Bishop, D. J., Girard, O., and Mendez-Villanueva, A. (2011). Repeated-sprint ability – Part II. Recommendations for training. *Sports Med.* 49, 741–756. doi: 10.2165/11590560-000000000-00000

Bowtell, J. L., Cooke, K., Turner, R., Mileva, K. N., and Sumners, D. P. (2014). Acute physiological and performance responses to repeated sprints in varying degrees of hypoxia. *J. Sci. Med. Sport* 17, 399–403. doi: 10.1016/j.jsams.2013.05.016

Brocherie, F., Girard, O., Faiss, R., and Millet, G. P. (2015a). High-intensity intermittent training in hypoxia: a double-blinded, placebo-controlled field study in youth football players. *J. Strength Cond. Res.* 29, 226–237. doi: 10.1519/JSC.0000000000000590

Brocherie, F., Millet, G. P., and Girard, O. (2015b). Neuro-mechanical and metabolic adjustments to the repeated anaerobic sprint test in professional football players. *Eur. J. Appl. Physiol.* 115, 891–903. doi: 10.1007/s00421-014-3070-z

Buckthorpe, M. W., Hannah, R., Pain, T. G., and Folland, J. P. (2012). Explosive isometric contractions, with special reference to electromyography normalization techniques. *Muscle Nerve* 46, 566–576. doi: 10.1002/mus.23322

Buckthorpe, M., Pain, M. T., and Folland, J. (2014). Central fatigue contributes to the greater reductions in explosive than maximal strength with high-intensity fatigue. *Exp. Physiol.* 99, 964–973. doi: 10.1113/expphysiol.2013.075614

Calbet, J. A., De Paz, J. A., Garatechea, N., Cabeza de Veca, S., and Chavarren, J. (2003). Anaerobic energy provision does not limit Wingate exercise performance in endurance-trained cyclists. *J Appl Physiol.* 94, 668–676. doi: 10.1152/japplphysiol.00128.2002

Christian, R. J., Bishop, D. J., Billaut, F., and Girard, O. (2014). The role of sense of effort on self-selected cycling power output. *Front. Physiol.* 5:115. doi: 10.3389/fphys.2014.00115

de Oliveira, F. B., Rizatto, G. F., and Denadai, B. S. (2013). Are early and late force development differently influenced by fast-velocity resistance training? *Clin. Physiol. Funct. Imaging* 33, 282–287. doi: 10.1111/cpf.12025

Duchateau, J., and Baudry, S. (2014). Maximal discharge rate of motor units determines the maximal rate of force development during ballistic contractions in human. *Front. Hum. Neurosci.* 8:234. doi: 10.3389/fnhum.2014.00234

Edman, K. A., and Josephson, R. K. (2007). Determinants of force rise time during isometric contraction of frog muscle fibres. *J. Physiol.* 580, 1007–1019. doi: 10.1113/jphysiol.2006.119982

Feriche, B., García-Ramos, A., Calderón-Soto, C., Drobnic, F., Bonitch-Gongóra, J. G., Galilea, P. A., et al. (2014). Effect of acute exposure to moderate altitude on muscle power: hypobaric hypoxia vs. normobaric hypoxia. *PLoS ONE* 9:e114072. doi: 10.1371/journal.pone.0114072

Folland, J. P., Buckthorpe, M. W., and Hannah, R. (2014). Human capacity for explosive force production: neural and contractile determinants. *Scand. J. Med. Sci. Sports* 24, 894–906. doi: 10.1111/sms.12131

Gandevia, S. C. (2001). Spinal and supraspinal factors in human muscle fatigue. *Physiol. Rev.* 81, 1725–1789.

Girard, O., Bishop, D. J., and Racinais, S. (2013). Hot conditions improve power output during repeated cycling sprints without modifying neuromuscular fatigue characteristics. *Eur. J. Appl. Physiol.* 113, 359–369. doi: 10.1007/s00421-012-2444-3

Girard, O., Brocherie, F., Morin, J. B., and Millet, G. P. (2015a). Neuro-mechanical determinants of repeated treadmill sprints - Usefulness of an "hypoxic to normoxic recovery" approach. *Front. Physiol.* 6:260. doi: 10.3389/fphys.2015.00260

Girard, O., Brocherie, F., Morin, J. B., and Millet, G. P. (2015b). Intra- and inter-session reliability of running mechanics during treadmill sprints. *Int. J. Sports Physiol. Perform.* doi: 10.1123/ijspp.2015-0145. [Epub ahead of print].

Girard, O., Mendez-Villanueva, A., and Bishop, D. J. (2011). Repeated-sprint ability-Part I. *Sports Med.* 41, 673–694. doi: 10.2165/11590550-000000000-00000

Girard, O., and Millet, G. (2009). Maximal rate of force development can represent a more functional measure of muscle activation. *J. Appl. Physiol.* 107, 359–360.

Girard, O., Nybo, L., Mohr, M., and Racinais, S. (2015c). Plantar flexor neuromuscular adjustments following match-play football in hot and cool conditions. *Scand. J. Med. Sci. Sports* 25, 154–163. doi: 10.1111/sms.12371

Girard, O., Racinais, S., and Périard, J. (2014). Tennis in hot and cool conditions decreases the rapid muscle torque production capacity of the knee extensors but not the plantar flexors. *Br. J. Sports Med.* 48, 52–58. doi: 10.1136/bjsports-2013-093286

Goodall, S., Charlton, K., Howatson, G., and Thomas, K. (2015). Neuromuscular fatigability during repeated-sprint exercise in male athletes. *Med. Sci. Sports Exerc.* 47, 528–536. doi: 10.1249/MSS.0000000000000443

Goodall, S., Ross, E. Z., and Romer, L. M. (2010). Effect of graded hypoxia on supraspinal contributions to fatigue with unilateral knee-extensor contractions. *J. Appl. Physiol.* 109, 1842–1851. doi: 10.1152/japplphysiol.00458.2010

Goods, P. S. R., Dawson, B. T., Landers, G. J., Gore, C. J., and Peeling, P. (2014). Effect of different simulated altitudes on repeat-sprint performance in team-sport athletes. *Int. J. Sports Physiol. Perform.* 9, 857–862. doi: 10.1123/ijspp.2013-0423

Griffin, L., and Cafarelli, E. (2005). Resistance training: cortical, spinal, and motor unit adaptations. *Can. J. Appl. Physiol.* 30, 328–340. doi: 10.1139/h05-125

Hamada, T., Sale, D. G., MacDougall, J. D., and Tarnopolsky, M. A. (2003). Interaction of fibre type, potentiation and fatigue in human knee extensor muscles. *Acta Physiol. Scand.* 178, 165–173. doi: 10.1046/j.1365-201X.2003.01121.x

Harridge, S. D., Bottinelli, R., Canepari, M., Pellegrino, M. A., Reggiani, C., Esbjornsson, M., et al. (1996). Whole-muscle and single-fibre contractile properties and myosin heavy chain isoforms in humans. *Pflugers Arch.* 432, 913–920. doi: 10.1007/s004240050215

Holtermann, A., Roeleveld, K., Vereijken, B., and Ettema, G. (2007). The effect of rate of force development on maximal force production: acute and training-related aspects. *Eur. J. Appl. Physiol.* 99, 605–613. doi: 10.1007/s00421-006-0380-9

Hureau, T. J., Olivier, N., Millet, G. Y., Meste, O., and Blain, G. M. (2014). Exercise performance is regulated during repeated sprints to limit the development of peripheral fatigue beyond a critical threshold. *Exp. Physiol.* 99, 951–963. doi: 10.1113/expphysiol.2014.077974

Krishnan, C., Allen, E. J., and Williams, G. N. (2011). Effect of knee position on quadriceps muscle force steadiness and activation strategies. *Muscle Nerve.* 43, 563–573. doi: 10.1002/mus.21981

Krivoshchekov, S. G., Balioz, N. V., Nekipelova, N. V., and Kapilevich, L. V. (2014). Age, gender, and individually-typological features of reaction to sharp hypoxic influence. *Hum. Physiol.* 40, 34–45. doi: 10.1134/S0362119714060061

Kuitunen, S., Komi, P. V., and Kyröläinen, H. (2002). Knee and ankle joint stiffness in sprint running. *Med. Sci. Sports Exerc.* 34, 166–173. doi: 10.1097/00005768-200201000-00025

Levine, B. D., Stray-Gundersen, J., and Mehta, R. D. (2008). Effect of altitude on football performance. *Scand. J. Med. Sci. Sports* 18, 76–84. doi: 10.1111/j.1600-0838.2008.00835.x

Luhtanen, P., and Komi, P. V. (1979). Mechanical power and segmental contribution to force impulses in long jump take-off. *Eur. J. Appl. Physiol. Occup. Physiol.* 41, 267–274. doi: 10.1007/BF00429743

Millet, G. P., Faiss, R., and Pialoux, V. (2012). Point: hypobaric hypoxia induces different physiological responses from normobaric hypoxia. *J. Appl. Physiol.* 112, 1783–1784. doi: 10.1152/japplphysiol.00067.2012

Morel, B., Rouffet, D. M., Saboul, D., Rota, S., Clémençon, M., and Hautier, C. (2015). Peak torque and rate of torque development influence on repeated maximal exercise performance: contractile and neural contributions. *PLoS ONE* 10:e0119719. doi: 10.1371/journal.pone.0119719

Morin, J. B., Gimenez, P., Edouard, P., Arnal, P., Jiménez-Reyes, P., Samozino, P., et al. (2015). Sprint acceleration mechanics: the major role of hamstrings in horizontal force production. *Front. Physiol.* 6:404. doi: 10.3389/fphys.2015.00404

Morin, J. B., Samozino, P., Bonnefoy, R., Edouard, P., and Belli, A. (2010). Direct measurement of power during one single sprint on treadmill. *J. Biomech.* 43, 1970–1975. doi: 10.1016/j.jbiomech.2010.03.012

Morris, M. G., Dawes, H., Howells, K., Scott, O. M., Cramp, M., and Izadi, H. (2010). Muscle contractile characteristics: relationship to high-intensity exercise. *Eur. J. Appl. Physiol.* 110, 295–300. doi: 10.1007/s00421-010-1496-5

Nelson, A. G. (1996). Supramaximal activation increases motor unit velocity of unloading. *J. Appl. Biomech.* 12, 285–291.

Pearcey, G. E., Murphy, J. R., Behm, D. G., Hay, D. C., Power, K. E., and Button, D. C. (2015). Neuromuscular fatigue of the knee extensors during repeated maximal intensity intermittent-sprints on a cycle ergometer. *Muscle Nerve* 51, 569–579. doi: 10.1002/mus.24342

Penailillo, L., Blazevich, A., Numazawa, H., and Nosaka, K. (2014). Rate of force development as a measure of muscle damage. *Scand. J. Med. Sci. Sports* 3, 417–427. doi: 10.1111/sms.12241

Perrey, S., Racinais, S., Saimouaa, K., and Girard, O. (2010). Neural and muscular adjustments following repeated running sprints. *Eur. J. Appl. Physiol.* 109, 1027–1036. doi: 10.1007/s00421-010-1445-3

Perrey, S., and Rupp, T. (2009). Altitude-induced changes in muscle contractile properties. *High Alt. Med. Biol.* 10, 175–182. doi: 10.1089/ham.2008.1093

Proske, U., and Morgan, D. L. (1987). Tendon stiffness: methods of measurement and significance for the control of movement. A review. *J. Biomech.* 20, 75–82. doi: 10.1016/0021-9290(87)90269-7

Racinais, S., Bishop, D., Denis, R., Lattier, G., Mendez-Villaneuva, A., and Perrey, S. (2007). Muscle deoxygenation and neural drive to the muscle during repeated sprint cycling. *Med. Sci. Sports Exerc.* 39, 268–274. doi: 10.1249/01.mss.0000251775.46460.cb

Racinais, S., Maffiuletti, N. A., and Girard, O. (2013). M-wave, H- and V-Reflex recruitment curves during maximal voluntary contraction. *J. Clin. Neurophysiol.* 30, 415–421. doi: 10.1097/WNP.0b013e31829ddcf1

Sahaly, R., Vandewalle, H., Driss, T., and Monod, H. (2003). Surface electromyograms of agonist and antagonist muscle during force development of maximal isometric exercises - effects of instruction. *Eur. J. Appl. Physiol.* 89, 79–84. doi: 10.1007/s00421-002-0762-6

Spencer, M., Bishop, D., Dawson, B., and Goodman, C. (2005). Physiological and metabolic responses of repeated-sprint activities: specific to field-based team sports. *Sports Med.* 35, 1025–1044. doi: 10.2165/00007256-200535120-00003

Suetta, C., Aagaard, P., Rosted, A., Jakobsen, A. K., Duus, B., Kjaer, M., et al. (2004). Training-induced changes in muscle CSA, muscle strength, EMG and rate of force development in elderly subjects after long-term unilateral disuse. *J. Appl. Physiol.* 97, 1954–1961. doi: 10.1152/japplphysiol.01307.2003

Thorlund, J. B., Aagaard, P., and Madsen, K. (2009). Rapid muscle force capacity changes after soccer match play. *Int. J. Sports Med.* 30, 273–278. doi: 10.1055/s-0028-1104587

Thorlund, J. B., Michalsik, L. B., Madsen, K., and Aagaard, P. (2008). Acute fatigue-induced changes in muscle mechanical properties and neuromuscular activity in elite handball players following a handball match. *Scand. J. Med. Sci. Sports* 18, 462–472. doi: 10.1111/j.1600-0838.2007.00710.x

Thorstensson, A., Karlsson, J., Viitasalo, J. H., Luhtanen, P., and Komi, P. V. (1976). Effect of strength training on EMG of human skeletal muscle. *Acta Physiol. Scand.* 98, 232–236. doi: 10.1111/j.1748-1716.1976.tb00241.x

Tillin, N. A., Pain, M. T., and Folland, J. (2013). Explosive force production during isometric squats correlates with athletic performance in rugby union players. *J. Sports Sci.* 31, 66–76. doi: 10.1080/02640414.2012.720704

14

Acute Mountain Sickness is Associated with a High Ratio of Endogenous Testosterone to Estradiol After High-Altitude Exposure at 3,700 m in Young Chinese Men

*Xiao-Han Ding[1,2], Yanchun Wang[1], Bin Cui[3], Jun Qin[3], Ji-Hang Zhang[3], Rong-Sheng Rao[4], Shi-Yong Yu[3], Xiao-Hui Zhao[3] and Lan Huang[3]**

[1] Department of Health Care and Geriatrics, Lanzhou General Hospital of Lanzhou Military Region, Lanzhou, China,
[2] Department of Geriatric Cardiology, Chinese PLA General Hospital, Beijing, China, [3] Department of Cardiology, Xinqiao Hospital, Army Medical University (Third Military Medical University), Chongqing, China, [4] Department of Ultrasonography, Xinqiao Hospital, Army Medical University (Third Military Medical University), Chongqing, China

***Correspondence:**
Lan Huang
huanglan260@126.com

Background: A large proportion of populations suffer from acute mountain sickness (AMS) after exposure at high altitude. AMS is closely related with age and gender implying that the sex hormones may play critical roles in AMS. Our observational study aimed to identify the association between the endogenous testosterone (T), estradiol (E2) and AMS.

Methods: A total of 113 subjects were recruited in 2012. The participants were evaluated at 500 m and after acute (1 day) and short-term (7 days) high-altitude exposure at 3,700 m. The subjects also completed a case report form questionnaire and underwent blood pressure measurements and an echocardiography examination. The red blood cell (RBC) count, Hb concentration ([Hb]), hematocrit (HCT), E2, T, and erythropoietin (EPO) were measured.

Results: Upon acute high-altitude exposure, E2 and EPO were significantly lower in AMS^+ group, and T/E2 and stroke volume were higher. On the 1st day, AMS score correlated positively with the T/E2 ratio while it negatively correlated with E2. After 7 days at 3,700 m, the AMS^+ subjects had higher erythropoietic parameters: EPO, T, and T/E2 were significantly higher in the AMS^+ group. [Hb], RBC count, HCT, EPO, T and T/E2 were also correlated with AMS score. EPO, HCT, and the RBC count were also correlated with T/E2. Regression analyses indicated that T/E2 significantly correlated to AMS score and T/E2 on the 1st day was an independent predictor for AMS on the 7th day.

Conclusion: AMS was correlated with T/E2 ratio and EPO. After short-term exposure, higher T/E2 may contribute to AMS together with EPO *via* erythropoiesis. Furthermore, T/E2 level at high altitude in the early stage was an independent predictor for AMS in the latter stage.

Keywords: testosterone, estradiol, acute mountain sickness, erythropoiesis, high-altitude exposure

INTRODUCTION

Acute mountain sickness (AMS) has been defined as a syndrome involving headache, dizziness, gastrointestinal symptoms, insomnia and fatigue after arrival at high-altitude (>2500 m) (Imray et al., 2010; Bartsch and Swenson, 2013). The underlying mechanisms of AMS, which may involve the ventilation response, circulatory alteration and disequilibrium in the endocrine system induced by hypobaric hypoxia, have not been fully elucidated (Hackett and Roach, 2001; Imray et al., 2010; Davis et al., 2011; Bartsch and Swenson, 2013). The respiratory and cardiovascular aspects of AMS have been studied for many years; however, attention should be given to the endocrine aspects, particularly the effects of sex hormones and hematopoiesis on AMS (Naeije, 2010; Oliver et al., 2012). The endocrine system has been proposed to be of critical importance for the high-altitude adaptation process, which involves regulation of the hemoglobin (Hb) level (Gonzales, 2011). Previous studies have identified that several genes are associated with high-altitude adaptation and three of them are associated with [Hb] indicating that high-altitude adaptation and diseases may be associated with hematopoiesis and genetic factors (Simonson et al., 2010; Lorenzo et al., 2014). Testosterone (T) and E2 are the two most active sex hormones and are suggested to participate in AMS, based on the gender differences in the incidence of AMS (Harris et al., 1966; Wu et al., 2012).

Erythropoiesis is a hormonally regulated process that involves at least two hormones, EPO and testosterone (Richmond et al., 2005; Bachman et al., 2013). The crucial regulator of erythrocyte production, EPO, is elevated after short-term high-altitude exposure and hypoxia treatment. However, EPO does not increase proportionally with exposure time, and it even shows a tendency to decrease after reaching a peak (Koury, 2005; Gunga et al., 2007). Testosterone also enhances hemopoiesis and participates in many physiological functions, including erythropoiesis (Congote et al., 1977; Coviello et al., 2008; Rochira et al., 2009; Gonzales et al., 2011; Oskui et al., 2013; Shin et al., 2016). Though it has been suggested that high T concentrations, could compromise adaptation to high altitude, an association between T and EE in CMS has also been demonstrated (Gonzales et al., 2009, 2011), which indicates that T may participate in mountain sickness through its effects on erythropoiesis. The possibility that the variation in the normal physiological range of T concentration modulates men's adaptation to hypobaric high-altitude hypoxia by stimulating Hb production and/or causing respiratory disturbances and exacerbating hypoxemia has been suggested (Gonzales, 2011, 2013; Gonzales et al., 2011b). E2 exhibits opposite effects that limit EPO and RBC production, and testosterone is converted to E2 by aromatase directly or after exerting its action. Both pathways of the conversion will reduce T biological actions. Thus, the T/E2 ratio may be used as a indicator of sex hormones balance in many diseases.

Numerous investigations have been performed on the acute responses in respiratory and cardiovascular systems and on EE in CMS (Ou et al., 1994; Cornolo et al., 2004; Iturriaga et al., 2005; Imray et al., 2010); however, fewer studies have given proper attention to erythropoiesis, which is balanced by sex hormones and EPO upon acute high-altitude exposure, and their roles in AMS. We postulate that the indicator of the sex hormone balance, ratio of T to E2, may participate the pathophysiological process of AMS. Furthermore, T/E2 represent the balance of T and E2 which may indicate diseases. The current study aimed to identify the relationship between endogenous T, E2, T/E2, and AMS upon acute and a short-term of high-altitude exposures.

MATERIALS AND METHODS

Participants and Procedures

Participants

Altogether, 113 subjects (6 were lost to follow-up) participated in the study according to the inclusion and exclusion criteria. The inclusion criteria were that the subjects be healthy males who were between 18 and 60 years old. The exclusion criteria were as follows: respiratory diseases, cardiovascular diseases, neuropsychosis, cerebrovascular diseases, malignant tumor, diseases of the liver, and diseases of the kidneys.

Subjects who participated in the study voluntarily were fully familiar with the purpose and procedures of this study and signed informed consent before the field trials. The study was reviewed and approved by the Ethics Committee of Xinqiao Hospital, the Third Military Medical University. The trials have been performed in accordance with the ethical standards laid down in an appropriate version of the Declaration of Helsinki.

Procedures

The participants were recruited in June 2012. The field trials were performed in June 2012 within 18–24 h after the participants arrived at 3,700 m by plane, which occurred within a 2-h window, and on the 7th day after their arrival. The baseline data were recorded at 500 m within 1 week prior to departure for the high-altitude trials.

Structured CRF questionnaires were used to record demographic data (age, BMI, smoking and alcohol consumption) and the symptoms of AMS including headache (0 = no headache; 1 = mild headache; 2 = moderate headache; 3 = severe headache), dizziness (0 = no dizziness; 1 = mild dizziness; 2 = moderate dizziness; 3 = severe dizziness), gastrointestinal symptoms (0 = without and 1 = with any gastrointestinal symptom), insomnia (0 = normal sleep pattern; 1 = worse than usual; 2 = wake up multiple times during the night and 3 = extreme difficulty sleeping) and fatigue (0 = without fatigue and 1 = with fatigue). AMS was diagnosed by the LLS. Subjects were diagnosed with AMS if they had a headache upon arriving at high altitude and recorded an LLS score > 3. The SpO_2 and

Abbreviations: AMS^+, with AMS; AMS^-, without AMS; AMS, acute mountain sickness; BMI, body mass index; CIn, cardiac index; CMS, chronic mountain sickness; CO, cardiac output; CRF, case report form; DBP, diastolic blood pressure; E2, estradiol; EE, excessive erythrocytosis; EF, ejection fraction; EPO, erythropoietin; [Hb], Hb concentration; HCT, hematocrit; HIF, hypoxia-inducible factor; HR, heart rate; LLS, Lake Louise self-assessment scoring system; PCT, plateletocrit; PLT, platelet count; RBC, red blood cell; SBP, systolic blood pressure; SpO_2, pulse oxygen saturation; SV, stroke volume; T, testosterone.

HR were measured by a pulse oximeter (NONIN-9550, Nonin Onyx, United States). The SV, EF, and CO were measured by ultrasonography using the S5-1 cardiac probe (CX50, Philips, United States). CIn were calculated using CO divided by body surface area.

The venous blood samples were obtained from all participants between 8 and 10 am after an overnight fast (at least 12 h). The measurements of RBC count, [Hb], HCT, PLT, PCT, E2, T, and EPO were as follow: Blood samples were obtained after a rest of 30 min by vein puncture and collected in tubes containing EDTA. Routine blood tests (RBC count, [Hb] and HCT) were performed using an automated hematology corpuscle analyzer (AU400; Olympus Optical, Co., Tokyo, Japan) at 3,700 m in the Laboratory Department in Army Brigade Hospital immediately after the blood samples were obtained. Routine blood tests [RBC count, [Hb] and HCT] were performed using an automated hematology corpuscle analyzer (AU400; Olympus Optical, Co., Tokyo, Japan). The venous blood samples were allowed to clot for 30–60 min and were then centrifuged at 1,000 *g* for 10 min at room temperature to obtain serum, which was immediately stored at −20°C until the assays for hormonal analysis. The E2, T, and EPO were measured in duplicate using commercially available ELISA kits (human E2, T and EPO kits, BlueGene Ltd., China). To measure the exact concentrations of E2, T, and EPO, each sample was assayed in duplicate. All of the biochemical variables (except blood routine examinations) were measured from the blood specimens in the Clinical Laboratory Department, Xinqiao Hospital, Army Medical University, following the criteria of the World Health Organization Lipid Reference Laboratories.

Statistical Analysis

The CRFs were excluded if the required items were not completed. The mean concentrations of E2, T, and EPO were calculated from duplicate wells in the ELISA plates. Because all variables (age, BMI, [Hb], RBC counts, HCT, E2, T, EPO, T/E2, HR, SV, EF, CO, and CIn) were normally distributed, they are expressed as mean ± standard deviation (SD). The changes in [Hb], RBC count, HCT, E2, T, EPO, T/E2, HR, SV, EF, CO, and CIn from sea level to 3,700 m (acute and short-term exposures) were evaluated by analyses of variance for repeated measurements. The variables mentioned above were compared between the AMS^+ and AMS^- groups by the independent-samples Student's *t*-test on the 1st and 7th days at 3,700 m, respectively. The enumerated data (smokers and AMS) are expressed as the rate of occurrence (%). Additionally, the relationships between the AMS score and the above-mentioned parameters at 3,700 m were obtained by Spearman's correlation analyses. Multiple regression analyses were also performed after the AMS scores were normalized by natural logarithm transformation. Variable with *p* less than 0.3 was selected for further adjusted analyses after each of them was analyzed by univariate Logistic regression. The statistical analyses were performed using SPSS 19.0 software for Windows. $P \leq 0.05$ was considered statistically significant. The detailed statistical methods and flow chart are summarized in **Figure 1**.

RESULTS

The age of the subjects in this study was 23.08 ± 4.17 years, and the BMI was 21.56 ± 2.19 kg/m^2. Overall, the incidences of AMS upon acute exposure and upon 1-week exposure at 3,700 m were 57.9%b (62/107) and 19.6% (21/107), respectively.

The alterations of SpO_2, HR, [Hb], RBC count and HCT after exposures to 3,700 m were revealed in **Figures 2A–E**. The erythrocytosis-regulated hormone EPO increased significantly after acute exposure (3.31 ± 1.20 and 3.85 ± 1.42 mIU/ml, $p = 0.045$) and increased even further after short-term exposure to 3,700 m (4.46 ± 1.44 mIU/ml, **Figure 2F**). Furthermore, the PLT and PCT were decreased on the 1st day and recovered on the 7th day (**Figures 2G,H**). E2 had a slight increase (72.11 ± 14.78 vs. 74.07 ± 16.00 pg/ml, but not significantly) and T (1713.16 ± 468.06 vs. 1992.29 ± 423.96 pg/ml) had a significant increase from baseline to the acute time point. Both fell to a lower level than baseline at 7 days (64.26 ± 15.41 and 1592.82 ± 330.55 pg/ml, respectively) (**Figures 2I,J**). Though T decreased after a sharp elevation and E decreased after 7 days, the ratio of T to E2 increased significantly (24.76 ± 8.91 vs. 28.96 ± 8.93) from baseline to 24 h, and it remained at a relatively high level on the 7th day (25.48 ± 6.34) (**Figure 2K**). We also found that EF and SV increased after arrival at 3,700 m remained significantly increased after 7 days (**Figures 2L,M**). Both CO and CIn increased at 24 h and remained significantly increased after 7 days (**Figures 2N,O**).

Upon acute high-altitude exposure, E2 and EPOwere significantly lower in the AMS^+ group than in the AMS^- group, while the T/E2 ratio was higher in the AMS^+ group without significant changes in T. SV was significantly lower in the AMS^+ group than the AMS^- group. However, SpO_2, HR, CO, [Hb], RBC count and HCT showed no significant differences between AMS^+ and AMS^- individuals, as indicated in **Table 1**.

After short-term exposure to 3,700 m, the AMS^+ group had higher erythrocytosis parameters. Specifically, the AMS^+ subjects showed significantly higher [Hb], RBC count and HCT (all *p*-values < 0.05). We also observed that T and T/E2 were higher in AMS^+ individuals than in AMS^- individuals, whereas E2 showed no differences between the two groups. In contrast to the data obtained after 24 h at high altitude, EPO was higher in the AMS^+ group than in the AMS^- group after 7 days. The hemodynamic parameters showed no differences between the AMS^+ and AMS^- groups (all *p*-values > 0.05, **Table 1**).

After a 24 h-exposure to 3,700 m, both T ($p < 0.05$) and T/E2 ($p < 0.05$) were highly correlated with the AMS score, and E2 ($p < 0.05$) was negatively correlated with the AMS score (**Table 2**). Additionally, the AMS score on the 1st day at 3,700 m was correlated with SV ($p < 0.05$) and HR ($p < 0.05$).

On the 7th day at 3,700 m, the AMS score was closely correlated with [Hb] ($r = 0.206$, $p = 0.033$), RBC ($r = 0.307$, $p = 0.001$) and HCT ($r = 0.275$, $p = 0.004$). Furthermore, T/E2 had a positive relationship with the AMS score ($r = 0.241$, $p = 0.012$). More importantly, the AMS score was correlated with EPO ($r = 0.210$, $p = 0.030$) (**Table 2**).

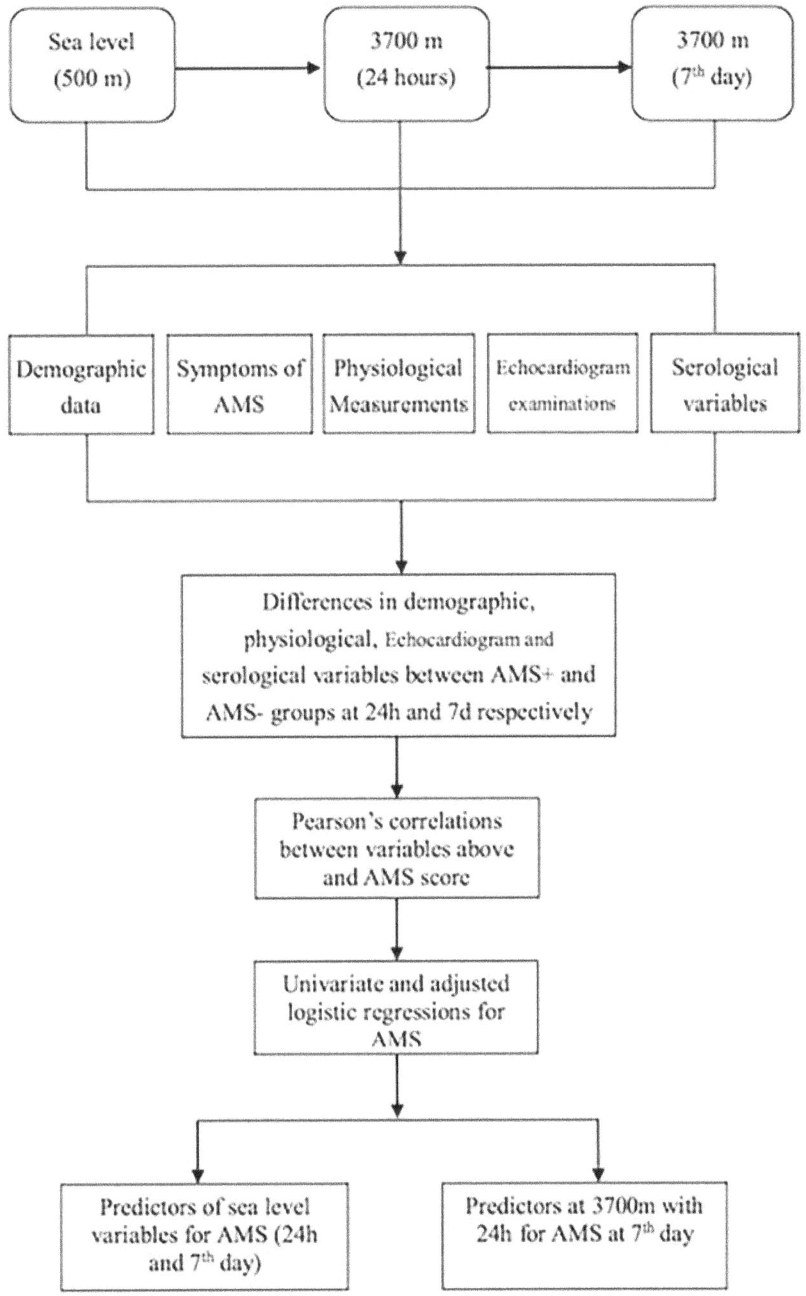

FIGURE 1 | The flow chart of this study.

Among the erythropoietic and hemodynamic parameters, SV was significantly correlated with EPO ($r = 0.199$, $p = 0.039$) and T/E2 ($r = -0.236$, $p = 0.015$) on the 1st day at 3,700 m. The RBC count had significant positive relationships with EPO ($r = 0.293$) and T/E2 ($r = 0.281$, $p = 0.003$) after 7 days of exposure to high altitude. A significant relationship between EPO and T/E2 ($r = 0.193$, $p = 0.046$) was also observed (**Table 3**).

Regression analyses demonstrated that EPO and T/E2 ($p < 0.001$) correlated with the AMS score after 24 h of exposure to 3,700 m, while HCT and T/E2 were related to the AMS after 7 days (**Table 4**). Univariate regressions showed that E2 and SV at sea level were associated with AMS on the 1st day whereas SpO_2, RBC and [Hb] can be included in the adjusted regression to identify the predictor for AMS on the 7th day (**Table 5**). Regarding to variables within 24 h at 3,700 m, only SV and T (T/E2) entered adjusted Logistic analyses. The adjusted Logistic regressions showed that baseline RBC count can predict AMS on the 7th day. Furthermore, T/E2 on the 1st day at 3,700 m is an independent predictor for AMS after 7 days' exposure (**Table 6**).

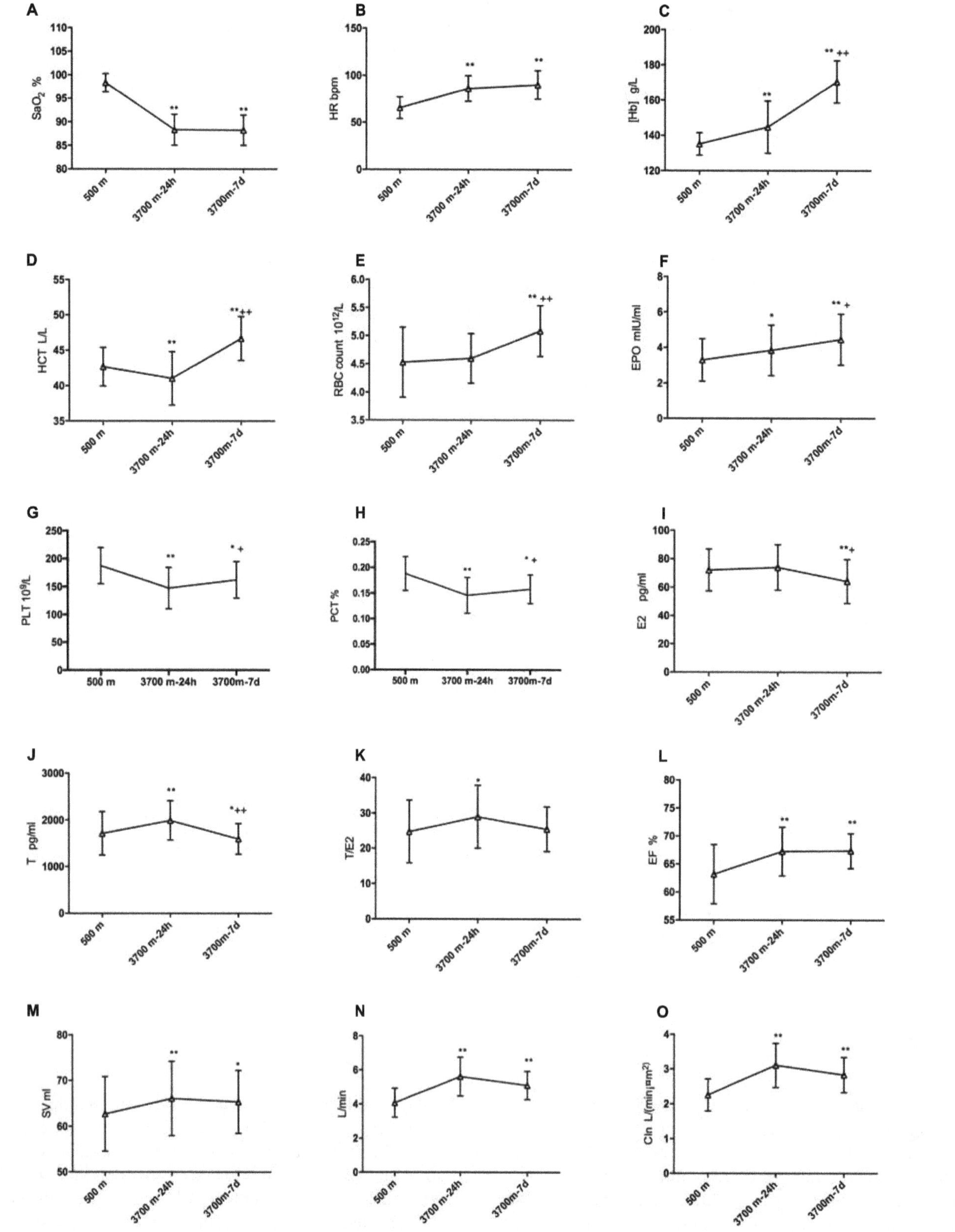

FIGURE 2 | Modifications of sex hormones, EPO and hematopoiesis after high-altitude exposure. Compared with baseline: $^{*}p$ is 0.05 or less; $^{**}p$ is 0.01 or less. Compared with 24-h level: ^{+}p is 0.05 or less; ^{++}p is 0.01 or less. **(A)** Modification of SpO_2; **(B)** Change of HR; **(C)** Modification of [Hb]; **(D)** Change of HCT; **(E)** Change of EBC count; **(F)** Change of EPO; **(G)** Change of E2; **(H)** Change of T; **(I)** Change of T/E2; **(J)** Change of EF; **(K)** Change of SV; **(L)** Change of CIn; **(M)** Change of SV after high altitude exposure; **(N)** Change of CO after high altitude exposure; and **(O)** Change of CIn after high altitude exposure.

TABLE 1 | Differences of sex hormones, EPO, cardiovascular, hematopoietic and erythropoiesis between AMS+ and AMS− groups.

	3,700 m-24 h			3,700 m -7 days		
	AMS− (45)	**AMS+ (62)**	***p***	**AMS− (86)**	**AMS+ (21)**	***p***
SpO_2	88.77 ± 2.80	87.98 ± 359	0.227	87.93 ± 2.50	88.50 ± 3.90	0.481
[Hb]	145.73 ± 15.43	144.00 ± 14.58	0.553	169.24 ± 12.29	175.71 ± 9.32	0.026
RBC	4.62 ± 0.40	4.59 ± 0.48	0.650	5.04 ± 0.45	5.56 ± 0.46	0.025
HCT	41.34 ± 3.85	40.84 ± 3.75	0.663	46.29 ± 3.12	48.27 ± 2.38	0.008
E2	78.26 ± 14.94	71.02 ± 16.17	0.020	62.65 ± 15.49	63.32 ± 15.10	0.872
T	1723.59 ± 557.55	170.59 ± 395.37	0.854	1537.00 ± 301.200	1821.45 ± 353.88	<0.001
T/E2	25.55 ± 13.01	31.32 ± 15.80	0.045	25.32 ± 6.45	29.49 ± 6.45	0.009
EPO	4.08 ± 1.63	3.68 ± 1.28	0.039	4.29 ± 1.38	5.12 ± 1.50	0.017
HR	84.66 ± 13.08	88.41 ± 13.42	0.156	90.74 ± 15.72	87.93 ± 11.09	0.444
EF	67.11 ± 3.57	67.37 ± 4.86	0.762	67.10 ± 3.19	68.48 ± 2.60	0.071
SV	68.78 ± 7.17	64.16 ± 7.94	0.002	64.91 ± 6.74	67.19 ± 7.13	0.172
Cln	3.06 ± 0.63	3.14 ± 0.65	0.646	2.80 ± 0.51	2.94 ± 0.46	0.266
CO	5.56 ± 1.15	5.66 ± 1.13	0.530	5.03 ± 0.82	5.40 ± 0.80	0.067

SpO_2, %; HR, beat per min; E2, pg/ml; EPO, mIU/ml; T, pg/ml; [Hb], g/L; RBC, 10^{12}/L; HCT, l/L; SV, ml; EF, %; CO, L/min and Cln, L/(min · m^2); PCT, l/L; PLT, 10^9/L.

TABLE 2 | Relationship between AMS score and sex hormones, EPO, echocardiography and erythropoiesis at 3,700 m.

	SpO_2	**T/E2**	**[Hb]**	**RBC**	**HCT**	**E2**	**EPO**	**T**	**HR**	**EF**	**SV**	**CO**	**Cln**
3,700 m-24 h													
r	−0.122	0.273	−0.036	−0.082	−0.038	−0.311	−0.110	0.029	0.289	−0.002	−0.304	0.083	0.061
p	0.215	0.005	0.713	0.403	0.695	0.001	0.258	0.767	0.003	0.978	0.001	0.396	0.533
3,700 m-7 days													
r	0.030	0.221	0.201	0.257	0.187	−0.009	0.201	0.171	−0.015	0.091	0.021	0.050	−0.025
p	0.760	0.015	0.030	0.004	0.054	0.905	0.038	0.077	0.877	0.351	0.734	0.613	0.799

T/E2 was the only variable significantly related to AMS score after 24 h and 7 days high-altitude exposure.

DISCUSSION

We have found that the AMS was closely associated with T/E2 and the T/E2 may predict AMS in a short term of time in this study.

Associations Between AMS and Sex Hormones, EPO, and Hematopoiesis

Few studies have examined the relationships among sex hormones, EPO, hematopoiesis, and AMS. Most reports have demonstrated that CMS is characterized by high T concentrations and erythropoiesis, mainly due to the relationships among the T level, erythropoiesis and the symptoms of headache and sleep disturbance (Ou et al., 1994; Gonzales et al., 2009, 2011; Gonzales, 2011, 2013; Ekart et al., 2013). This evidence suggests that T and erythropoiesis may also participate in the pathogenesis of AMS. Hence, we observed that AMS was characterized by higher T, EPO, HCT, RBC count and [Hb] after 7 days at high altitude, though the T, HCT, RBC count and [Hb] were not significantly different between the AMS+ and AMS− groups following acute exposure.

These results partly agree with the previous findings that high serum T and Hb are adequate for acclimatization due to the improvement of oxygen transport, while even higher levels of T and Hb are associated with EE (Gonzales, 2011; Ekart et al., 2013), which may account for the positive relationships between T/E2 ratio and AMS score on the 1st day as well as association of after 7 days of exposure. However, E2 was higher in the AMS− group than in the AMS+ group, which may suggest that E2 may play a protective role in AMS upon acute exposure. EPO was also higher in the AMS− group upon acute exposure, which suggests that in the acute phase, higher E2 and EPO may be the primary protective factors against AMS, perhaps due to the respiratory action of E2 and the non-hematopoietic effect of EPO (see below). Furthermore, E2 may protect individuals from AMS *via* the relief of pulmonary artery contraction through its depressive effect on pulmonary endothelin-1 induced by hypoxia (Earley and Resta, 2002). Though both EPO and E2 appear to protect against AMS, E2 downregulates HIF response genes, including *EPO* (Earley and Resta, 2002). It is possible that the depression of EPO by E2 is attenuated by acute hypoxia. Thus, the preventive effect of E2 may also be ascribed to its indirect role in polycythemia and right ventricular functions in the acute phase.

High T and T/E2 are correlated with hypoventilation, sleep disturbances, EE and, in turn, the etiopathogenesis of CMS in natives (Gonzales et al., 2011b). E2 prevents CMS *via* its protective effects on cardiovascular and respiratory functions

TABLE 3 | Associations among erythropoiesis, EPO, echocardiography, and sex hormones.

	EPO		E2		T		T/E2	
	r	*p*	*r*	*p*	*r*	*p*	*r*	*p*
3,700 m-24 h								
EPO	/	/	−0.171	0.078	−0.044	0.652	0.162	0.099
Hb	−0.005	0.960	0.044	0.651	0.170	0.079	−0.007	0.940
RBC	−0.006	0.955	0.039	0.687	0.085	0.385	0.045	0.646
HCT	−0.018	0.856	0.043	0.662	0.093	0.342	0.052	0.598
EF	−0.132	0.174	−0.094	0.335	−0.071	0.468	0.096	0.330
SV	0.199	0.039	0.061	0.533	−0.037	0.707	−0.236	0.015
CO	0.029	0.765	−0.005	0.958	−0.010	0.916	−0.072	0.465
CIn	0.026	0.789	−0.052	0.596	−0.036	0.713	−0.070	0.476
3,700 m-7 days								
EPO	/	/	−0.026	0.789	0.148	0.129	0.193	0.046
Hb	0.105	0.281	−0.097	0.323	0.087	0.372	0.161	0.098
RBC	0.293	0.002	−0.146	0.133	0.164	0.092	0.281	0.003
HCT	0.099	0.309	−0.104	0.287	0.127	0.194	0.203	0.036
EF	0.023	0.810	0.084	0.390	0.098	0.317	−0.068	0.485
SV	−0.057	0.557	0.045	0.644	0.092	0.346	0.026	0.792
CO	−0.017	0.862	0.034	0.731	0.138	0.155	< 0.0001	0.999
CIn	−0.030	0.757	0.031	0.754	0.120	0.218	−0.018	0.855

TABLE 4 | Multiple linear regressions at 3,700 m.

AMS score#	β	*t*	*p*-value	95%CI lower bound	95%CI upper bound
3,700 m-24 h					
T/E2	0.044	3.131	0.003	0.017	0.076
SV	−0.075	−2.525	0.008	−0.131	−0.021
EPO	−0.345	−2.152	0.022	−0.684	−0.054
3,700 m-7 days					
T/E2	0.063	2.040	0.047	0.004	0.127
HCT	0.158	2.476	0.018	0.031	0.285

#Normalized by natural logarithm transformation.
95%CI lower bound and 95%CI upper bound are the upper and lower limits of the 95% confidence interval.
β, regression coefficient.
t, statistic of T-test for the regression.

(Zabka et al., 2006; Mattingly et al., 2008). Thus, it is reasonable to postulate that T and E2 play opposing roles in AMS, including the hematopoietic and respiratory effects.

Though T/E2 at sea level cannot be used as independent predictors for AMS neither on the 1st day nor the 7th day, T/E2 values upon acute exposure at 3,700 m was shown to be an independent predictor for AMS after a short-time exposure.

Sex Hormones May Participate in AMS via Hematopoietic or Non-hematopoietic Effect of EPO

The production of erythrocytes by erythropoiesis requires time, which is in accordance with our result that the RBC count was unchanged in the acute phase followed by a rise at 7 days. Previous study showed that the plasma volume and blood volume were decreased about 10–12% after acute high altitude exposure. However, they will be recovered in few days to 1 or 2 weeks at high altitude or after return to sea level. There was an interesting result that the HCT and PCT were decreased on the 1st day following by PCT remained significantly reduced after 7 days while HCT increased, which may be caused by the water-sodium retention in acute phase. This have been also reported in few studies which were not completely coincident with other researches. Also, in the days at high altitude, the HCT were significantly increased combined with the increased of [Hb] and RBC, may revealed that the decreases of plasma volume and blood volume have emerged. However, on the 7th day, the mean increase percentages of [Hb] and RBC were 24 and 12%, whilst the HCT evaluated only 9% compared with sea level. This mismatching of [Hb] or RBC with HCT may not be explained by the decrease of PV completely. Which may indicate the erythropoiesis process have started by EPO (peak level appeared on 2–4 days at high altitude). Indeed, it is important to measure the plasma volume and blood volume directly to evaluate the changes of them. However, we searched the published papers and note that the simplest and easily get methods as follow: PV = BV − RCV; BV = RCV*100/Hct; RCV = tHb/MCHC*100. In our study, it is difficult for us to measure the total tHb due the difficult of flied study at high altitude. Thus, we cannot directly evaluate PV in this study. Therefore, the following explanation of our results dependent on the increased amplitudes in [Hb], RBC count and HCT indirectly. That is, in the short terms of high altitude exposure, both of PV decrease and erythropoiesis have emerged. Further analysis showed that the erythropoiesis may be preponderant in our study, which needs further precise studies.

Acute mountain sickness was characterized by higher erythropoiesis after 7 days of exposure, but it was not associated with [Hb] or RBC count upon acute exposure to high altitude. What are the underlying mechanisms by which EPO participates in AMS during acute exposure, if not by promoting erythropoiesis? The non-hematopoietic effect of EPO has been revealed by studies that have reported its inotropic effect on the myocardium, which results in elevated EF (Riksen et al., 2008). This observation may be interpreted as a protective effect of EPO in the acute exposure phase, before erythropoiesis plays a major role, as indicated by the relationship between SV and EPO in the present study.

E2 *per se* has a protective effect on the cardiovascular system and a stimulatory effect on the respiratory system (Mattingly et al., 2008; Smith et al., 2014). Combined with the enhanced respiration effects of EPO, we can suggest that the regulation of the respiratory and cardiovascular systems by E2 and EPO may account for their roles in preventing AMS in the case of acute exposure.

However, after a short time, the modifications of RBC, HCT, and [Hb] induced by the synergism of T and EPO were of critical importance in AMS. The RBC count had a positive correlation with EPO, which was also positively correlated with T. T also has a direct erythropoiesis effect (Gonzales et al.,

TABLE 5 | Univariate Logistic regression for AMS.

	AMS (3,700 m-24 h)					AMS (3,700 m-7 days)				
	β	OR	95%CI		*p*	β	OR	95%CI		*p*
Variable at sea level										
SBP	0.017	1.016	0.983	1.054	0.299	−0.007	0.991	0.876	1.018	0.765
DBP	0.004	1.004	0.966	1.043	0.834	−0.015	0.980	0.940	1.022	0.375
HR	0.002	1.002	0.966	1.040	0.982	−0.006	0.994	0.956	1.034	0.788
SpO_2	0.073	1.077	0.690	1.681	0.831	−0.259	0.772	0.482	1.236	0.281
E2	0.003	1.003	0.998	1.009	0.250	0.001	1.001	0.995	1.007	0.767
EPO	−0.001	0.999	0.933	1.068	0.968	−0.070	0.932	0.866	1.004	0.063
T	0.010	1.010	0.851	1.199	0.912	0.097	1.102	0.908	1.336	0.325
T/E2	−0.010	0.990	0.947	1.036	0.670	0.019	1.020	0.972	1.070	0.430
RBC	0.127	1.136	0.592	2.179	0.701	0.918	2.503	1.157	5.414	0.020
HB	0.015	1.016	0.955	1.081	0.619	−0.052	0.949	0.890	1.012	0.112
HCT	0.034	1.039	0.897	1.204	0.606	−0.065	0.938	0.801	1.097	0.420
EF	0.010	1.011	0.937	1.091	0.772	0.029	1.029	0.946	1.119	0.503
SV	0.044	1.051	0.993	1.112	0.088	−0.163	0.849	0.503	1.436	0.542
Variable at 3,700 m (24 h)										
SBP	0.015	1.016	0.977	1.055	0.429	0.008	1.008	0.969	1.049	0.697
DBP	0.017	1.017	0.975	1.060	0.434	0.018	1.018	0.974	1.064	0.419
HR	0.023	1.024	0.991	1.057	0.156	0.004	1.004	0.972	1.037	0.809
SpO_2	−0.101	0.904	0.791	1.034	0.142	−0.030	0.970	0.851	1.105	0.647
E2	−0.006	0.994	0.989	1.000	0.035	0.000	1.000	0.995	1.005	0.996
EPO	−0.064	0.938	0.882	0.997	0.039	−0.016	0.984	0.925	1.046	0.606
T	0.089	1.093	0.963	1.242	0.169	0.119	1.126	0.999	1.269	0.052
T/E2	0.037	1.038	0.999	1.078	0.053	0.024	1.024	0.996	1.054	0.090
RBC	−0.001	0.999	0.399	2.501	0.998	−0.297	0.743	0.280	1.968	0.550
HB	−0.007	0.993	0.965	1.021	0.609	0.004	1.004	0.975	1.034	0.805
HCT	−0.023	0.977	0.877	1.088	0.670	0.024	1.024	0.912	1.151	0.685
EF	0.043	1.044	0.950	1.148	0.373	−0.024	0.976	0.882	1.079	0.636
SV	−0.091	0.913	0.861	0.968	0.002	−0.043	0.958	0.907	1.012	0.126

The variable with p-value less than 0.3 was selected for the adjusted Logistic regression.
β, regression coefficient.
OR, odds ratio.

TABLE 6 | Predictive roles of sex hormones in AMS (adjusted regression).

	β	OR	95%CI		*p*
For AMS (7 days)					
RBC	0.840	2.030	1.005	5.012	0.033
Variables at 3,700 m (24 h)					
For AMS (7 days)					
T/E2	0.128	1.124	1.004	1.23	0.045

RBC at sea level predicts AMS independently while T/E2 at 3,700 m on the 1st day is the independent predictor for AMS after 7 days.

2009; Gonzales, 2011), which was revealed here by the positive associations of the RBC count and HCT with the T level. Furthermore, our novel observation that EPO was higher in the AMS^+ group after 7 days of exposure but that it was lower in AMS^+ individuals upon acute exposure may further indicate that EPO has a diphasic role in AMS, depending on the duration of hypoxic exposure. Thus, in the short-term condition, T on its own and in combination with EPO induced erythropoiesis, perhaps enhancing the viscosity of the blood, which is harmful for acclimating to high-altitude hypoxia (Heinicke et al., 2003; Bachman et al., 2013; Ekart et al., 2013). Though previous studies indicate that EPO does not play a further important role in EE (Koury, 2005; Gunga et al., 2007), it may stimulate erythrocytosis when its effects are combined with the effects of T. T induces erythrocytosis via direct effects on bone marrow and indirect effects on EPO (Gonzales et al., 2009; Maggio et al., 2013), which finally results in the augmentation of [Hb], HCT, and RBC count that aggravate AMS.

We may conclude that E2 and EPO prevent AMS via the non-hematopoietic effect (inotropic effect on the myocardium, alterations in hemodynamics) in the acute phase, while T and EPO aggravated AMS through erythropoiesis (alterations in the hematological system) after short-term exposure (**Figure 3**). Additionally, E2 was still beneficial to individuals through the stimulation of ventilation in the latter phase.

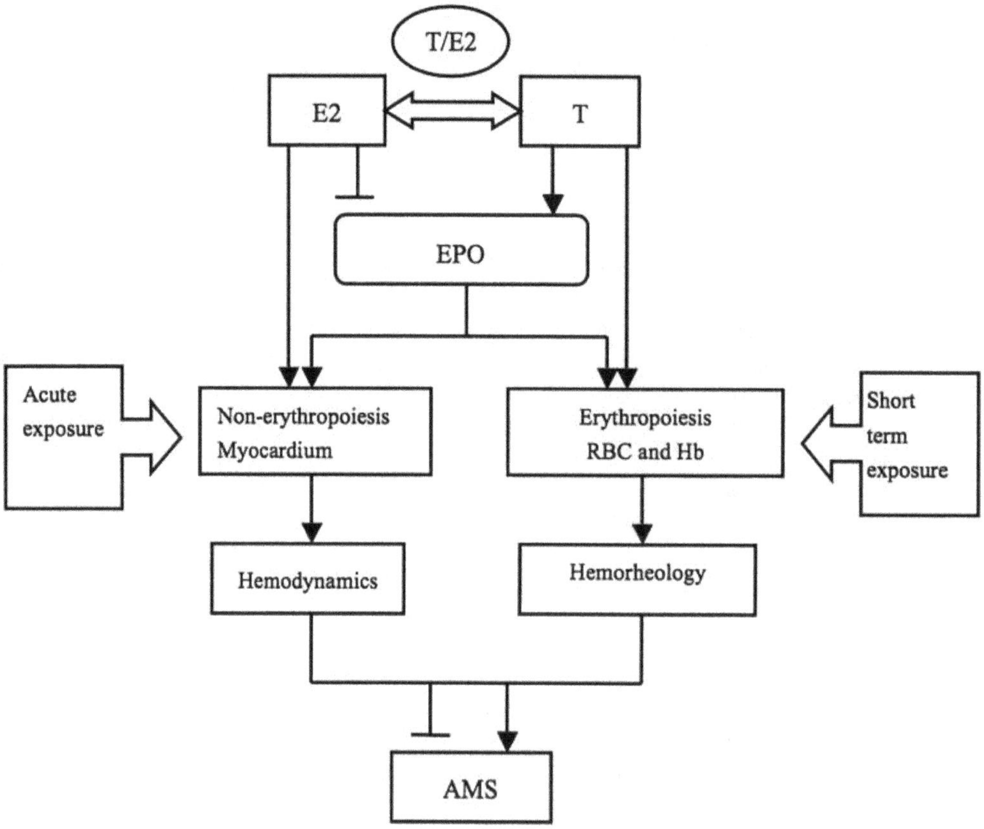

FIGURE 3 | The potential mechanisms of sex hormones in AMS during different exposure durations. T and E2 may play various roles in AMS through different pathophysiological processes in a time dependent way.

Disequilibrium of Endogenous E2 and T May Be Involved in AMS

T and E2 are the most active sex hormones in the human body. They play opposite roles in respiratory regulation and erythropoiesis (Ou et al., 1994). T is converted to E2 by aromatase after acting on erythrocytosis (Jiang et al., 2010). Thus, the ratio of T/E2, which is determined by the levels of T and E2 as well as aromatase, is more important than the absolute value of each sex hormone.

Though the effects of T/E2 on SpO_2 have been reported, which our results do not corroborate the relationship between SpO_2 and T/E2 (Gonzales and Villena, 2000) (which our results do not corroborate), as have the effects of T/E2 on respiratory regulation, erythrocytosis, and even CMS, few studies have focused on AMS. Our observations reveal that T/E2 was closely associated with the AMS score, which indicates the importance of T/E2 in the pathophysiological process of AMS. The erythropoietic effect of T occurred before aromatase could convert it into E2, which had no effect on erythropoiesis (even with a reverse action) (Zabka et al., 2006). On the other hand, T enhanced EPO production and erythropoiesis and induced hypoventilation, while E2 enhanced ventilation, increased SpO_2 and inhibited EPO and RBC production. However, T may reduce these effects by down regulating the estradiol and progesterone receptors in response to ventilation, favoring hypoventilation and stimulating erythropoiesis (Ou et al., 1994; Zabka et al., 2006; Jiang et al., 2010).

Based on the evidence described above for CMS and our observations, it may be possible to regulate the T/E2 ratio by increasing the aromatization of T into E2, increasing aromatase expression or even applying E2 exogenously to prevent and treat AMS. Furthermore, T/E2 may participate in AMS *via* erythropoiesis, as indicated by the associations among T/E2, EPO, and RBC. The precise mechanisms by which T/E2 participates in AMS warrant further basic research.

The Predictive Roles of T/E2 in AMS at High Altitude

The T/E2 at sea level was on an independent predictor for AMS on the 1st day or the 7th day at 3,700 m indicated by both univariate or adjusted regressions. However, the T/E2 on the 1st day at 3,700 m can predict AMS after 7 days indicating that the role of T/E2 was in progressing pathophysiological progress. Though, the sea level T/E2 failed to predict AMS, its association between AMS has been revealed in our present study. In addition, the predictive of T/E2 may be dependent on other risk factors that warrant further study.

CONCLUSION

Acute mountain sickness was correlated with the ratio of T to E2 and the level of EPO. Our observations suggest that higher T/E2 may promote AMS by acting through or combining with EPO to affect erythropoiesis, however, the mechanisms by which this may occur warrant further study. Furthermore, though T/E2 at sea level was not an independent predictor for AMS, the T/E2 on the 1st day at 3,700 m was an independent predictor for AMS on the 7th day.

Limitations

The subjects of this study were all young male workers, mostly aged between 16 and 40 years, which could perhaps generate a bias due to age or gender. The current study is an observational study with a small sample size, and larger sample sizes and mechanistic studies are needed.

AUTHOR CONTRIBUTIONS

LH and X-HD participated in the design of this research. X-HD, YW, and LH drafted the manuscript and performed the statistical analyses. LH, J-HZ, and JQ reviewed and revised this manuscript critically for important intellectual content. X-HD, J-HZ, BC, and X-HZ completed the collection of clinical data and performed the measurements of BP, HR, and the biomarkers (T, E2, and blood routine tests). R-SR and S-YY performed the echocardiography examinations.

FUNDING

This work was supported by the Ministry of Health of the People's Republic of China (Grant No. 201002012) and People's Liberation Army China (Grant No. BWS14J040).

ACKNOWLEDGMENTS

We would like to thank all of the individuals who participated in this study for their support. We are also grateful to Mr. Can Chen, Bai-Da Xu, Guo-Zhu Chen, Xu-Gang Tang, and Cheng-Rong Zheng and Miss. Wen-Yun Guo, Shuang-Fei Li, and Yang Liu for their helps in the data collection.

REFERENCES

Bachman, E., Travison, T. G., Basaria, S., Davda, M. N., Guo, W., Li, M., et al. (2013). Testosterone induces erythrocytosis via increased erythropoietin and suppressed hepcidin: evidence for a new erythropoietin/hemoglobin set point. *J. Gerontol. A Biol. Sci. Med. Sci.* 69, 725–735. doi: 10.1093/gerona/glt154

Bartsch, P., and Swenson, E. R. (2013). Acute high-altitude illnesses. *N. Engl. J. Med.* 369, 1666–1667. doi: 10.1056/NEJMcp1214870

Congote, L. F., Bruno, F., and Solomon, S. (1977). Effects of testosterone and estradiol on ratios of adult to fetal hemoglobin in cell cultures of human fetal liver. *Biol. Neonate* 32, 310–318. doi: 10.1159/000241034

Cornolo, J., Mollard, P., Brugniaux, J. V., Robach, P., and Richalet, J.-P. (2004). Autonomic control of the cardiovascular system during acclimatization to high altitude: effects of sildenafil. *J. Appl. Physiol.* 97, 935–940. doi: 10.1152/japplphysiol.00239.2004

Coviello, A. D., Kaplan, B., Lakshman, K. M., Chen, T., Singh, A. B., and Bhasin, S. (2008). Effects of graded doses of testosterone on erythropoiesis in healthy young and older men. *J. Clin. Endocrinol. Metab.* 93, 914–919. doi: 10.1210/jc.2007-1692

Davis, P. R., Pattinson, K. T., Mason, N. P., Richards, P., and Hillebrandt, D. (2011). High altitude illness. *J. R. Army Med. Corps* 157, 12–17. doi: 10.1136/jramc-157-01-03

Earley, S., and Resta, T. C. (2002). Estradiol attenuates hypoxia-induced pulmonary endothelin-1 gene expression. *Am. J. Physiol. Lung Cell. Mol. Physiol.* 283, L86–L93. doi: 10.1152/ajplung.00476.2001

Ekart, R., Taskovska, M., Hojs, N., Bevc, S., and Hojs, R. (2013). Testosterone and hemoglobin in hemodialysis male and female patients. *Artif. Organs* 38, 598–603. doi: 10.1111/aor.12218

Gonzales, G. F. (2011). Hemoglobin and testosterone: importance on high altitude acclimatization and adaptation. *Rev. Peru. Med. Exp. Salud Publica* 28, 92–100. doi: 10.1590/S1726-46342011000100015

Gonzales, G. F. (2013). Serum testosterone levels and excessive erythrocytosis during the process of adaptation to high altitudes. *Asian J. Androl.* 15, 368–374. doi: 10.1038/aja.2012.170

Gonzales, G. F., Gasco, M., Tapia, V., and Gonzales-Castaneda, C. (2009). High serum testosterone levels are associated with excessive erythrocytosis of chronic mountain sickness in men. *Am. J. Physiol. Endocrinol. Metabol.* 296, E1319–E1325. doi: 10.1152/ajpendo.90940.2008

Gonzales, G. F., Tapia, V., Gasco, M., and Gonzales-Castañeda, C. (2011). Serum testosterone levels and score of chronic mountain sickness in Peruvian men natives at 4340 m. *Andrologia* 43, 189–195. doi: 10.1111/j.1439-0272.2010.01046.x

Gonzales, G. F., and Villena, A. (2000). Low pulse oxygen saturation in post-menopausal women at high altitude is related to a high serum testosterone/estradiol ratio. *Int. J. Gynaecol. Obstet.* 71, 147–154. doi: 10.1016/S0020-7292(00)00270-8

Gunga, H. C., Kirsch, K. A., Roecker, L., Kohlberg, E., Tiedemann, J., Steinach, M., et al. (2007). Erythropoietin regulations in humans under different environmental and experimental conditions. *Respir. Physiol. Neurobiol.* 158, 287–297. doi: 10.1016/j.resp.2007.03.006

Hackett, P. H., and Roach, R. C. (2001). High-altitude illness. *N. Engl. J. Med.* 345, 107–114. doi: 10.1056/NEJM200107123450206

Harris, C. W., Shields, J. L., and Hannon, J. P. (1966). Acute mountain sickness in female. *Aerosp. Med.* 37, 1163–1167.

Heinicke, K., Prommer, N., Cajigal, J., Viola, T., Behn, C., and Schmidt, W. (2003). Long-term exposure to intermittent hypoxia results in increased hemoglobin mass, reduced plasma volume, and elevated erythropoietin plasma levels in man. *Eur. J. Appl. Physiol.* 88, 535–543. doi: 10.1007/s00421-002-0732-z

Imray, C., Wright, A., Subudhi, A., and Roach, R. (2010). Acute mountain sickness: pathophysiology, prevention, and treatment. *Prog. Cardiovasc. Dis.* 52, 467–484. doi: 10.1016/j.pcad.2010.02.003

Iturriaga, R., Rey, S., and Del Rio, R. (2005). Cardiovascular and ventilatory acclimatization induced by chronic intermittent hypoxia: a role for the carotid body in the pathophysiology of sleep apnea. *Biol. Res.* 38, 335–340. doi: 10.4067/S0716-97602005000400004

Jiang, J., Tang, N. L., Ohlsson, C., Eriksson, A. L., Vandenput, L., Chan, F. W., et al. (2010). Association of genetic variations in aromatase gene with serum estrogen and estrogen/testosterone ratio in Chinese elderly men. *Clin. Chim. Acta* 411, 53–58. doi: 10.1016/j.cca.2009.09.039

Koury, M. J. (2005). Erythropoietin: the story of hypoxia and a finely regulated hematopoietic hormone. *Exp. Hematol.* 33, 1263–1270. doi: 10.1016/j.exphem.2005.06.031

Lorenzo, F. R., Huff, C., Myllymaki, M., Olenchock, B., Swierczek, S., Tashi, T., et al. (2014). A genetic mechanism for Tibetan high-altitude adaptation. *Nat. Genet.* 46, 951–956. doi: 10.1038/ng.3067

Maggio, M., Snyder, P. J., Ceda, G. P., Milaneschi, Y., Luci, M., Cattabiani, C., et al. (2013). Is the haematopoietic effect of testosterone mediated by erythropoietin?

The results of a clinical trial in older men. *Andrology* 1, 24–28. doi: 10.1111/j.2047-2927.2012.00009.x

Mattingly, K. A., Ivanova, M. M., Riggs, K. A., Wickramasinghe, N. S., Barch, M. J., and Klinge, C. M. (2008). Estradiol stimulates transcription of nuclear respiratory factor-1 and increases mitochondrial biogenesis. *Mol. Endocrinol.* 22, 609–622. doi: 10.1210/me.2007-0029

Naeije, R. (2010). Physiological adaptation of the cardiovascular system to high altitude. *Prog. Cardiovasc. Dis.* 52, 456–466. doi: 10.1016/j.pcad.2010.03.004

Oliver, S. J., Sanders, S. J., Williams, C. J., Smith, Z. A., Lloyd-Davies, E., Roberts, R., et al. (2012). Physiological and psychological illness symptoms at high altitude and their relationship with acute mountain sickness: a prospective cohort study. *J. Travel Med.* 19, 210–219. doi: 10.1111/j.1708-8305.2012.00609.x

Oskui, P. M., French, W. J., Herring, M. J., Mayeda, G. S., Burstein, S., and Kloner, R. A. (2013). Testosterone and the cardiovascular system: a comprehensive review of the clinical literature. *J. Am. Heart Assoc.* 2:e000272. doi: 10.1161/JAHA.113.000272

Ou, L. C., Sardella, G. L., Leiter, J. C., Brinck-Johnsen, T., and Smith, R. P. (1994). Role of sex hormones in development of chronic mountain sickness in rats. *J. Appl. Physiol.* 77, 427–433. doi: 10.1152/jappl.1994.77.1.427

Richmond, T. D., Chohan, M., and Barber, D. L. (2005). Turning cells red: signal transduction mediated by erythropoietin. *Trends Cell Biol.* 15, 146–155. doi: 10.1016/j.tcb.2005.01.007

Riksen, N. P., Hausenloy, D. J., and Yellon, D. M. (2008). Erythropoietin: ready for prime-time cardioprotection. *Trends Pharmacol. Sci.* 29, 258–267. doi: 10.1016/j.tips.2008.02.002

Rochira, V., Zirilli, L., Madeo, B., Maffei, L., and Carania, C. (2009). Testosterone action on erythropoiesis does not require its aromatization to estrogen: insights from the testosterone and estrogen treatment of two aromatase-deficient men. *J. Steroid Biochem. Mol. Biol.* 113, 189–194. doi: 10.1016/j.jsbmb.2008.12.007

Shin, Y. S., You, J. H., Cha, J. S., and Park, J. K. (2016). The relationship between serum total testosterone and free testosterone levels with serum hemoglobin and hematocrit levels: a study in 1221 men. *Aging Male* 19, 209–214. doi: 10.1080/13685538.2016.1229764

Simonson, T. S., Yang, Y., Huff, C. D., Yun, H., Qin, G., Witherspoon, D. J., et al. (2010). Genetic evidence for high-altitude adaptation in Tibet. *Science* 329, 72–75. doi: 10.1126/science.1189406

Smith, N. L., Blondon, M., Wiggins, K. L., Harrington, L. B., van Hylckama Vlieg, A., Floyd, J. S., et al. (2014). Lower risk of cardiovascular events in postmenopausal women taking oral estradiol compared with oral conjugated equine estrogens. *JAMA Intern. Med.* 174, 25–31. doi: 10.1001/jamainternmed.2013.11074

Wu, T. Y., Ding, S. Q., Liu, J. L., Jia, J. H., Chai, Z. C., and Dai, R. C. (2012). Who are more at risk for acute mountain sickness:a prospective study in Qinghai-Tibet railroad construction workers on Mt Tanggula. *Chin. Med. J.* 2012, 1393–1400.

Zabka, A. G., Mitchell, G. S., and Behan, M. (2006). Conversion from testosterone to oestradiol is required to modulate respiratory long-term facilitation in male rats. *J. Physiol.* 576(Pt 3), 903–912. doi: 10.1113/jphysiol.2006.114850

Heavy Resistance Training in Hypoxia Enhances 1RM Squat Performance

*Mathew W. H. Inness[1, 2], François Billaut[1, 3], Emily J. Walker[1, 4], Aaron C. Petersen[1], Alice J. Sweeting[1] and Robert J. Aughey[1]**

[1] Institute of Sport, Exercise and Active Living, Victoria University, Melbourne, VIC, Australia, [2] Western Bulldogs Football Club, Melbourne, VIC, Australia, [3] Département de Kinesiologie, Université Laval, Quebec City, QC, Canada, [4] Collingwood Football Club, Melbourne, VIC, Australia

***Correspondence:**
Robert J. Aughey
robert.aughey@vu.edu.au

Purpose: To determine if heavy resistance training in hypoxia (IHRT) is more effective at improving strength, power, and increasing lean mass than the same training in normoxia.

Methods: A pair-matched, placebo-controlled study design included 20 resistance-trained participants assigned to IHRT (FIO2 0.143) or placebo (FIO2 0.20), (n = 10 per group). Participants were matched for strength and training. Both groups performed 20 sessions over 7 weeks either with IHRT or placebo. All participants were tested for 1RM, 20-m sprint, body composition, and countermovement jump pre-, mid-, and post-training and compared via magnitude-based inferences.

Presentation of Results: Groups were not clearly different for any test at baseline. Training improved both absolute (IHRT: 13.1 ± 3.9%, effect size (ES) 0.60, placebo 9.8 ± 4.7%, ES 0.31) and relative 1RM (IHRT: 13.4 ± 5.1%, ES 0.76, placebo 9.7 ± 5.3%, ES 0.48) at mid. Similarly, at post both groups increased absolute (IHRT: 20.7 ± 7.6%, ES 0.74, placebo 14.1 ± 6.0%, ES 0.58) and relative 1RM (IHRT: 21.6 ± 8.5%, ES 1.08, placebo 13.2 ± 6.4%, ES 0.78). Importantly, the change in IHRT was greater than placebo at mid for both absolute [4.4% greater change, 90% Confidence Interval (CI) 1.0:8.0%, ES 0.21, and relative strength (5.6% greater change, 90% CI 1.0:9.4%, ES 0.31 (relative)]. There was also a greater change for IHRT at post for both absolute (7.0% greater change, 90% CI 1.3:13%, ES 0.33), and relative 1RM (9.2% greater change, 90% CI 1.6:14.9%, ES 0.49). Only IHRT increased countermovement jump peak power at Post (4.9%, ES 0.35), however the difference between IHRT and placebo was unclear (2.7, 90% CI –2.0:7.6%, ES 0.20) with no clear differences in speed or body composition throughout.

Conclusion: Heavy resistance training in hypoxia is more effective than placebo for improving absolute and relative strength.

Keywords: hypoxia, resistance training, strength, 1RM squat, power, hypertrophy

INTRODUCTION

Hypoxia has long been used in combination with endurance training (Terrados et al., 1988). The benefits of endurance training in hypoxia include increased intermittent running performance (Inness et al., 2016), glycolytic enzyme activity (Faiss et al., 2013), and rates of phosphocreatine regeneration (Holliss et al., 2013). Hypoxia may also improve performance in time trials

(Czuba et al., 2011), although this is less conclusive (Inness et al., 2016). These benefits are potentially important to enhance team-sport athlete performance.

The development of strength and power is also important for team-sport athletes due to the physical involvements in collision sports including Australian football and the Rugby codes (Dawson et al., 2004; Roberts et al., 2008). Therefore, resistance training plays an integral part in the physical preparation of team-sport athletes. The positive effects of resistance training in hypoxia are becoming evident (Takarada et al., 2000b). When used in combination with resistance training, hypoxia is commonly achieved in two ways, blood flow restriction, and intermittent hypoxic resistance training (IHRT) With blood flow restriction, a pressure cuff is applied to the limb, restricting blood flow, participants then perform resistance training exercises (Takarada et al., 2000b). Blood flow restriction causes many perturbations in the muscle, only one of which is hypoxia. Restricting blood flow to the muscle places the restricted tissue in an ischemic state, leading to hypoxia. Some of the possible mechanisms behind increased strength and hypertrophy through blood flow restriction include increased type ii fiber type recruitment (Yasuda et al., 2010), accumulation of metabolites (Loenneke et al., 2010), increases in plasma growth hormone (Takarada et al., 2000a), and muscle cell swelling (Loenneke et al., 2012).

There are practical limitations to blood flow restriction when using traditional resistance training exercises such as squats, deadlifts, and bench press. Firstly, it is only possible to restrict blood flow to the limbs; therefore a large proportion of musculature used during these exercises is not in a hypoxic state. This causes a disassociation in muscle hypertrophy between the muscles of the limb, which is exposed to blood flow restriction, and the muscles of the trunk, which is not exposed to blood flow restriction (Yasuda et al., 2011). Since blood flow restriction is usually matched with low intensity resistance training, the changes in cross sectional area and strength may not be accompanied by a concomitant increase in connective tissue strength. This is due to decreased mechanical loading through low intensity resistance training used with blood flow restriction (Scott et al., 2015a), therefore the strength of muscles and connective tissue will adapt disproportionately. Increased tensile strength of the tendon might be expected to maintain the safety of the tendon under increasing loads (Buchanan and Marsh, 2002). Although currently unknown, there is a possibility that increasing the strength of the muscle without allowing the tendons time to adapt to this increased force production of the muscle may result in an increased risk of musculotendinous injuries. Due to these limitations in blood flow restriction, it is possible IHRT may be more suited for athletes and strength-trained individuals, as it allows high force production during training that also strengthens connective tissue to aid in injury prevention.

With IHRT, participants perform resistance training in hypoxia, induced by either a normobaric reduction of oxygen content in the mixture (Friedmann et al., 2003; Nishimura et al., 2010), or decreased partial pressure of air as evident at moderate to high altitude (Feriche et al., 2014). There is very little research on IHRT, with conflicting findings on its the effectiveness for increasing 1RM. One of the earliest studies using IHRT showed increased strength and hypertrophy compared to the same training in normoxia (Nishimura et al., 2010). For two sessions per week for 6 weeks, French press and arm curls were performed at 70% 1RM. The IHRT group showed greater hypertrophy and strength than the control group. To further support the use of IHRT, netball athletes undertaking low intensity IHRT had a greater improvement in maximal voluntary contraction than a control group (Manimmanakorn et al., 2013). Similarly, in previously untrained participants, using a moderate intensity resistance training protocol, only the IHRT group improved muscular endurance as measured by maximal repetitions at 70% 1RM (Kon et al., 2014). However, the IHRT group showed no greater improvement in 1RM compared to control (Kon et al., 2014). This is interesting considering a moderate training intensity of 70% 1RM, using 5 sets of 10 reps was used throughout the study.

In the aforementioned study, both groups had similar increases in lean mass and decreases in fat mass (Kon et al., 2014). A low intensity IHRT protocol with previously untrained participants did not have the same effect on muscular endurance (Friedmann et al., 2003). Maximal strength, as measured through a maximal voluntary contraction, did not increase. It is clear the current research is conflicting, and further investigations are required to deduce the best training combinations.

There is currently no research using a high intensity resistance training protocol. The effects of IHRT on strength-trained participants have also not been determined. This study will therefore investigate if heavy IHRT is more effective at developing maximal strength in resistance-trained participants. A secondary aim is to determine whether IHRT aids changes in body composition, sprint performance, and power production during the countermovement jump.

METHODS

Participants

Twenty strength-trained male participants aged between 18 and 34 volunteered as participants. Participants were required to record a training diary, and qualified as strength trained by achieving at least 12 months continuous resistance training history immediately prior to the study. Resistance training prior to the study needed to include squats and deadlifts as part of their regular training program. The study was approved by the University Human Research Ethics Committee and conformed to the Declaration of Helsinki. All participants provided written informed consent. Participants completed a training log of their current resistance training, including frequency, exercises, sets, repetitions, and intensity to ensure they qualified as strength trained for the purpose of the study. Participants were then pair-matched on absolute 1RM squat strength and training history, and assigned to either the hypoxic (IHRT) or placebo groups.

Testing

Pre-, mid-, and post-study, participants were scanned using dual energy x-ray absorptiometry (DXA) to assess changes in body composition, tested for 1RM squat strength, countermovement jump, and 20-m sprint time with 5 and 10-m splits.

All participants were familiar with the 1RM squat, a warm up set of five repetitions at 50% predicted 1RM was performed, followed by three repetitions at 80% predicted 1RM, then a single repetition at 90% predicted 1RM. The weight was then increased in small increments until failure, with the goal of achieving a 1RM in a further 3–4 attempts. For the lift to be successful, a depth was required whereby the crease of the hips was below the top of the patella. The same Australian Strength and Conditioning Association Level 3 qualified coach assessed 1RM depth throughout the study. A linear position transducer was connected to the bar, and during the warm-up sets, participants were instructed as to the required depth for 1RM testing by the assessor. This depth was recorded via minimum displacement from the linear position transducer. A failed attempt was recorded if the participant failed to lift the weight, or if adequate depth was not achieved.

The 20-m sprint was performed pre- and post-intervention on the same indoor basketball court using Swift timing gates (Swift, http://www.spe.com.au. Wacol, Queensland, Australia). Participants were instructed to place their toe on a line between the two starting gates, with their weight over their front foot to ensure acceleration occurs from a stationary start with no rock back. Timing gates were placed at 0, 5, 10, and 20-m to record split times. A minimum of three attempts was allowed, with a fourth attempt given if the third trial was the fastest. Participants were offered as much rest as required to ensure each effort was maximal, with a minimum of 3 min given.

A countermovement jump using a force plate, linear position transducer, and corresponding Ballistic Measurement System Software (Fitness Technologies, http://www.fittech.com.au, Adelaide, South Australia, Australia) was used to assess jump qualities. The force plate and linear position transducer were calibrated prior to each testing session according to manufacturer's instructions. Participants performed a familiarization session for the countermovement jump prior to baseline testing. At each testing session, participants performed four single jumps with ~30 s between each jump, with the jump that achieved the highest power output being used for analysis.

Body mass was measured on calibrated scales and height was measured on a calibrated stadiometer. A DXA scan was performed to assess change in body composition measures including fat mass, lean tissue, and bone mass. The DXA scanner used was a Discovery W version 13.4.2. It was calibrated prior to each testing session according to manufacturer's instructions. A standard scanning protocol was used to ensure measurement reliability (Nana et al., 2013). Two experienced technicians performed the scans throughout the study, however each participant was scanned and analyzed by the same technician at pre, mid, and post to remove any inter-tester differences. The protocol for the DXA scan is described in detail elsewhere (Nana et al., 2013). Briefly, participants were positioned on their back in the supine position with hands pronated and legs positioned slightly apart with the femur rotated inwards.

Participants were instructed to maintain a food diary for the first week of the study, and told to replicate this eating plan as closely as possible for the duration of the study. This was to minimize the likelihood that any changes in body composition were due to a change in diet. Participants were instructed not to start taking any supplements.

Training

During the training sessions, all participants wore a face-mask connected to a hypoxic simulator (Altitude Training Systems, http://www.ats-altitude.com, Lidcombe, NSW, 2141). The hypoxic simulator exposed the participants to simulated altitude by increasing the percentage of nitrogen in the inspired air. The simulator was set at one of two altitudes. The placebo group was exposed to air with an FiO_2 of 0.20, simulating an altitude of 400-m above sea level, while the hypoxic group was exposed to air with an FiO_2 of 0.145 for the first 4 weeks, simulating an altitude of 3100-m, and FiO_2 of 0.141 for the last 3 weeks, simulating 3400-m above sea level. Groups were blinded to their group allocation until the completion of all testing post-study. Participants completed 7 weeks of heavy resistance training three times per week, with sessions performed on non-consecutive days. Each session consisted of squats, deadlifts, and lunges, with repetitions ranging from 3 to 6, and sets ranging from 2 to 4 (**Table 1**). Rest periods were set at 3 min throughout the study. For squats, starting weight was 75% 1RM for session 1. This weight was chosen after pilot testing, as it was the heaviest weight that could be lifted whereby participants remained blinded to the simulated altitude. During pilot testing, when loads above 75% were used for six repetitions participants were able to correctly guess whether they were in the IHRT or placebo trial. We wanted to ensure participants remained blinded to their groups while still using heavy loads. The placebo effect may play a part in determining endurance changes due to altitude (Lundby et al., 2012), however it is unknown if the placebo effect plays a part in resistance training strength changes through altitude. To control for a possible placebo effect, it was important participants remained blinded to the group allocation. The starting weight for deadlift was the same as squat, while lunge started at 50% squat 1RM. If participants lifted the weight to the predetermined repetition goal, they were encouraged to increase the weight. Participants were asked for a rating of perceived exertion (RPE, Borg 6-20 scale) immediately post-set, and this, combined with the judgment of the researcher was used to determine whether the participant should increase the weight for the next set. This method of increasing the load each session was chosen over a set increase per session or week to allow for individual variations in adaptation over time. For squats and lunges, the bar was positioned on the back across the superior trapezius, with participants instructed to achieve a depth of crease of hips below the top of the patella, as for 1RM testing. For deadlift, the weight was lowered to the ground between each rep. As participants were experienced in these exercises, a degree of flexibility was allowed regarding placement of feet, with some choosing a wider stance, and others a narrower stance.

The hypoxic mask was worn for the last warm up set and all working sets. Once applied, the hypoxic mask was not removed until the completion of the session (~45 min).

TABLE 1 | Repetitions (Reps) and sets each week for squats, deadlifts, and lunges (3 lunges each leg per set) and percentage 1RM for squat lifted and post-set RPE for each group each week.

Week	Sets	Squat reps	Deadlift reps	Lunge reps	Squat %1RM IHRT load	Squat %1RM placebo load	Post-set IHRT RPE	Post-set placebo RPE
1	3	6	6	6	77.5 ± 3.7	78.2 ± 3.9	6.74 ± 1.63	6.02 ± 2.19
2	3	5	5	6	85.4 ± 5.3	83.8 ± 4.0	7.39 ± 2.14	7.03 ± 1.90
3	3	4	4	6	94.4 ± 5.6#	90.5 ± 4.1	7.80 ± 2.28	7.38 ± 2.13
4	2	4	4	6	99.2 ± 5.4#	94.2 ± 4.5	6.98 ± 2.44	6.71 ± 2.16
5	3	5	5	6	100.4 ± 6.5#	94.7 ± 5.9	8.14 ± 2.49	7.66 ± 2.10
6	4	4	4	6	104.2 ± 7.8#	98.6 ± 6.5	7.86 ± 2.80	7.71 ± 1.87
7	4	3	3	6	109.9 ± 8.2#	104.5 ± 5.9	7.60 ± 2.80	7.83 ± 2.15

 # Likely Large effect in the difference of 1RM lifted between groups. All data is Mean ± SD.

Prior to hypoxic exposure, baseline SpO_2 and heart rate were taken via pulse-oximetry. These values were also taken pre- and post-each working set, with the values immediately prior to the set used as the pre-set value, and the lowest value of SpO_2 and highest value for heart rate used as the post-set value. Post-set values were usually achieved 15–30 s post-set. As well as the 6–20 Borg scale post each working set, the Borg 1–10 RPE scale was used post-session. After the first session, and regularly throughout the 7 weeks, participants were asked which group they thought they were in.

Statistical Analysis

A contemporary statistical approach was used to analyse all data, and expressed as mean ± *SD* and effect size [ES ± 90% confidence limits (CL)]. Percentage change was determined in comparison to baseline. The difference in the change between groups was determined using both ES and % changes ± 90% CL. Where the difference in between group change for 90% CL crossed from positive to negative (across 0%), this was interpreted as unclear at 90% CL. Standards for measuring ES were as previously described (Hopkins et al., 2009).

RESULTS

Participants were blinded to condition, with only one participant guessing their group allocation. **Table 2** gives details of the participants. Of the 20 volunteers, 18 completed the study (9 per group), while the other two completed the mid testing. One participant withdrew due to illness, and the other through injury, both unrelated to the training study. Only the 18 who finished the study were included for post-analysis, while all 20 participants were included in the mid testing analysis. Groups were not clearly different for any of the testing procedures at baseline.

Baseline

Absolute strength was 121.4 ± 22.1 kg for IHRT and 125.5 ± 30.7 kg for placebo. Relative strength was 1.46 ± 0.19 $kg.bm^{-1}$ for IHRT and 1.56 ± 0.30 $kg.bm^{-1}$ for placebo. Differences between groups for strength, or any other testing parameter at baseline were unclear (**Table 2**).

Training Data

Pre-training SpO_2values were not different between groups (98.3 ± 1.3% for IHRT and 98.4 ± 1.3% for placebo; **Table 3**). During the session, oxygen desaturation occurred in IHRT only, with a *likely* large effect in the difference between groups pre-set (90.0 ± 2.5% for IHRT vs. 97.3 ± 1.3% for placebo. ES −5.61, 90% CL for ES −5.7 to −5.5). There was also greater desaturation post-set for IHRT with a *most likely* large effect in the difference between groups (84.1 ± 3.5% for IHRT vs. 96.5 ± 1.7% for placebo, ES −7.3, CL for ES −7.4 to −7.2; **Table 3**). Neither session RPE (IHRT 7.5 ± 1.3 vs. placebo 7.3 ± 1.6), nor post-set RPE (IHRT 15.4 ± 2.5 vs. placebo 15.2 ± 2.3) were different between groups.

Heart rate was higher post-set compared to pre in both groups (pre- to post-set HR 103.7 ± 19.6 to 144.8 ± 19.0 bpm for IHRT, and 104.0 ± 18.3 to 144.9 ± 18.2 bpm for placebo), with no clear difference between groups (**Table 3**). Load lifted when reported as percentage of squat 1RM was not different between groups during week 1 (77.5. ± 3.7% for IHRT vs. 78.2 ± 3.9 for placebo). For squat, there was a trend toward IHRT lifting a greater percentage of baseline 1RM compared to placebo throughout the study (**Table 3**). By week 3, IHRT was lifting a greater percentage of starting 1RM for squat compared to placebo, with a *likely* large effect (3.9%, ES 0.94, 90% CL 0.65–1.24). This greater percentage of 1RM lifted in training for IHRT compared to placebo remained through to week 7 (5.4%, ES 0.91, 90% CL 0.61–1.20).

Mid

Compared to baseline, both groups improved both absolute (12.7 ± 3.9% for IHRT vs. 8.7 ± 4.7% for placebo) and relative (12.9 ± 5.1% for IHRT vs. 8.2 ± 5.3% for placebo) 1RM squat (**Figure 1**). Compared to placebo, the IHRT group had a *possibly* greater change for absolute (4.4% greater change, CL 1.0–8.0%, ES 0.21, 90% CL 0.05–0.37) and a *likely* greater change for relative 1RM (5.1% greater change, CL 1.0–9.4%, ES 0.31, 90% CL 0.06–0.57). There was no change for lean mass or countermovement jump parameters either between or within groups.

Post

Compared to baseline both groups improved both absolute (22.2 ± 7.6% for IHRT vs. 14.2 ± 6.0% for placebo) and relative

TABLE 2 | Testing results for all performance tests for both IHRT and Placebo groups.

Test	IHRT group			Placebo group		
	Pre (*n* = 10)	Mid (*n* = 10)	Post (*n* = 9)	Pre (*n* = 10)	Mid (*n* = 10)	Post (*n* = 9)
Height (cm)	183.1 ± 4.5	183.1 ± 4.5	184.1 ± 4.5	181.0 ± 5.8	181.0 ± 5.8	180.8 ± 5.8
Body mass (kg)	83.1 ± 7.5	83.0 ± 7.5	83.7 ± 7.9	80.2 ± 12.0	80.5 ± 11.2	78.7 ± 9.8
Absolute 1RM strength (kg)	121.4 ± 22.1	138.2 ± 27.8	148.4 ± 32.7**	125.5 ± 30.7	135.7 ± 29.5	141.8 ± 28.8#
Relative squat strength ($kg.bm^{-1}$)	1.46 ± 0.19	1.66 ± 0.22	1.76 ± 0.26**	1.56 ± 0.30	1.69 ± 0.29	1.80 ± 0.25#
5 m split time (s)	1.17 ± 0.08		1.17 ± 0.03	1.13 ± 0.08		1.12 ± 0.07
10 m split time (s)	1.94 ± 0.11		1.94 ± 0.06	1.89 ± 0.09		1.88 ± 0.08
20 m split time (s)	3.25 ± 0.15		3.27 ± 0.10	3.21 ± 0.14		3.18 ± 0.09
Absolute Peak Power (W)	4360 ± 602		4676 ± 463*	4333 ± 656		4299 ± 527

**Possibly greater pre-post change than placebo. **Likely greater change than placebo. #Likely greater than pre. All data is Mean ± SD.*

TABLE 3 | Average SpO_2 and Heart Rate values pre and post all sets for the duration of the training study and post-set RPE for each group.

	IHRT pre-session	IHRT pre-set	IHRT post-set	Placebo pre-session	Placebo pre-set	Placebo post-set
SpO_2%	98.29 ± 1.3	89.97 ± 2.5*	84.13 ± 3.5*#	98.38 ± 1.3	97.26 ± 1.3	96.51 ± 1.7
Heart Rate (BPM)	93.8 ± 19.1	103.7 ± 19.6	144.8 ± 19.0**	93.8 ± 17.2	104.0 ± 18.3	144.9 ± 18.2**
RPE (au)			15.43 ± 2.5			15.16 ± 2.3
Post-session RPE (au)			7.53 ± 1.28			7.27 ± 1.61

**Most likely less than placebo. #Most likely less than pre. **Most likely greater than pre-set. All Data is Mean ± SD.*

(20.5 ± 8.5% for IHRT vs. 13.6 ± 6.4% for placebo). The IHRT group had a *likely* greater change than placebo from pre to post for both absolute (7.0% greater change, CL 1.3–13.0%, ES 0.33, 90% CL 0.06–0.59) and relative (8.0% greater change, 90% CL 1.6–14.9%, ES 0.49, 90% CL 0.10–0.87) 1RM. At post, only IHRT improved countermovement jump peak power, however this change was unclear in comparison to placebo (2.7% greater change, 90% CL −2.0–7.6%, ES 0.20, 90% CL −0.15–0.54). There was no difference between or within groups compared to pre for 20-m sprint or body composition.

DISCUSSION

Hypoxia improved both absolute and relative 1RM compared to the same training using a placebo despite no change in lean mass. The placebo group also improved 1RM strength, however the IHRT change was 5.8 and 9.2% greater than placebo in absolute and relative 1RM strength, respectively. Considering participants were already strength trained with a moderate to high level of strength, this is a meaningful change between groups after only 7 weeks.

This is the first study to use heavy resistance training combined with hypoxia. Only an acute resistance exercise bout has been previously used (Scott et al., 2015b), therefore the present study reports original findings using heavy resistance training and hypoxia in a training study. The majority of resistance and systemic hypoxia studies used low to moderate intensity resistance training of ∼30–70% 1RM. However, the present study used 75% 1RM for the first session, increasing to 104% starting 1RM for placebo and 109% for IHRT. Unlike high-intensity interval training in hypoxia, which shows a decrease in maximal work (Balsom et al., 1994), hypoxia does not appear to impact on physical performance during high-load resistance exercise. This is shown by no differences in RPE and heart rate between groups, and is in agreement with the only other research using heavy resistance exercise and hypoxia. Using five repetitions of squat and deadlift in three different conditions (FiO_2 of 0.21, 0.16, and 0.13), heart rate, and post-set RPE were not different in the conditions with an FiO_2 of 0.21 and 0.16 despite using the same load. However, at the more extreme hypoxia, heart rate was higher than the other two conditions (Scott et al., 2015b). This, combined with our findings, confirms resistance training exercise intensity is not affected by moderate hypoxia, at least in trained individuals.

While increased strength and hypertrophy is consistently achieved through resistance training combined with blood flow restriction (Takarada et al., 2000b; Scott et al., 2014), there are conflicting findings whether systemic hypoxia increases strength to a greater extent than resistance training alone. The inconsistent findings can be partly attributed to differences in study design. For example, studies of moderate volume and intensity (3–4 sets of ∼70% 1RM) generally show greater changes in muscle hypertrophy using hypoxia (Nishimura et al., 2010; Kurobe et al., 2015), although one showed no difference between groups (Kon et al., 2014). There are also inconsistent results regarding changes in 1RM between groups when using IHRT with submaximal loads. Studies show increases in 1RM using both moderate (Nishimura et al., 2010) and very light loads (Manimmanakorn et al., 2013), while others show no benefit on 1RM through hypoxia compared to control (Kon et al., 2014). Unfortunately, the study by Nishimura et al. used a predictive equation to determine 1RM from a 10RM test. Therefore, although authors concluded an increase in muscular strength, it is rather likely that, because of the non-specific testing (Reynolds

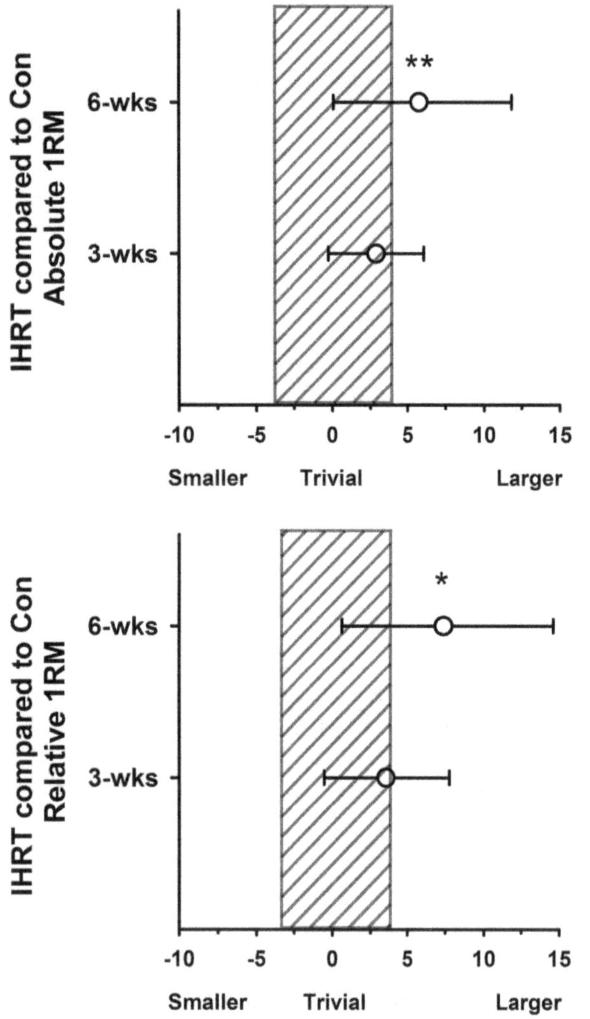

FIGURE 1 | Percentage difference in the change in performance from baseline for intermittent hypoxic resistance training (IHRT) compared with placebo with 90% CI. (A) Between-groups change in Absolute 1RM strength. **(B)** Between-groups change in Relative 1RM strength. Shaded bar represents uncertainty in the measure. **Possibly* small effect in the difference in change between groups, ***Likely* small effect in the difference in the change between groups.

et al., 2006; Tanner and Gore, 2013), an increase in muscular endurance explained the change in predicted 1RM.

Two studies have used tests of moderate intensities to test for muscular endurance, similar to the load used during training, with hypoxic groups showing both a benefit (Kon et al., 2014), and no change in performance (Kurobe et al., 2015). In the Kon et al. study, systemic hypoxia showed no greater change in 1RM compared to control, however when testing using the same intensity as training, muscular endurance improved more in the hypoxic group (Kon et al., 2014), showing the importance of the testing protocol matching the training protocol.

As all hypoxia and resistance training studies to date have used moderate intensities more suited to hypertrophy and muscular endurance gains (Fleck and Kraemer, 2014), combined with the differences in methodology for determining 1RM, it is not surprising that changes in 1RM through systemic hypoxia are conflicting. Therefore, it is important to ensure the testing battery is appropriate to reflect the nature of the training intervention (Tanner and Gore, 2013). Systemic hypoxia may merely magnify the expected outcome from a given training program, with specificity of the stimulus and testing protocol important to test the outcome of training.

It is possible there were no increases in lean mass due to our study employing a lower volume, high intensity program designed to increase maximal strength more so than muscle hypertrophy. This type of protocol is more likely to see changes in strength as opposed to muscle hypertrophy (Kraemer and Ratamess, 2004). This change in strength despite a lack of change in lean mass is an important finding, as many athletes, including team-sport athletes with a high running demand in their sport, athletes competing in weight classes, and many endurance athletes want to increase strength without an increase in mass.

Other researchers have concluded that the placebo effect may be at least partly responsible for performance changes through hypoxia (Siebenmann et al., 2012), however this was not the case in our study. As participants were successfully blinded to the environmental condition, the greater changes in strength observed in IHRT in the present study cannot be attributed to a placebo effect. Due to no placebo effect, and no changes in lean mass, we cannot fully explain the mechanisms responsible for the differences between groups. When beginning strength training, most of the early strength changes can be attributed to neural adaptations (Moritani and deVries, 1979). Such early changes include adaptations in agonist, antagonist, and stabilizer muscle activation, increased firing frequency, motor unit synchronization, and agonist co-activation (Folland and Williams, 2007). As all participants were strength trained, matched for training status and 1RM, any neural adaptations could be expected to be minimal.

When undertaking endurance training in hypoxia, intermittent hypoxic training maintains the proportion of type II fibers to a greater extent to the same training in normoxia (Zoll et al., 2006). After 6 weeks, an intermittent hypoxic training group had the same percentage of type II fibers (29.4 $\pm$ 7.4 at pre, and 29.9 $\pm$ 6.2 at post), whereas the same training in normoxia saw type II fibers decrease (41.0 $\pm$ 8.1% at pre, to 33.9 $\pm$ 6.6% at post; Zoll et al., 2006). Type II muscle fibers have a greater force production than type I fibers (Bottinelli et al., 1999). As intermittent hypoxic training maintains type II fibers, if this maintenance of type II fibers is also apparent with IHRT, it is possible there was a greater strength adaptation in the IHRT group compared to placebo despite no changes in muscle mass due to type II fiber maintenance.

The decreases in SpO_2 in IHRT are similar to other systemic hypoxic studies (Kon et al., 2010; Scott et al., 2015b). A decrease in SpO_2 occurs with hypoxia, and this activates a cascade of events that eventually lead to changes in endurance performance (Rusko et al., 2004). It is yet to be determined what effect a decrease in SpO_2 has on changes seen through IHRT. There is reduced central fatigue following adaptation to hypoxia (Amann et al., 2013). Enhanced cerebral O_2 delivery to compensate for hypoxia could enhance neurotransmitter turnover, thus enhancing skeletal muscle fiber firing rate (Amann et al., 2013), which is a typical neural adaptation seen through resistance training. The heavy resistance training used in the current study increases the level of neural activity (Tan, 1999). Whether these changes are evident following IHRT is unknown, however if apparent, this would possibly explain an adaptation to hypoxia that may increase strength through neural changes including muscle fiber firing rate. Although there are possible neural changes that could explain increases in 1RM through IHRT, most changes in neural adaptation occur quite early in a resistance-training program (Moritani and deVries, 1979). As we used resistance-trained participants, most of the neural changes would have already occurred. Therefore, it is quite surprising that there were changes in 1RM despite no change in muscle mass. Because of this, the mechanisms behind increased 1RM are not known. Neural changes should be analyzed in further IHRT studies to determine whether neural changes are responsible for the change in performance following IHRT.

We found no change in 20-m sprint performance for either group, despite a change in 1RM. Although only IHRT improved CMJ peak power, the difference in the change between groups was unclear. There is a strong correlation between maximal squat strength and sprint performance (Wisløff et al., 2004; McBride et al., 2009), this correlation is also apparent between maximal squat strength and CMJ performance (Wisløff et al., 2004). It is also generally believed that improving 1RM directly increases sprint performance. In soccer athletes, there was a small change in 20-m sprint times after improvements in 1RM squat strength (Styles et al., 2016). A low volume, heavy resistance training protocol was used. Although not stated, the Styles et al. study was performed during the competition season and it is assumed these athletes would have been exposed to maximal running velocity during training and matches. Therefore, strength changes through resistance training, combined with the sprint training during the on pitch training may have combined to increase 20-m sprint performance. To support this, strength training only, and sprint training only displayed the same changes in 30-m sprint times, while a combination of strength and sprint training had a greater enhancement in 30-m sprint times (Marques et al., 2015).

As our study was heavy resistance training only, and the participants were not performing sprint training as part of their normal activity outside of the study, a possible reason for the lack of change in 20-m sprint times and CMJ performance in our study is due to no explosive training being performed as part of training. In a study on team-sport athletes, a group that performed plyometric exercises improved sprint times, while a control group showed no change (Marques et al., 2013), however it should be noted that neither group performed resistance training as part of the study. The addition of sprint or plyometric training combined with maximal strength training may therefore be important to improve sprint times, with resistance training alone insufficient to increase speed and power.

In a normal periodized resistance-training program for athletes, high velocity resistance training either follows, or is completed in conjunction with heavy strength training. This change in strength could well be transferred into changes in power with appropriate subsequent training.

PRACTICAL APPLICATIONS

- IHRT increases relative and absolute 1RM in comparison to a strength and training matched control group.
- Increases in 1RM occurred despite no changes in muscle mass, 20-m sprint or CMJ parameters.
- Athletes wanting to increase strength without increasing muscle mass are advised to undertake heavy resistance training in systemic hypoxia.

AUTHOR CONTRIBUTIONS

MI, FB, RA responsible for study design, recruitment of participants, data collection, data analysis, manuscript drafting and editing. EW, AP, AS responsible for some data collection, some data analysis and editing manuscript.

ACKNOWLEDGMENTS

The authors would like to acknowledge the help of all the lab staff and participants. We would also like to thank Amber Rowell, Brendan Lazarus, James McMahon, Jan Lemon, Kristal Hammond, and Raku Shimakawa for supervising the training sessions.

REFERENCES

Amann, M., Goodall, S., Twomey, R., Subudhi, A. W., Lovering, A. T., and Roach, R. C. (2013). AltitudeOmics: on the consequences of high-altitude acclimatization for the development of fatigue during locomotor exercise in humans. *J. Appl. Physiol.* 115, 634–642. doi: 10.1152/japplphysiol.00606.2013

Balsom, P. D., Gaitanos, G. C., Ekblom, B., and SjÖDin, B. (1994). Reduced oxygen availability during high intensity intermittent exercise impairs performance. *Acta Physiol. Scand.* 152, 279–285. doi: 10.1111/j.1748-1716.1994.tb09807.x

Bottinelli, R., Pellegrino, M. A., Canepari, M., Rossi, R., and Reggiani, C. (1999). Specific Contributions of various muscle fibre types to human muscle performance: an *in vitro* study. *J. Electromyogr. Kinesiol.* 9, 87–95. doi: 10.1016/S1050-6411(98)00040-6

Buchanan, C. I., and Marsh, R. L. (2002). Effects of exercise on the biomechanical, biochemical and structural properties of tendons. *Comp. Biochem. Physiol.* 133, 1101–1107. doi: 10.1016/S1095-6433(02)00139-3

Czuba, M., Waskiewicz, Z., Zajac, A., Poprzecki, S., Cholewa, J., and Roczniok, R. (2011). The effects of intermittent hypoxic training on aerobic capacity and endurance performance in cyclists. *J. Sport Sci. Med.* 10, 175–183.

Dawson, B., Hopkinson, R., Appleby, B., Stewart, G., and Roberts, C. (2004). Player movement patterns and game activities in the Australian Football League. *J. Sci. Med. Sport* 7, 278–291. doi: 10.1016/S1440-2440(04)80023-9

Faiss, R., Léger, B., Vesin, J.-M., Fournier, P.-E., Eggel, Y., Dériaz, O., et al. (2013). Significant molecular and systemic adaptations after repeated sprint training in hypoxia. *PLoS ONE* 8:e56522. doi: 10.1371/journal.pone.0056522

Feriche, B., Garcia-Ramos, A., Calderon-Soto, C., Drobnic, F., Bonitch-Gongora, J., Galilea, P., et al. (2014). Effects of acute exposure to moderate altitude on muscle power: hypobaric hypoxia vs. normobaric hypoxia. *PLoS ONE* 9:e114072. doi: 10.1371/journal.pone.0114072

Fleck, S. J., and Kraemer, W. (2014). *Designing Resistance Training Programs*. Champaign, IL: Human Kinetics.

Folland, J. P., and Williams, A. G. (2007). The adaptations to strength training: morphological and neurological contributions to increased strength. *Sports Med.* 37, 145–168. doi: 10.2165/00007256-200737020-00004

Friedmann, B., Kinscherf, R., Borisch, S., Richter, G., Bärtsch, P., and Billeter, R. (2003). Effects of low-resistance/high-repetition strength training in hypoxia on muscle structure and gene expression. *Pflügers Arch.* 446, 742–751. doi: 10.1007/s00424-003-1133-9

Holliss, B. A., Fulford, J., Vanhatalo, A., Pedlar, C. R., and Jones, A. M. (2013). Influence of intermittent hypoxic training on muscle energetics and exercise tolerance. *J. Appl. Physiol.* 114, 611–619. doi: 10.1152/japplphysiol.01331.2012

Hopkins, W. G., Marshall, S. W., Batterham, A. M., and Hanin, J. (2009). Progressive statistics for studies in sports medicine and exercise science. *Med. Sci. Sport Exerc.* 41, 3–12. doi: 10.1249/MSS.0b013e31818cb278

Inness, M., Aughey, R., and Billaut, F. (2016). Team-Sport Athletes' improvement of performance on the yo-yo intermittent recovery test level 2, but not of time-trial performance, with intermittent hypoxic training. *Int. J. Sport Physiol. Perform.* 11, 15–21. doi: 10.1123/ijspp.2014-0246

Kon, M., Ikeda, T., Homma, T., Akimoto, T., Suzuki, Y., and Kawahara, T. (2010). Effects of acute hypoxia on metabolic and hormonal responses to resistance exercise. *Med. Sci. Sport Exerc.* 42, 1279–1285. doi: 10.1249/MSS.0b013e3181ce61a5

Kon, M., Ohiwa, N., Honda, A., Matsubayashi, T., Ikeda, T., Akimoto, T., et al. (2014). Effects of systemic hypoxia on human muscular adaptations to resistance exercise training. *Physiol. Rep.* 2:e12033. doi: 10.14814/phy2.12033

Kraemer, W. J., and Ratamess, N. A. (2004). Fundamentals of resistance training: progression and exercise prescription. *Med. Sci. Sport Exerc.* 36, 674–688. doi: 10.1249/01.MSS.0000121945.36635.61

Kurobe, K., Huang, Z., Nishiwaki, M., Yamamoto, M., Kanehisa, H., and Ogita, F. (2015). Effects of resistance training under hypoxic conditions on muscle hypertrophy and strength. *Clin. Physiol. Funct. Imaging* 35, 197–202. doi: 10.1111/cpf.12147

Loenneke, J. P., Fahs, C. A., Rossow, L. M., Abe, T., and Bemben, M. G. (2012). The anabolic benefits of venous blood flow restriction training may be induced by muscle cell swelling. *Med. Hypotheses.* 78, 151–154. doi: 10.1016/j.mehy.2011.10.014

Loenneke, J. P., Wilson, G. J., and Wilson, J. M. (2010). A mechanistic approach to blood flow occlusion. *Int. J. Sport Sci.* 31, 1–4. doi: 10.1055/s-0029-1239499

Lundby, C., Millet, G. P., Calbet, J. A., Bärtsch, P., and Subudhi, A. W. (2012). Does 'altitude training' increase exercise performance in elite athletes? *Br. J. Sports Med.* 46, 792–795. doi: 10.1136/bjsports-2012-091231

Manimmanakorn, A., Hamlin, M. J., Ross, J. J., Taylor, R., and Manimmanakorn, N. (2013). Effects of low-load resistance training combined with blood flow restriction or hypoxia on muscle function and performance in netball athletes. *J. Sci. Med. Sport* 16, 337–342. doi: 10.1016/j.jsams.2012.08.009

Marques, M. C., Gabbett, T. J., Marinho, D. A., Blazevich, A. J., Sousa, A., van den Tillaar, R., et al. (2015). Influence of strength, sprint running, and combined strength and sprint running training on short sprint performance in young adults. *Int. J. Sport Sci.* 36, 789–795. doi: 10.1055/s-0035-1547284

Marques, M. C., Pereira, A., Reis, I. G., and van den Tillaar, R. (2013). Does an in-Season 6-Week combined sprint and jump training program improve strength-speed abilities and kicking performance in young soccer players? *J. Hum. Kinet.* 39, 157–166. doi: 10.2478/hukin-2013-0078

McBride, J. M., Blow, D., Kirby, T. J., Haines, T. L., Dayne, A. M., and Triplett, N. T. (2009). Relationship between maximal squat strength and five, ten, and forty yard sprint times. *J. Strength Cond. Res.* 23, 1633–1636. doi: 10.1519/JSC.0b013e3181b2b8aa

Moritani, T., and deVries, H. (1979). Neural factors versus hypertrophy in the time course of muscle strength gain. *Am. J. Physiol. Med.* 58, 115–130.

Nana, A., Slater, G. J., Hopkins, W. G., and Burke, L. M. (2013). Effects of exercise sessions of DXA measurements of body composition and active people. *Med. Sci. Sport Exerc.* 45, 178–185. doi: 10.1249/MSS.0b013e31826c9cfd

Nishimura, A., Sugita, M., Kato, K., Fukuda, A., Sudo, A., and Uchida, A. (2010). Hypoxia increases muscle hypertrophy induced by resistance training. *Int. J. Sport Physiol. Perform.* 5, 497–508. doi: 10.1123/ijspp.5.4.497

Reynolds, J. M., Gordon, T. J., and Robergs, R. A. (2006). Prediction of one repetition maximum strength from multiple repetition maximum testing and anthropometry. *J. Strength Cond. Res.* 20, 584–592. doi: 10.1519/R-15304.1

Roberts, S. P., Trewartha, G., Higgitt, R. J., El-Abd, J., and Stokes, K. A. (2008). The physical demands of elite English rugby union. *J. Sport Sci.* 26, 825–833. doi: 10.1080/02640410801942122

Rusko, H., Tikkanen, H., and Peltonen, J. (2004). Altitude and endurance training. *J. Sport Sci.* 22, 928–945. doi: 10.1080/02640410400005933

Scott, B. R., Slattery, K. M., and Dascombe, B. J. (2015a). Intermittent hypoxic resistance training: is metabolic stress the key moderator? *Med. Hypotheses* 84, 145–149. doi: 10.1016/j.mehy.2014.12.001

Scott, B. R., Slattery, K. M., Sculley, D. V., and Dascombe, B. J. (2014). Hypoxia and resistance exercise: a comparison of localized and systemic methods. *Sports Med.* 44, 1037–1054. doi: 10.1007/s40279-014-0177-7

Scott, B. R., Slattery, K. M., Sculley, D. V., Hodson, J. A., and Dascombe, B. J. (2015b). Physical performance during high-intensity resistance exercise in normoxic and hypoxic conditions. *J. Strength Cond. Res.* 29, 807–815. doi: 10.1519/JSC.0000000000000680

Siebenmann, C., Robach, P., Jacobs, R. A., Rasmussen, P., Nordsborg, N., Diaz, V., et al. (2012). Live high-train low using normobaric hypoxia: a double-blinded, placebo-controlled study. *J. Appl. Physiol.* 112, 106–117. doi: 10.1152/japplphysiol.00388.2011

Styles, W. J., Matthews, M. J., and Comfort, P. (2016). Effects of strength training on squat and sprint performance in soccer players. *J. Strength Cond. Res.* 30, 1534–1539. doi: 10.1519/JSC.0000000000001243

Takarada, Y., Nakamura, Y., Aruga, S., Onda, T., Miyazaki, S., and Ishii, N. (2000a). Rapid increase in plasma growth hormone after low-intensity resistance exercise with vascular occlusion. *J. Appl. Physiol.* 88, 61–65.

Takarada, Y., Takazawa, H., Sato, Y., Takebayashi, S., Tanaka, Y., and Ishii, N. (2000b). Effects of resistance exercise combined with moderate vascular occlusion on muscular function in humans. *J. Appl. Physiol.* 88, 2097–2106.

Tan, B. (1999). Manipulating resistance training program variables to optimize maximum strength in men: a review. *J. Strength Cond. Res.* 13, 289–304. doi: 10.1519/00124278-199908000-00019

Tanner, R., and Gore, C. J. (2013). *Physiological Tests for Elite Athletes*. Champaign, IL: Human Kinetics.

Terrados, N., Melichna, J., Sylvën, C., Jansson, E., and Kaijser, L. (1988). Effects of traning at simulated altitude on performance and muscle metabolic capacity in competitive road cyclists. *Eur. J. Appl. Physiol. Occup. Physiol.* 57, 203–209. doi: 10.1007/BF00640664

Wisløff, U., Castagna, C., Helgerud, J., Jones, R., and Hoff, J. (2004). Strong correlation of maximal squat strength with sprint performance and vertical jump height in elite soccer players. *Br. J. Sports Med.* 38, 285–288. doi: 10.1136/bjsm.2002.002071

Yasuda, T., Abe, T., Brechue, W. F., Iida, H., Takano, H., Meguro, K., et al. (2010). Venous blood gas and metabolite response to low-intensity muscle contractions with external limb compression. *Metabolism* 59, 1510–1519. doi: 10.1016/j.metabol.2010.01.016

Yasuda, T., Ogasawara, R., Sakamaki, M., Bemben, M. G., and Abe, T. (2011). Relationship between limb and trunk muscle hypertrophy following high-intensity resistance training and blood flow-restricted low-intensity resistance training. *Clin. Physiol. Funct. Imaging* 31, 347–351. doi: 10.1111/j.1475-097X.2011.01022.x

Zoll, J., Ponsot, E., Dufour, S., Doutreleau, S., Ventura-Clapier, R., Vogt, M., et al. (2006). Exercise training in normobaric hypoxia in endurance runners. III. Muscular adjustments of selected gene transcripts. *J. Appl. Physiol.* 100, 1258–1266. doi: 10.1152/japplphysiol.00359.2005

16

Twin Resemblance in Muscle HIF-1α Responses to Hypoxia and Exercise

Ruud Van Thienen[1†], Evi Masschelein[1†], Gommaar D'Hulst[1], Martine Thomis[2] and Peter Hespel[1]*

[1] Exercise Physiology Research Group, Department of Kinesiology, KU Leuven, Leuven, Belgium, [2] Physical Activity, Sports and Health Research Group, Department of Kinesiology, KU Leuven, Leuven, Belgium

***Correspondence:**
Peter Hespel
peter.hespel@faber.kuleuven.be

† These authors have contributed equally to this work.*

Hypoxia-inducible factor-1 (HIF-1) is a master regulator of myocellular adaptation to exercise and hypoxia. However, the role of genetic factors in regulation of HIF-1 responses to exercise and hypoxia is unknown. We hypothesized that hypoxia at rest and during exercise stimulates the HIF-1 pathway and its downstream targets in energy metabolism regulation in a genotype-dependent manner. Eleven monozygotic twin (MZ) pairs performed an experimental trial in both normoxia and hypoxia (FiO_2 10.7%). Biopsies were taken from m. vastus lateralis before and after a 20-min submaximal cycling bout @∼30% of sea-level VO_2max. Key-markers of the HIF-1 pathway and glycolytic and oxidative metabolism were analyzed using real-time PCR and Western Blot. Hypoxia increased HIF-1α protein expression by ∼120% at rest vs. +150% during exercise ($p < 0.05$). Furthermore, hypoxia but not exercise increased muscle mRNA content of HIF-1α (+50%), PHD2 (+45%), pVHL (+45%; $p < 0.05$), PDK4 (+1200%), as well as PFK-M (+20%) and PPAR-γ1 (+60%; $p < 0.05$). Neither hypoxia nor exercise altered PHD1, LDH-A, PDH-A1, COX-4, and CS mRNA expressions. The hypoxic, but not normoxic exercise-induced increment of muscle HIF-1α mRNA content was about 10-fold more similar within MZ twins than between the twins ($p < 0.05$). Furthermore, in resting muscle the hypoxia-induced increments of muscle HIF-1α protein content, and HIF-1α and PDK4 mRNA content were about 3–4-fold more homogeneous within than between the twins pairs ($p < 0.05$). The present observations in monozygotic twins for the first time clearly indicate that the HIF-1α protein as well as mRNA responses to submaximal exercise in acute hypoxia are at least partly regulated by genetic factors.

Keywords: monozygotic twin design, HIF-1, exercise, hypoxia, muscle biopsies

INTRODUCTION

Whenever the human body is exposed to oxygen deficiency, numerous physiological responses are initiated. Adaptations at both the cardiovascular, respiratory, neurological and skeletal muscle level (Petousi and Robbins, 2014) aim to maintain adequate oxygen uptake and delivery so as to preserve cellular energy homeostasis and tissue integrity. At the level of skeletal muscles, differential mechanisms are involved in the response to either acute or chronic hypoxia. For instance, in acute hypoxic stress fuel selection is shifted from fatty acids to carbohydrates, which increases the ATP yield per molecule of oxygen consumed. Such mechanism not only facilitates energy homeostasis (Hoppeler and Vogt, 2001; Hoppeler et al., 2008; Murray, 2009) but also protects against excessive mitochondrial production of reactive oxygen species (Zhang et al., 2008; Murray, 2009; Edwards et al., 2010). Furthermore, acute hypoxia also regulates gene expression of several rate-limiting enzymes in the primary energy pathways, i.e., glycolysis, the Krebs cycle, as well as oxidative phosphorylation (Zoll et al., 2006; Murray and Horscroft, 2016). These alterations eventually result in a downregulation of oxidative energy production, vs. upregulation of anaerobic ATP production via glycolysis, aiming to assure adequate rates of sustained ATP-production whenever abundant oxygen supply is lacking, most prominently during exercise (Murray, 2009). The effects of chronic hypoxia on skeletal muscle on the other hand serve to facilitate oxygen diffusion in muscle tissue by stimulation of neovascularization vs. decrease of muscle fiber cross-sectional area, which reduces oxygen diffusion distance (Hoppeler and Vogt, 2001; Deldicque and Francaux, 2013). Furthermore, loss of mitochondrial density and mitochondrial uncoupling decreased ROS production, which might otherwise be exaggerated especially during hypoxic exercise (Murray and Horscroft, 2016).

It is the prevailing opinion that hypoxia-inducible factor 1 (HIF-1) plays a pivotal role in myocellular adaptations to hypoxia (Vogt et al., 2001). HIF-1 is a heterodimeric transcription factor, built of a HIF-1α and a HIF-1β subunit, and serves as an intracellular oxygen-sensor to trigger cellular responses needed to cope with any drop of intramyocellular oxygen tension (Ameln et al., 2005; Mason and Johnson, 2007). In normoxic conditions, in contrast to hypoxia, the HIF-1α subunit is not hydroxylated and is immediately degraded. Conversely, in hypoxia, HIF-1α accumulates in the cytosol and migrates to the nucleus to dimerize with the HIF-1β subunit. The heterodimer so formed can bind to the regulatory domain of different target genes which in turn initiate the concerted cellular response to the hypoxic stress. The importance of HIF-1 in regulation of metabolic genes, including all glycolytic enzymes, *pyruvate dehydrogenase kinase 1* (PDK1) and subunit 4-2 of *cytochrome c oxidase* (COX), but also regulation of angiogenesis is well established (Ameln et al., 2005; Papandreou et al., 2006; Mason and Johnson, 2007; Murray, 2009). Activation of HIF-1 in hypoxic conditions also leads to enhanced mitochondrial autophagy and a decrease in mitochondrial biogenesis and respiration (Zhang et al., 2008). However, data on the inter-individual variability of HIF-1 responses to hypoxia and the role of heritability in HIF-1 regulation in muscle are lacking. Nonetheless, we previously found genetic variants to be important in explaining some specific muscular responses to hypoxia (regulation of maximal oxygen uptake and protein metabolism) (Masschelein et al., 2014, 2015a). Furthermore, epidemiological studies in high-altitude natives to explore the incidence of gene polymorphisms that may be beneficial for survival at high altitude, have provided evidence to indicate that the HIF transcriptional system is associated with some specific loci encoding the erythropoietin and hemoglobin proteins (Simonson et al., 2010; Yi et al., 2010; Petousi and Robbins, 2014). In contrast, the role of genetic factors in modulating the response of HIF-1 in *lowlanders* ascending to altitude is unknown. In fact, qualitative studies on the contribution of genetic factors in exercise performance in hypoxia are scarce (Hennis et al., 2015). To date published literature only supports a potential role of the *angiotensin-converting enzyme insertion* (ACE-I) and *endothelial PAS domain-containing protein 1* (EPAS1) alleles in exercise performance in hypoxia (Montgomery et al., 1998; Masschelein et al., 2015a).

Against this background, the hypothesis driving the current study was that the variability in response of myocellular HIF-1 and its downstream targets implicated in regulation of glycolysis as well as oxidative metabolism, is at least partly explained by genetic factors. To test this hypothesis, we conducted a well-controlled cross-over study (Masschelein et al., 2014, 2015b) in which monozygotic (MZ) twins were exposed to normoxia vs. hypoxia equivalent to ~5300 m altitude, both at rest and during submaximal exercise. The data presented in this paper for the first time demonstrate that both HIF-1 mRNA and protein expression are upregulated by acute normobaric hypoxia and/or exercise in a genotype-dependent manner.

METHODS

Subjects

The data presented in this paper are original and are part of a larger study in which 13 monozygotic twin brothers ($n = 26$) were enrolled (Masschelein et al., 2014, 2015b). Inclusion criteria on admission were: non-smoking, no history of cardiovascular or respiratory disease, similar physical activity levels within twins, and no residence at altitude >1500 m during 6 months before the study. Mono-zygosity of the twin pairs was confirmed via 8 polymorphic markers (chromosome (chr) 13, GATA30H01 and GATA85D03; chr 18, GATA2E06, GATA64H04, and GATA88A12; and chr 21, GATA163G03, GATA24H09, and GATA71H10). Only 11 of the 13 twin pairs agreed to have muscle biopsies taken during the experiments and were eventually included in the current analyses ($n = 22$; age, 24.4 ± 0.8 years; body weight, 75.9 ± 1.7 kg; VO_2max 55.3 ± 2.1 ml O_2 kg^{-1} min^{-1}). The study protocol was approved by the local ethics committee and was performed in accordance with the Declaration of Helsinki. Subjects gave written consent after being informed in detail of all experimental procedures and passed an a priori medical examination. The twins were instructed to maintain their habitual diet and physical activity levels during the study and to omit exercise for 24 h before each experimental day.

Study Design

Details of the study design have been described previously as this study is part of a greater research project (Masschelein et al., 2014, 2015b). Subjects participated in two experimental days in a normobaric hypoxic facility at 20°C and 50% relative humidity (Sporting Edge, Sherfield on Loddon, UK) with a 2-wk washout period in between. The first experimental trial was in normoxia (NOR; $FIO_2 = 0.209$) and the second one in hypoxia (HYP; $FIO_2 = 0.107$) (see **Figure 1**). The NOR experiment was always done first to exclude possible "memory" effects due to an earlier hypoxic exposure. Breakfast (700 kcal from 84% carbohydrates, 9% fat, and 7% protein) and all later meals and snacks (1880 kcal from 76% carbohydrates, 12% fat,

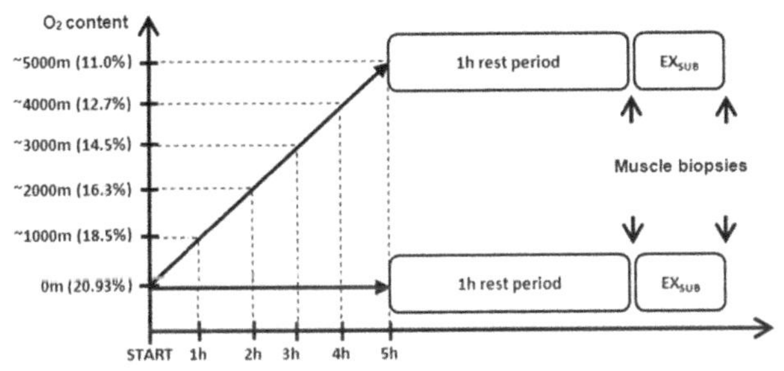

FIGURE 1 | Schematic overview of the experimental study design. Subjects rested for 5 h in either 0.209 FIO_2 (NOR), or while FIO_2 was gradually decreased from 0.209 to 0.107 (HYP). Sixty min after the target FIO_2 was established a needle biopsy sample was taken from the left m. vastus lateralis (pre-ex biopsy, see subsequent figures). Subjects then performed a 20-min submaximal constant-load (1.2 W/kg) exercise (EX_{SUB}) bout on a cycle ergometer after which a second biopsy sample was obtained (post-ex biopsy, see subsequent figures). See Methods for further details.

and 12% protein) and drinks (500 ml of water per 2 h) during both the experimental days were standardized. On each day, twins reported to the 50 m^2 hypoxic facility at 8:00 am and were put in separated compartments within the chamber in order to keep them both ignorant about the experimental events and outcomes occurring in their twin brother. They first rested for 5 h in a comfortable chair in either 0.209 FIO_2 (NOR), or while FIO_2 was gradually decreased from 0.209 to 0.107 (HYP). Thereafter they stayed for an additional 3 h at the target FIO_2 of either 0.209 (NOR) or 0.107 (HYP). Sixty min after the target FIO_2 was established a needle biopsy sample was taken from the left m. vastus lateralis under local anesthesia (1 ml of lidocaine 2 % without adrenaline) through a 5-mm incision in the skin and with the needle tip pointing proximally. Subjects then performed a 20-min submaximal constant-load (1.2 W/kg) exercise (EX) bout on a cycle ergometer (Cyclus II; Avantronic, Leipzig, Germany), corresponding to 50.7 ± 2.3% of VO_2max in normoxia vs. 81.4 ± 3.2% of VO_2max in hypoxia. These exercise modalities (load and duration) were selected after preliminary experiments had shown that 1.2 W/kg for 20 min in similar subjects corresponded to near-maximal exercise tolerance at 0.107 FIO_2. Such workload (~100 W) corresponds to a normal ascent rate of 300 m per hour in mountaineers (Burtscher, 2004). We also wanted to compare responses to an absolute workload rather than a relative workload. Immediately after exercise (post-ex), another muscle biopsy sample was taken through the same incision as the pre-ex biopsy sample but with the needle pointing distally in the muscle. All muscle samples were quickly frozen in liquid nitrogen and stored at −80°C until biochemical assays were performed.

Western Blot

Details of the immunoblotting procedures were described previously (Deldicque et al., 2010). Briefly, frozen muscle tissue (~20 mg) was homogenized 3 times for 5 s each with a Polytron mixer (Polytron Technologies, Taoyuan City, Taiwan) in ice-cold buffer [1:10, w/v; 50 mM Tris-HCl, pH 7.0; 270 mM sucrose; 5 mM EGTA; 1 mM EDTA; 1 mM sodium orthovanadate; 50 mM glycerophosphate; 5 mM sodium pyrophosphate; 50 mM sodium fluoride; 1 mM dithiothreitol; 0.1% Triton X-100; and a complete protease inhibitor tablet (Roche Applied Science, Vilvoorde, Belgium)]. Homogenates were then centrifuged at 10,000 g for 10 min at 4°C. The supernatant was collected and immediately stored at −80°C. The protein concentration was measured using a DC protein assay kit (Bio-Rad Laboratories, Nazareth, Belgium). Proteins (30–80 g) were separated by SDS-PAGE (8–12% gels) and transferred to polyvinylidene difluoride membranes. Subsequently, membranes were blocked with 5% nonfat milk for 1 h and then incubated overnight (4°C) with the following antibodies (1:1000): total eukaryotic elongation factor 2 (eEF2) (Cell Signaling, Leiden, The Netherlands) and hypoxia-inducible factor-1α (HIF-1α). Horseradish peroxidase-conjugated anti-rabbit (1:5000) and anti-guinea pig (1:5000) secondary antibodies (Sigma-Aldrich, Bornem, Belgium) were used for chemiluminescent detection of proteins. Membranes were scanned and quantified with GeneSnap and Gene Tools software (Syngene, Cambridge, UK), respectively. The results are presented as the ratio protein of interest/eEF2. All values from the respective condition were reported to the mean value of the first sample (pre-ex) in NOR. One subject was excluded from analysis due to lack of sample.

RNA Extraction and Reverse Transcription

The method used for reverse transcription is described in detail elsewhere (Vincent et al., 2010; Jamart et al., 2011). In brief, total RNA was extracted using TRIzol (Invitrogen, Vilvoorde, Belgium) from 20 to 25 mg of frozen muscle tissue. Total RNA was extracted only in 19 subjects because of the lack of material in 3 individuals. RNA quality and quantity were assessed by spectrophotometry with a NanoDrop (Thermo Scientific, Erembodegem, Belgium). Then 1 g of RNA was reverse-transcribed using a High-Capacity cDNA Reverse Transcription kit (Applied Biosystems, Gent, Belgium) according to the manufacturer's instructions.

Real-Time Quantitative PCR Analysis

A SYBR Green-based master mix (Applied Biosystems) was used for real-time PCR analyses using the ABI PRISM 7300 system (Applied Biosystems). Real-time PCR primers were designed for the genes of interest. Thermal cycling conditions consisted of 40 3-step cycles including denaturation for 30 s at 95°C, annealing for 30 s at 58°C, and extension for 30 s at 72°C. All reactions were performed in triplicate. To compensate for variations in input RNA amounts and efficiency of reverse transcription, glyceraldehyde-3-phosphate dehydrogenase (GAPDH) and ribosomal protein L4 (RPL4) mRNA were quantified, and results were normalized to these values. These genes were chosen out of 3 normalization genes using the GeNorm applet according to the guidelines and theoretical framework described elsewhere as the Vandesompele-method (Vandesompele et al., 2002). All values from the respective condition were reported to the mean value of the first sample (pre-ex) in NOR.

Statistical Analysis

A 2-way repeated-measures analysis of variance (ANOVA) was used to assess the statistical significance of differences between mean values over time and between conditions (Systat Software, San Jose, CA, USA). When appropriate, a Bonferroni *t*-test was used as a *post hoc* test. In addition, the correlated observations at the level of the twins, together with the individual repeated measures of the oxygen level conditions (NOR vs. HYP) and exercise response (time), were also analyzed using a multilevel mixed-model approach (random effects for time level nested in condition level, nested in twin level; SAS 9.3; SAS Institute, Cary, NC, USA). Because the multilevel mixed-model approach gave the same significant results as the ANOVA, it was chosen to present all data according to the results of the 2-way repeated-measures ANOVA analyses. When the latter analyses revealed a significant difference in protein or mRNA expression, the genetic influence was determined by 2-way repeated-measures ANOVA on one factor, with the twins nested in pairs, and by intra-class correlation coefficients (ICC's; SAS Enterprise Guide 4.3, SAS Institute). F-ratios thus obtained represent the ratio of between-pair over within-pair variability in the induced responses, whereas ICCs provide a quantitative estimate of the similarity within MZ twin pairs and an upper-limit estimate of the genetic component in these responses (genotype × hypoxia and genotype × exercise interaction) (Bouchard et al., 1990). A probability level of $P < 0.05$ was considered statistically significant. All data are presented as means ± standard of the mean (SEM).

RESULTS

Hif-1α Pathway (Table 1 and Figures 2–4)

Compared to NOR, HYP increased HIF-1α protein expression by ~120% at rest, and by an additional 35% post exercise ($p < 0.05$). Compared to the resting condition in NOR, exercise in HYP raised HIF-1α protein expression about 2.5-fold ($p < 0.05$). HYP, but not exercise, increased HIF-1α mRNA expression by about 30–50% ($p < 0.05$). Irrespective of rest and exercise, HYP stimulated PHD2 as well as pVHL mRNA content by ~40–50% ($p < 0.05$), whilst PHD1 mRNA content was affected neither by HYP, nor by exercise. Compared to NOR, HYP slightly elevated VEGF-2A mRNA content post ($p < 0.05$) but not pre exercise.

Some of the above average responses were not randomly distributed between subjects. Conversely, some responses were significantly more homogeneous within the twins than between the twins (**Table 1**). Most strikingly, stimulation of HIF-1α mRNA content by the combination of exercise and HYP yielded high similarity between twin brothers (see **Figure 4**). The effect of HYP to stimulate the exercise-induced increment in HIF-1α mRNA content was about 10-fold more homogeneous within twin pairs than between twin pairs ($p < 0.05$), with an ICC as high as 0.91 ($p < 0.05$). By analogy, the effect of exercise to stimulate HIF-1α in HYP, showed about 8-fold higher similarity within the twin pairs (ICC: 0.89, $p < 0.05$) than between the twins. Significant twin resemblance was also found for the effect of HYP to raise HIF-1α protein (ICC = 0.72, $p = 0.05$, **Figure 2**) and mRNA (ICC = 0.79, $p < 0.05$, **Figure 2**) content in resting

TABLE 1 | MZ twin resemblance for muscle protein and mRNA responses to hypoxia and/or exercise.

	Effect of hypoxia				Effect of exercise			
	Pre-ex NOR vs. pre-ex HYP		Post-ex NOR vs. post-ex HYP		Pre-ex NOR vs. post-ex NOR		Pre-ex HYP vs. post-ex HYP	
	ICC	*F*	ICC	*F*	ICC	*F*	ICC	*F*
HIF-1α PATHWAY								
HIF-1α (protein)	0.72*	2.53*	0.45	0.82	0.23	0.29	0.58	1.37
HIF-1α (mRNA)	0.79*	3.77*	0.91*	9.80*	0.44	0.78	0.89*	8.29*
PHD1	0.46	0.86	0.51	1.03	0.85*	5.50*	0.51	1.04
PHD2	0.63	1.68	0.58	1.38	0.70	2.30	0.48	0.94
pVHL	0.52	1.07	0.74#	2.84#	0.52	1.10	0.83*	4.81*
VEGF-2a	0.79*	3.82*	0.67	2.04	0.49	0.94	0.76#	3.10#
GLYCOLYTIC METABOLISM								
PFK-M	0.60	1.50	0.56	1.29	0.67	2.04	0.61	1.58
PDH-A1	0.62	1.63	0.49	0.95	0.77#	3.30#	0.62	1.65
PDK4	0.77#	3.43#	0.78*	3.56*	0.68	2.08	0.11	0.13
LDH-A	0.72#	2.62#	0.45	0.82	0.46	0.85	0.84*	5.17*
OXIDATIVE METABOLISM								
CS	0.48	0.93	0.58	1.39	0.69	2.18	0.70	2.29
COX-4	0.44	0.80	0.59	1.45	0.55	1.20	0.59	1.42
PGC-1α	0.33	0.50	0.74#	2.89#	0.75#	2.98#	0.82*	4.46*
PPAR- γ1	0.77#	3.37#	0.42	0.73	0.46	0.85	0.78#	3.65#
TFAM	0.64	1.77	0.27	0.37	0.59	1.42	0.53	1.13

ICC's and corresponding F-ratios (between/within pair's variance; n = 11) represent similarity within twin pairs for the hypoxia response either pre or post exercise (ex), or similarity within twin pairs for the exercise response during either NOR or HYP. Individual twin-pair responses for the underscored results are presented in ***Figure 4****. *P < 0.05; #P < 0.10.*

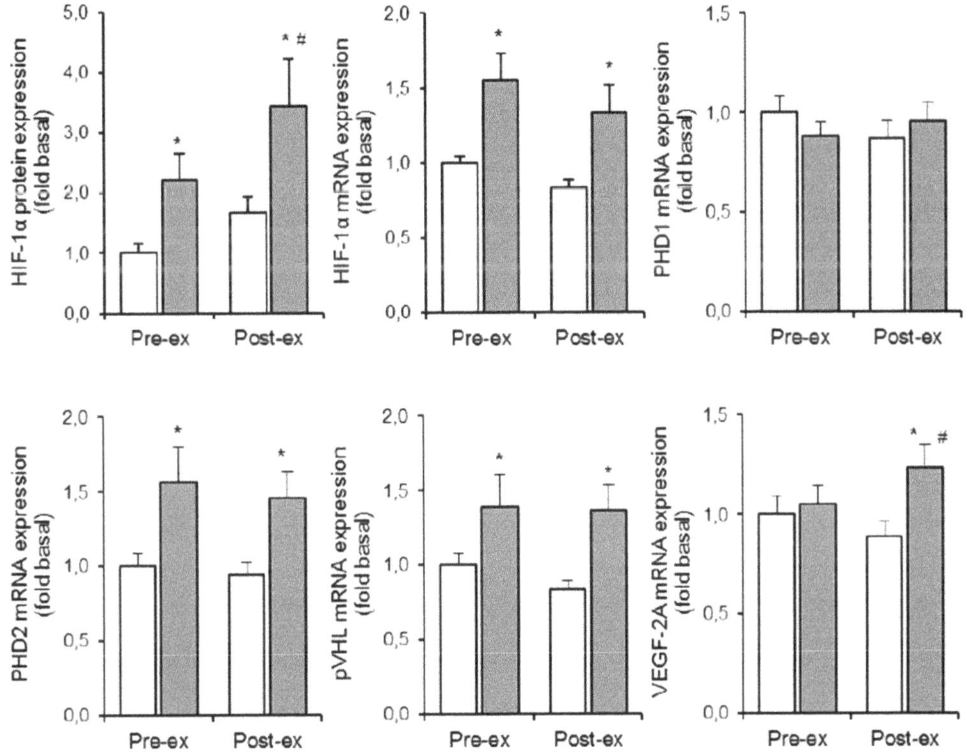

FIGURE 2 | Effect of hypoxia and exercise on the HIF-1α pathway. Data are means ± SEM of 11 twin pairs ($n = 22$) before (pre-ex) and immediately after (post-ex) a 20-min submaximal exercise bout in either normoxia (empty bars) or hypoxia equivalent to ~5300 m altitude (full bars). HIF-1α, hypoxia-inducible factor 1α; PHD1-2, prolyl hydroxylase domains 1-2; pVHL, Von Lippel-Hindau protein; VEGF-2A, vascular endothelial growth factor-2A. See Methods for further details.*$P < 0.05$ vs. NOR #$P < 0.05$ vs. pre-ex.

muscle. However, the effect of exercise, alone or in combination with HYP, to stimulate HIF-1α protein content did not yield significant twin resemblance. Furthermore, the exercise-induced increment of pVHL mRNA content in HYP, but not in NOR, was ~5-fold more similar within twins than between twins (ICC = 0.83, $p < 0.05$).

Glycolytic Metabolism (Table 1 and Figure 5)

Compared to NOR, HYP increased PDK4 mRNA expression ~12-fold both pre and post exercise ($p < 0.05$; **Figure 3**). In the resting condition in HYP, mRNA levels of PFK-M were ~20% higher compared to NOR with no additional effect of exercise ($p < 0.05$; **Figure 3**). Neither LDH-A nor PDH-A1 mRNA expression was affected by either exercise or hypoxia (**Figure 5**).

The HYP-induced increased PDK4 gene expression was ~3.5-fold more similar within twin brothers than between the different twin pairs ($p < 0.05$). Furthermore, exercise in HYP on average did not significantly increase LDH-A mRNA content indeed, yet responses were ~5-fold more similar within twins than between twins. Overall variability in PFK-M mRNA expression on the other hand, was comparable between subjects with no significant twin resemblance.

Oxidative Metabolism (Table 1 and Figure 6)

HYP increased PPAR-γ1 mRNA expression to the same degree (+60%, $p < 0.05$, **Figure 6**) both at rest and during exercise. Pre exercise PGC-1α mRNA levels were identical in NOR and HYP. However, exercise decreased PGC-1α mRNA expression by ~15% in NOR ($p < 0.05$), vs. increased PGC-1α mRNA content by ~15% in HYP ($p < 0.05$, **Figure 4**). TFAM responses to exercise in hypoxia were comparable, which resulted in higher TFAM mRNA content post exercise in HYP compared with NOR ($p < 0.05$, **Figure 4**). Neither exercise nor HYP affected either COX-4 or CS (**Figure 6**) mRNA contents.

The response of PGC-1α mRNA expression to exercise was about 3 to 5-fold more similar within twin pairs than between twin pairs, particularly during exercise in HYP ($p < 0.05$). Conversely, variability of either exercise-induced or hypoxia-induced changes of citrate synthase, COX-4, PPAR-γ, and TFAM mRNA expressions were not significantly different between twins than within twin pairs.

DISCUSSION

In this study we explored the contribution of genetic factors in the myocellular responses of HIF-1α and its downstream targets to acute hypoxia. We exposed monozygotic twin brothers to high altitude (~5300 m) simulated by means of normobaric

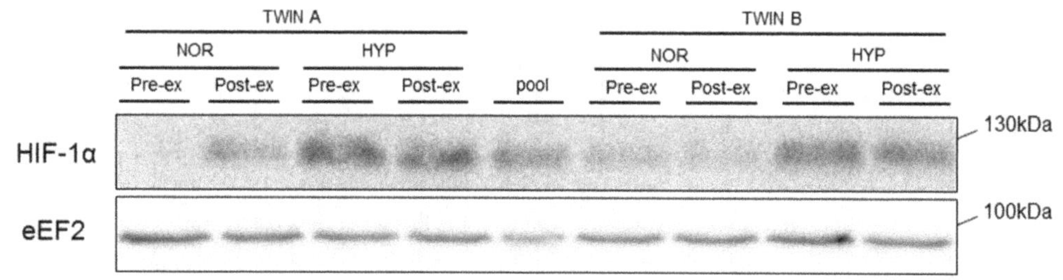

FIGURE 3 | Representative blot of HIF-1α protein. Representative blot of HIF1-α in one monozygotic twin pair before (pre-ex) and immediately after (post-ex) exercise in either normoxia (NOR) or hypoxia (HYP). eEF2 is shown as loading control.

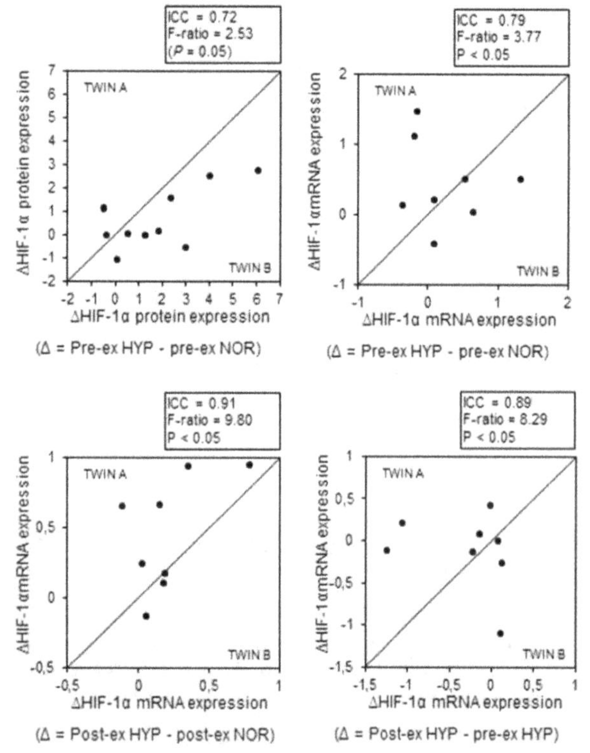

FIGURE 4 | MZ twin resemblance for the effects of hypoxia and exercise on the HIF-1α pathway. Each data point represents the values for one pair of twins (twin A vs. twin B) before (pre-ex) and after (post-ex) a 20-min submaximal exercise bout. Data are hypoxia-induced changes (Δ) and exercise-induced changes for either HIF-1α protein or mRNA expression. Intra-class correlations and corresponding F-ratios (between/within pair's variance) are given in the figure. See Methods for further details.

hypoxia (FIO_2 0.107) and compared the responses with normoxia (FIO_2 20.9%), both at rest and during submaximal exercise. We have previously reported that the current protocol on average decreased VO_2max by ~40% (range: 25–55%), yet with very high twin resemblance (Masschelein et al., 2015b). Furthermore, we also found hypoxia to modulate protein metabolism at rest and after moderate exercise by increasing markers of protein breakdown, more specifically markers of the autophagy-lysosomal system, including a significant genetic contribution for both hypoxia-induced regulation of REDD1 and microtubule-associated protein 1 light chain 3 (LC3) lipidation (Masschelein et al., 2014). Here we postulated that if heritability is an important determinant of myocellular adaptation to hypoxia, then this must translate into genotype-dependent regulation of HIF-1α during an acute hypoxic challenge. In support of such contention, our current data for the first time clearly demonstrate that acute hypoxia, alone or in conjunction with exercise, substantially increased both muscle HIF-1α mRNA and protein content. Moreover, the HIF-1α increments yielded much higher within-twin than between-twin resemblance, indicating significant genotype impact.

Hypoxia-inducible factor-1α (HIF-1α) plays an important role in the acute responses as well as in the long-term cellular adaptations to oxygen deficiency (Stroka et al., 2001). Upon decreasing intracellular PO_2, HIF-1α translocates to the nucleus to dimerize with the constitutively active HIF-1β. The HIF1 complex so formed eventually acts as a transcription factor for a larger number of genes implicated in regulation of muscle energy metabolism and morphology (Zhang et al., 2008; Luo et al., 2011). In tumor cells, ATP production was impaired and HIF-1α-dependent genes were upregulated whenever intracellular PO_2 dropped below ~10 mmHg (Richardson et al., 2006; Flueck, 2009). Conversely, muscle cells appear to be more resistant to oxygen deficit because the rate of ATP production is well maintained even at <10 mmHg intracellular PO_2 values inherent to high-intensity muscle contractions (Richardson et al., 1995, 2006; Favier et al., 2015). Conversely, at the very low rates of ATP turnover existing in resting muscle a net arterial PO_2 drop by at least 30 mmHg is needed to significantly decrease intramyocellular PO_2 (Johnson et al., 2005; Richardson et al., 2006). Accordingly, even at an inspired PO_2 as low as ~75 mmHg corresponding to ~5500 m altitude, muscle PO_2 is maintained at ~20–25 mmHg, which is still manifold higher than during maximal exercise in normoxia (<5 mmHg) (Richardson et al., 1995, 2006). Based on the above observations it has been postulated that passive exposure to a low-oxygen environment cannot elicit HIF stabilization (D'Hulst et al., 2013; Favier et al., 2015). Our current observations clearly contradict such conclusion. We did not measure intracellular PO_2, indeed, yet in line with earlier observations (Richardson et al., 2006; Rissanen et al., 2012; D'Hulst et al., 2013) resting arterial oxygen saturation on average decreased from ~98% in normoxia to

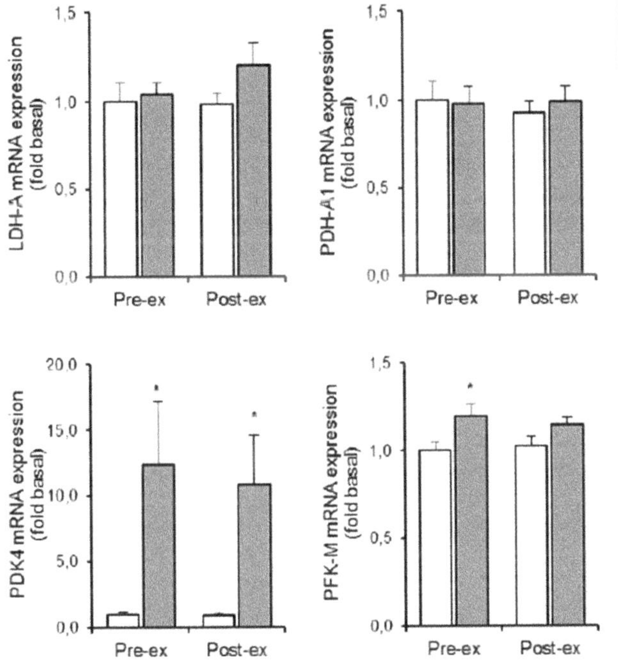

FIGURE 5 | Effect of hypoxia and exercise on glycolytic metabolism. Data are means ± SEM of 11 twin pairs ($n = 22$) before (pre-ex) and immediately after (post-ex) a 20-min submaximal exercise bout in either normoxia (empty bars) or hypoxia equivalent to ~5300 m altitude (full bars). LDH-A, lactate dehydrogenase-A; PDH-A1, pyruvate dehydrogenase-A1; PDK4, pyruvate dehydrogenase kinase-4; PFK-M, phosphofructokinase muscle-type. See Methods for further details. *$P < 0.05$ vs. NOR.

~78% in 0.107 FIO_2 (Masschelein et al., 2015b), which should yield intracellular PO_2 values in the range of ~20–25 mmHg (Richardson et al., 2006). Nonetheless, HIF-1α protein expression on average increased ~ 2-fold and further increased during exercise (20 min @1.2 W/kg; see **Figure 2**). This submaximal exercise alone did not stimulate HIF-1α protein expression. To the best of our knowledge, this is the first experiment documenting HIF-1α stabilization due to ambient hypoxia in healthy humans at rest. It is difficult to explain the discrepancy between our current and previous observations (D'Hulst et al., 2013). However, besides the rate and magnitude of effected intramyocellular PO_2 decrease, also training status (Lindholm et al., 2014) and history of hypoxic exposure conceivably play a role in regulation of HIF-1α stabilization.

We have previously shown by using near-infrared spectroscopy that normobaric hypoxia equivalent to 5300 m decreased muscle tissue oxygenation by no more than ~8% compared to normoxic conditions (Masschelein et al., 2014; Van Thienen and Hespel, 2016). Addition of a submaximal cycling exercise bout similar to the present protocol, decreased oxygenation status by an additional ~12 vs. 5% in normoxia (Masschelein et al., 2014; Van Thienen and Hespel, 2016). These data indicate that the effects of hypoxia and exercise on muscular oxygenation status are additive. Still, tissue oxygenation status measured by near-infrared spectroscopy only partially reflects intramyocellular oxygen tension, which is critical to regulation of HIF-1α. It has been shown that stabilization and expression of HIF-1α is tightly regulated by decreases in intramyocellular PO_2 within the physiological range. Acute exercise reduces myocellular PO_2 to 1/40th of that of inhaled air (PIO_2) while intramyocellular PO_2 values at rest remain at ~1/5th of the PIO_2 (Richardson et al., 1995). In the conditions of the current study, PIO_2 in hypoxia was ~75 mmHg which conceivably made intramyocellular PO_2 to drop below 2 mmHg, which is ample to elicit HIF-1α stabilization (Richardson et al., 1995, 2006; Fong and Takeda, 2008). Indeed, due to the specific value of the Michaelis constant of ~240 μM, the hydroxylase activity of PHD2 is dependent and sensitive to oxygen partial pressures in the range of 0.1–30 mmHg typically occurring in muscle cells at rest and during exercise (Richardson et al., 1995). As the inhibition of PHD2, and thus stabilization of HIF-1α is proportional to the degree of intracellular PO_2 drop (Fong and Takeda, 2008), hypoxia and exercise logically act as additive agents to stimulate HIF-1α protein stabilization and expression via inhibition of PHD2 activity. Furthermore, literature data indicate that HIF-1 is not only regulated by decrease in myocellular PO_2 but also through some humoral factors such as α-ketoglutarate. Plasma α-ketoglutarate concentration increases due to elevated Krebs cycle activity during exercise (Leibowitz et al., 2012). Available evidence indicates that α-ketoglutarate can stabilize HIF-1, probably via inhibition of the PHD2 enzyme (Hou et al., 2014). This provides a mechanism by which exercise *per se*, but not hypoxia, can stimulate HIF-1 activity. Thus, exercise in hypoxia will stimulate HIF-1 activity more than exercise or hypoxia alone, due to Ameln et al. (2005) the synergistic effects of exercise and hypoxia in decreasing myocellular PO_2 and thus activation of PHD2 and (Aragonés et al., 2009) the additional effect of exercise-induced α-ketoglutarate over hypoxia-induced HIF-1 stabilization.

The current hypoxic protocol caused a consistent stimulation of HIF-1α, indeed, yet the responses were highly variable between individuals. Individual changes ranged from −100 to +600% for HIF-1α protein content, vs. no change to +150% for mRNA expression. Interestingly, however, the HIF-1α responses exhibited high twin resemblance. F-ratios indicate that inter-pair variability was about 10-fold greater than intra-pair variability (see **Figure 4**), and hypoxia-induced changes of both muscle HIF-1α protein (ICC = 0.72) and mRNA (ICC = 0.91) contents yielded high MZ twin correlations. In addition, ICCs were substantially higher for the hypoxia effects compared to the exercise effects. This clearly indicates genetic modulation of muscular HIF-1α responses during acute hypoxic stress. Further support for such statement comes from the observation that the hypoxia-induced, but not the exercise-induced changes in mRNA expression of VEGF-2α, a primary downstream target of HIF-1α, were highly similar within twin brothers (ICC = 0.76). In addition, the responses of VEGF-2α were ~3-fold more variable between twin-pairs than within the pairs. In line with published literature data (Ke and Costa, 2006; Fong and Takeda, 2008), we also observed hypoxia-induced stabilization of muscle HIF-1α to be associated with increased mRNA expression of PHD2 and pVHL. However, for these regulators of HIF-1α degradation we

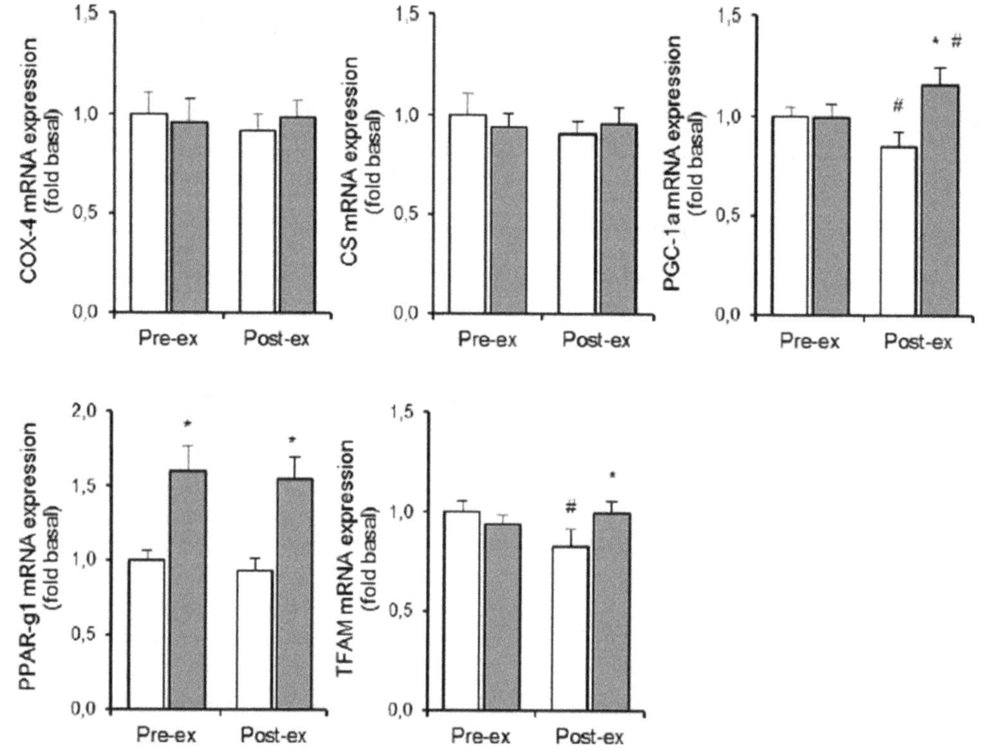

FIGURE 6 | Effect of hypoxia and exercise on oxidative metabolism. Data are means ± SEM of 11 twin pairs ($n = 22$) before (pre-ex) and immediately after (post-ex) a 20-min submaximal exercise bout in either normoxia (empty bars) or hypoxia equivalent to ~5300 m altitude (full bars). COX-4, cytochrome c oxidase-4; CS, citrate synthase; PGC-1A, peroxisome proliferator-activated receptor gamma, coactivator 1A; PPAR-γ1, peroxisome proliferator-activated receptor gamma-1; TFAM, mitochondrial transcription factor-A. See Methods for further details. *$P < 0.05$ vs. NOR #$P < 0.05$ vs. pre-ex.

could not demonstrate genotype-dependence, which may be at least partly explained by predominant regulation of the HIF-1 pathway at the post-transcriptional level (Aragonés et al., 2009; Formenti et al., 2010). The increase in the mRNA expression of PHD2 and pVHL may seem counter intuitive. However, it has been shown before that acute hypoxia selectively increases expression of both PHD2 mRNA and protein levels in rat glioma cells and in cell cultures (Berra et al., 2003; D'Angelo et al., 2003). This hypoxic upregulation of PHD2 probably acts as a negative feedback loop to immediately stop hypoxic and thus HIF-1 responses in cells once they are re-oxygenated again (Berra et al., 2003; D'Angelo et al., 2003).

Long-term acclimatization to altitude/hypoxia a.o. involves metabolic reprogramming yielding higher glycolytic capacity to compensate for reduced rate of oxidative phosphorylation during episodes of explicit O_2-deficiency, e.g., during contractions (Harris et al., 2002). The pyruvate dehydrogenase (PDH) enzyme-complex channels the output of pyruvate units from glycolysis into either acetyl-CoA formation, or into the lactate dehydrogenase reaction to produce ATP via lactate production. PDK4 inhibits muscle PDH activity by phosphorylation (Harris et al., 2002; Kim et al., 2006; Lee et al., 2012). It has been demonstrated that HIF-1α stimulates PDK4 gene transcription via regulation of the estrogen-related nuclear receptor (Lee et al., 2012). We did not measure ERR activation, yet in keeping with the above pathway of PDK4 activation we found hypoxia-induced HIF-1α stabilization to be associated with a substantial increment of muscle PDK4 gene transcription rate (~10-fold increased mRNA content; see **Figure 5**). Assuming that repeated hypoxic exposures eventually will upregulate PDK4 enzyme activity, energy provision via anaerobic glycolysis is likely to be facilitated due to inhibition of PDH-A1 activity. Interestingly, the hypoxia-induced change in PDK4 mRNA expression also exhibited high MZ twin resemblance (ICC= 0.77), indicating that PDK4 also is a site of genotype-dependent regulation of acute hypoxic adaptation. Additional support for upregulation of the glycolytic pathway comes from our observation that hypoxia *per se* also slightly elevated muscle PFK mRNA content.

The PGC-1 family of regulated coactivators plays a pivotal role in the control of mitochondrial biogenesis and respiratory function. PGC-1-induced upregulation of mitochondrial mass increases the capacity for oxygen consumption, which in turn leads to drop of intracellular oxygen availability and stabilization of HIF-1 (O'Hagan et al., 2009). However, such chronic adaptive mechanism is irrelevant during acute hypoxia, which in the conditions of the current study did not even elevated muscle PGC-1α mRNA content. However, PGC-1 activity which is largely regulated by posttranslational modifications which in turn tune the activity of a series of downstream targets, including peroxisome proliferator-activated receptor-γ, which also modulates PDK4 protein expression (Wende et al., 2005). Acute hypoxia here raised PPAR-γ1 mRNA level by ~60% (**Figure 6**), and again changes were highly similar within the MZ twins (ICC = 0.78, F-ratio = 3.65; $p < 0.05$). This finding adds evidence to indicate that genetic background plays a role in upregulation of anaerobic glycolysis via stimulation of the PPAR-γ ~PDK4~PDH pathway in hypoxia.

Because long-term exposure to sever hypoxia decreases mitochondrial volume density in muscle cells (Hoppeler et al., 2003), we also measure some key-enzymes and nuclear transcription factors that are implicated in mitochondrial metabolism and biogenesis. However, 5 h of acute exposure to simulated ~5300 m altitude changed neither CS nor COX-4 mRNA expression, which is in line with published literature (Edwards et al., 2010; Horscroft and Murray, 2014; Murray and Horscroft, 2016). Also muscle mRNA contents of PGC-1 and TFAM were unchanged, and in addition data variability was small. Hence our current set-up does not allow to evaluate the genetic contribution in hypoxia-induced regulation of oxidative metabolism. Moreover, the timing of the muscle biopsies may have been inadequate to detect elevated mRNA expressions for some of the aforementioned variables.

Because of obvious limitations in finding twin pairs eligible to participate in our invasive study, we chose to recruit only monozygotic twins in order to accumulate a significant number of observations within this specific group. Similar monozygotic twin study designs previously were successful to explore genotype~environment interactions in phenotype adaptation (Bouchard et al., 1986, 1990). Nonetheless, because we did not include dizygotic twins in the study design, it is not possible to discriminate here between genetic and shared environmental similarity-inducing factors (Bouchard et al., 1990). For MZ twin resemblance results from both true genetic and shared family environmental effects, at least if both members of the pair were raised/lived together. Therefore, twin resemblances reported here probably reflect the upper-limit of heritability. Nonetheless, one should also recognize that data variability inherent to the muscle biopsy procedure *per se* (Van Thienen et al., 2014) as well as rtPCR and Western Blotting assays, confound the true physiological variabilities within and between twins. Therefore, the physiological significance of some upper-limit heritability coefficients may be even higher than could appear from the numerical statistical output. Accordingly, the absence of statistically significant ICC's and/or F-ratio's does not exclude genotype-dependent regulation. For the average effect-size and concurrent data variability for some variables might have been too small, indeed, to allow pertinent correlational analyses to compare within-twin and between-twin variabilities. This study has shown genotype*exercise and genotype*hypoxia interactions to exist for the HIF-1α pathway as well for its downstream transcriptional targets. Future research should aim to identify specific gene variants using genome-wide association studies.

In conclusion, our study provides novel data to prove that genetic factors play an important role in the muscular responses to acute hypoxic stress at rest and during exercise in young healthy individuals. We for the first time clearly show that regulation of HIF-1α stabilization in acute hypoxia is genotype-dependent. This report therefore contributes to a better understanding of the variation in the integrated response to altitude/hypoxia in humans.

AUTHOR CONTRIBUTIONS

RVT and EM: Conception and design of research, prepared figures and manuscript, edited and revised manuscript, approved final version of manuscript. GD: Analyzed results of experiments, edited and revised manuscript, approved final version of manuscript. MT and PH: Conception and design of research, edited and revised manuscript, approved final version of manuscript.

FUNDING

This study was supported by grant OT/09/033 from the Katholieke Universiteit Leuven.

ACKNOWLEDGMENTS

The authors thank all subjects for participating in this study.

REFERENCES

Ameln, H., Gustafsson, T., Sundberg, C. J., Okamoto, K., Jansson, E., Poellinger, L., et al. (2005). Physiological activation of hypoxia inducible factor-1 in human skeletal muscle. *FASEB J.* 19, 1009–1011. doi: 10.1096/fj.04-2304fje

Aragonés, J., Fraisl, P., Baes, M., and Carmeliet, P. (2009). Oxygen sensors at the crossroad of metabolism. *Cell Metab.* 9, 11–22. doi: 10.1016/j.cmet.2008.10.001

Berra, E., Benizri, E., Ginouvès, A., Volmat, V., Roux, D., and Pouysségur, J. (2003). HIF prolyl-hydroxylase 2 is the key oxygen sensor setting low steady-state levels of HIF-1alpha in normoxia. *EMBO J.* 22, 4082–4090. doi: 10.1093/emboj/cdg392

Bouchard, C., Lesage, R., Lortie, G., Simoneau, J. A., Hamel, P., Boulay, M. R., et al. (1986). Aerobic performance in brothers, dizygotic and monozygotic twins. *Med. Sci. Sports Exerc.* 18, 639–646. doi: 10.1249/00005768-198612000-00006

Bouchard, C., Pérusse, L., and Leblanc, C. (1990). Using MZ twins in experimental research to test for the presence of a genotype-environment interaction effect. *Acta Genet. Med. Gemellol. (Roma).* 39, 85–89. doi: 10.1017/S0001566000005596

Burtscher, M. (2004). Endurance performance of the elderly mountaineer: requirements, limitations, testing, and training. *Wien. Klin. Wochenschr.* 116, 703–714. doi: 10.1007/s00508-004-0258-y

D'Angelo, G., Duplan, E., Boyer, N., Vigne, P., and Frelin, C. (2003). Hypoxia up-regulates prolyl hydroxylase activity: a feedback mechanism that limits HIF-1 responses during reoxygenation. *J. Biol. Chem.* 278, 38183–38187. doi: 10.1074/jbc.M302244200

D'Hulst, G., Jamart, C., Van, T. R., Hespel, P., Francaux, M., and Deldicque, L. (2013). Effect of acute environmental hypoxia on protein metabolism in human skeletal muscle. *Acta Physiol.* 208, 251–264. doi: 10.1111/apha.12086

Deldicque, L., De, B. K., Maris, M., Ramaekers, M., Nielens, H., Francaux, M., et al. (2010). Increased p70s6k phosphorylation during intake of a protein-carbohydrate drink following resistance exercise in the fasted state. *Eur. J. Appl. Physiol.* 108, 791–800. doi: 10.1007/s00421-009-1289-x

Deldicque, L., and Francaux, M. (2013). Acute vs. chronic hypoxia: what are the consequences for skeletal muscle mass? *Cell. Mol. Exerc. Physiol.* 2:e5. doi: 10.7457/cmep.v2i1.e5

Edwards, L. M., Murray, A. J., Tyler, D. J., Kemp, G. J., Holloway, C. J., Robbins, P. A., et al. (2010). The effect of high-altitude on human skeletal muscle energetics: P-MRS results from the Caudwell Xtreme Everest expedition. *PLoS ONE* 5:e10681. doi: 10.1371/journal.pone.0010681

Favier, F. B., Britto, F. A., Freyssenet, D. G., Bigard, X. A., and Benoit, H. (2015). HIF-1-driven skeletal muscle adaptations to chronic hypoxia: molecular insights into muscle physiology. *Cell. Mol. Life Sci.* 72, 4681–4696. doi: 10.1007/s00018-015-2025-9

Flueck, M. (2009). Plasticity of the muscle proteome to exercise at altitude. *High Alt. Med. Biol.* 10, 183–193. doi: 10.1089/ham.2008.1104

Fong, G. H., and Takeda, K. (2008). Role and regulation of prolyl hydroxylase domain proteins. *Cell Death Differ.* 15, 635–641. doi: 10.1038/cdd.2008.10

Formenti, F., Constantin-Teodosiu, D., Emmanuel, Y., Cheeseman, J., Dorrington, K. L., Edwards, L. M., et al. (2010). Regulation of human metabolism by hypoxia-inducible factor. *Proc. Natl. Acad. Sci. U.S.A.* 107, 12722–12727. doi: 10.1073/pnas.1002339107

Harris, R. A., Bowker-Kinley, M. M., Huang, B., and Wu, P. (2002). Regulation of the activity of the pyruvate dehydrogenase complex. *Adv. Enzyme Regul.* 42, 249–259. doi: 10.1016/S0065-2571(01)00061-9

Hennis, P. J., O'Doherty, A. F., Levett, D. Z., Grocott, M. P., and Montgomery, H. M. (2015). Genetic factors associated with exercise performance in atmospheric hypoxia. *Sports Med.* 45, 745–761. doi: 10.1007/s40279-015-0309-8

Hoppeler, H., Klossner, S., and Vogt, M. (2008). Training in hypoxia and its effects on skeletal muscle tissue. *Scand. J. Med. Sci. Sports* 18(Suppl. 1), 38–49. doi: 10.1111/j.1600-0838.2008.00831.x

Hoppeler, H., and Vogt, M. (2001). Muscle tissue adaptations to hypoxia. *J. Exp. Biol.* 204, 3133–3139.

Hoppeler, H., Vogt, M., Weibel, E. R., and Flück, M. (2003). Response of skeletal muscle mitochondria to hypoxia. *Exp. Physiol.* 88, 109–119. doi: 10.1113/eph8802513

Horscroft, J. A., and Murray, A. J. (2014). Skeletal muscle energy metabolism in environmental hypoxia: climbing towards consensus. *Extrem. Physiol. Med.* 3:19. doi: 10.1186/2046-7648-3-19

Hou, P., Kuo, C. Y., Cheng, C. T., Liou, J. P., Ann, D. K., and Chen, Q. (2014). Intermediary metabolite precursor dimethyl-2-ketoglutarate stabilizes hypoxia-inducible factor-1alpha by inhibiting prolyl-4-hydroxylase PHD2. *PLoS ONE* 9:e113865. doi: 10.1371/journal.pone.0113865

Jamart, C., Raymackers, J. M., Li, A. G., Deldicque, L., and Francaux, M. (2011). Prevention of muscle disuse atrophy by MG132 proteasome inhibitor. *Muscle Nerve* 43, 708–716. doi: 10.1002/mus.21949

Johnson, P. C., Vandegriff, K., Tsai, A. G., and Intaglietta, M. (2005). Effect of acute hypoxia on microcirculatory and tissue oxygen levels in rat cremaster muscle. *J. Appl. Physiol.* 98, 1177–1184. doi: 10.1152/japplphysiol.00591.2004

Ke, Q., and Costa, M. (2006). Hypoxia-inducible factor-1 (HIF-1). *Mol. Pharmacol.* 70, 1469–1480. doi: 10.1124/mol.106.027029

Kim, J. W., Tchernyshyov, I., Semenza, G. L., and Dang, C. V. (2006). HIF-1-mediated expression of pyruvate dehydrogenase kinase: a metabolic switch required for cellular adaptation to hypoxia. *Cell Metab.* 3, 177–185. doi: 10.1016/j.cmet.2006.02.002

Lee, J. H., Kim, E. J., Kim, D. K., Lee, J. M., Park, S. B., Lee, I. K., et al. (2012). Hypoxia induces PDK4 gene expression through induction of the orphan nuclear receptor ERRγ. *PLoS ONE* 7:e46324. doi: 10.1371/journal.pone.0046324

Leibowitz, A., Klin, Y., Gruenbaum, B. F., Gruenbaum, S. E., Kuts, R., Dubilet, M., et al. (2012). Effects of strong physical exercise on blood glutamate and its metabolite 2-ketoglutarate levels in healthy volunteers. *Acta Neurobiol. Exp. (Wars).* 72, 385–396.

Lindholm, M. E., Fischer, H., Poellinger, L., Johnson, R. S., Gustafsson, T., Sundberg, C. J., et al. (2014). Negative regulation of HIF in skeletal muscle of elite endurance athletes: a tentative mechanism promoting oxidative metabolism. *Am. J. Physiol. Regul. Integr. Comp. Physiol.* 307, R248–R255. doi: 10.1152/ajpregu.00036.2013

Luo, W., Hu, H., Chang, R., Zhong, J., Knabel, M., O'Meally, R., et al. (2011). Pyruvate kinase M2 is a PHD3-stimulated coactivator for hypoxia-inducible factor 1. *Cell* 145, 732–744. doi: 10.1016/j.cell.2011.03.054

Mason, S., and Johnson, R. S. (2007). The role of HIF-1 in hypoxic response in the skeletal muscle. *Adv. Exp. Med. Biol.* 618, 229–244. doi: 10.1007/978-0-387-75434-5_18

Masschelein, E., Puype, J., Broos, S., Van Thienen, R., Deldicque, L., Lambrechts, D., et al. (2015a). A genetic predisposition score associates with reduced aerobic capacity in response to acute normobaric hypoxia in lowlanders. *High Alt. Med. Biol.* 16, 34–42. doi: 10.1089/ham.2014.1083

Masschelein, E., Van Thienen, R., D'Hulst, G., Hespel, P., Thomis, M., and Deldicque, L. (2014). Acute environmental hypoxia induces LC3 lipidation in a genotype-dependent manner. *FASEB J.* 28, 1022–1034. doi: 10.1096/fj.13-239863

Masschelein, E., Van Thienen, R., Thomis, M., and Hespel, P. (2015b). High twin resemblance for sensitivity to hypoxia. *Med. Sci. Sports Exerc.* 47, 74–81. doi: 10.1249/MSS.0000000000000386

Montgomery, H. E., Marshall, R., Hemingway, H., Myerson, S., Clarkson, P., Dollery, C., et al. (1998). Human gene for physical performance. *Nature* 393, 221–222. doi: 10.1038/30374

Murray, A. J. (2009). Metabolic adaptation of skeletal muscle to high altitude hypoxia: how new technologies could resolve the controversies. *Genome Med.* 1:117. doi: 10.1186/gm117

Murray, A. J., and Horscroft, J. A. (2016). Mitochondrial function at extreme high altitude. *J. Physiol.* 594, 1137–1149. doi: 10.1113/JP270079

O'Hagan, K. A., Cocchiglia, S., Zhdanov, A. V., Tambuwala, M. M., Cummins, E. P., Monfared, M., et al. (2009). PGC-1α is coupled to HIF-1α-dependent gene expression by increasing mitochondrial oxygen consumption in skeletal muscle cells. *Proc. Natl. Acad. Sci. U.S.A.* 106, 2188–2193. doi: 10.1073/pnas.0808801106

Papandreou, I., Cairns, R. A., Fontana, L., Lim, A. L., and Denko, N. C. (2006). HIF-1 mediates adaptation to hypoxia by actively downregulating mitochondrial oxygen consumption. *Cell Metab.* 3, 187–197. doi: 10.1016/j.cmet.2006.01.012

Petousi, N., and Robbins, P. A. (2014). Human adaptation to the hypoxia of high altitude: the Tibetan paradigm from the pregenomic to the postgenomic era. *J. Appl. Physiol.* 116, 875–884. doi: 10.1152/japplphysiol.00605.2013

Richardson, R. S., Duteil, S., Wary, C., Wray, D. W., Hoff, J., and Carlier, P. G. (2006). Human skeletal muscle intracellular oxygenation: the impact of ambient oxygen availability. *J. Physiol.* 571, 415–424. doi: 10.1113/jphysiol.2005.102327

Richardson, R. S., Noyszewski, E. A., Kendrick, K. F., Leigh, J. S., and Wagner, P. D. (1995). Myoglobin O2 desaturation during exercise. Evidence of limited O2 transport. *J. Clin. Invest.* 96, 1916–1926. doi: 10.1172/JCI118237

Rissanen, A. P., Tikkanen, H. O., Koponen, A. S., Aho, J. M., Hägglund, H., Lindholm, H., et al. (2012). Alveolar gas exchange and tissue oxygenation during incremental treadmill exercise, and their associations with blood O_2 carrying capacity. *Front. Physiol.* 3:265. doi: 10.3389/fphys.2012.00265

Simonson, T. S., Yang, Y., Huff, C. D., Yun, H., Qin, G., Witherspoon, D. J., et al. (2010). Genetic evidence for high-altitude adaptation in Tibet. *Science* 329, 72–75. doi: 10.1126/science.1189406

Stroka, D. M., Burkhardt, T., Desbaillets, I., Wenger, R. H., Neil, D. A., Bauer, C., et al. (2001). HIF-1 is expressed in normoxic tissue and displays an organ-specific regulation under systemic hypoxia. *FASEB J.* 15, 2445–2453.

Van Thienen, R., D'Hulst, G., Deldicque, L., and Hespel, P. (2014). Biochemical artifacts in experiments involving repeated biopsies in the same muscle. *Physiol. Rep.* 2:e00286. doi: 10.14814/phy2.286

Van Thienen, R., and Hespel, P. (2016). Enhanced muscular oxygen extraction in athletes exaggerates hypoxemia during exercise in hypoxia. *J. Appl. Physiol.* 120, 351–361. doi: 10.1152/japplphysiol.00210.2015

Vandesompele, J., De, P. K., Pattyn, F., Poppe, B., Van, R. N., De, P. A., et al. (2002). Accurate normalization of real-time quantitative RT-PCR data by geometric averaging of multiple internal control genes. *Genome Biol.* 3:RESEARCH0034.

Vincent, B., Windelinckx, A., Nielens, H., Ramaekers, M., Van Leemputte, M., Hespel, P., et al. (2010). Protective role of alpha-actinin-3 in the response to an acute eccentric exercise bout. *J. Appl. Physiol.* 109, 564–573. doi: 10.1152/japplphysiol.01007.2009

Vogt, M., Puntschart, A., Geiser, J., Zuleger, C., Billeter, R., and Hoppeler, H. (2001). Molecular adaptations in human skeletal muscle to endurance training under simulated hypoxic conditions. *J. Appl. Physiol.* 91, 173–182.

Wende, A. R., Huss, J. M., Schaeffer, P. J., Giguère, V., and Kelly, D. P. (2005). PGC-1α coactivates PDK4 gene expression via the orphan nuclear receptor ERRα: a mechanism for transcriptional control of muscle glucose metabolism. *Mol. Cell. Biol.* 25, 10684–10694. doi: 10.1128/MCB.25.24.10684-10694.2005

Yi, X., Liang, Y., Huerta-Sanchez, E., Jin, X., Cuo, Z. X., Pool, J. E., et al. (2010). Sequencing of 50 human exomes reveals adaptation to high altitude. *Science* 329, 75–78. doi: 10.1126/science.1190371

Zhang, H., Bosch-Marce, M., Shimoda, L. A., Tan, Y. S., Baek, J. H., Wesley, J. B., et al. (2008). Mitochondrial autophagy is an HIF-1-dependent adaptive metabolic response to hypoxia. *J. Biol. Chem.* 283, 10892–10903. doi: 10.1074/jbc.M800102200

Zoll, J., Ponsot, E., Dufour, S., Doutreleau, S., Ventura-Clapier, R., Vogt, M., et al. (2006). Exercise training in normobaric hypoxia in endurance runners. III. Muscular adjustments of selected gene transcripts. *J. Appl. Physiol.* 100, 1258–1266. doi: 10.1152/japplphysiol.00359.2005

17

Divergent Mitochondrial Antioxidant Activities and Lung Alveolar Architecture in the Lungs of Rats and Mice at High Altitude

*Alexandra Jochmans-Lemoine[1], Susana Revollo[1], Gabriella Villalpando[2], Ibana Valverde[2], Marcelino Gonzales[2], Sofien Laouafa[1,3], Jorge Soliz[1] and Vincent Joseph[1]**

[1] Centre de Recherche de l'Institut Universitaire de Cardiologie et de Pneumologie de Québec, Université Laval, Quebec City, QC, Canada, [2] Instituto Boliviano de Biologia de Altura, Universidad Mayor de San Andrés, La Paz, Bolivia, [3] Centre National de la Recherche Scientifique, UMR 5023, Université Claude Bernard Lyon 1, Villeurbanne, France

***Correspondence:**
Vincent Joseph
vincent.joseph@fmed.ulaval.ca

Compared with mice, adult rats living at 3,600 m above sea level (SL—La Paz, Bolivia) have high hematocrit, signs of pulmonary hypertension, and low lung volume with reduced alveolar surface area. This phenotype is associated with chronic mountain sickness in humans living at high altitude (HA). We tested the hypothesis that this phenotype is associated with impaired gas exchange and oxidative stress in the lungs. We used rats and mice (3 months old) living at HA (La Paz) and SL (Quebec City, Canada) to measure arterial oxygen saturation under graded levels of hypoxia (by pulse oximetry), the alveolar surface area in lung slices and the activity of pro- (NADPH and xanthine oxidases—NOX and XO) and anti- (superoxide dismutase, and glutathione peroxidase—SOD and GPx) oxidant enzymes in cytosolic and mitochondrial lung protein extracts. HA rats have a lower arterial oxygen saturation and reduced alveolar surface area compared to HA mice and SL rats. Enzymatic activities (NOX, XO, SOD, and GPx) in the cytosol were similar between HA and SL animals, but SOD and GPx activities in the mitochondria were 2–3 times higher in HA vs. SL rats, and only marginally higher in HA mice vs. SL mice. Furthermore, the maximum activity of cytochrome oxidase-c (COX) measured in mitochondrial lung extracts was also 2 times higher in HA rats compared with SL rats, while there was only a small increase in HA mice vs. SL mice. Interestingly, compared with SL controls, alterations in lung morphology are not observed for young rats at HA (15 days after birth), and enzymatic activities are only slightly altered. These results suggest that rats living at HA have a gradual reduction of their alveolar surface area beyond the postnatal period. We can speculate that the elevation of SOD, GPx, and COX activities in the lung mitochondria are not sufficient to compensate for oxidative stress, leading to damage of the lung tissue in rats.

Keywords: oxidative stress, mitochondria, high altitude, lung, postnatal hypoxia

INTRODUCTION

Mammals living at high altitude (HA) can deploy several strategies to counteract ambient hypoxia, and it is noteworthy that different types of genetic adaptations or physiological acclimatization to low ambient O_2 can be observed. Several studies have focused on rodent (Cheviron et al., 2012; Lau et al., 2017) or lagomorph (Li et al., 2009; Bai et al., 2015) species that are endemic to HA in order to understand the genetic mechanisms and signatures underlying HA adaptation. However, recent migration of lowland native species to HA regions offers unique opportunities to document adaptive strategies that can operate on a much shorter time-frame (Storz et al., 2007; Jochmans-Lemoine et al., 2016). Striking examples of this are found in the HA regions of South-America, where new animal species such as rats or mice have migrated over the past five centuries, following the European conquests (Guenet and Bonhomme, 2003; Storz et al., 2007). We recently described key differences between rats and mice that have been living in La Paz (Bolivia, 3,600 m above sea level—SL) under laboratory conditions for several generations (Jochmans-Lemoine et al., 2015). While mice maintained low hematocrit, high ventilation, and larger lung volumes, rats had high hematocrit, lower ventilation, signs of severe pulmonary hypertension, and lower arterial oxygen saturations when challenged with high or low levels of inspired O_2. Overall, the phenotype observed in rats is strikingly similar to the pathological features of chronic mountain sickness, a syndrome of de-adaptation to hypoxia with chronic hypoventilation, high hematocrit levels, pulmonary hypertension, and reduced diffusion capacity within the lungs (Julian et al., 2015; Villafuerte and Corante, 2016). We also reported that it was possible to partially revert this phenotype by a simple exposure to an enriched O_2 environment during the first 2-weeks following birth (Lumbroso et al., 2012). HA rats exposed to inspired SL O_2 pressure during postnatal development had lower hematocrit, signs of reduced pulmonary pressure, and lungs with reduced airspaces suggesting improved alveolar development.

The large surface area of the lungs and continuous contact of the lung epithelium with environmental O_2 predispose to oxidative damage (Santus et al., 2014), and oxidative stress in the lung is a potent cause of injury and inflammation (Salama et al., 2014). Furthermore, it is well acknowledged that chronic hypoxia (Turrens, 2003) and HA (Dosek et al., 2007) lead to excessive reactive oxygen species (ROS) production and oxidative stress. A recent study showed that delayed alveolar formation following exposure to postnatal hyperoxia (used as a model of bronchopulmonary dysplasia) is linked to the mitochondrial-dependent generation of ROS (Datta et al., 2015). Accordingly, we performed the present study to assess the hypothesis that the typical low alveolar surface area in the lungs of rats living at HA is associated with impaired gas exchange and oxidative stress in the lungs. We compared arterial oxygen saturation under graded levels of hypoxia, lung histology, and the activity of pro- and anti-oxidant enzymes in homogenized lung tissue from adult rats living at SL or HA. Similar experiments were performed in mice, which represented a control group of animals with successful physiological adaptations to HA. In addition, we tested the hypothesis that altered lung histology and oxidative stress are already present during postnatal development in rats at HA by using newborn rats (2 weeks-old) exposed to HA or SL. Finally, we tested the effects of postnatal hypoxia in rats living at SL, or postnatal O_2 enrichment in rats living at HA during postnatal days 4–14 (P4–P14—the timeframe corresponding to lung alveolar formation in rats—Burri et al., 1974) on arterial oxygen saturation during graded levels of hypoxia, alveolar morphology and oxidative stress balance.

MATERIALS AND METHODS

Animals and Experimental Groups

Animals

This study was carried out in accordance with the recommendations of the Canadian Council of Animal Care. The protocols were approved by the Committee on Animal Care and Use for Laval University in Canada, or by the scientific committee of the Instituto Boliviano de Biologa de Altura (IBBA) in Bolivia. In both countries, animals were housed under standard conditions, had access to food and water ad-libitum, and were exposed to a 12:12 h light/dark cycle.

In Canada

Adult Sprague Dawley male rats and FVB mice around 2 months old were ordered from Charles-Rivers (Charles-River—St-Constant, Québec), and left undisturbed at least for 7 days before being used. Newborn rats were obtained from 8 Sprague Dawley female rats (Charles-River—St-Constant, Québec) that were housed with males for mating for at least 7 consecutive days. Once pregnancy was confirmed by weight gain, the females were isolated in a separate cage. At birth, all litters were culled to 12 pups with an equal number of males and females.

In Bolivia

All rats were obtained from the Instituto Boliviano de Biologia de Altura (IBBA, La Paz, Bolivia, 3,600 m). These are Sprague-Dawley rats that were originally imported from France (IFFA-CREDO) in 1992, and continuously bred at the IBBA. Males and females were left together until pregnancy was confirmed, and at birth all pups were kept alive (litters generally have less than 12 pups). Adult mice were obtained from the Instituto Nacional de Laboratorios de Salud (INLASA, La Paz, Bolivia). These mice are descended from a lineage of animals that were originally imported from France (IFFA-CREDO) 20–25 years ago and have 73.11% homology with the FVB strain, suggesting that they are either a mix of FVB with 2 other strains or an outbred strain (Jochmans-Lemoine et al., 2015).

Exposure to Postnatal Hypoxia in Canada

Four days after birth, animals were placed under normobaric hypoxia in a 50 L plexiglass chamber, connected to an Oxycycler (A84XOV, BioSpherix, Redfield, NY, USA). On the 1st day of exposure, the O_2 level in the chamber was progressively decreased to 13.5% (1% O_2 every 20 min) and kept constant at this level for 10 consecutive days (until postnatal day 14). This corresponds to an inspired PO_2 around 100 mmHg, which is the inspired PO_2 found in La Paz. To avoid humidity and CO_2 accumulation, Drierite (anhydrous calcium sulfate; Hammond Drierite, Xenia, OH, USA) and Amsorb Plus (calcium hydroxide; Armstrong Medical, Coleraine, North Ireland) were placed inside the chamber. Control animals were kept in the same room and left undisturbed (except for normal cage cleaning—once a week).

At postnatal day 14 (P14), the O_2 level inside the chamber was progressively returned to 21% (at the rate of 1% O_2 every 15 min), the animals were sacrificed 24 h later for lung tissue sampling.

Exposure to Postnatal O_2 Enrichment in Bolivia

Four days after birth, animals were placed under hypobaric normoxia in a 50 liter plexiglass chamber or left in ambient room air. The O_2 level was continuously measured in the chamber, and maintained at $\approx$ 32% O_2 (corresponding to an inspired PO_2 of 160 mmHg, the normal SL inspired PO_2) by a continuous flow from a calibrated gas tank. The CO_2 level was controlled twice daily with a dedicated CO_2 sensor and never exceeded 0.3%. The air inside the chamber was continuously mixed with a small fan, and there was no apparent humidity inside the chamber. At P14, the chamber was opened, and the animals were returned to ambient air. These animals were sacrificed 24 h later for lung tissue sampling.

Pulse Oximetry Recordings

Pulse oximetry recordings were performed in sealed chambers (adapted to the size of the animals and constantly flushed with fresh room air). *In Canada*, animals were equipped with a neck collar (Mouse OX® STARR Life Sciences Corp, USA) and *in Bolivia*, animals were equipped with a limb sensor (MouseSTAT—Kent Scientific, Torrington, CT, USA) allowing recordings of pulse oximetry capillary O_2 saturation (SpO_2). We have verified that at SL, the two systems gave similar SpO_2 values under graded hypoxia. Each animal was placed in the chamber for a period of acclimatization (10–15 min), then the inflowing tube was switched to a nitrogen gas line calibrated to obtain the desired O_2%. *In Canada*, animals were subsequently exposed to 18, 15, 12, and 9% O_2, each for 10 min and *in Bolivia*, animals were exposed to 32% O_2-corresponding to the inspired air at SL—followed by 18, 15, 12% O_2 for 10 min each. In the present work, we report values that have been collected under comparable pressures of inspired O_2 at 160 mmHg (SL room and 32% O_2 at HA) and 90 mmHg (12% O_2 at SL and 18% O_2 at HA).

Lung Dissection, Histology, and Morphology

In both countries, we used 2 males from each litter of newborn rats (4 litters per group) and 4 adult males of each species (rats and mice). Animals were deeply anesthetized and perfused through the heart with ice-cold PBS solution. Next, a catheter was fixed in the trachea, the lungs were inflated with 4% PFA for 30 min at a constant pressure of 24 cm H_2O, then the trachea was ligated and the lungs dissected. The total volume of the inflated lungs was measured by liquid displacement. Dissected lungs were kept in 4% PFA for 24 h at room temperature. The next day, the lungs were separated into left and right lungs (for newborn rats and adult mice) or into 5 lobes (for adult rats), which were automatically embedded in paraffin (*in Canada*, using the Tissue-Tek VIP, Miles scientific) or manually (*in Bolivia* as previously described; Jochmans-Lemoine et al., 2015). Twenty-four hours later, the samples were included in paraffin and stored until they were processed for lung histology as previously described (Jochmans-Lemoine et al., 2015). We have verified the two embedding approaches gave similar morphological results on a sample of SL lung for both species. In another 4 newborn male rats and 6 adult rats and mice, the lungs were immediately removed from the chest after the cardiac PBS perfusion, weighed, frozen on dry ice and stored until they were processed to determine enzymatic activity.

Lung Morphology

After deparaffinization and coloration (Hematoxylin), images of each lung section were captured (magnification: x100; see Jochmans-Lemoine et al., 2015, for details). We analyzed 3 slides per animal, and randomly selected 3 non-overlapping images from each slide (we used a total of 4 adult male rats and mice in each group, and 8 P15 male rats in each group). The Mean Linear Intercept (Lm) was determined by overlapping a grid of 20 horizontal and vertical lines (189 μm each) on each image and by counting the number of intersections with alveolar walls (Hsia et al., 2010). When a line crossed a vessel wall rather than an alveolar wall it was counted as 0.5 intersections. Lm was calculated by using the following equation: $Lm = (N.d)/m$, with N being the number of lines (20), d the length of each line (189 μm), and m the number of intersections with alveolar walls. From Lm values, we calculated the relative alveolar surface area as $S\ (m^2/cm^3) = 4\ V/Lm$, with V being the volume of one image (Hsia et al., 2010). An estimation of the total alveolar surface area was calculated as the product of the relative alveolar surface area and lung volume.

To compare lung morphology between adult rats vs. mice, and between P15 rats living at SL vs. HA, we used allometric scaling parameters as previously described (Jochmans-Lemoine et al., 2015), with the corresponding units: lung weight (g/g), lung volume (ml/g), and relative alveolar surface area ($m^2/cm^3/g^{-0.13}$).

Biochemical Analysis

Protein Extraction

Protein was extracted from frozen lungs (50–100 mg) as follows: after homogenization in 1 ml of PBS-EDTA (0.5 mM), the samples were centrifuged for 4 min at 1,500 g and then for 10 min at 12,000 g (all centrifugations at 4°C). Four aliquots (200 μl) of the cytosolic fraction were recovered from the second centrifugation and stored until further analysis. The remaining pellet was homogenized in 1.5 ml of mitochondrial isolation buffer (250 mM sucrose, 1 mM EGTA and 20 mM Tris-base pH 7.3) and centrifuged for 10 min at 1,500 g. We collected the supernatant in a new tube and centrifuged it once more at 9,000 g for 11 min. The supernatant was eliminated and the pellet (containing the mitochondrial protein fraction) homogenized with 300 μl of the mitochondrial isolation buffer and stored at −80°C until further analysis. The concentration of proteins in each fraction was determined using the BCA protein assay kit (ThermoFisher Scientific, catalog #23225) and all subsequent measurements were normalized to protein concentration.

Xanthine Oxidase (XO) Activity

XO activity was assessed in the cytosolic protein fraction using a cocktail containing nitroblue tetrazolium (NTB—2.2 mM in water), Tris-HCl pH 8 (2.8 mM), NaCN 1 mM (to inhibit the degradation of superoxide anions by cytosolic SOD_{Cu-Zn}), and diethylene-triamine-penta-acetic acid (DTPA—1.3 mM in Tris-HCl) combined with a fresh solution of hypoxanthine (500 μM per well in Tris-HCl). Fifty microliter of sample, 200 μl of cocktail and 30 μl of hypoxanthine solution was added to each well, and the plate was gently shaken for 40 min at room temperature. The wavelength absorbance of the complex (formazan blue) formed by NTB and the superoxide anion produced by XO in the sample was read at 560 nm every 5 min for 1 h; XO activity corresponded to the slope of the formation of formazan blue by time.

NADPH Oxidase (NOX) Activity

NOX activity was assessed in the cytosolic protein fraction using the same cocktail solution as XO and a fresh solution of NADPH (1 mM). Twenty microliter of sample, 250 μl of cocktail, and 30 μl (100 μM/well) of NADPH were added to each well, the plate was shaken for 2 min at room temperature and absorbance was read at 560 nm every 50 s for 10 min. NOX activity corresponded to the slope of the formation of formazan blue by time.

Cytosolic and Mitochondrial Superoxide Dismutase (SOD_{Cu-Zn} and SOD_{Mn})

SOD activity was measured in the cytosolic and mitochondrial protein fractions. SOD_{Cu-Zn} activity was determined in the cytosolic protein fraction by the degree of inhibition of the reaction between the reactive O_2 anion superoxide ($O_2\cdot^-$: produced by a hypoxanthine-xanthine oxidase system) and NTB. We used the same cocktail described for XO and NOX activities combined with hypoxanthine (0.19 mM) and prepared a fresh solution of xanthine oxidase (1.02 units/ml). We added 20 μl of sample, 250 μl of cocktail and 20 μl of XO to each well, and mixed the plate for 4–5 s at room temperature. The absorbance was quickly read at 450 nm every 50 s for 5 min. SOD_{Mn} activity was similarly determined in the mitochondrial protein fraction. For this assay, 4 wells containing 20 μl of PBS 1X (rather than samples) were used as blanks, and 1 mM of NaCN was added in all wells to inhibit SOD_{Cu-Zn}. SOD_{Mn} activity corresponded to the difference between the slopes of the formation of formazan blue by time between the blank and each sample.

Glutathione Peroxidase (GPx)

GPx activity was determined in the mitochondrial protein fraction as the rate of oxidation of NADPH to NADP+ in a cocktail solution containing glutathione reductase, NADPH (1.7 mM) and reduced glutathione (1.6 mM in water) using H_2O_2 (0.036% in water) as a substrate (Paglia and Valentine, 1967). We added 20 μl of sample, 200 μl of PBS 1X, 30 μl of cocktail solution and 30 μl of H_2O_2 to each well and mixed the plate for 4–5 s at room temperature. The absorbance was quickly read at 340 nm every 50 s for 5 min. GPx activity was measured as the slope of the NADPH extinction by time.

Cytochrome c Oxidase Assay

Complex IV is the last enzyme of the mitochondrial electron transport chain and catalyzes oxidation of the reduced cytochrome c by O_2. We measured the maximum activity of cytochrome c oxidase (COX—complex IV of the mitochondrial respiratory chain) by measuring O_2 consumption in the mitochondrial protein fraction using a high-resolution respirometer system (Oroboros oxygraph-2k). We used 50–150 μl of sample, with 1 μl of Antimycin A, 5 μl of ascorbate and 5 μl of Tétraméthyl-paraphénylènediamine (TMPD) in 2 ml of mitochondrial respiratory buffer (0.5 mM EGTA, 3 mM $MgCl_2$, 60 mM potassium lactobionate, 10 mM KH_2PO_4, 20 mM Hepes, 110 mM sucrose, 1 g/l BSA). The maximal activity of COX was read when O_2 consumption rate was stable (typically a few minutes after starting the recording).

Statistical Analysis

All values are reported as mean ± s.e.m., and the significant *P*-value was set at 0.05. We used GraphPad Prism 6.0c for all analysis. We analyzed arterial oxygen saturation at 160 mmHg and 90 mmHg, lung morphology and the protein assays using a two-way ANOVA with species and altitude as grouping variables. When significant effects or a significant interaction between species and PiO_2 appeared, a *post-hoc* analysis was performed (Fisher's LSD).

P-values are reported in the figures with the following general pattern: *, **, ***, and **** are used to report $P < 0.05, 0.01, 0.001$, and 0.0001, respectively. Main ANOVA results are reported in the text whereas Ficher's LSD results are found in the figures.

RESULTS

Lung Architecture Is Preserved at HA in Adult Mice but Impaired in Rats

Representative images of lung slices in adult rats and mice living at SL and HA are presented in **Figure 1**, along with the results of the morphometric analysis. Adult mice living at HA have significantly increased (over 3-fold) lung volume compared with their SL counterparts, and this is not observed in rats (*P*-value for altitude <0.0001, *P*-value for altitude x species <0.0001). The mean linear intercept (Lm) was significantly lower in mice living at HA compared with SL and tended to be higher in rats living at HA compared with SL (*P*-value for species x altitude = 0.01—*post-hoc P*-value for altitude in rats = 0.067). Comparisons between HA and SL revealed that rats had a reduced mass-corrected relative alveolar surface area (in $m^2/cm^3/g^{-0.13}$) at HA; but when compared with mice at HA, the mass-corrected relative alveolar surface area was lower in rats (*P*-value for species x altitude = 0.02). These results suggest that the lung morphology of HA rats does not facilitate improved gas exchange.

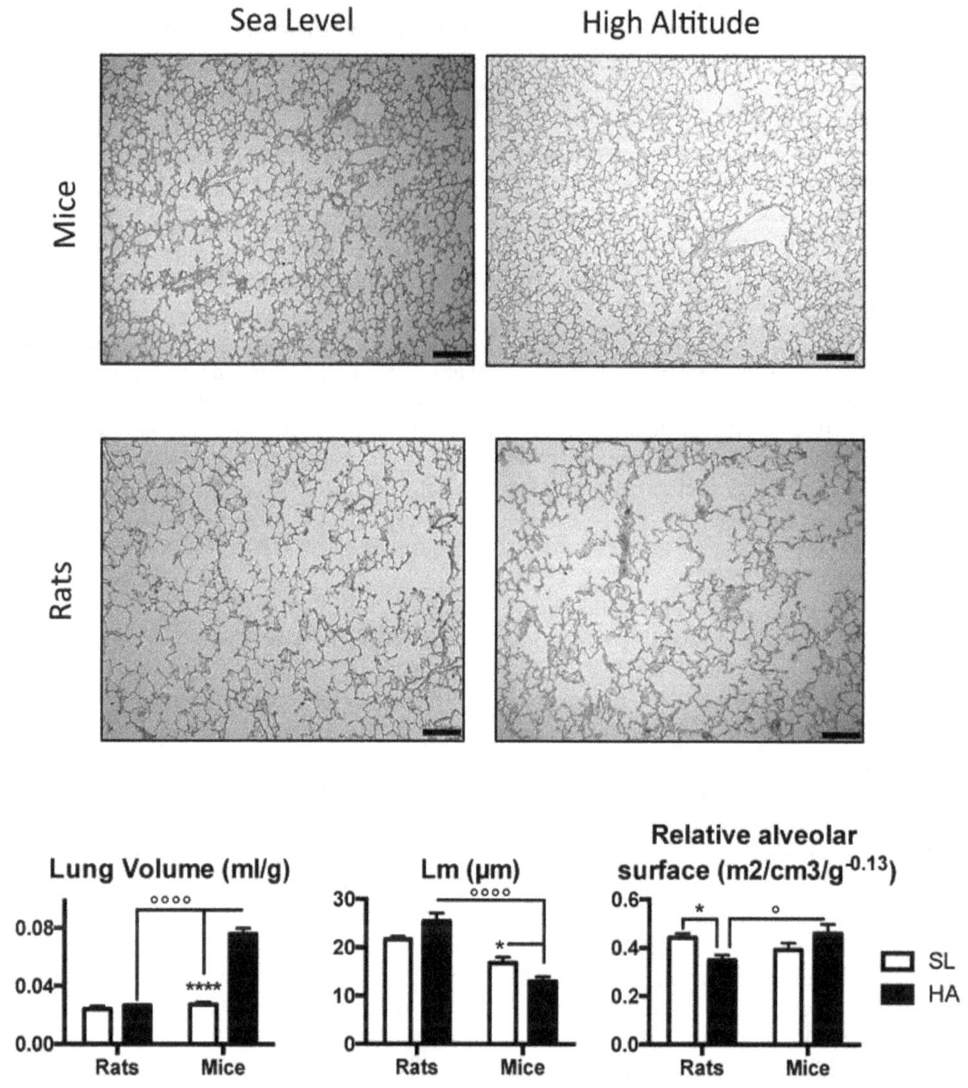

FIGURE 1 | Representative microphotographs showing lung and alveolar structures in adult rats and mice living at sea level (SL—Quebec-city, Canada), and at high altitude (HA—La Paz, Bolivia, 3,600 m). Lower panels show lung volume, mean linear intercept (Lm), and relative alveolar surface in rats and mice at SL and HA. All values are mean + s.e.m. Number of animals in each group: $n = 4$. Scale bars: 50 μm. $^{*}P < 0.05$, and $^{****}P < 0.0001$ HA vs. SL. $^{\circ}P < 0.05$, and $^{\circ\circ\circ\circ}P < 0.0001$ mice vs. rats.

HA Mice Maintain a Higher Arterial Oxygen Saturation in Response to Graded Hypoxia

In rats, SpO_2 was lower at HA than at SL for normoxic O_2 levels (160 mmHg), but was similar between the two altitudes for a PiO_2 of 90 mmHg (**Figure 2**). In mice at HA, SpO_2 was higher than HA rats under PiO_2's of 160 and 90 mmHg. At 90 mmHg, HA mice had a significantly higher SpO_2 than SL mice.

Mitochondrial Antioxidant Activities Are Increased in the Lungs of Adult Rats at HA

The activities of NOX, XO, GPx, and SOD_{Cu-Zn} in the cytosolic protein fraction from the lungs of adult rats and mice are similar between SL and HA (**Figure 3**). In the mitochondrial protein fraction, there was increased SOD_{Mn} and GPx activity (around 2-fold) in HA adult rats compared with SL. The activity of Complex IV of the mitochondrial respiratory chain (or cytochrome c oxidase—COX) was also increased in rats living at HA compared with SL. In mice, the activity of mitochondrial SOD_{Mn} and COX were slightly increased at HA compared with SL. Overall this suggests that important changes in mitochondrial oxidative reactions occur in the lungs of rats living at HA compared with SL control animals, while this does not occur in mice.

The Alveolar Surface Area in Young Rats Is Impaired by Postnatal Hypoxia at SL, but Preserved at HA

Representative images of lung slices along with the results of the morphometric analysis in SL and HA P15 rats exposed to room air, postnatal hypoxia (at SL), or postnatal O_2 enrichment (at HA) are presented in **Figure 4**. At P15, SL rats exposed to

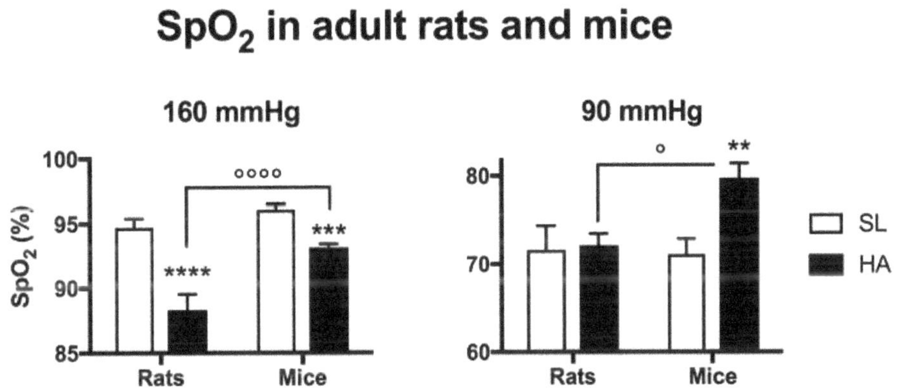

FIGURE 2 | Arterial O_2 saturation recorded in adult rats and mice living at sea level (SL—Quebec-city, Canada), and at high altitude (HA—La Paz, Bolivia, 3,600 m) during exposure to 160 or 90 mmHg. All values are mean + s.e.m. Number of animals in each group at SL: $n = 10$ mice, 6 rats. Number of animals in each group at HA: $n = 9$ mice, 6 rats. $^{**}P < 0.01$, $^{***}P < 0.001$, and $^{****}P < 0.0001$ HA vs. SL. $^{\circ}P < 0.05$, and $^{\circ\circ\circ\circ}P < 0.0001$ mice vs. rats.

postnatal hypoxia have a similar lung volume to control rats, but a higher value of Lm and reduced mass-corrected relative alveolar surface area. At HA, P15 rats have higher lung volumes compared with SL P15 rats, and a similar Lm and alveolar surface area. At HA, postnatal O_2 enrichment reduced Lm and increased the mass-corrected relative alveolar surface area.

Arterial Oxygen Saturation in Young Rats Is Impaired by Postnatal Exposure to Hypoxia at SL

At SL, postnatal exposure to hypoxia significantly reduced SpO_2 in young rats during a PiO_2 of 90 mmHg (**Figure 5**). Interestingly, when young control rats maintained at HA were exposed to 90 mmHg, the observed SpO_2 was lower than for control SL rats, but was higher than SL rats exposed to postnatal hypoxia.

Cytosolic SOD Activity in the Lungs Is Reduced by Postnatal Hypoxia at SL, but Increased by Postnatal O_2 Enrichment at HA

NOX and XO enzymatic activities were lower at HA than at SL (*P*-value for altitude = 0.0003 and 0.038 respectively—**Figure 6**), but there was no effect resulting from exposure to postnatal hypoxia (at SL), or O_2 enrichment (at HA). At SL, exposure to postnatal hypoxia significantly reduced SOD activity, while at HA postnatal O_2 enrichment had the opposite effect (*P*-value for altitude × O_2 level = 0.002). These results suggest reduced production of ROS by NADPH, and greater anti-oxidant capacity by GPx in P15 control HA rats compared with SL controls. In the mitochondrial protein fraction, there was no change in enzyme activities (**Figure 6**) due to postnatal O_2 level or altitude.

DISCUSSION

In the present study, we reported that compared to SL controls, in mice, exposure to HA for several generations led to larger lungs with a higher relative alveolar surface area. The opposite response was observed in rats: at HA, lung volume was not increased compared with SL, and the relative alveolar surface area was reduced. In line with this, mice exposed to low O_2 levels at HA had higher SpO_2 values than rats, but remarkably HA mice also had higher SpO_2 values than SL mice, indicating highly efficient gas exchange functions. Because previous studies demonstrated that chronic hypoxia (Turrens, 2003) and HA (Dosek et al., 2007) lead to excessive ROS production and oxidative stress, a well-known cause of lung injury and inflammation (Salama et al., 2014), we hypothesized that such damage could occur in rats. We measured the activities of pro- and anti-oxidant enzymes in cytosolic and mitochondrial protein extracts in the lungs. Our data showed that HA had no effect on the activity of pro- or anti-oxidant enzymes in the cytosol. However, antioxidant enzyme activities in the mitochondrial protein fraction were about 2 times higher in HA rats compared with SL rats, whereas in mice there was a smaller increase only for the SOD_{Mn} and COX activities (1.25 times higher).

Several studies have shown that postnatal hypoxia reduced lung alveolarization in rats (Blanco et al., 1991; Truog et al., 2008); we thus tested the hypothesis that at HA, young rats (P15) would present early signs of altered lung alveolarization. Surprisingly, this was not the case as our data showed that at HA, young rats had lung volumes, Lm, and relative alveolar surface areas similar to SL young rats. Interestingly, SpO_2 values during a PiO_2 of 90 mmHg were higher in control rats at HA than in SL rats exposed to postnatal hypoxia, therefore indicating more efficient gas exchange function at HA in the former group. Furthermore, our data indicated that O_2 enrichment between postnatal days 4–14 at HA can further increase the alveolar surface area at P15, but this was not associated with improved SpO_2 values. In previous studies, however, we showed that at HA, O_2 enrichment during postnatal development has long-term effects including improved lung alveolar architecture, reduced pulmonary hypertension and lower hematocrit in adult rats (Lumbroso et al., 2012), likely indicating long-term improvement in arterial O_2 saturation. Young rats at HA had lower activity of NADPH and XO (two

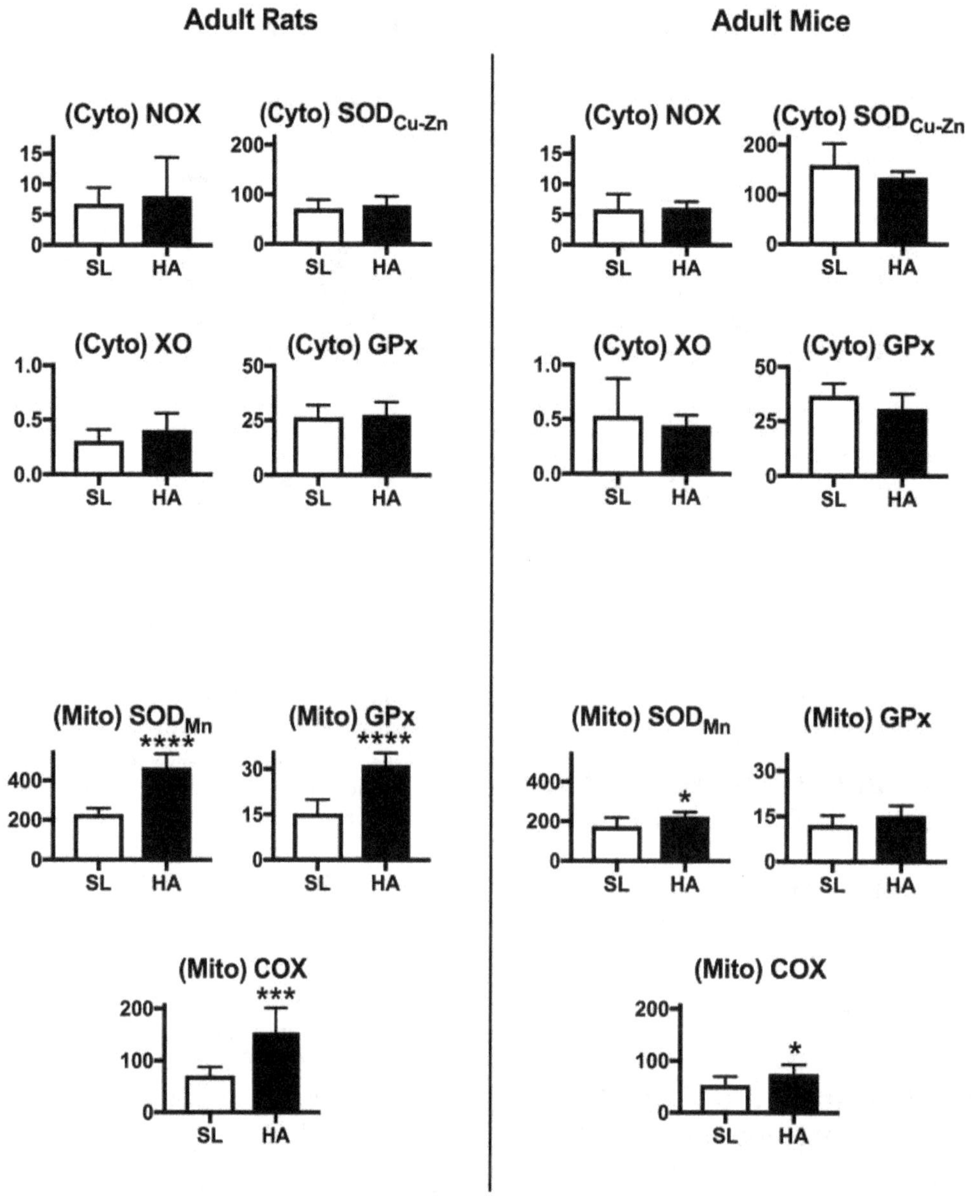

FIGURE 3 | Upper panels: Activity of NADPH oxidase (NOX), xanthine oxidase (XO), copper-zinc superoxide dismutase (SOD_{Cu-Zn}), and glutathione peroxidase (GPx) measured in cytosolic (Cyto) lung extracts. **Lower panels**: Activity of manganese superoxide dismutase (SOD_{Mn}), glutathione peroxidase (GPx), and cytochrome-c oxidase (COX) measured in mitochondrial (Mito) lung extracts in rats and mice living at sea level (SL), or high altitude (HA). All values are mean + s.e.m. Values for NOX, XO, GPx, and SOD are in nmol/min/μg protein, and for COX in pmol O_2/sec/mg protein (see text for further details). Number of animals in each group: SL rats and mice $n = 9$ and 10, HA rats and mice $n = 6$ and 6. $^{*}P < 0.05$, $^{***}P < 0.001$, and $^{****}P < 0.0001$. HA vs. SL.

major sources of cytosolic ROS production) compared with SL rats, while O_2 enrichment during postnatal development increased SOD activity in the cytosol, and hypoxic exposure during the same period at SL had the opposite effect.

Overall, these findings suggest that in adult HA rats, the high activities of SOD, GPx, and COX could be a strategy to buffer excessive mitochondrial ROS production. In contrast, antioxidant enzyme activities are increased in young HA rats, and pro-oxidant enzymes are concurrently decreased as a strategy to maintain ROS equilibrium.

Alterations of Lung Morphology Are Present in Adult Rats at HA Despite High Mitochondrial Anti-oxidant Activity

Hypoxic exposure induces ROS production in the mitochondria (Jezek and Hlavata, 2005), and excessive ROS production induces pro-inflammatory responses and has cytotoxic effects including lipid membrane peroxidation, DNA damage, oxidation of amino acids and oxidative cleavage of peptide bonds in proteins. A previous study showed that iron supplementation induced lung

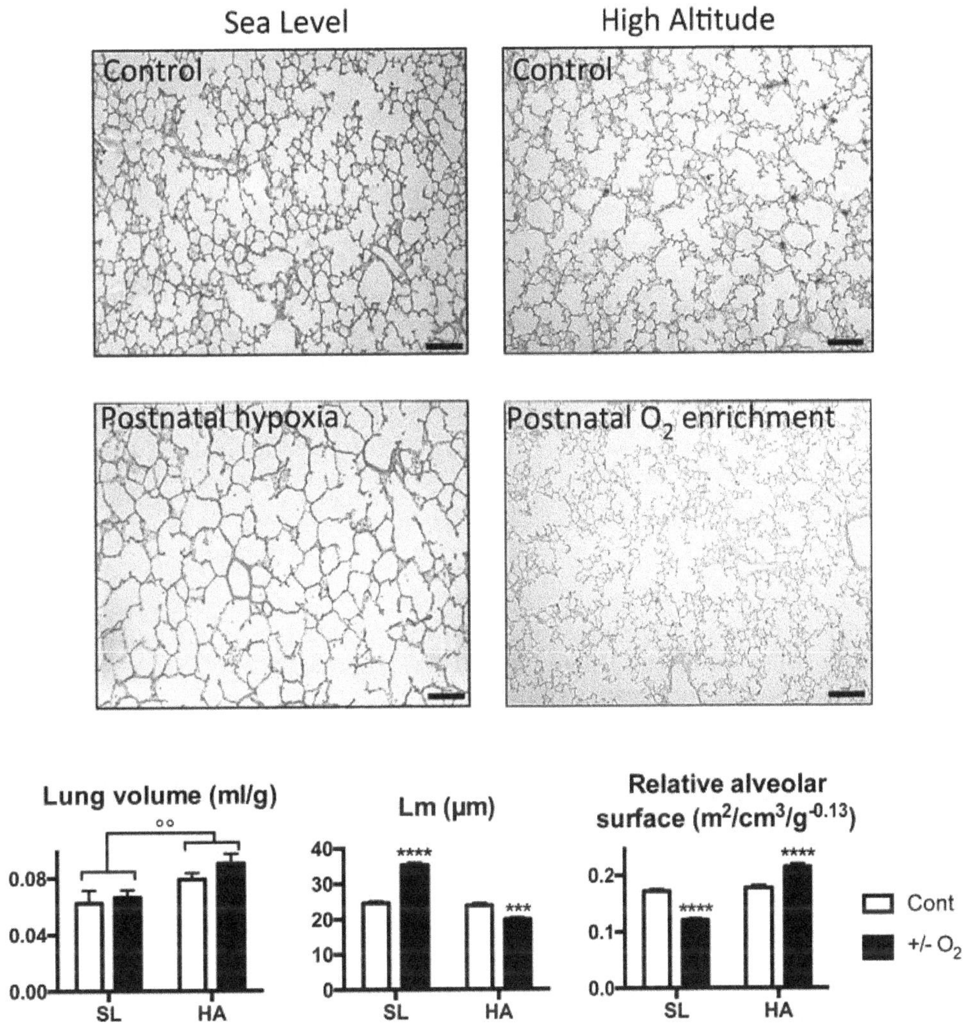

FIGURE 4 | Representative microphotographs showing lung and alveolar structures in young (postnatal day 15) rats living at sea level (SL—Quebec-city, Canada), and at high altitude (HA—La Paz, Bolivia, 3,600 m), following exposure to ambient O_2 level (control), hypoxia (at SL–13.5% O_2), or O_2 enrichment (at HA–32% O_2) between postnatal days 4–14. Lower panels show lung volume, mean linear intercept (Lm), and relative alveolar surface in control (Cont) rats and in rats exposed to hypoxia (at SL), or normoxia (at HA). All values are mean + s.e.m. Number of animals in each group: SL control and hypoxic rats $n = 9$ and 12, HA control and O_2 enriched rats $n = 8$ and 8. Scale bars: 50 µm. $^{***}P < 0.001$, and $^{****}P < 0.0001 \pm O_2$ vs. Cont. $^{\circ\circ}P < 0.01$ HA vs. SL.

injuries in rats at HA through excessive production of ROS and induction of inflammatory responses (Salama et al., 2014). Moreover, a role for oxidative stress has been proposed in the development of chronic obstructive lung diseases (van Eeden and Sin, 2013). Since adult rats at HA had elevated activity of mitochondrial antioxidant enzymes, we can hypothesize that there was elevated ROS production in the mitochondria of lung cells in rats, but not mice. Indeed, even if ROS can be produced in cells by diverse mechanisms and in several compartments, up to 90% are produced at complexes I and III of the electron transfer chain in mitochondria (Adam-Vizi, 2005). Due to the fact that ROS play a key role in lung diseases, it is possible that the elevated anti-oxidant activity we observed in the lungs of rats living at HA is not sufficient to completely protect against oxidative stress, and this could in part explain why HA rats had low alveolar surface areas. Using the same line of evidence, this implies that mice at HA were not subjected to excessive mitochondrial oxidative stress in the lung, and while we cannot infer a direct causal link, it is striking to observe that in parallel mice had increased relative alveolar surface area.

Cytochrome-c oxidase (COX—complex IV of the electron transfer chain) catalyzes the final step of the electron transport chain and the production of H_2O from O_2, thus accounting for mitochondrial O_2 consumption. COX activity is also important for mitochondrial ROS production, and it is well established that low COX activity, which increases mitochondrial ROS production by complexes I and III of the electron transfer chain, is involved in several pathological conditions (Srinivasan and Avadhani, 2012). Our results showed higher maximum COX activity in rats living at HA than at SL, while this effect

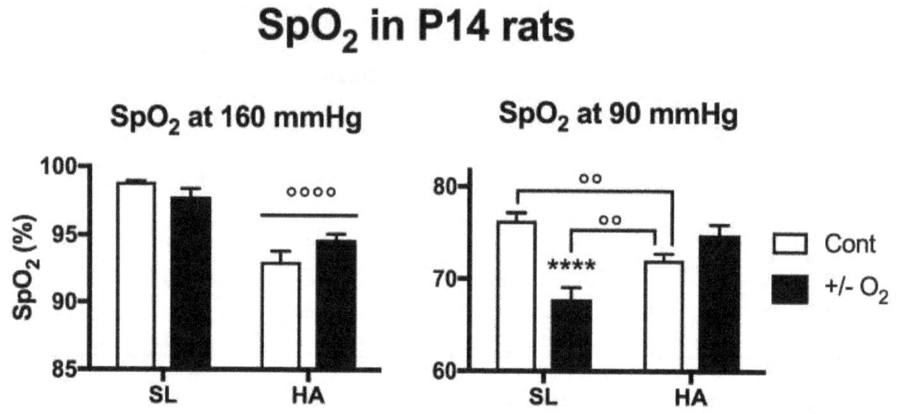

FIGURE 5 | Arterial O_2 saturation recorded in young (postnatal day 14) rats living at sea level (SL—Quebec-city, Canada), and at high altitude (HA—La Paz, Bolivia, 3,600 m), during exposure to ambient O_2 levels (control), hypoxia (at SL−13.5% O_2), or O_2 enrichment (at HA−32% O_2) between postnatal days 4–14. All values are mean + s.e.m. Number of animals in each group at SL: control and hypoxic rats $n = 15$ and 17, and at HA: control and O_2 enriched rats $n = 10$ and 12. ****$P < 0.0001 \pm O_2$ vs. Cont. $^{\circ\circ}P < 0.01$, and $^{\circ\circ\circ\circ}P < 0.0001$ HA vs. SL.

of altitude residence was minimal in mice. This is surprising because acute hypoxic exposure reduces COX activity, directly contributing to increasing ROS production in hypoxia (Prabu et al., 2006; Fukuda et al., 2007; Srinivasan and Avadhani, 2012). In the cardiac myocytes of bar-headed geese (a bird species adapted to flight at extreme altitude), maximum COX activity is reduced, but the affinity of COX for reduced cytochrome-c is higher (Scott et al., 2011). A higher affinity for substrates could ensure higher COX activity at a low or normal concentration of reduced cytochrome-c, thus allowing lower ROS production in the electron transport chain (Scott et al., 2011; Cheviron and Brumfield, 2012). Similarly, increased activity of COX was associated with hypoxia tolerance in Tibetan locusts (Zhang et al., 2013). We can, therefore, hypothesize that in HA rats that have been bred at 3,600 m above SL for 25 years, the increased COX activity could contribute to reduced mitochondrial ROS production, which would be in line with the increased SOD_{Mn} and mitochondrial GPx activities. However, these increased enzymatic activities are apparently not sufficient to buffer the deleterious consequences of oxidative stress, leading to pathological responses such as the altered architecture observed in the lungs of HA rats.

A summary of these findings is presented in **Figure 7**, incorporating a hypothetical mechanism underlying our results. Interestingly, we previously reported that, compared with HA mice, HA rats have lower whole body O_2 consumption and higher glycolytic metabolism as reported by an elevated respiratory exchange ratio (Jochmans-Lemoine et al., 2015). Translated at the cellular level, it is possible to speculate that mitochondrial O_2 consumption and ATP production are lower in HA rats compared with mice. A state of low mitochondrial respiration increases the production of superoxide anion (O_2•-) by complexes I and III of the mitochondrial electron transport chain (Murphy, 2009), and in HA rats this can be partially overcome by the high activities of mitochondrial SOD_{Mn} and GPx that reduce O_2•- to H_2O_2 and water. High levels of H_2O_2, however, would lead to the production of hydroxyl radicals (HO•) through the Fenton reaction (Thomas et al., 2009), and this highly reactive ROS could interact with biomolecules to cause oxidative damage (Halliwell, 2001). As alveolar lung morphology is altered in rats at HA, we hypothesize that the elevated antioxidant activity is not sufficient to abolish oxidative stress.

Alteration of Lung Morphology and Elevated Mitochondrial Anti-oxidant Activity Are Not Present in Young Rats at HA

The fact that HA rats at P15 had a similar Lm and relative alveolar surface area as SL rats was a surprising finding, and was in contrast with the effect of postnatal hypoxia in rats at SL that induced a delay in alveolar formation (the latter results being in line with previous data; Blanco et al., 1991; Truog et al., 2008). In addition, when young rats were exposed to low O_2, SpO_2 was higher in HA rats than in SL rats that had been exposed to postnatal hypoxia. Therefore, our results suggest that young HA rats were able to acquire mechanisms to maintain alveolar development in the lungs similar to that of SL rats, and this might have beneficial long-term effects. Indeed, we reported that exposure of HA rats to SL O_2 levels between postnatal days 4–14 induces a persistent increase in alveolar surface area for adults (Lumbroso et al., 2012), and we have unpublished observations indicating that the alterations induced by postnatal hypoxia at SL persist in adult rats.

We previously reported that the physiological responses observed in rats at HA could be correlated with symptoms reported in chronic mountain sickness (Lumbroso et al., 2012; Jochmans-Lemoine et al., 2015). Interestingly, it has been suggested that chronic mountain sickness is linked to altered perinatal oxygenation (Moore et al., 2007; Julian et al., 2015), and that excessive erythrocytosis (a preclinical state of

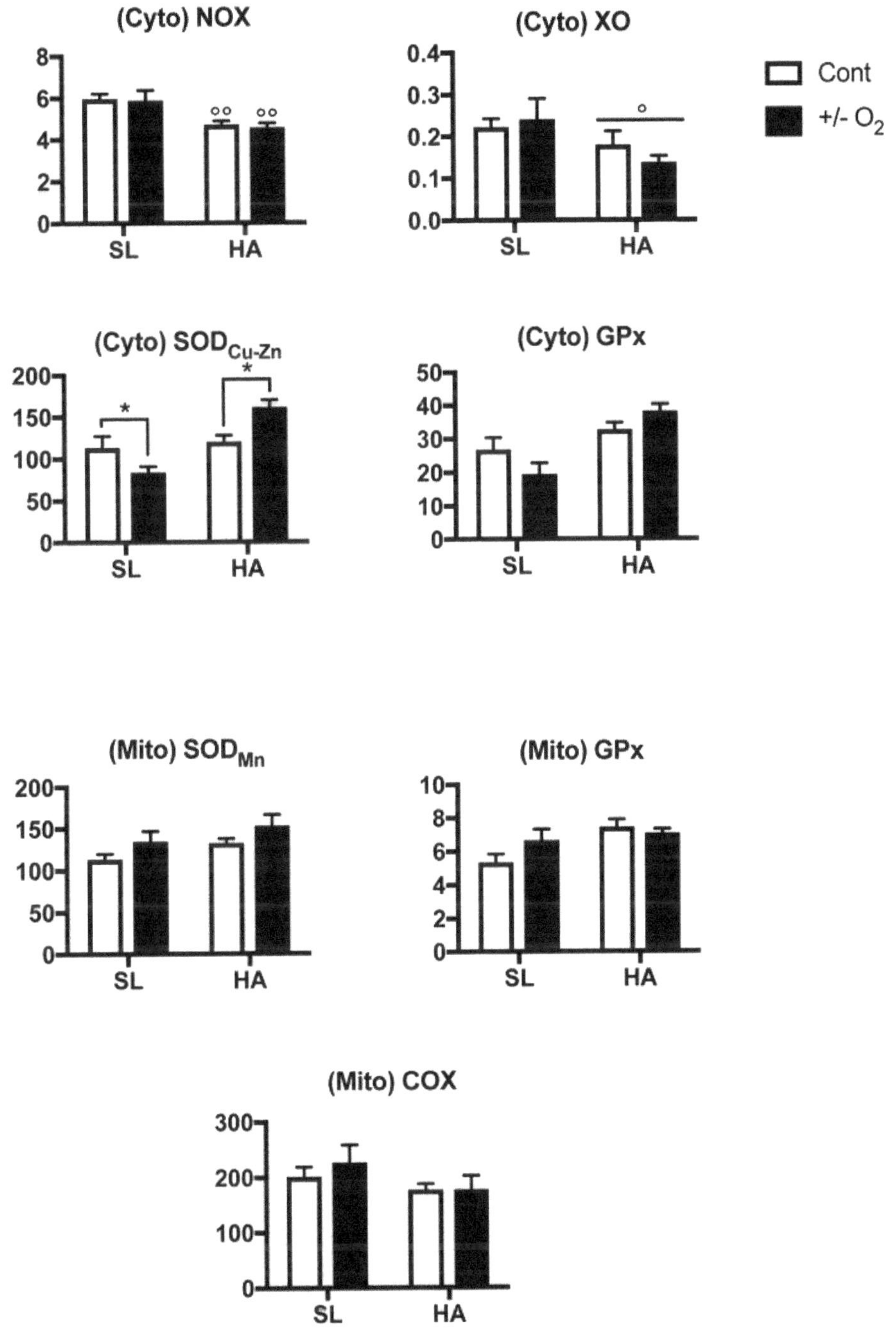

FIGURE 6 | Upper panels: Activity of NADPH oxidase (NOX), xanthine oxidase (XO), copper-zinc superoxide dismutase (SOD_{Cu-Zn}), and glutathione peroxidase (GPx) measured in cytosolic (Cyto) lung extracts. **Lower panels**: Activity of manganese superoxide dismutase (SOD_{Mn}), glutathione peroxidase (GPx), and cytochrome-c oxidase (COX) measured in mitochondrial (Mito) lung extracts in young (postnatal day 15) rats living at sea level (SL—Quebec-city, Canada), and at high altitude (HA—La Paz, Bolivia, 3,600 m), following exposure to ambient O_2 level (control), hypoxia (at SL—13.5% O_2), or O_2 enrichment (at HA—32% O_2) between postnatal days 4–14. All values are mean + s.e.m. Values for NOX, XO, GPx, and SOD are in nmol/min/μg protein, and for COX in pmol O_2/sec/mg protein (see text for further details). Number of animals in each group at SL: control and hypoxic rats $n = 9$ and 8, and at HA: control and O_2 enrichment rats $n = 8$ and 6. $^*P < 0.05$ ± O_2 vs. Cont. $^{\circ}P < 0.05$, and $^{\circ\circ}P < 0.01$ HA vs. SL.

chronic mountain sickness) at HA is associated with elevated oxidative stress (Julian et al., 2013). Contrasting with the results for adult rats, in young HA rats the cytosolic activity of the pro-oxidant enzymes (NOX and XO) is decreased compared with SL rats. These findings are interesting, because chronic pulmonary hypertension in newborn rats exposed to

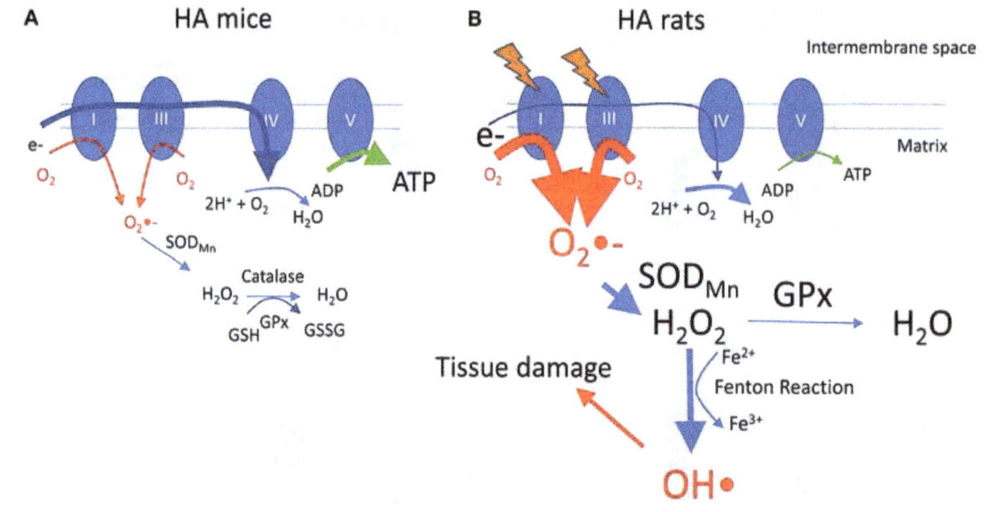

FIGURE 7 | Hypothetical model showing differences between adult rats and mice at HA. In mice **(A)**, the transfer of electrons in mitochondrial complexes is normal (for clarity electron supply is shown only at complex I through oxidation of NADH), resulting in normal production of superoxide ($O_2\bullet$-), that can be reduced first to hydrogen peroxide (H_2O_2) and then to water by SOD_{Mn} and GPx. In rats **(B)**, exposure to HA alters mitochondrial functions and reduces the activity of complexes I and/or III, leading to a reduced flow of electrons that then become available to generate $O_2\bullet$-. High activity of mitochondrial SOD and GPx helps to reduce $O_2\bullet$- to H_2O_2 and water, but high levels of H_2O_2 leads to accumulation of hydroxyl radicals (OH•) through the Fenton reaction. OH•, being a highly reactive ROS, causes accumulation of oxidative damage in the lung tissue, altering the alveolar architecture. High activity of complex IV might contribute to accelerate electron transfer and avoid superoxide accumulation. See text for references.

hypoxia has been associated with ROS generated by xanthine oxidase in the lungs (Jankov et al., 2008). Furthermore, in a study where young mice were exposed to hyperoxia for 72 h between postnatal days 0–3, developmental defects in the lungs were observed at P15 and linked to an exaggerated mitochondrial oxidative stress response and amplification of ROS signaling via NOX-1 (a member of the NOX family of NADPH oxidases; Bedard and Krause, 2007) activity (Datta et al., 2015). Thus, it might be possible that the reduced activity of NOX is in part responsible for the maintenance of lung architecture observed in HA young rats compared with those at SL.

Study Limitations

One of the potential limitations of these studies is the particular nature of the HA species and the fact that they have been genetically isolated for several generations. Aside from the overwhelming influence of constant hypoxic exposure, we cannot completely rule out that these animals have been subjected to genetic drift resulting in a specific phenotype. However, because Charles-River maintains a program to avoid genetic drift between their different stocks of SD rats, we can assume that the original breeders of the HA population and the SD rats used in Quebec are similar. A second limitation is that newborn rats at SL or HA were exposed to room air for 24 h before sacrifice and tissue harvesting. While it is highly unlikely that this short time frame alters lung morphology, it is still possible that it might affect the biochemical analysis, and could contribute to discrepancies in some of our results. As such, the results of the biochemical analysis obtained when animals were exposed to hypoxia at SL or enriched oxygen at HA should be considered cautiously. However, it is striking that there are only limited differences for NOX and XO between newborn rats at SL and HA, while differences are much more substantial in adults. Finally, one should keep in mind that, unfortunately, samples from female rats were not included in these studies. However, despite the fact that ovarian steroids could have potent anti-oxidant effects in mitochondria (Laouafa et al., 2017), we have not detected sex-specific alterations in lung morphology in HA rats (Jochmans-Lemoine et al., 2015).

CONCLUSION

We conclude from this study that rats living at HA present an unusually elevated mitochondrial anti-oxidant capacity in the lungs, possibly as a compensatory response to high mitochondrial ROS production. Rats also presented morphological alterations in the lung tissue and a low alveolar surface area—a phenotype known to be induced by high oxidative stress in the lungs. Therefore, our data suggest that the high activities of antioxidant enzymes might not be efficient to adequately protect the lungs. Mice at HA had normal anti-oxidant enzymatic activities in the lungs and were able to develop a higher lung volume, alveolar surface area, and high arterial O_2 saturation at HA.

Since mitochondrial anti-oxidant enzyme activities and alveolar surface area were normal in young rats at HA, alteration of lung alveolar morphology and oxidative stress balance occur beyond the second postnatal week in rats living at HA. Finally, the phenotype reported in HA rats is strikingly similar to what is observed in patients affected by chronic mountain sickness (Julian et al., 2015; Villafuerte and Corante, 2016). The present findings might thus have clinical relevance for HA residents and provide evidence that targeting mitochondrial ROS production with selective mitochondrial anti-oxidant agents could be an interesting therapeutic opportunity.

AUTHOR CONTRIBUTIONS

AJ-L, GV, IV, MG: Contributed to sampling and processing tissue samples in Bolivia. AJ-L, SR, SL: Contributed to sampling and processing tissue samples in Canada. AJ-L, JS, VJ: Contributed to initial study design. AJ-L, VJ: Analyzed data, drafted the figures and manuscript, wrote and edited the manuscript. All authors: Commented early drafts of the paper and data presentation, read and approved the final version.

ACKNOWLEDGMENTS

This study was funded by the Natural Sciences and Engineering Research Council of Canada (VJ, JS: grant # RGPGP-2014-00083). AJ-L has been supported by a training grant in respiratory physiology from Réseau en Santé Réspiratoire (Fonds de Recherche du Québec—Santé, and Canadian Institute for Health Research). The authors acknowledge Dr. Tara Adele Janes for careful editorial revision of the paper.

REFERENCES

Adam-Vizi, V. (2005). Production of reactive oxygen species in brain mitochondria: contribution by electron transport chain and non-electron transport chain sources. *Antioxid. Redox Signal.* 7, 1140–1149. doi: 10.1089/ars.2005.7.1140

Bai, Z., Voituron, N., Wuren, T., Jeton, F., Jin, G., Marchant, D., et al. (2015). Role of glutamate and serotonin on the hypoxic ventilatory response in high-altitude-adapted plateau Pika. *Respir. Physiol. Neurobiol.* 212–214, 39–45. doi: 10.1016/j.resp.2015.03.006

Bedard, K., and Krause, K. H. (2007). The NOX family of ROS-generating NADPH oxidases: physiology and pathophysiology. *Physiol. Rev.* 87, 245–313. doi: 10.1152/physrev.00044.2005

Blanco, L. N., Massaro, D., and Massaro, G. D. (1991). Alveolar size, number, and surface area: developmentally dependent response to 13% O_2. *Am. J. Physiol.* 261, L370–L377. doi: 10.1152/ajplung.1991.261.6.L370

Burri, P. H., Dbaly, J., and Weibel, E. R. (1974). The postnatal growth of the rat lung. *I. Morphometry. Anat. Rec.* 178, 711–730. doi: 10.1002/ar.1091780405

Cheviron, Z. A., Bachman, G. C., Connaty, A. D., McClelland, G. B., and Storz, J. F. (2012). Regulatory changes contribute to the adaptive enhancement of thermogenic capacity in high-altitude deer mice. *Proc. Natl. Acad. Sci. U.S.A.* 109, 8635–8640. doi: 10.1073/pnas.1120523109

Cheviron, Z. A., and Brumfield, R. T. (2012). Genomic insights into adaptation to high-altitude environments. *Heredity* 108, 354–361. doi: 10.1038/hdy.2011.85

Datta, A., Kim, G. A., Taylor, J. M., Gugino, S. F., Farrow, K. N., Schumacker, P. T., et al. (2015). Mouse lung development and NOX1 induction during hyperoxia are developmentally regulated and mitochondrial ROS dependent. *Am. J. Physiol. Lung Cell. Mol. Physiol.* 309, L369–L377. doi: 10.1152/ajplung.00176.2014

Dosek, A., Ohno, H., Acs, Z., Taylor, A. W., and Radak, Z. (2007). High altitude and oxidative stress. *Respir. Physiol. Neurobiol.* 158, 128–131. doi: 10.1016/j.resp.2007.03.013

Fukuda, R., Zhang, H., Kim, J. W., Shimoda, L., Dang, C. V., and Semenza, G. L. (2007). HIF-1 regulates cytochrome oxidase subunits to optimize efficiency of respiration in hypoxic cells. *Cell* 129, 111–122. doi: 10.1016/j.cell.2007.01.047

Guenet, J. L., and Bonhomme, F. (2003). Wild mice: an ever-increasing contribution to a popular mammalian model. *Trends Genet.* 19, 24–31. doi: 10.1016/S0168-9525(02)00007-0

Halliwell, B. (2001). Role of free radicals in the neurodegenerative diseases: therapeutic implications for antioxidant treatment. *Drugs Aging* 18, 685–716. doi: 10.2165/00002512-200118090-00004

Hsia, C. C., Hyde, D. M., Ochs, M., Weibel, E. R., Albertine, K. H., Burri, P. H., et al. (2010). An official research policy statement of the American Thoracic Society/European Respiratory Society: standards for quantitative assessment of lung structure. *Am. J. Respir. Crit. Care Med.* 181, 394–418. doi: 10.1164/rccm.200809-1522ST

Jankov, R. P., Kantores, C., Pan, J., and Belik, J. (2008). Contribution of xanthine oxidase-derived superoxide to chronic hypoxic pulmonary hypertension in neonatal rats. *Am. J. Physiol. Lung Cell. Mol. Physiol.* 294, L233–L245. doi: 10.1152/ajplung.00166.2007

Jezek, P., and Hlavatá, L. (2005). Mitochondria in homeostasis of reactive oxygen species in cell, tissues, and organism. *Int. J. Biochem. Cell Biol.* 37, 2478–2503. doi: 10.1016/j.biocel.2005.05.013

Jochmans-Lemoine, A., Shahare, M., Soliz, J., and Joseph, V. (2016). HIF1alpha and physiological responses to hypoxia are correlated in mice but not in rats. *J. Exp. Biol.* 219, 3952–3961. doi: 10.1242/jeb.142869

Jochmans-Lemoine, A., Villalpando, G., Gonzales, M., Valverde, I., Soria, R., and Joseph, V. (2015). Divergent physiological responses in laboratory rats and mice raised at high altitude. *J. Exp. Biol.* 218, 1035–1043. doi: 10.1242/jeb.112862

Julian, C. G., Gonzales, M., Rodriguez, A., Bellido, D., Salmon, C. S., Ladenburger, A., et al. (2015). Perinatal hypoxia increases susceptibility to high-altitude polycythemia and attendant pulmonary vascular dysfunction. *Am. J. Physiol. Heart Circ. Physiol.* 309, H565–H573. doi: 10.1152/ajpheart.00296.2015

Julian, C. G., Vargas, E., Gonzales, M., Dávila, R. D., Ladenburger, A., Reardon, L., et al. (2013). Sleep-disordered breathing and oxidative stress in preclinical chronic mountain sickness (excessive erythrocytosis). *Respir. Physiol. Neurobiol.* 186, 188–196. doi: 10.1016/j.resp.2013.01.016

Laouafa, S., Ribon-Demars, A., Marcouiller, F., Roussel, D., Bairam, A., Pialoux, V., et al. (2017). Estradiol protects against cardiorespiratory dysfunctions and oxidative stress in intermittent hypoxia. *Sleep* 40:zsx104. doi: 10.1093/sleep/zsx104. Available online at: https://academic.oup.com/sleep/article/40/8/zsx104/3871076

Lau, D. S., Connaty, A. D., Mahalingam, S., Wall, N., Cheviron, Z. A., Storz, J. F., et al. (2017). Acclimation to hypoxia increases carbohydrate use during exercise in high-altitude deer mice. *Am. J. Physiol. Regul. Integr. Comp. Physiol.* 312, R400–R411. doi: 10.1152/ajpregu.00365.2016

Li, H. G., Ren, Y. M., Guo, S. C., Cheng, L., Wang, D. P., Yang, J., et al. (2009). The protein level of hypoxia-inducible factor-1α is increased in the plateau pika (Ochotona curzoniae) inhabiting high altitudes. *J. Exp. Zool. A Ecol. Genet. Physiol.* 311, 134–141. doi: 10.1002/jez.510

Lumbroso, D., Lemoine, A., Gonzales, M., Villalpando, G., Seaborn, T., and Joseph, V. (2012). Life-long consequences of postnatal normoxia exposure in rats raised at high altitude. *J. Appl. Physiol.* 112, 33–41.

Moore, L. G., Niermeyer, S., and Vargas, E. (2007). Does chronic mountain sickness (CMS) have perinatal origins? *Respir. Physiol. Neurobiol.* 158, 180–189. doi: 10.1016/j.resp.2007.06.016

Murphy, M. P. (2009). How mitochondria produce reactive oxygen species. *Biochem. J.* 417, 1–13. doi: 10.1042/BJ20081386

Paglia, D. E., and Valentine, W. N. (1967). Studies on the quantitative and qualitative characterization of erythrocyte glutathione peroxidase. *J. Lab. Clin. Med.* 70, 158–169.

Prabu, S. K., Anandatheerthavarada, H. K., Raza, H., Srinivasan, S., Spear, J. F., and Avadhani, N. G. (2006). Protein kinase A-mediated phosphorylation modulates cytochrome c oxidase function and augments hypoxia and myocardial ischemia-related injury. *J. Biol. Chem.* 281, 2061–2070. doi: 10.1074/jbc.M507741200

Salama, S. A., Omar, H. A., Maghrabi, I. A., AlSaeed, M. S., and EL-Tarras, A. E. (2014). Iron supplementation at high altitudes induces inflammation and oxidative injury to lung tissues in rats. *Toxicol. Appl. Pharmacol.* 274, 1–6. doi: 10.1016/j.taap.2013.10.034

Santus, P., Corsico, A., Solidoro, P., Braido, F., Di Marco, F., and Scichilone, N. (2014). Oxidative stress and respiratory system: pharmacological and clinical reappraisal of N-acetylcysteine. *COPD* 11, 705–717. doi: 10.3109/15412555.2014.898040

Scott, G. R., Schulte, P. M., Egginton, S., Scott, A. L., Richards, J. G., and Milsom, W. K. (2011). Molecular evolution of cytochrome C oxidase underlies high-altitude adaptation in the bar-headed goose. *Mol. Biol. Evol.* 28, 351–363. doi: 10.1093/molbev/msq205

Srinivasan, S., and Avadhani, N. G. (2012). Cytochromec oxidase dysfunction in oxidative stress. *Free Radic. Biol. Med.* 53, 1252–1263. doi: 10.1016/j.freeradbiomed.2012.07.021

Storz, J. F., Baze, M., Waite, J. L., Hoffmann, F. G., Opazo, J. C., and Hayes, J. P. (2007). Complex signatures of selection and gene conversion in the duplicated globin genes of house mice. *Genetics* 177, 481–500. doi: 10.1534/genetics.107.078550

Thomas, C., Mackey, M. M., Diaz, A. A., and Cox, D. P. (2009). Hydroxyl radical is produced via the Fenton reaction in submitochondrial particles under oxidative stress: implications for diseases associated with iron accumulation. *Redox Rep.* 14, 102–108. doi: 10.1179/135100009X3 92566

Truog, W. E., Xu, D., Ekekezie, I. I., Mabry, S., Rezaiekhaligh, M., Svojanovsky, S., et al. (2008). Chronic hypoxia and rat lung development: analysis by morphometry and directed microarray. *Pediatr. Res.* 64, 56–62. doi: 10.1203/PDR.0b013e31817289f2

Turrens, J. F. (2003). Mitochondrial formation of reactive oxygen species. *J. Physiol.* 552, 335–344. doi: 10.1113/jphysiol.2003.049478

van Eeden, S. F., and Sin, D. D. (2013). Oxidative stress in chronic obstructive pulmonary disease: a lung and systemic process. *Can. Respir. J.* 20, 27–29. doi: 10.1155/2013/509130

Villafuerte, F. C., and Corante, N. (2016). Chronic mountain sickness: clinical aspects, etiology, management, and treatment. *High Alt. Med. Biol.* 17, 61–69. doi: 10.1089/ham.2016.0031

Zhang, Z. Y., Chen, B., Zhao, D. J., and Kang, L. (2013). Functional modulation of mitochondrial cytochrome c oxidase underlies adaptation to high-altitude hypoxia in a Tibetan migratory locust. *Proc. Biol. Sci.* 280:20122758. doi: 10.1098/rspb.2012.2758

18

Maximal Oxygen Uptake is Achieved in Hypoxia but not Normoxia during an Exhaustive Severe Intensity Run

Matthew I. Black[1], Christopher R. Potter[2], Jo Corbett[3], Cain C. T. Clark[2] and Stephen B. Draper[2]*

[1] School of Sport, Exercise and Health Sciences, Loughborough University, Loughborough, UK, [2] HE Sport, University Centre, Hartpury College, Gloucestershire, UK, [3] Department of Sport and Exercise Science, University of Portsmouth, Portsmouth, UK

***Correspondence:**
Matthew I. Black
m.i.black@lboro.ac.uk

Highly aerobically trained individuals are unable to achieve maximal oxygen uptake ($\dot{V}O_{2max}$) during exhaustive running lasting ~2 min, instead $\dot{V}O_2$ plateaus below $\dot{V}O_{2max}$ after ~1 min. Hypoxia offers the opportunity to study the ($\dot{V}O_2$) response to an exhaustive run relative to a hypoxia induced reduction in $\dot{V}O_{2max}$. The aim of this study was to explore whether there is a difference in the percentage of $\dot{V}O_{2max}$ achieved (during a 2 min exhaustive run) in normoxia and hypoxia. Fourteen competitive middle distance runners (normoxic $\dot{V}O_{2max}$ 67.0 ± 5.2 ml.kg^{-1}.min^{-1}) completed exhaustive treadmill ramp tests and constant work rate (CWR) tests in normoxia and hypoxia (F_iO_2 0.13). The $\dot{V}O_2$ data from the CWR tests were modeled using a single exponential function. End exercise normoxic CWR $\dot{V}O_2$ was less than normoxic $\dot{V}O_{2max}$ (86 ± 6% ramp, $P < 0.001$). During the hypoxic CWR test, hypoxic $\dot{V}O_{2max}$ was achieved (102 ± 8% ramp, $P = 0.490$). The phase II time constant was greater in hypoxia (12.7 ± 2.8 s) relative to normoxia (10.4 ± 2.6 s) ($P = 0.029$). The results demonstrate that highly aerobically trained individuals cannot achieve $\dot{V}O_{2max}$ during exhaustive severe intensity treadmill running in normoxia, but can achieve the lower $\dot{V}O_{2max}$ in hypoxia despite a slightly slower $\dot{V}O_2$ response.

Keywords: $\dot{V}O_2$, $\dot{V}O_2$ kinetics, severe intensity, hypoxia, treadmill running

INTRODUCTION

Middle distance (800–3000 m) running performance is dependent on the speed that an athlete can sustain for the duration of the event. This speed is dependent on the ability of the locomotor muscles to produce power and resist fatigue (di Prampero et al., 1986; Lacour et al., 1990). The relatively high speed sustained throughout middle distance running events results in an energy demand in excess of the maximal aerobic energy yield (~110–120%), as assessed via pulmonary oxygen uptake ($\dot{V}O_2$) and, thus necessitates the integrative contribution from both aerobic and anaerobic pathways (Lacour et al., 1990; Craig and Morgan, 1998; Spencer and Gastin, 2001; Duffield et al., 2005). The 800 m event, for example, requires an ~66 and 34% relative contribution from aerobic and anaerobic metabolism, respectively (Spencer and Gastin, 2001).

The overall energy demand of middle distance running events places these events within the severe, or possibly the extreme intensity domain (Jones and Burnley, 2009). It is assumed that during exercise within the severe or extreme intensity domain, $\dot{V}O_2$ will project exponentially toward the maximal rate of pulmonary oxygen uptake ($\dot{V}O_{2max}$) until $\dot{V}O_{2max}$ is achieved, or exhaustion occurs (Whipp, 1994; Gaesser and Poole, 1996; Poole and Richardson, 1997; Hill and Ferguson, 1999; Jones and Burnley, 2009). However, research utilizing exhaustive constant work rate (CWR) treadmill running of ~2 min and highly aerobically trained middle distance runners ($\dot{V}O_{2max} \geq 60$ ml.kg^{-1}.min^{-1}) has found that $\dot{V}O_2$ does not achieve $\dot{V}O_{2max}$ despite sufficient time for the full response to develop (Draper and Wood, 2005a,b; Sandals et al., 2006; James et al., 2007a,b, 2008). Instead, a submaximal steady state $\dot{V}O_2$ is achieved following ~1 min of exercise with no evidence of a further increase in $\dot{V}O_2$ (Draper and Wood, 2005b).

Previous studies using cross-sectional designs have shown that individuals with a greater $\dot{V}O_{2max}$ achieve a lower percentage of $\dot{V}O_{2max}$ (%$\dot{V}O_{2max}$) during exhaustive CWR treadmill running of ~2 min (Draper and Wood, 2005a; James et al., 2007a). However, it should be recognized that individuals with a larger $\dot{V}O_{2max}$ typically have faster $\dot{V}O_2$ kinetics (Draper and Wood, 2005b; Kilding et al., 2006; Ingham et al., 2007; Marwood et al., 2010). It is therefore unclear why individuals whom possess a large $\dot{V}O_{2max}$ and faster $\dot{V}O_2$ kinetics achieve a lower %$\dot{V}O_{2max}$ than lesser aerobically trained individuals during exercise of this type.

It is well-known that acute hypoxic exposure results in significant reductions in $\dot{V}O_{2max}$ relative to values obtained in normoxic conditions (Dill et al., 1966; Dill and Adams, 1971; Engelen et al., 1996; Woorons et al., 2005; Calbet et al., 2015), and the decrement in $\dot{V}O_{2max}$ is linearly associated to the fraction of inspired oxygen (FiO_2) (Lawler et al., 1988). Acute hypoxic exposure, therefore, allows the $\dot{V}O_{2max}$ of highly aerobically trained individuals to be artificially and temporarily reduced. Whilst it is recognized that hypoxia may slow $\dot{V}O_2$ kinetics relative to normoxia (Engelen et al., 1996), the magnitude of slowing suggests that $\dot{V}O_2$ kinetics will remain sufficiently fast to permit the manifestation of its full response within <1 min, although evidence from exercise within the severe intensity domain is limited (Heubert et al., 2005). Therefore, hypoxia might provide the opportunity to explore whether highly aerobically trained individuals who are unable to achieve $\dot{V}O_{2max}$ during an exhaustive (~2 min) CWR treadmill run in normoxia can achieve a hypoxia reduced $\dot{V}O_{2max}$ during a time matched, thus relative intensity matched CWR treadmill run performed in hypoxia.

The purpose of this study, therefore, was to investigate the effect of artificially lowering $\dot{V}O_{2max}$ in trained individuals on their ability to attain $\dot{V}O_{2max}$ during an exhaustive treadmill run. We hypothesized that highly aerobically trained individuals would be unable to attain $\dot{V}O_{2max}$ during a CWR run lasting ~2 min performed in normoxia, but would be able to achieve a hypoxic reduced $\dot{V}O_{2max}$.

METHODS

Subjects

Thirteen males and one female (mean ± SD: age 21 ± 3 y, height 1.76 ± 0.06 m, mass 66.0 ± 7.0 kg) volunteered for the study. All were trained middle distance runners with an 800 m seasonal best of <130 s. Written and informed consent was obtained prior to data collection. Subjects were instructed to report to all testing sessions in a similar state, following their usual pre-competition routine. The study was approved by the institutional ethics committee.

General Procedures

Subjects completed a laboratory familiarization session which was also used to determine appropriate speeds for the CWR tests. The speeds of the CWR tests were adjusted to ensure exhaustion between 105 and 135 s. All tests were performed in an environmental chamber (Sanyo Gallenkamp, PLC, Loughborough), on the same motorized treadmill (ELG 55, Woodway Gmbh, Weil am Rhein, Germany). Air temperature and humidity were controlled at ~16°C and ~40%, respectively. FiO_2 was manipulated to reflect normoxia (FiO_2 0.21) or hypoxia (FiO_2 0.13) by a hypoxic unit (Sporting Edge UK Ltd, Sherfield-on-Lodden).

Following familiarization, subjects visited the laboratory on four occasions to a complete ramp incremental tests and CWR tests, in normoxia and hypoxia. The speed of the treadmill was increased by 0.1 km.h^{-1} every 5 s (1.2 km.h^{-1}.min^{-1}) during the ramp incremental tests, the starting speeds were selected to elicit exhaustion in 8–12 min (Buchfuhrer et al., 1983) in both conditions. The speeds of the CWR tests were based on trial runs completed during the familiarization sessions. If exhaustion was not achieved between 105 and 135 s, the treadmill speed was adjusted and subjects repeated the test on a different day. Trials were randomized to minimize any order effects.

Prior to each CWR run, subjects performed a warm-up on an identical treadmill outside of the environmental chamber. Subjects ran for 5 min at 12 km.h^{-1}, 2 min at 15 km.h^{-1}, and performed 3 × 10 s runs at the speed of the subsequent CWR test interspersed with 30 s of rest. Following the warm-up the subject entered the environmental chamber. Subjects were encouraged to perform light stretching for 2 min. Following the warm-up and stretching routine, subjects straddled the treadmill for 5 min, allowing the belt to move at the required speed for the test. Heart rate (HR) (recorded every 5 s) and breath-by-breath ($\dot{V}O_2$) data were recorded during this period to determine baseline values.

All tests started with the subjects lowering themselves onto the moving treadmill belt. The treadmill was fitted with two handrails, which subjects used to lift themselves onto or clear of the belt. The subject remained in contact with these rails at the start of the test for as long as necessary to reach the required leg speed (typically 2–3 s). The test was stopped when subjects were unable to continue and lifted themselves clear of the treadmill belt.

Data Acquisition

Throughout testing, subjects wore a chest strap and HR was measured using short-range telemetry (810i; Polar Electro Oy, Kempele, Finland), and breathed through a low-dead space (90 ml), low resistance (5.5 cm H_2O at 510 L.min^{-1}) mouthpiece and turbine assembly. Gases were collected continuously from the mouthpiece through a 2 m sampling line (0.5 mm internal diameter) to a quadrupole mass spectrometer (MSX 671: Ferraris

Respiratory Europe Ltd, Hertford, UK) where they were analyzed for O_2, CO_2, Ar and N_2. Expired volumes were determined using a turbine volume transducer (Interface Associates, Alifovieja, US). The mass spectrometer and turbine were calibrated before each test using mixtures of known composition (Linde Gas, London, UK), and a 3 L calibration syringe (Hans Rundolf, KS), respectively. Two identical quadrupole mass spectrometers were used; one was placed outside the environmental chamber to accurately determine the internal environmental conditions, this system was calibrated against outside atmospheric air (20.94% O_2, 0.04% CO_2, 0.93% Argon, and 78.08% N_2) and a normoxic gas bottle (14.99% O_2, 5.01% CO_2, 5.02% Argon, and 74.98% N_2). The second system was placed inside the environmental chamber and was calibrated against the environmental conditions provided by the other mass spectrometer and a gas bottle of known composition; the normoxic gas bottle was used during normoxic testing, and a gas bottle composed of 5% O_2, 5.01% CO_2, 5.02% Argon, and 84.97% N_2 was used in hypoxia. The volume and concentration signals were time aligned, accounting for transit delay in capillary gas and analyser rise time relative to the volume signal. $\dot{V}O_2$, $\dot{V}CO_2$, $\dot{V}_E$ were calculated for each breath.

Data Analysis

Moving 15 s averages were used to calculate $\dot{V}O_2$, $\dot{V}CO_2$, and $\dot{V}_E$ for every complete 15 s period throughout all tests. $\dot{V}O_{2max}$ was defined as the highest 15 s $\dot{V}O_2$ value attained during the ramp incremental tests, and $\dot{V}O_{2peak}$ was the highest 15 s $\dot{V}O_2$ value achieved during the CWR tests. HR was recorded every 5 s and the highest value achieved during the ramp incremental test was taken as maximum HR (HR_{max}) and the highest value recorded during the CWR exercise was the peak HR (HR_{peak}).

The breath-by-breath $\dot{V}O_2$ data from the CWR tests were initially examined to exclude errant breaths caused by coughing, swallowing, etc., and values lying more than 4 SD from the local mean were removed. Subsequently, the breath-by-breath data were converted to second-by-second data using linear interpolation and time aligned to the start of the test. The first 15 s of data were removed to account for the cardio-dynamic phase (Murias et al., 2011). A single exponential model was used to characterize $\dot{V}O_2$ kinetics as described in the following equation:

$$\dot{V}O_2(t) = \dot{V}O_2 \text{ baseline} + A(1 - (e^{-(t-\delta)/\tau})) \qquad (1)$$

where $\dot{V}O_2$ (t) represents the absolute $\dot{V}O_2$ at a given time (t), $\dot{V}O_2$ baseline is the average of the $\dot{V}O_2$ measured over the final 120 s of quiet standing, A is the asymptotic amplitude, τ is the time constant of the exponential response and δ is a delay. No parameters were constrained.

Statistical Analysis

Data were tested for normality (Duffy and Jacobsen, 2001) and was found to be normally distributed. Two-way (test × condition) repeated measures ANOVA was employed to determine the effect of hypoxia on $\dot{V}O_2$, minute ventilation ($\dot{V}_E$), ventilatory equivalents (i.e., $\dot{V}_E/\dot{V}O_2$, $\dot{V}_E/\dot{V}CO_2$) and HR. *Post hoc t*-tests with Bonferroni correction were used to explore the origin of any significant interaction effect. Paired *t*-tests were used to explore differences in estimates of the modeled $\dot{V}O_2$ data in normoxia and hypoxia. Pearson's Product Moment Correlation was used to investigate the relationship between $\dot{V}O_{2max}$, CWR running speed, and the % $\dot{V}O_{2max}$ achieved during the CWR tests. The relationship between the difference in running speed and the difference in % $\dot{V}O_{2max}$ achieved during the normoxic and hypoxic CWR tests was also investigated. Statistical significance was set at $P < 0.05$. Data are presented as mean ± SD unless otherwise stated.

RESULTS

The $\dot{V}O_{2max}$ measured in the normoxic ramp incremental test was 4.40 ± 0.42 $L.min^{-1}$ (67.0 ± 5.2 $ml.kg^{-1}.min^{-1}$) and HR_{max} was 185 ± 7 bpm. Hypoxia reduced $\dot{V}O_{2max}$ to 2.97 ± 0.27 $L.min^{-1}$ (45.1 ± 3.0 $ml.kg^{-1}.min^{-1}$; $P < 0.001$) and HR_{max} to 181 ± 6 bpm; $P < 0.05$).

The average speed utilized for the normoxic CWR trials was 22.0 ± 1.0 $km.h^{-1}$ which resulted in a trial duration of 114 ± 11 s (range: 100 s to 130 s). The speed of the hypoxic CWR trial was performed at a significantly slower speed (20.5 ± 1.0 $km.h^{-1}$; $P < 0.001$) to ensure a similar duration of trial between conditions. The duration of the hypoxic CWR trial (114 ± 11 s, range: 105 s to 135 s) was not significantly different to the duration of the normoxic CWR trial (114 ± 5 s, range: 105 s to 125 s) ($P > 0.05$). Normoxic $\dot{V}O_{2max}$ was not achieved during the normoxic CWR trial (3.79 ± 0.47 $L.min^{-1}$; 86 ± 6% $\dot{V}O_{2max}$; $P < 0.05$; **Figure 1**).However, subjects attained hypoxic $\dot{V}O_{2max}$ during the hypoxic CWR trial (3.02 ± 0.30 $L.min^{-1}$; 102 ± 8%; $P > 0.05$; **Figure 1**). $\dot{V}O_{2max}$ was inversely associated with %$\dot{V}O_{2max}$ achieved during the normoxic ($r = -0.64$, $P < 0.05$) and hypoxic ($r = -0.68$, $P < 0.01$) CWR trials, and when the normoxic and hypoxic trials were combined ($r = -0.85$, $P < 0.001$; **Figure 2**). Condition-specific HR_{max} was attained during normoxic (189 ± 7 bpm) and hypoxic (181 ± 7 bpm) CWR trials ($P > 0.05$). The parameters of the modeled $\dot{V}O_2$ data are presented in **Table 1**. No relationships were observed between speed and % $\dot{V}O_2$ achieved during the CWR trials performed in normoxia ($r = 0.34$, $P > 0.05$), hypoxia ($r = -0.16$, $P > 0.05$), or the difference in speed and $\dot{V}O_2$ between the normoxic and hypoxic CWR trials ($r = -0.05$, $P > 0.05$).

No significant interaction effect was observed for $\dot{V}_E$ ($P > 0.05$) with no significant main effect for condition (normoxia, 137.3 ± 17.5 $L.min^{-1}$; hypoxia 130 ± 16.2 $L.min^{-1}$; $P > 0.05$), but a significant main effect for test (ramp, 128.0 ± 16.6 $L.min^{-1}$; CWR, 139.2 ± 16.0 $L.min^{-1}$; $P < 0.001$). There was a significant interaction effect for $\dot{V}_E/\dot{V}O_2$ ($P < 0.05$) with significant main effects for condition (normoxia, 35.3 ± 6.7 $L.min^{-1}$; hypoxia 43.7 ± 4.7 $L.min^{-1}$; $P < 0.001$) and test (ramp, 128.0 ± 16.6 $L.min^{-1}$; CWR, 139.2 ± 16.0 $L.min^{-1}$; $P < 0.001$). There was a significant interaction effect for $\dot{V}_E/\dot{V}CO_2$ ($P < 0.01$) with significant main effects for condition (normoxia, 28.2 ± 3.7 $L.min^{-1}$; hypoxia 31.6 ± 6.0 $L.min^{-1}$; $P < 0.05$), but no significant difference for test (ramp, 29.8 ± 5.0 $L.min^{-1}$; CWR, 26.2 ± 3.4 $L.min^{-1}$; $P > 0.05$).

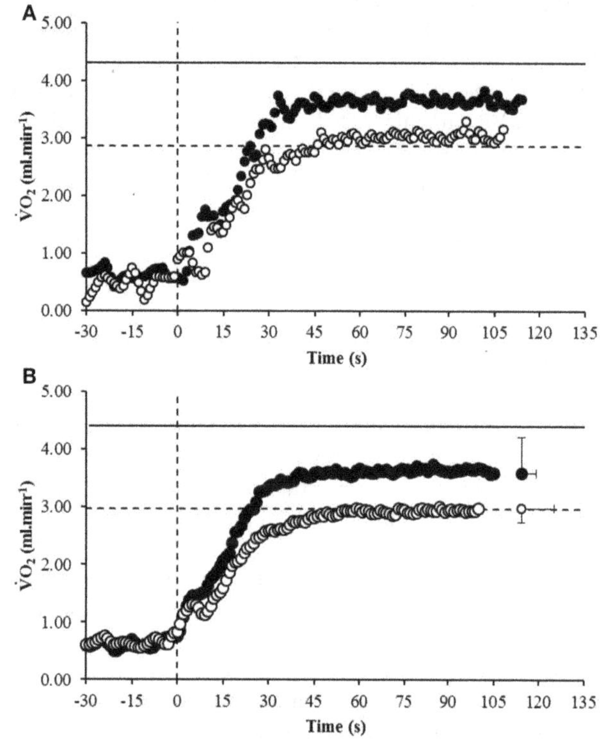

FIGURE 1 | The $\dot{V}O_2$ response of a representative participant (A) and the group mean **(B)** to the normoxic CWR test (black circles) and hypoxic CWR test (white circles). The $\dot{V}O_{2max}$ to the normoxic ramp (solid line) and hypoxic ramp (broken line) is also provided. Error bars represent the standard error of measurement. For clarity the error bars are omitted for all but the final data point.

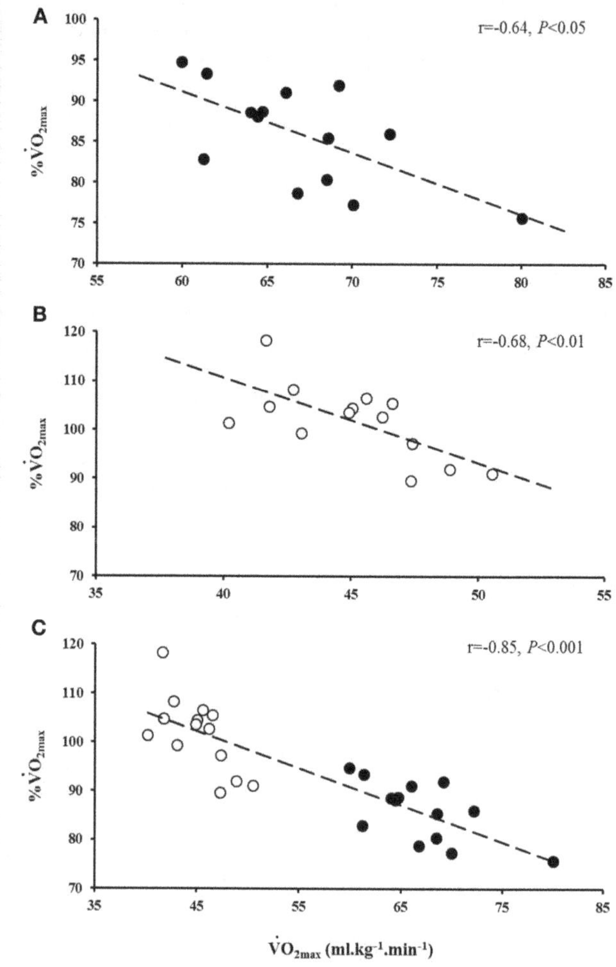

FIGURE 2 | The relationship between $\dot{V}O_{2max}$ and the percentage $\dot{V}O_{2max}$ (%$\dot{V}O_{2max}$) achieved during the normoxic (A, black circles) and hypoxic (**B**, white circles) CWR tests. The combined relationship between $\dot{V}O_{2max}$ and the % $\dot{V}O_{2max}$ achieved in normoxia and hypoxia is also provided **(C)**.

DISCUSSION

The principle novel finding of the current study was that despite being unable to attain $\dot{V}O_{2max}$ during normoxic CWR running lasting ~2 min, highly aerobically trained individuals could achieve a hypoxia reduced $\dot{V}O_{2max}$ during CWR running of a matched duration, thus of a similar relative intensity. This is the first study to demonstrate that subjects whose $\dot{V}O_2$ plateaued below $\dot{V}O_{2max}$ during an exhaustive CWR run, were subsequently able to attain $\dot{V}O_{2max}$ when the exercise bout was replicated in hypoxic conditions despite a slowed $\dot{V}O_2$ response.

Previous research has demonstrated that during normoxic CWR running lasting ~2 min, more highly aerobically trained individuals achieved a lower %$\dot{V}O_{2max}$ (Draper and Wood, 2005a; James et al., 2007a). In agreement with these findings, the current study reported an inverse association between $\dot{V}O_{2max}$ and the %$\dot{V}O_{2max}$ achieved during the normoxic CWR trial (**Figure 2**). To gain further insight into the relationship between $\dot{V}O_{2max}$ and %$\dot{V}O_{2max}$ achieved the present study investigated whether a hypoxia induced reduction in $\dot{V}O_{2max}$ may permit highly aerobically trained individuals to attain $\dot{V}O_{2max}$ during exhaustive CWR running at a matched relative intensity. The acute hypoxic exposure reduced $\dot{V}O_{2max}$ by ~32%, consistent with previous reports (Engelen et al., 1996; Martin and O'Kroy, 1993; Woorons et al., 2005), and subject to this reduction $\dot{V}O_{2max}$ was achieved (**Figure 1B**). No relationship was observed between % $\dot{V}O_{2max}$ achieved and the running speed during the CWR tests in normoxia or hypoxia, nor the difference in speed between conditions (i.e., normoxia and hypoxia) and the difference in %VO_{2max} achieved (all $P > 0.05$), suggesting that $\dot{V}O_{2max}$ may be an important parameter in determining whether an individual may be able to achieve their $\dot{V}O_{2max}$ during this type of exercise. Furthermore, these findings highlight that further improvements in $\dot{V}O_{2max}$ are of less benefit to high-intensity exercise performance compared to similar gains in anaerobic capability. These findings perhaps seem incongruous with the high $\dot{V}O_{2max}$ values typically reported in elite 800 m runners (Svedenhag and Sjödin, 1984; Ingham et al., 2008) that they are apparently unable to fully utilize. However, such a high $\dot{V}O_{2max}$ value may be due to the high volume of interval training performed by these athletes (Helgerud et al.,

TABLE 1 | The parameters of the modeled $\dot{V}O_2$ response to CWR exercise in normoxia and hypoxia.

	Normoxia	Hypoxia	*P*-value
Ramp $\dot{V}O_{2max}$ ($L.min^{-1}$)	4.40 ± 0.42	2.97 ± 0.27	<0.001
CWR $\dot{V}O_{2peak}$ ($L.min^{-1}$)	3.79 ± 0.47	3.02 ± 0.30	<0.001
Baseline O_2 ($L.min^{-1}$)	0.60 ± 0.11	0.67 ± 0.15	>0.05
A ($L.min^{-1}$)	2.45 ± 0.50	1.61 ± 0.27	<0.001
Baseline + A ($L.min^{-1}$)	3.05 ± 0.51	2.28 ± 0.21	<0.001
τ (s)	10.4 ± 2.6	12.7 ± 2.8	<0.05
δ (s)	7.6 ± 2.6	7.4 ± 3.3	>0.05

2007). There have certainly been instances where performance at altitude would indicate that the decrement in $\dot{V}O_{2max}$ may not substantially impair performance. For example, Ralph Doubell equalled the World Record at the 1968 Mexico Olympics which was performed at an altitude of 2,240 m above sea level; a feat that would seem implausible if one's $\dot{V}O_{2max}$ was a necessity for optimum performance.

The $\dot{V}O_2$ kinetics were similar to values previously reported during investigations utilizing similarly highly aerobically trained runners during CWR running lasting ~2 min (Draper and Wood, 2005a,b; Draper et al., 2008). The phase I time delays are also similar to those reported by Wilkerson et al. (2004). Consistent with Engelen et al. (1996), we found a slower phase II τ in the hypoxic condition (**Table 1**). However, it should be noted that despite a slower phase II τ, resulting in ~10 s difference in the attainment of the $\dot{V}O_2$ amplitude, hypoxic $\dot{V}O_{2max}$ was achieved. Conversely, despite faster $\dot{V}O_2$ kinetics normoxic $\dot{V}O_{2max}$ was not attained. Instead, there was an evident $\dot{V}O_2$ plateau in normoxia at ~86% normoxic $\dot{V}O_{2max}$.The occurrence of a $\dot{V}O_2$ plateau, rather than a continued trajectory toward $\dot{V}O_{2max}$ and indeed the energy demands of the exercise, questions contemporary models of $\dot{V}O_2$ kinetics during CWR exercise lasting ~2 min in this highly aerobically trained group. Interestingly, this same response is not evident during exhaustive cycle ergometry of a similar duration whereby $\dot{V}O_2$ continues to increase throughout, although maximum values are not attained (Draper et al., 2003). At present the reasons for the differences between exercise modes in $\dot{V}O_2$ response to severe intensity exercise are unclear. Increasing oxygen uptake has been associated with reduced efficiency arising from factors, such as metabolite accumulation, limitations in substrate availability, pH disturbance, increased muscle temperature, and altered motor unit recruitment (Grassi et al., 2015). Indeed, it is well established that the patterns of muscle action, including the relative proportion of eccentric and concentric contraction and the contribution of the stretch-shortening cycle differ between running and cycling (van Ingen-Schenau et al., 1997; Bijker et al., 2002). These effects might, at least in part, contribute to the between mode differences in $\dot{V}O_2$ kinetics, particularly for higher work rates where the use of elastic energy is optimized (Dalleau et al., 1998); whether or not increased stored energy during the stretch shortening cycle can help maintain efficiency despite increased metabolic fatigue warrants further investigation.

Consistent with previous investigations, we found that HR_{max} was greater in normoxia than hypoxia (Benoit et al., 1995; Mollard et al., 2007). However, similar to our $\dot{V}O_2$ findings normoxic HR_{max} was not achieved during the normoxic CWR test (Draper and Wood, 2005a,b), but hypoxic HR_{max} could be achieved during the hypoxic CWR trial. Assuming HR_{max} is needed to achieve maximal cardiac output (Q_{max}), these findings suggest that Q_{max} was not achieved during the normoxic CWR test. Despite a lower HR_{max} in hypoxia relative to normoxia, previous findings have shown that hypoxia has no effect on Q_{max} (Mollard et al., 2007), implying a compensatory increase in maximal stroke volume in hypoxia. Therefore, the inability to achieve $\dot{V}O_{2max}$ in the normoxic CWR trial may be associated with submaximal cardiac output. However, further investigation that assesses cardiac output and blood flow is necessary to gain insight into Q_{max} as a potential limiting factor in the attainment of $\dot{V}O_{2max}$ during this type of exercise.

Although end exercise $\dot{V}_E$ was greater during the CWR trials relative to the ramp incremental tests, this was not different between normoxia and hypoxia. Furthermore, we observed no differences in ventilatory equivalents between conditions (i.e., normoxia and hypoxia). These similar ventilatory responses might serve to attenuate or prevent the exercise induced arterial hypoxemia that has been described in highly aerobically trained individuals (Dempsey et al., 1984; Powers et al., 1988, 1992; Caillaud et al., 1993; review Prefaut et al., 2000). In normoxia, the increased $\dot{V}_E$ during CWR exercise would likely increase the work of breathing thereby compromising limb muscle blood flow (Wetter et al., 1999). In hypoxia, the PO_2 is in the steep portion of the oxygen-hemoglobin dissociation curve and increased $\dot{V}_E$ could have pronounced effects on arterial oxygen concentration and may help to preserve muscle $\dot{V}O_2$ despite reduced limb blood flow. However, in normoxia the PO_2 is in the flatter region of the oxygen-hemoglobin dissociation curve and the same increases in $\dot{V}_E$ would be less effective in altering arterial oxygen concentration relative to hypoxia. As a consequence the increased work associated with breathing would result in little/small increases in arterial oxygen concentration and reduce muscle blood flow and thus muscle $\dot{V}O_2$. However, it should be noted that exercise induced arterial hypoxemia has also been reported during different exercise modalities, such as cycling (Powers et al., 1988), whereas the phenomenon whereby $\dot{V}O_2$ attains a plateau below $\dot{V}O_{2max}$ has only been reported in highly aerobically trained individuals during CWR running exercise lasting ~2 min. The mechanistic origin(s) for this phenomenon is currently unknown and requires further research.

Despite only one transition to the CWR trial in each condition, due to the large amplitude of the $\dot{V}O_2$ response during this intensity of exercise there is a much greater signal/noise ratio when compared to exercise of a lower intensity (Lamarra et al., 1987). In lesser trained individuals with smaller $\dot{V}O_2$ amplitude, thus smaller signal to noise ratio, Draper et al. (2008) demonstrated that two transitions would at worst (i.e., smallest signal to noise ratio) provide 95% confidence intervals of 1 s. Given that the current study recruited more highly aerobically trained individuals than Draper et al. (2008), thus a greater signal to noise ratio, it would be reasonable to expect 95% confidence intervals of better than 2 s for τ. Furthermore, the current study design was sufficiently sensitive and had adequate power to detect differences in τ between conditions.

In conclusion, the results of the present study demonstrate that highly aerobically trained individuals whom are unable to achieve $\dot{V}O_{2max}$ during an exhaustive CWR run lasting ~2 min, are able to achieve a hypoxia reduced $\dot{V}O_{2max}$ despite exhibiting slower $\dot{V}O_2$ kinetics. These data further support the notion that $\dot{V}O_{2max}$ is an important determinant of the %$\dot{V}O_{2max}$ that can be achieved during a short duration exhaustive CWR run. The present data demonstrate that ventilatory differences are unable to explain the inability to attain $\dot{V}O_{2max}$ during normoxic CWR trials. Future research should explore the possibility of an O_2 delivery or blood perfusion limitation during this type of exercise in highly aerobically trained runners. Future research should also consider utilizing an experimental condition in normoxia which uses gradient on the treadmill (or weighted vest) instead of hypoxia to slow the running speed down and induce task failure in ~2 min. This would aid in deciphering the novel finding of this study.

AUTHOR CONTRIBUTIONS

MB, CP, SD, JC, and CC were involved in conceptual design, data collection, interpretation, and manuscript preparation. All authors approve the submission of this work and agree to be accountable for all aspects of the work.

REFERENCES

Benoit, H., Busso, T., Castells, J., Denis, C., and Geyssant, A. (1995). Influence of hypoxic ventilatory response on arterial O_2 saturation during maximal exercise in acute hypoxia. *Eur. J. Appl. Physiol. Occup. Physiol.* 72, 101–105. doi: 10.1007/BF00964122

Bijker, K. E., de Groot, G., and Hollander, A. P. (2002). Differences in leg muscle activity during running and cycling in humans. *Eur. J. Appl. Physiol.* 87, 556–561. doi: 10.1007/s00421-002-0663-8

Buchfuhrer, M. J., Hansen, J. E., Robinson, T. E., Sue, D. Y., Wasserman, K., and Whipp, B. J. (1983). Optimizing the exercise protocol for cardiopulmonary assessment. *J. Appl. Physiol.* 55, 1558–1564.

Caillaud, C., Anselme, F., Mercier, J., and Préfaut, C. (1993). Pulmonary gas exchange and breathing pattern during and after exercise in highly trained athletes. *Eur. J. Appl. Physiol. Occup. Physiol.* 67, 431–437. doi: 10.1007/BF 00376460

Calbet, J. A. L., Gonzalez-Alonso, J., Helge, J. W., Sondergaard, H., Munch-Andersen, T., Saltin, B., et al. (2015). Central and peripheral hemodynamics in exercising humans: leg vs arm exercise. *Scand. J. Med. Sci. Sports* 25, 144–157. doi: 10.1111/sms.12604

Craig, I. S., and Morgan, D. W. (1998). Relationship between 800-m running performance and accumulated oxygen deficit in middle-distance runners. *Med. Sci. Sports Exerc.* 30, 1631–1636. doi: 10.1097/00005768-199811000-00012

Dalleau, G., Belli, A., Bourdin, M., Lacour, J. (1998). The spring-mass model and the energy cost of running. *Eur. J. Appl. Physiol. Occup. Physiol.* 77, 257–263. doi: 10.1007/s004210050330

Dempsey, J. A., Hanson, P. G., and Henderson, K. S. (1984). Exercise-induced arterial hypoxemia in healthy human subjects at sea-level. *J. Physiol.* 355, 161–175. doi: 10.1113/jphysiol.1984.sp015412

Dill, D. B., and Adams, W. C. (1971). Maximal oxygen uptake at sea level and at 3,090-m altitude in high school champion runners. *J. Appl. Physiol.* 30, 854–859.

Dill, D. B., Myhre, G., Phillips, E. E., and Brown, D. K. (1966). Work capacity in acute exposure to altitude. *J. Appl. Physiol.* 21, 1168–1176.

di Prampero, P. E., Atchou, G., Brückner, J. C., and Moia, C. (1986). The energetics of endurance running. *Eur. J. Appl. Physiol.* 55, 259–266. doi: 10.1007/BF02343797

Draper, S. B., and Wood, D. M. (2005a). The VO_2 response for an exhaustive treadmill run at 800-m pace: a breath-by-breath analysis. *Eur. J. Appl. Physiol.* 93, 381–389. doi: 10.1007/s00421-004-1278-z

Draper, S. B., and Wood, D. M. (2005b). The oxygen uptake response of sprint- vs. endurance-trained runners to severe intensity running. *J. Sci. Med. Sport* 8, 233–243. doi: 10.1016/S1440-2440(05)80014-3

Draper, S. B., Wood, D. M., Corbett, J., James, D. V., and Potter, C. R. (2008). The effect of prior moderate- and heavy-intensity running on the VO2 response to exhaustive severe-intensity running. *Int. J. Sports Physiol. Perform.* 1, 361–374. doi: 10.1123/ijspp.1.4.361

Draper, S. B., Wood, D. M., and Fallowfiled, J. L. (2003). The $\dot{V}O2$ response to exhaustive square-wave exercise: influence of intensity and mode. *Eur. J. Appl. Physiol.* 90, 92–100. doi: 10.1007/s00421-003-0877-4

Duffield, R., Dawson, B., and Goodman, C. (2005). Energy system contribution to 400-metre and 800-metre track running. *J. Sports Sci.* 23, 299–307. doi: 10.1080/02640410410001730043

Duffy, J., and Jacobsen, B. (2001). "Univariate descriptive statistics," in *Statistical Methods for Health Care Research*, ed B. H. Munro (Philiadelphia, PA: Lippincott Williams and Wilkins), 29–62.

Engelen, M., Porszasz, J., Riley, M., Wasserman, K., Maehara, K., and Barstow, T. J. (1996). Effects of hypoxic hypoxia on O_2 uptake and heart rate kinetics during heavy exercise. *J. Appl. Physiol.* 81, 2500–2508.

Gaesser, G. A., and Poole, D. C. (1996). The slow component of oxygen uptake kinetics in humans. *Exerc. Sport Sci. Rev.* 24, 35–71. doi: 10.1249/0000 3677-199600240-00004

Grassi, B., Rossiter, H. B., and Zoladz, J. A. (2015). Skeletal muscle fatigue and decreased efficiency: two sides of the same coin?. *Exerc. Sport Sci. Rev.* 43, 75–83. doi: 10.1249/JES.0000000000000043

Helgerud, J., Hoydal, K., Wang, E., Karlsen, T., Berg, P., Bjerkaas, M., et al. (2007). Aerobic high-intensity intervals improve O_{2max} more than moderate training. *Med. Sci. Sports Exerc.* 39, 665–671. doi: 10.1249/mss.0b013e3180304570

Heubert, R. A. P., Quaresima, V., Laffite, L. P., Koralsztein, J. P., and Billat, V. L. (2005). Acute moderate hypoxia affects the oxygen desaturation and the performance but not the oxygen uptake response. *Int. J. Sports Med.* 26, 542–551 doi: 10.1055/s-2004-821329

Hill, D. W., and Ferguson, C. S. (1999). A physiological description of critical velocity. *Eur. J. Appl. Physiol. Occup. Physiol.* 79, 290–293. doi: 10.1007/s004210050509

Ingham, S. A., Carter, H., Whyte, G. P., and Doust, J. H. (2007). Comparison of the oxygen uptake kinetics of club and olympic champion rowers. *Med. Sci. Sports Exerc.* 39, 865–871. doi: 10.1249/mss.0b013e31803350c7

Ingham, S. A., Whyte, G. P., Pedlar, C., Bailey, D. M., Dunman, N., and Nevill, A. M. (2008). Determinants of 800-m and 1500-m running performance using allometric models. *Med. Sci. Sports Exerc.* 40, 345–350. doi: 10.1249/mss.0b013e31815a83dc

James, D. V., Sandals, L. E., Draper, S. B., Maldonado-Martin, S., and Wood, D. M. (2008). Influence of test duration on oxygen uptake attained during treadmill running. *Euro. J. Sport Sci.* 8, 225–230. doi: 10.1080/17461390802116708

James, D. V., Sandals, L. E., Draper, S. B., and Wood, D. M. (2007b). Relationship between maximal oxygen uptake and oxygen uptake attained during treadmill middle-distance running. *J. Sports Sci.* 25, 851–858. doi: 10.1080/02640410600875226

James, D. V., Sandals, L. E., Draper, S. B., Maldonado-Martin, S., and Wood, D. M. (2007a). VO_2 attained during treadmill running: the influence of a specialist (400-m or 800-m) event. *Int. J. Sports Physiol. Perform.* 2, 128–136. doi: 10.1123/ijspp.2.2.128

Jones, A. M., and Burnley, M. (2009). Oxygen uptake kinetics: an underappreciated determinant of exercise performance. *Int. J. Sports Physiol. Perform.* 4, 524–532. doi: 10.1123/ijspp.4.4.524

Kilding, A. E., Winter, E. M., and Fysh, M. (2006). A comparison of pulmonary oxygen uptake kinetics in middle- and long-distance runners. *Int. J. Sports Med.* 27, 419–426. doi: 10.1055/s-2005-865778

Lacour, J. R., Magunacelaya, S., Barthélémy, J. C., and Dormois, D. (1990). The energetics of middle distance running. *Eur. J. Appl. Physiol.* 60, 38–43. doi: 10.1007/BF00572183

Lamarra, N., Whipp, B. J., Ward, S. A., and Wasserman, K. (1987). Effect of interbreath fluctuations on characterizing exercise gas exchange kinetics. *J. Appl. Physiol.* 62, 2003–2012.

Lawler, J., Power, S. K., and Thompson, D. (1988). Linear relationship between VO_{2max} and VO_{2max} decrement during exposure to acute hypoxia. *J. Appl. Physiol.* 64, 1486–1492.

Martin, D., and O'Kroy, J. (1993). Effects of acute hypoxia on the VO_{2max} of trained and untrained subjects. *J. Sports Sci.* 11, 37–42. doi: 10.1080/02640419308729961

Marwood, S., Roche, D., Rowland, T., Garrard, M., and Unnithan, V. B. (2010). Faster pulmonary oxygen uptake kinetics in trained versus untrained male adolescents. *Med. Sci. Sports Exerc.* 42, 127–134. doi: 10.1249/MSS.0b013e3181af20d0

Mollard, P., Woorons, X., Letournel, M., Lamberto, C., Favret, F., Pichon, A., et al. (2007). Determinants of maximal oxygen uptake in moderate acute hypoxia in endurance athletes. *Eur. J. Appl. Physiol.* 100, 663–673. doi: 10.1007/s00421-007-0457-0

Murias, J. M., Spencer, M. D., Kowalchuk, J. M., and Paterson, D. H. (2011). Influence of phase I duration on phase II VO_2 kinetics parameter estimates in older and young adults. *Am. J. Physiol. Regul. Integr. Comp. Physiol.* 301, R218–R224. doi: 10.1152/ajpregu.00060.2011

Poole, D. C., and Richardson, R. S. (1997). Determinants of oxygen uptake. Implications for exercise testing. *Sports Med.* 24, 308–320. doi: 10.2165/00007256-199724050-00003

Powers, S. K., Dodd, S., Lawler, J., Landry, G., Kirtley, M., McKnight, T., et al. (1988). Incidence of exercise induced hypoxemia in elite endurance athletes at sea level. *Eur. J. Appl. Physiol. Occup. Physiol.* 58, 298–302. doi: 10.1007/BF00417266

Powers, S. K., Martin, D., Cicale, M., Collop, N., Huang, D., and Criswell, D. (1992). Exercise-induced hypoxemia in athletes: role of inadequate hyperventilation. *Eur. J. Appl. Physiol. Occup. Physiol.* 65, 37–42. doi: 10.1007/BF01466272

Prefaut, C., Durand, F., Mucci, P., and Caillaud, C. (2000). Exercise-induced arterial hypoxemia in athletes A review. *Sports Med.* 30, 47–61. doi: 10.2165/00007256-200030010-00005

Sandals, L. E., Wood, D. M., Draper, S. B., and James, D. V. (2006). Influence of pacing strategy on oxygen uptake kinetics during treadmill middle-distance running. *Int. J. Sports Med.* 27, 37–42. doi: 10.1055/s-2005-837468

Spencer, M. R., and Gastin, P. B. (2001). Energy system contribution during 200- to 1500-m running in highly trained athletes. *Med. Sci. Sports Exerc.* 33, 157–162. doi: 10.1097/00005768-200101000-00024

Svedenhag, J., and Sjödin, B. (1984). Maximal and submaximal oxygen uptakes and blood lactate levels in elite male middle- and long-distance runners. *Int. J. Sports Med.* 5, 255–261. doi: 10.1055/s-2008-1025916

van Ingen-Schenau, G. J., Bobbert, M. F., and de Haan, A. (1997). Does elastic energy enhance work and efficiency in the stretch-shortening cycle? *J. Appl. Biomech.* 13, 389–415.

Wetter, T. J., Harms, C. A., Nelson, W. B., Pegelow, D. F., and Dempsey, J. A. (1999). Influence of respiratory muscle work on VO_2 and leg blood flow during submaximal exercise. *J. Appl. Physiol.* 87, 643–651.

Whipp, B. J. (1994). The slow component of O_2 uptake kinetics during heavy exercise. *Med. Sci. Sports Exerc.* 26, 1319–1326. doi: 10.1249/00005768-199411000-00005

Wilkerson, D. P., Koppo, K., Barstow, T. J., and Jones, A. M. (2004). Effect of work rate on the functional 'gain' of Phase II pulmonary O_2 uptake response to exercise. *Respir. Physiol. Neurobiol.* 142, 211–223. doi: 10.1016/j.resp.2004.06.001

Woorons, X., Mollard, P., Lamberto, C., Letournel, M., and Richalet, J. P. (2005). Effect of acute hypoxia on maximal exercise in trained and sedentary women. *Med. Sci. Sports Exerc.* 37, 147–154. doi: 10.1249/01.MSS.0000150020.25153.34

19

Increased P_IO_2 at Exhaustion in Hypoxia Enhances Muscle Activation and Swiftly Relieves Fatigue: A Placebo or a P_IO_2 Dependent Effect?

*Rafael Torres-Peralta[1,2], José Losa-Reyna[1,2], David Morales-Alamo[1,2], Miriam González-Izal[3], Ismael Pérez-Suárez[1,2], Jesús G. Ponce-González[1], Mikel Izquierdo[3] and José A. L. Calbet[1,2]**

[1] Department of Physical Education, University of Las Palmas de Gran Canaria, Las Palmas, Spain, [2] Research Institute of Biomedical and Health Sciences, Instituto Universitario de Investigaciones Biomédicas y Sanitarias, Las Palmas, Spain, [3] Department of Health Sciences, Public University of Navarra, Tudela, Spain

***Correspondence:**
José A. L. Calbet
lopezcalbet@gmail.com

To determine the level of hypoxia from which muscle activation (MA) is reduced during incremental exercise to exhaustion (IE), and the role played by P_IO_2 in this process, ten volunteers (21 ± 2 years) performed four IE in severe acute hypoxia (SAH) (P_IO_2 = 73 mmHg). Upon exhaustion, subjects were asked to continue exercising while the breathing gas mixture was swiftly changed to a placebo (73 mmHg) or to a higher P_IO_2 (82, 92, 99, and 142 mmHg), and the IE continued until a new exhaustion. At the second exhaustion, the breathing gas was changed to room air (normoxia) and the IE continued until the final exhaustion. MA, as reflected by the *vastus medialis* (VM) and *lateralis* (VL) EMG raw and normalized root mean square (RMSraw, and RMSNz, respectively), normalized total activation index (TAINz), and burst duration were 8–20% lower at exhaustion in SAH than in normoxia ($P < 0.05$). The switch to a placebo or higher P_IO_2 allowed for the continuation of exercise in all instances. RMSraw, RMSNz, and TAINz were increased by 5–11% when the P_IO_2 was raised from 73 to 92, or 99 mmHg, and VL and VM averaged RMSraw by 7% when the P_IO_2 was elevated from 73 to 142 mmHg ($P < 0.05$). The increase of VM-VL average RMSraw was linearly related to the increase in P_IO_2, during the transition from SAH to higher P_IO_2 ($R^2 = 0.915$, $P < 0.05$). In conclusion, increased P_IO_2 at exhaustion reduces fatigue and allows for the continuation of exercise in moderate and SAH, regardless of the effects of P_IO_2 on MA. At task failure, MA is increased during the first 10 s of increased P_IO_2 when the IE is performed at a P_IO_2 close to 73 mmHg and the P_IO_2 is increased to 92 mmHg or higher. Overall, these findings indicate that one of the central mechanisms by which severe hypoxia may cause central fatigue and task failure is by reducing the capacity for reaching the appropriate level of MA to sustain the task. The fact that at exhaustion in severe hypoxia the exercise was continued with the placebo-gas mixture demonstrates that this central mechanism has a cognitive component.

Keywords: fatigue, performance, hypoxia, altitude, muscle activation, human experimentation, exercise, oxygenation

INTRODUCTION

Muscle activation, as reflected by the root mean square of the electromyographic signal (EMG_{RMS}), is higher in severe acute hypoxia (SAH) than normoxia at the same absolute intensity, but lower in hypoxia than in normoxia at the same relative intensity (Torres-Peralta et al., 2014). Close to exhaustion, the surface integrated electromyographic (iEMG) activity is higher during constant-intensity exercise in hyperoxia ($F_IO_2 = 0.30$) than in SAH ($F_IO_2 = 0.10$) (Amann et al., 2007). This could mean that hypoxia limits the motor drive output from the central nervous system (CNS) leading to reduced muscle activation (MA) and task failure. In agreement with this idea, during exercise in severe hypoxia, fatigue is rapidly relieved by oxygenation with normoxic (Calbet et al., 2003a) or hyperoxic gas (Amann et al., 2007). If hypoxia depresses muscle activation, oxygenation should be accompanied by an immediate increase in MA while the intensity of exercise remains at the same absolute level. However, it remains unknown whether the ergogenic effect of an increase in oxygenation requires a concomitant elevation of muscle activation.

During exercise in severe acute (Calbet et al., 2003a, 2015a; Amann et al., 2007; Morales-Alamo et al., 2015) and chronic hypoxia (Kayser et al., 1994; Calbet et al., 2003b) task failure is thought to be predominantly caused by central mechanisms sensitive to reduced O_2 delivery to the brain (Goodall et al., 2012, 2014) and to reduced interstitial brain PO_2 (Amann and Calbet, 2008). A fundamental difference between exercise in severe and moderate hypoxia is the region of the hemoglobin oxygen dissociation curve (ODC) at which the gas exchange occurs in the lungs. In severe hypoxia, pulmonary gas exchange occurs in the straight region of the ODC, implying that a small increase in arterial oxygen pressure (PaO_2) would result in a greater elevation of arterial hemoglobin saturation (SaO_2) (Calbet et al., 2003a; Calbet and Lundby, 2009). In moderate hypoxia, pulmonary gas exchange occurs at the upper and flatter region of the ODC, where an improvement in PaO_2 translates into a smaller elevation of SaO_2 (Amann et al., 2007). The fact that increasing inspiratory oxygen pressure (P_IO_2) to hyperoxic levels only relieved fatigue when applied at exhaustion in severe hypoxia could indicate that a substantial elevation of arterial oxygen content (CaO_2) is required (Amann et al., 2007). However, the observation by Amann et al. (2007) that increased P_IO_2 does not relieve fatigue during moderate hypoxia could indicate that the increase in SaO_2 is even more critical than the elevation of PaO_2, since in the flatter region of the ODC the improvement of SaO_2 for a given increase of PaO_2 is smaller. It remains unknown what levels of improvement in PaO_2 and CaO_2 are required to relieve fatigue and enhance the neural activation of muscles upon exhaustion in hypoxia.

Therefore, the aims of this study were to (a) determine the influence of the level of hypoxia on a potential reduction of MA at exhaustion; (b) determine the minimum increase in P_IO_2 needed to enhance muscle activation at exhaustion in hypoxia; and (c) find out if the ergogenic effect of increasing P_IO_2 is always accompanied by enhanced muscle activation, which would be an indication of a predominantly central mechanism.

We hypothesized that an increase of P_IO_2 upon exhaustion would rapidly increase MA depending on the level of hypoxia at exhaustion and the inspiratory O_2 pressure of the breathing gas.

MATERIALS AND METHODS

Subjects

Ten healthy men (age: 21.1 ± 2.1 years, height: 173 ± 8 cm, body mass: 71 ± 9 kg, body fat: 16.6 ± 4.5%, VO_2max: 50.4 ± 4.7 $mL.kg^{-1}.min^{-1}$) agreed to participate in this investigation. After being informed about the experiments and the possible risks associated with participation they provided written consent. The study was performed by the Helsinki Declaration and was approved by the Ethical Committee of the University of Las Palmas de Gran Canaria (CEIH-2010-01 and CEIH-2009-01).

General Overview

This study was a part of a larger project that included several experiments designed to address the mechanisms limiting whole body exercise performance in humans. The results focusing on muscle metabolism and O_2 transport have been published (Calbet et al., 2015a; Morales-Alamo et al., 2015). Body composition was determined by dual-energy x-ray absorptiometry (DEXA) (Hologic QDR-1500, Hologic Corp., software version 7.10, Waltham, MA), during the familiarization sessions. The leg muscle mass was calculated from the DEXA scans using the model of Wang et al. (1999). Subjects reported to the laboratory to familiarize with maximal exercise tests in normoxia and normobaric hypoxia ($Altitrainer_{200}$, SMTEC, Switzerland) on separate days. For experimental purposes, subjects performed two sets of IE tests, here called *invasive* and *deception* test. On the first experimental day, all subjects performed the invasive tests as previously described (Calbet et al., 2015a) and on the second and third day, they completed the deception protocol. The exercise tests were carried out on a cycle ergometer (Lode Excalibur Sport 925900, Groningen, The Netherlands) and subjects were instructed to pedal at 80 revolutions per minute (rpm). To facilitate the maintenance of the targeted pedaling cadence, subjects received visual feedback, and verbal instructions when deviations of 5 or more rpm occurred.

Exercise Protocol

Invasive Experiments

Subjects reported to the laboratory at 07.00 after an overnight fast from 22.00 h. After catheterization (see below), subjects were assigned to either an IE test to exhaustion in normoxia (30 W/2 min) or hypoxia ($P_IO_2 = 73$ mmHg; 20 W/2 min; Altitrainer200, SMTEC, Switzerland), in random order and separated by 90 min rest. Before the start of the IE in hypoxia, subjects were breathing the hypoxic gas for 3 min while they were pedaling 20–40 rpm with the ergometer unloaded. At exhaustion (Exh1), the subjects were rapidly switched to breath room air (normoxia) and requested to continue the exercise at the same load for 2 min, then the load was increased by 20 W every 2 min until exhaustion (Exh2). This was followed by a lunch break (a sandwich and 200 mL of apple or pineapple juice) and a 120 min resting period. Thereafter, the IE in hypoxia was repeated. At Exh1 the subjects were requested to keep pedaling while a valve deviated the inspired flow to a 30 L anesthesia bag pre-filled with hypoxic gas (F_IO_2 = ~13.3, P_IO_2 = ~91 mmHg) and a small amount of CO (7 mL·kg^{-1} body mass). The gas was breathed in an open circuit system in a well-ventilated room until the bag was almost emptied. The valve was then returned to the previous position such that the subjects continued the incremental test at this level of hypoxia (F_IO_2: ~13.3, P_IO_2: ~91 mmHg). After 2 min at the load eliciting exhaustion, the intensity was increased by 20 W/2 min until a new exhaustion (Exh2). Again, subjects were requested to keep pedaling while they were switched to breath room air (normoxia). After 2 min, the load was increased by 20 W/2 min until exhaustion (Exh3). The invasive experiments were used to study the influence of different levels of oxygenation on the hemodynamic responses and fatigue mechanisms in hypoxia, as reported previously (Calbet et al., 2015a).

Deception Protocol (Noninvasive)

Subjects performed four IE tests on 2 different days, separated by at least 1 week. A 90 min recovery period was established between the two tests carried out on the same day (**Figure 1**), as previously done (Calbet et al., 2003a). This resting period is sufficient to allow for a full recovery of peak power output and VO_2max, as previously reported (Scharhag-Rosenberger et al., 2014; Calbet et al., 2015a). Each deception test was composed of an initial phase in severe hypoxia (P_IO_2 = 73 mmHg) (HYP1), followed by a second phase with a similar or a less severe level of hypoxia (HYP2), which continued with a final phase in normoxia (NX3). HYP1 started with an intensity of 60 or 70 W which, after 2 min was increased by 20 or 30 W every 2 min until exhaustion (Exh1). The 70 W starting load and the steps of 30 W were used in one of the subjects who was a well-trained triathlete, so the duration of his test was similar to the duration of the tests performed by the other subjects. Like during the invasive experiments, before the start of the IE in hypoxia, subjects were breathing the hypoxic gas for 3 min while they were pedaling at 20–40 rpm with the ergometer unloaded. At Exh1, the inspired gas mixture was rapidly changed to one of four different gas mixtures [P_IO_2 = 73 (placebo), 82, 92, and 99 mmHg, equivalent to 5200, 4400, 3600, and 3100 m above sea level, respectively]. Subjects were told and believed that they were getting normoxic gas at exhaustion. These gas mixtures were administered in random order and with a double-blind design. After 2 min at the load eliciting Exh1, the load was increased by 20 or 30 W every 2 min until exhaustion (Exh2). At Exh2, the gas mixture was rapidly changed to room air (P_IO_2 = 142 mmHg) while the subjects were strongly encouraged to continue pedaling. After 2 min at the load eliciting Exh2, the load was increased by 20 or 30 W every 2 min until exhaustion (Exh3). Although the change of P_IO_2 upon exhaustion was intended to be maintained for 2 min before increasing the load, in some instances, for example during the placebo experiments, subjects fatigued before reaching 2 min in the new oxygenation condition. In these cases, the breathing gas mixture was rapidly changed to normoxia, maintained for 2 min in normoxia, and then increased by 20 or 30 W every 2 min until exhaustion. Exhaustion during the IE tests was defined by either the subject stopping pedaling or dropping pedaling rate below 60 rpm during 5 s (or earlier if the cadence was dropping very fast), despite strong verbal encouragement. A 30 L anesthesia bag was prefilled with the target F_IO_2 and used as a buffer in the transition to HYP2, to gain few seconds to adjust the Altitrainer in such a way that the target F_IO_2 was instantaneously administered at the start of the transition. During the first 10–12 s of the transitions the subjects breathed from the anesthesia bag, then a four-way valve was used to direct the inspiratory port to either the Altitrainer or room air. These 10 s (bag breathing) were used to stabilize the Altitrainer at the target F_IO_2 corresponding to each HYP2 phase.

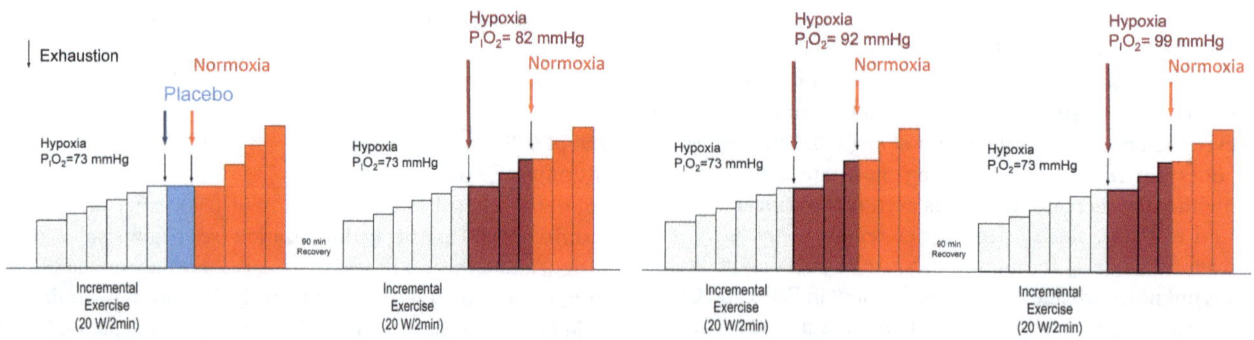

FIGURE 1 | Experimental protocol. Each experimental day the subjects performed two incremental exercise tests in random order. The incremental exercise test always began in severe hypoxia (P_IO_2 = 73 mmHg). At exhaustion (Exh1) the breathing gas mixture was swiftly changed to another one with a greater oxygen PO_2, except in one instance that the gas administered was the same one the subjects were breathing in severe acute hypoxia, i.e., P_IO_2 = 73 mmHg, to create a placebo condition. Subjects were asked to continue the exercise and after 2 min at the load eliciting Exh1, the load was increased by 20 or 30 W/2 min until exhaustion (Exh2). Once again, subjects were asked to keep pedaling while the gas mixture was swiftly changed to normoxia. After 2 min at the load eliciting Exh2, the intensity was increased by 20 or 30 W/2 min until the final exhaustion (Exh 3). Between Exh1 and Exh2, the breathing gas mixtures used corresponded to P_IO_2 of 73, 82, 92, 99, and 142 mmHg (Normoxia) and were administered following a double-blind design. Subjects were asked to pedal close to 80 rpm. However, when approaching exhaustion, the pedaling rate was always reduced.

Oxygen Uptake and Hemoglobin Oxygen Saturation

Oxygen uptake was measured with a metabolic cart (Vmax N29; Sensormedics, California, USA), calibrated before each test according to the manufacturer instructions. Respiratory variables were analyzed breath-by-breath and averaged every 10 s for the analysis of transitions at exhaustion. Hemoglobin oxygen saturation was estimated with a finger pulse oximeter (SpO_2) (OEM III module, 4549-000, Plymouth, MN).

Electromyography

Electrical MA was monitored using surface electromyography (EMG) (**Figure 2**). EMG signals were continuously recorded from the *vastus medialis* and *vastus lateralis*, as previously reported (Torres-Peralta et al., 2016). Before the application of the EMG electrodes, the skin surface was carefully shaved, and wiped with ethanol to reduce skin impedance. Bipolar single differential electrodes were placed longitudinally on the muscles following the SENIAM recommendations (Merletti and Hermens, 2000) and taped on the skin to minimize movement artifacts. The reference electrode was placed on the skin over the acromion. The position of the electrodes was marked on the skin with indelible ink, and these references were used for precise electrode placement in repeated experiments.

The EMG signals were acquired using a 16-channel recording system (Myomonitor IV, Delsys Inc., Boston, MA) at a sampling rate of 1000 Hz using rectangular shaped (19.8 mm wide and 35 mm long) bipolar surface electrodes with 1×10 mm 99.9% Ag conductors, and with an inter-conductor distance of 10 mm (DE-2.3 Delsys Inc.). The EMG data were filtered with a high-pass filter of 20 Hz and a low-pass filter of 450 Hz using a fifth-order Butterworth filter. The system has an input impedance of $>10^{15}\Omega$ per 0.2pF of input capacitance, a common mode rejection ratio of >80 dB, signal-to-noise ratio $< 1.2\ \mu V$, and a pre-amplifier gain 1000 V/V ±1 %. Each pedal revolution was detected using an electrogoniometer (Goniometer Biosignal Sensor S700 Joint Angle Shape Sensor; Delsys Inc. Boston) fixed on the left knee and sampled at 500 Hz. The electrogoniometer was individually calibrated taking as references the knee angles in fully extended and flexed positions. EMG and joint movement were simultaneously recorded by a portable device (Myomonitor IV, Delsys Inc. Boston) and wirelessly transmitted to a computer

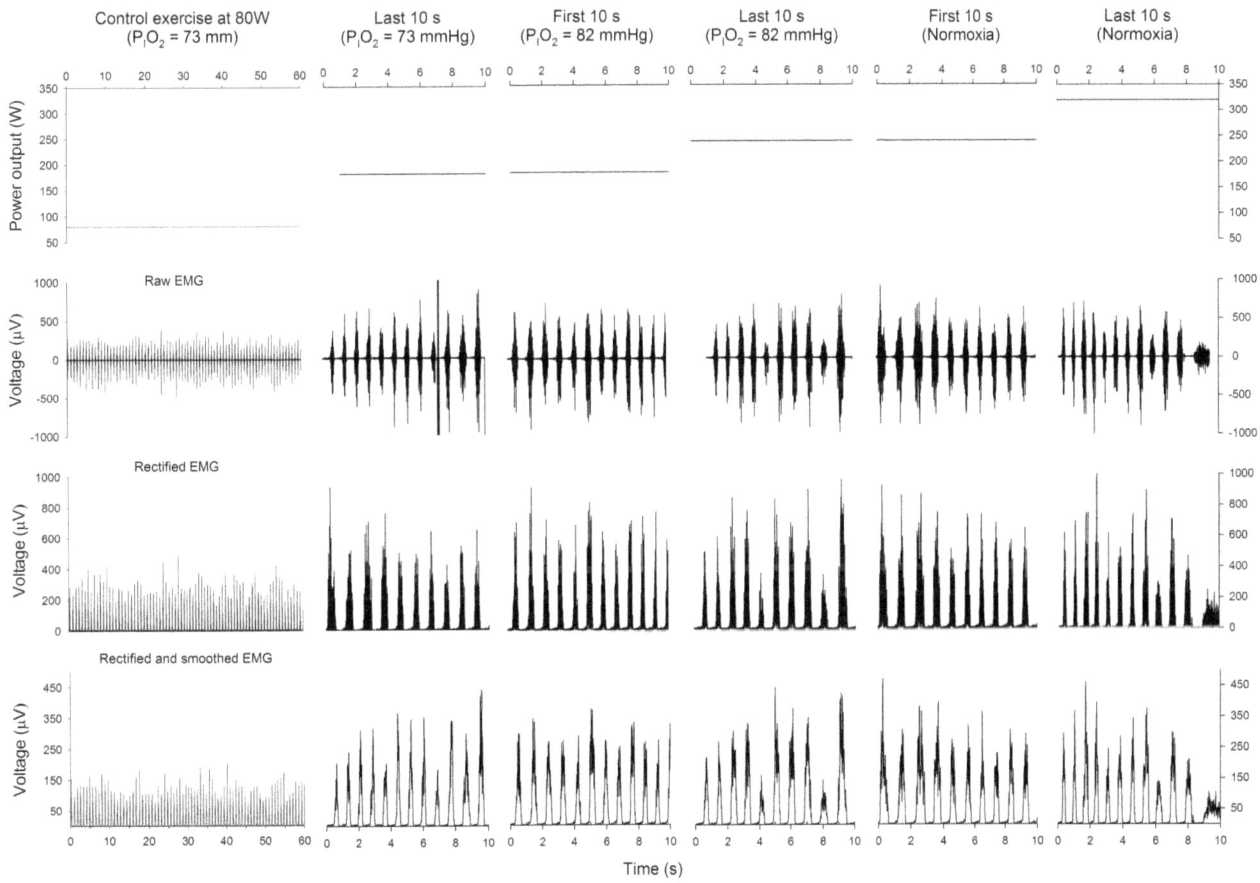

FIGURE 2 | Power output and EMG. Schematic representation of the power output (upper panels), raw EMG (2nd row), rectified EMG (3th row), and rectified and smoothed EMG (lower panels), during the last 60 s of the control submaximal exercise at 80 W in hypoxia (P_IO_2 = 73 mmHg), the last 10 s of the incremental exercise (IE) in severe hypoxia (P_IO_2 = 73 mmHg), the first 10 s of the transition from a P_IO_2 of 73 to 82 mmHg, the last 10 s of the IE at a P_IO_2 of 82 mmHg, the first 10 s in normoxia and the last 10 s before task failure in normoxia.

(EMGWorks Wireless application and EMGWorks Acquisition 3.7.1.3; Delsys, Inc. Boston).

The EMG signal corresponding to each muscle contraction was analyzed using code developed "in house" (Matlab R2012b, MathWorks, Natick, MA, USA). The EMG recordings were full-wave rectified and smoothed to provide an index of muscle activation; the amplitude characteristics were analyzed via average RMS of a 25-ms moving window for the duration of the contraction burst. Contraction burst onset and offset detection were determined using 20% of the maximal EMG_{RMS} activity of each contraction burst as a reference (Baum and Li, 2003; Hug and Dorel, 2009; Torres-Peralta et al., 2014), rather than a mean threshold value from 15 consecutive contraction bursts (Ozgunen et al., 2010). This approach yielded the same result as direct, simple visual discrimination, with 100% detection of all contraction bursts. Contraction timing was defined as the time elapsed from the knee at is greatest extension to the start of the contraction burst, expressed as a percentage of the full duration of each revolution. The EMG_{RMS} recorded during the last minute of a 2 min 80 W load (in hypoxia, $P_IO_2 = 73$ mmHg) was used to normalize the remaining EMG_{RMS} data. Besides, we defined a total activity index (TAI) as TAI = EMG_{RMS} × burst duration (ms) × number of pedal strokes during the period of time analyzed. The total activity index is similar to the integrated EMG signal, but was computed separately for each contraction burst and excluded the baseline EMG between contraction bursts (Torres-Peralta et al., 2014). The TAI recorded during the last minute of a 2 min 80 W load (in hypoxia) was used to normalize the rest of the TAI values.

The mean (MPF) and median (MdPF) power spectrum frequencies were calculated using Fast Fourier Transform (Solomonow et al., 1990). All variables were reported as the mean values of the pedal strokes recorded during the last 10 and 30 s of the incremental exercise. EMG data are reported separately for *vastus medialis* (VM) and *lateralis* (VL), and also as the average of the two muscles.

Calculation of the Improvement in SaO_2 during the First 10 s of the Transitions

The mean change in SaO_2 needed to explain the mean improvement in VO_2 observed during the first 10 s of the transition from hypoxia to higher a P_IO_2 was calculated by solving the Fick equation, using arterial blood gasses and thermodilution cardiac output data obtained in normoxia and hypoxia ($P_IO_2 = 73$ mmHg) in parallel invasive experiments performed by the same subjects (Calbet et al., 2015a). Since similar levels of peak cardiac output were reached in severe hypoxia and normoxia, it was assumed that the level of cardiac output reached at exhaustion at intermediate P_IO_2 levels (i.e., 82, 92, and 99 mmHg) must have been similar to that measured in normoxia. It was also assumed that cardiac output remained unchanged during the first 10 s of the transition, given the stability of heart rate during the transitions and the high dependency of cardiac output on the absolute exercise intensity (Calbet and Lundby, 2009; Calbet et al., 2009a, 2015b), which remained unchanged during the first 10 s of the transition.

Statistics

Normal distribution of variables was checked using the Shapiro-Wilks test. Since variables were normally distributed, differences between tests at Exh1 were determined using one-way repeated measures analysis of variance (ANOVA). The Mauchly's test of sphericity was run before the ANOVA and in the case of violation of the sphericity assumption the degrees of freedom were adjusted according to the Huynh and Feldt test. Pairwise comparisons at specific time points were performed with Student's paired *t*-tests and adjusted for multiple comparisons with the Holm–Bonferroni method. Since no significant differences were observed at exhaustion between the four tests in severe hypoxia ($P_IO_2 = 73$ mmHg), these four tests were averaged to obtain a representative value for exhaustion at a P_IO_2 of 73 mmHg. The same procedure was used to test for differences between the four IE tests ending in normoxia (Exh3). Similar results were obtained in the four tests at exhaustion in normoxia (Exh3) and hence, the values obtained in these four tests were also averaged to generate a single value representing normoxia. These two averages were compared with Student's paired *t*-tests. The effect of increasing P_IO_2 at exhaustion on all dependent variables was assessed using a two-way ANOVA for repeated measures with two factors: breathing gas (two levels: pre- vs. post-switch to the new breathing gas) and P_IO_2 (four levels), followed by pairwise comparisons using Student's paired *t*-tests adjusted for multiple comparisons with the Holm–Bonferroni method. The relationships between changes in P_IO_2 and the changes in the dependent variables were tested using linear regression analysis. To compare the first 10 s of the transition between the first and the second transition, an average value for the four conditions of each transition was calculated. This generated a single value per subject for the first and another unique value per subject for the second transition. The two transitions were compared with a paired Student's *t*-test. Values are reported as the mean ± standard deviation (unless otherwise stated). $P \leq 0.05$ was considered statistically significant. All statistical analyses were performed using SPSS v.15.0 for Windows (SPSS Inc., Chicago, IL) and Excel 2011 (Microsoft, Redmond, WA, USA).

RESULTS

Maximal Exercise in Severe Acute Hypoxia ($P_IO_2 = 73$ mmHg) and Normoxia ($P_IO_2 = 142$ mmHg)

As shown in **Table 1**, SpO_2, power output at exhaustion (Wmax), VO_2peak, pulmonary ventilation at exhaustion (V_E), respiratory rate (RR), heart rate at exhaustion (HR), end-tidal O_2 pressure ($P_{ET}O_2$), end-tidal CO_2 pressure ($P_{ET}CO_2$), and carbon dioxide production (VCO_2) were lower during the last 30 s of exercise in severe hypoxia than in normoxia, while the respiratory exchange ratio (RER) was higher in hypoxia than in normoxia (all $P \leq 0.05$).

TABLE 1 | Ergospirometric and electromyographic responses during the last 30 s of the incremental exercise to exhaustion in normoxia ($P_IO_2 \approx$ 142 mmHg) and severe hypoxia ($P_IO_2 \approx$ 73 mmHg).

	Hypoxia (P_IO_2= 73 mmHg)	Normoxia	P
F_IO_2 (%)	10.8 ± 0.07	20.8 ± 0.04	< 0.001
SpO_2 (%)	63.8 ± 5.7	92.8 ± 3.1	< 0.001
Wmax (W)	170.5 ± 17.9	213 ± 19.7	< 0.001
VO_2peak (L.min^{-1})	2.28 ± 0.19	3.44 ± 0.43	< 0.001
V_E (L.min^{-1})	115.2 ± 18.6	124.8 ± 15.6	< 0.001
RR (breaths.min^{-1})	50.6 ± 7.0	55.9 ± 7.1	< 0.001
HR (beats.min^{-1})	179.0 ± 8.4	184.8 ± 5.2	< 0.001
$P_{ET}O_2$ (mmHg)	51.3 ± 2.3	108.2 ± 7.4	< 0.001
$P_{ET}CO_2$ (mmHg)	28.1 ± 2.5	30.8 ± 3.1	< 0.001
RER	1.34 ± 0.13	1.05 ± 0.06	< 0.001
VCO_2 (L.min^{-1})	3.06 ± 0.36	3.55 ± 0.41	< 0.001
RPM	71.9 ± 4.1	68.4 ± 4.2	0.08
VM RMSraw (μV)	111.2 ± 38.6	128.3 ± 42.4	< 0.01
VL RMSraw (μV)	97.5 ± 30.8	110.4 ± 28.0	< 0.01
Average RMSraw (μV)	104.4 ± 29.0	119.4 ± 28.8	< 0.005
VM RMSNz (A.U.)	178.1 ± 35.2	209.2 ± 58.4	< 0.05
VL RMSNz (A.U.)	173.3 ± 35.4	200.0 ± 49.1	< 0.005
Average RMSNz (A.U.)	175.4 ± 31.2	204.6 ± 50.3	< 0.01
VM TAINz (A.U.)	111.5 ± 33.5	138.7 ± 47.8	< 0.005
VL TAINz (A.U.)	97.3 ± 21.0	117.4 ± 22.7	< 0.001
Average TAINz (A.U.)	102.9 ± 25.5	126.7 ± 30.9	< 0.001
VM MPF (Hz)	89.8 ± 16.9	85.2 ± 16.6	< 0.001
VL MPF (Hz)	89.6 ± 16.5	85.5 ± 17.1	< 0.001
Average MPF (Hz)	89.7 ± 16.7	85.4 ± 16.9	< 0.001
VM MdPF (Hz)	71.3 ± 12.1	69.2 ± 11.8	0.06
VL MdPF (Hz)	70.6 ± 12.1	68.9 ± 12.2	0.06
Average MdPF (Hz)	70.9 ± 12.1	69.0 ± 12.0	0.06
VM Burst (ms)	305.4 ± 51.5	334.3 ± 34.8	< 0.05
VL Burst (ms)	283.0 ± 34.5	306.2 ± 26.7	< 0.05
Average Burst (ms)	294.2 ± 42.1	320.2 ± 29.6	< 0.05

F_IO_2, inspiratory oxygen fraction; SpO_2, hemoglobin saturation in capillary blood measured by pulse oximetry; Wmax, power output at exhaustion; VO_2, oxygen consumption; V_E, pulmonary ventilation; RR, respiratory rate; HR, heart rate; $P_{ET}O_2$, end-tidal O_2 pressure; $P_{ET}CO_2$, end-tidal CO_2 pressure; RER, respiratory exchange ratio; VCO_2, CO_2 production; RPM, revolutions per minute; VL, vastus lateralis; VM, vastus medialis; RMSraw, raw root mean square; RMSNz, normalized root mean square; TAINz, normalized total activation index (arbitrary units, A.U.); MPF, mean power frequency; MdPF, median power frequency; Burst, contraction burst duration. n = 10.

Muscle activation, as reflected by VM and VL raw and normalized RMS, total activation index and contraction burst duration was 8–20% lower in hypoxia than normoxia ($P < 0.05$) (**Table 1**). In contrast, MPF was 5% lower in normoxia than hypoxia ($P < 0.001$) and a similar trend was observed for MdPF (**Table 1**).

Effect of Increased P_IO_2 on cardiorespiratory and EMG Variables

Increased P_IO_2 allowed for the continuation of exercise during 41.9 ± 19.8, 60.7 ± 30.2, 72.9 ± 52.0, and 170.5 ± 70.8 s for the transition from a P_IO_2 of 73 mmHg to placebo, 82, 92, and 99 mmHg, respectively, (all $P < 0.05$, compared to the end exercise in severe acute hypoxia). There was a linear relationship between the duration of the new oxygenation phases and the increase of P_IO_2 (time (s) = 35.1+ 4.86· ΔP_IO_2; $R^2 = 0.955$, $P < 0.001$, $n = 8$), where ΔP_IO_2 represents the increase in P_IO_2 in mmHg (**Figure 3A**). A similar relationship was obtained between endurance time and the estimated improvement in SaO_2 (time (s) $= 21.1 + 9.17 \cdot \Delta S_aO_2$; $R^2 = 0.973$, $P < 0.001$, $n = 8$) (**Figure 3B**).

Compared to the mean values observed during the last 10 s of exercise in severe hypoxia ($P_IO_2 = 73$ mmHg), $P_{ET}O_2$, and VO_2 were increased, and RER reduced during the first 10 s following the increase in oxygenation (**Tables 2** and **3**). SpO_2 was only significantly increased in transitions to normoxia (**Table 3**), in part due to the slow response time of the pulse oximeter. These effects were more accentuated the greater the difference in P_IO_2 between the hypoxic and the increased P_IO_2 condition.

Transition from Severe Hypoxia (P_IO_2 of 73 mmHg) to Higher Levels of P_IO_2

VL and VM RMSraw, RMSNz and TAINz were all enhanced by increasing the P_IO_2 at exhaustion (ANOVA main breathing gas effect $P < 0.05$) (**Table 2**). VM and VL RMSraw, as well as the VM-VL average RMSraw, were increased by 5–10% when the P_IO_2 was raised from 73 to 92, or 99 mmHg (**Table 2**). VL RMSraw and the VM-VL average RMSraw were also increased when the P_IO_2 was raised from 73 to 142 mmHg (**Table 3**). MPF and MdPF remained at the same level with the increase of P_IO_2.

Transition to Normoxia

As depicted in **Table 3**, increasing P_IO_2 from different hypoxia conditions to normoxia was also associated to increased VM and VL RMSraw and RMSNz, as well at VM TAINz and VM-VL Average TAINz (ANOVA breathing gas main effect $P < 0.05$) (**Table 3**). When the data from the two conditions with greater levels of hypoxia (P_IO_2 of 73 and 82 mmHg) were averaged, increasing P_IO_2 at exhaustion to normoxia significantly increased MA (RMSraw and RMSNz) and the normalized TAI ($P < 0.05$). However, this was not the case when the data from the less hypoxic conditions (P_IO_2 of 92 and 99 mmHg) were averaged, for which the transition to higher P_IO_2 did not result in significantly greater muscle activation. In general, MPF and MdPF remained at the same level or changed slightly with the transition to an increased P_IO_2.

We also analyzed the 10 s comprised between the 5th and the 15th second after the start of the transition and compared these 10 s with the last 10 s of the preceding exercise phase. The results of this analysis were essentially similar to those described above, i.e., increasing P_IO_2 at exhaustion resulted in increased MA (RMSraw and RMSNz), particularly when fatigue occurred at high levels of hypoxia (P_IO_2 of 73 and 82 mmHg).

In general, the pedaling rate was augmented with increased oxygenation at the transition from different levels of hypoxia to normoxia, and consequently, the duration of the contraction bursts was reduced (**Table 3**). At the same time, the start of the

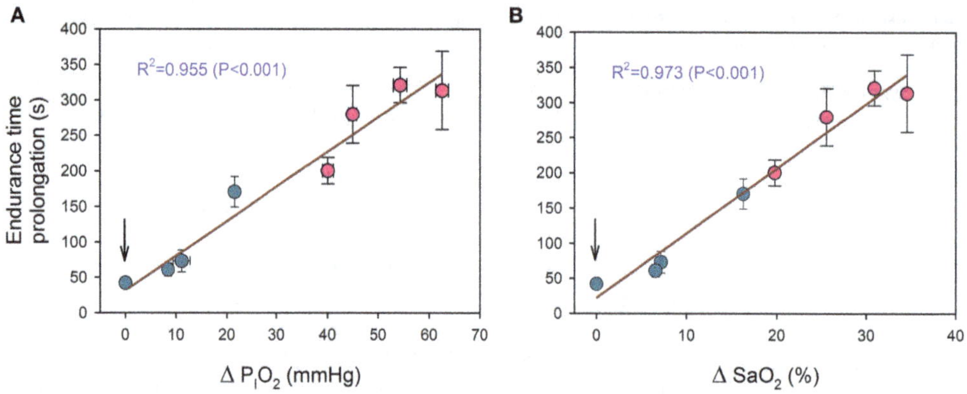

FIGURE 3 | Relationship between the duration of new oxygenation phases with: (A) the increase of P_IO_2 (ΔP_IO_2) and (B) the estimated improvement in arterial saturation (ΔSaO_2). Green circles: transitions from severe hypoxia (P_IO_2 = 73 mmHg) to placebo (vertical arrow) and moderate hypoxia; red circles: transitions from different levels of hypoxia (P_IO_2 of 73, 82, 92, and 99 mmHg) to normoxia. Each point corresponds to the mean of 10 subjects.

contraction bursts occurred slightly earlier with an increase in oxygenation from a P_IO_2 of 73 mmHg to normoxia.

The First Transition Compared with the Second Transition

In the first transition, the P_IO_2 was increased from severe hypoxia (P_IO_2 = 73 mmHg) to less hypoxic levels, while during the second transition the P_IO_2 was increased from different levels of hypoxia to normoxia. We calculated a mean value for the four P_IO_2 conditions of the first transition and compared it with the mean value calculated using the four conditions of the second transition, including in the analysis only the breath-by-breath data collected during the first 10 s of each transition. The mean P_IO_2 during the first and second transition was 84.3 ± 2.1, and 137.5 ± 3.0 mmHg, respectively, ($P < 0.001$); while SpO_2 was 64.1 ± 4.8 and 72.0 ± 4.7%, respectively, ($P < 0.001$). The mean exercise intensity at which the first and second transitions occurred was 170.5 ± 17.9 and 173.5 ± 16.3 W ($P = 0.08$). The mean response of heart rate, pulmonary ventilation, respiratory rate and tidal volume were similar in both transitions (**Figures 4A–D**, respectively). In contrast, the $P_{ET}CO_2$, $P_{ET}O_2$, VO_2, and VCO_2 were higher during the second transition (**Figures 4E–H**, respectively).

Muscle activation was 6% higher during second compared to the first transition, as reflected by the VM, VL, and VM-VL average RMSraw values (P <0.05) (**Figure 5A**). Similar results were obtained for the VM and VM-VL average RMSNz, which were 8 and 7% higher during the second compared to the first transition, respectively ($P < 0.05$) (**Figure 5B**). The VM, VL, and VM-VL average TAINz values were 8-10% higher during the second than the first transition ($P < 0.05$) (**Figure 5C**). VM, VL, and VM-VL average mean and median power frequencies were 4–6% lower during the second than the first transition ($P < 0.001$) (**Figures 5D** and **E**). The start of the burst occurred slightly earlier in the pedaling cycle during the second compared to the first transition for the VM and VM-VL average values, respectively, ($P < 0.05$) (**Figure 5F**). The duration of the burst and the mean pedaling rates were similar during both transitions ($P > 0.56$) (**Figures 5G** and **H**).

Importance of the Magnitude of the Change in P_IO_2 and the Pre-existing Level of Hypoxia on the Response to an Increase in P_IO_2

As reflected in **Figure 6**, the changes of $P_{ET}O_2$, VO_2, the duration of the bursts and pedaling rate (PR) were linearly related to the increase in P_IO_2 as shown in the equations:

$$\Delta VO_2 = 0.0277 \cdot \Delta P_IO_2 - 0.0514 (R^2 = 0.990; P < 0.001; n = 8); \quad \text{Equation 1, (Figure 6A)}$$

$$\Delta P_{ET}O_2 = 0.654 \cdot \Delta P_IO_2 - 0.852 (R^2 = 0.997; P < 0.001; n = 8); \quad \text{Equation 2, (Figure 6B)}$$

$$\Delta BD = 16.33 - 1.127 \cdot \Delta P_IO_2 (R^2 = 0.941; P < 0.001; n = 8); \quad \text{Equation 3, (Figure 6E)}$$

$$\Delta PR = 0.082 - 1.122 \cdot \Delta P_IO_2 (R^2 = 0.917; P < 0.001; n = 8); \quad \text{Equation 4, (Figure 6F)}$$

Where ΔVO_2 is expressed in L·min^{-1}; $\Delta P_{ET}O_2$ and ΔP_IO_2 in mmHg; BD in ms, and PR in rpm.

The VM-VL average RMSraw was linearly related to the increase in P_IO_2, but only in the transitions from a P_IO_2 of 73 mmHg to a higher P_IO_2 [Δ RMSraw (μV) = 1.945 + 0.449 · ΔP_IO_2 ($R^2 = 0.915$; $P < 0.05$, $n = 4$)] (**Figure 6C**). This relationship was lost after normalization of the RMS (**Figure 6D**).

Placebo Effects

In the placebo transition, subjects believed that they were receiving normoxia upon exhaustion in severe hypoxia; however, they were maintained at the same level of hypoxia. No significant changes were observed in MA (RMSNz and TAINz) as a consequence of this placebo treatment (**Table 2**).

TABLE 2 | Cardiorespiratory responses during the last 10 s of an incremental exercise to exhaustion in severe hypoxia (P_IO_2 = 73 mmHg) and during the first 10 s of oxygenation with different gas mixtures.

	Exhaustion P_IO_2 = 73 mmHg	Start of P_IO_2 = 99 mmHg	Exhaustion P_IO_2 = 73 mmHg	Start of P_IO_2 = 92 mmHg	Exhaustion P_IO_2 = 73 mmHg	Start of P_IO_2 = 82 mmHg	Exhaustion P_IO_2 = 73 mmHg	Start of P_IO_2 = 73 mmHg
F_IO_2 (%)	10.78 ± 0.10	13.92 ± 0.23^{c}	10.82 ± 0.12	12.45 ± 0.75^{c}	10.78 ± 0.06	12.01 ± 0.25^{c}	10.79 ± 0.08	10.79 ± 0.20¶§‡
SpO_2 (%)	62.4 ± 5.2	63.1 ± 5.5	64.3 ± 5.5	65.1 ± 5.7	63.5 ± 5.8	63.6 ± 5.9	64.7 ± 4.9	64.4 ± 5.7‡
Wmax (W)	172.0 ± 23.5	172.0 ± 23.5	170.0 ± 21.6	170.0 ± 21.6	168.0 ± 16.9	168.0 ± 16.9	172.0 ± 21.5	172.0 ± 21.5
VO_2peak (L.min^{-1})	2.32 ± 0.17	2.81 ± 0.46^{b}	2.23 ± 0.25	2.53 ± 0.34^{a}	2.33 ± 0.15	2.45 ± 0.27^{T}	2.27 ± 0.29	2.29 ± 0.32¶§‡
V_E (L.min^{-1})	118.2 ± 23.7	111.8 ± 20.8	114.8 ± 26.3	116.8 ± 22.6	117.5 ± 16.4	116.4 ± 15.1	114.8 ± 14.7	116.8 ± 15.6
RR (breaths.min^{-1})	51.7 ± 9.2	48.1 ± 7.2	51.3 ± 8.5	50.7 ± 8.2	51.5 ± 8.4	51.1 ± 7.6	51.3 ± 7.0	52.3 ± 7.7
HR (beats.min^{-1})	179.0 ± 10.2	179.3 ± 10.1	180.5 ± 8.2	181.0 ± 7.4	177.3 ± 7.4	177.5 ± 7.2	180.6 ± 7.9	180.8 ± 8.3¶
$P_{ET}O_2$ (mmHg)	51.4 ± 3.0	62.9 ± 5.1^{c}	51.7 ± 3.1	58.1 ± 6.3^{c}	51.4 ± 2.9	56.1 ± 3.9^{c}	51.6 ± 2.0	51.9 ± 2.0¶§‡
$P_{ET}CO_2$ (mmHg)	27.3 ± 2.9	27.3 ± 4.3	28.3 ± 2.9	28.4 ± 2.7	27.4 ± 3.7	27.6 ± 3.0	28.5 ± 2.3	28.2 ± 2.4
RER	1.32 ± 0.17	1.16 ± 0.15^{T}	1.36 ± 0.15	1.28 ± 0.13	1.32 ± 0.15	1.28 ± 0.15	1.36 ± 0.14	1.37 ± 0.17§
VCO_2 (L.min^{-1})	3.06 ± 0.42	3.01 ± 0.44	3.03 ± 0.48	3.12 ± 0.41	3.07 ± 0.29	3.06 ± 0.28	3.08 ± 0.41	3.11 ± 0.39
RPM	63.6 ± 9.4	66.3 ± 10.3	68.5 ± 7.0	71.3 ± 11.4	67.1 ± 9.5	68.2 ± 12.0	71.2 ± 7.8	70.0 ± 9.3
VM RMSraw (μV)	105.9 ± 37.2	119.3 ± 43.5^{c}	106.3 ± 42.6	112.2 ± 38.1^{a}	113.5 ± 42.7	120.6 ± 50.2^{T}	97.2 ± 43.0	99.7 ± 42.6¶‡
VL RMSraw (μV)	108.8 ± 38.4	119.1 ± 39.9^{c}	97.3 ± 48.9	102.0 ± 49.2^{a}	115.8 ± 49.9	114.1 ± 45.1	85.9 ± 35.5	87.4 ± 40.6¶
Average RMSraw (μV)	107.4 ± 29.1	119.2 ± 33.4^{c}	101.8 ± 41.5	107.1 ± 39.1^{b}	114.7 ± 39.2	117.3 ± 40.6	91.5 ± 34.9	93.6 ± 38.0¶‡
VM RMSNz (A.U.)	176.2 ± 48.1	195.8 ± 56.9^{c}	178.0 ± 58.4	191.2 ± 57.2^{a}	180.9 ± 50.4	187.6 ± 41.7	164.8 ± 67.2	168.6 ± 64.2¶
VL RMSNz (A.U.)	182.5 ± 55.5	199.6 ± 52.2^{c}	160.2 ± 38.8	171.1 ± 35.5^{a}	189.6 ± 67.0	185.6 ± 45.4	151.7 ± 49.2	152.3 ± 51.7¶‡
Average RMSNz (A.U.)	179.4 ± 49.8	197.7 ± 52.5^{c}	169.1 ± 47.0	181.2 ± 45.0^{a}	185.2 ± 56.4	186.6 ± 40.2	158.2 ± 56.8	160.5 ± 56.9¶‡
VM TAINz (A.U.)	39.6 ± 17.6	44.5 ± 19.5^{b}	35.6 ± 14.8	38.0 ± 12.5	37.1 ± 14.1	37.6 ± 11.1	33.5 ± 13.3	35.5 ± 14.1¶
VL TAINz (A.U.)	36.8 ± 13.5	41.2 ± 14.4^{c}	30.2 ± 9.7	32.8 ± 7.1	37.1 ± 12.6	35.8 ± 8.7	29.3 ± 8.8	31.6 ± 14.0¶
Average TAINz (A.U.)	38.2 ± 15.4	42.8 ± 16.9^{c}	32.9 ± 11.8	35.4 ± 9.5	37.1 ± 13.2	36.7 ± 9.6	31.4 ± 10.6	33.6 ± 13.3¶
VM MPF (Hz)	96.0 ± 24.8	95.1 ± 24.2	89.2 ± 22.8	91.5 ± 23.9	91.2 ± 17.3	89.8 ± 15.0	84.9 ± 15.5	83.6 ± 13.8
VL MPF (Hz)	97.0 ± 27.0	96.0 ± 27.5	88.9 ± 22.6	90.2 ± 23.2	91.2 ± 17.3	89.5 ± 15.5	84.9 ± 15.9	83.5 ± 14.4
Average MPF (Hz)	96.5 ± 25.9	95.5 ± 25.7	89.1 ± 22.7	90.9 ± 23.5	91.2 ± 17.3	89.6 ± 15.3	84.9 ± 15.7	83.5 ± 14.1
VM MdPF (Hz)	76.3 ± 17.1	76.9 ± 17.1	70.3 ± 15.7	72.7 ± 14.7	70.8 ± 13.2	71.8 ± 11.6	66.9 ± 10.3	66.2 ± 10.5
VL MdPF (Hz)	77.8 ± 19.7	77.6 ± 20.0	69.8 ± 15.9	70.9 ± 15.0	70.7 ± 13.2	71.4 ± 12.0	66.4 ± 10.8	65.6 ± 10.2
Average MdPF (Hz)	77.0 ± 18.3	77.3 ± 18.4	70.0 ± 15.8	71.8 ± 14.7	70.8 ± 13.2	71.6 ± 11.7	66.7 ± 10.5	65.9 ± 10.3§
VM Burst (ms)	361.5 ± 110.1	349.9 ± 85.9	310.7 ± 88.3	305.1 ± 81.2	310.3 ± 62.5	304.9 ± 94.7	309.3 ± 80.7	318.2 ± 74.7
VL Burst (ms)	343.2 ± 91.7	324.8 ± 81.7	297.8 ± 55.6	300.1 ± 70.7	310.2 ± 59.7	303.9 ± 91.5	300.0 ± 63.7	316.5 ± 86.6
Average Burst (ms)	352.4 ± 95.3	337.3 ± 79.0	304.3 ± 71.3	302.6 ± 75.4	310.2 ± 60.8	304.4 ± 93.0	304.7 ± 71.0	317.4 ± 76.5
VM Timing (%)	48.8 ± 3.8	47.6 ± 4.2^{a}	49.4 ± 2.5	49.1 ± 3.2	49.4 ± 2.3	49.3 ± 2.9	47.9 ± 3.9	48.3 ± 4.2‡
VL Timing (%)	50.7 ± 2.1	50.0 ± 2.3	50.2 ± 2.3	49.9 ± 2.5	50.3 ± 2.1	50.3 ± 2.4	49.5 ± 2.9	49.6 ± 3.0
Average Timing (%)	49.7 ± 2.6	48.8 ± 2.7	49.8 ± 2.3	49.5 ± 2.7	49.8 ± 2.2	49.8 ± 2.6	48.7 ± 3.4	49.0 ± 3.5

F_IO_2, inspiratory oxygen fraction; SpO_2, hemoglobin saturation in capillary blood measured by pulse oximetry; Wmax, power output at exhaustion; VO_2, oxygen consumption; V_E, pulmonary ventilation; RR, respiratory rate; HR, heart rate; $P_{ET}O_2$, end-tidal O_2 pressure; $P_{ET}CO_2$, end-tidal CO_2 pressure; RER, respiratory exchange ratio; VCO_2, CO_2 production; RPM, revolutions per minute; VL, vastus lateralis; VM, vastus medialis; RMSraw, raw root mean square; RMSNz, normalized root mean square; TAINz: normalized total activation index (arbitrary units, A.U.); MPF, mean power frequency; MdPF, median power frequency; Burst, contraction burst duration; Timing: start of activation expressed as percentage of total revolution duration. $^{a}P < 0.05$; $^{b}P < 0.01$; $^{c}P < 0.001$; and $^{T}P < 0.1$ (F_IO_2 = 73 mmHg vs. new gas mixture). $^{\P}P < 0.05$ ANOVA breathing gas switch main effect; $^{\S}P < 0.05$ ANOVA oxygenation level main effect; $^{\ddagger}P < 0.05$ ANOVA breathing gas switch x oxygenation level interaction; $n = 10$.

DISCUSSION

This study shows that MA during the last 10–30 s of an IE to exhaustion is lower in SAH than in normoxia, while at exhaustion in moderate hypoxia MA was similar to that observed at exhaustion in normoxia. We have shown that during exercise at different levels of hypoxia, increasing P_IO_2 at exhaustion with normoxic or less hypoxic gas mixtures rapidly relieves fatigue and allows for the continuation of exercise. This effect is accompanied by increased MA only when the level of hypoxia during the exercise eliciting exhaustion was severe (P_IO_2 of 73 mmHg, equivalent to an altitude close to 5200 m) and the P_IO_2 was increased to 92 mmHg or higher and the estimated SaO_2 to 70% or higher. Nevertheless, the close linear relationship between the increase in MA (average of VM and VL RMSraw) and the increase in P_IO_2 (**Figure 6C**) indicates that during exercise in SAH any small increase in P_IO_2 could have a positive effect on muscle activation. This is also supported by the fact that during the first 10 s of the transitions, MA was higher during the second than the first transition, despite the fact

TABLE 3 | Cardiorespiratory responses during the last 10 s of an incremental exercise to exhaustion in different levels of hypoxia (P_IO_2 = 73, 82, 92, and 99 mmHg) and during the first 10 s of oxygenation to normoxia (P_IO_2 = 142 mmHg).

	Exhaustion P_IO_2 = 99 mmHg	Start of Normoxia	Exhaustion P_IO_2 = 92 mmHg	Start of Normoxia	Exhaustion P_IO_2 = 82 mmHg	Start of Normoxia	Exhaustion P_IO_2 = 73 mmHg	Start of Normoxia
F_IO_2 (%)	14.42 ± 0.12	20.26 ± 0.46[c]	13.41 ± 0.39	19.99 ± 0.53[c]	11.98 ± 0.21	19.90 ± 0.62[c]	10.91 ± 0.44	20.02 ± 0.74[c¶§‡]
SpO_2 (%)	78.2 ± 4.1	80.2 ± 5.3[a]	70.4 ± 6.7	73.4 ± 6.8[c]	67.6 ± 4.5	68.2 ± 4.2[b]	64.7 ± 4.8	66.3 ± 6.20[a¶§‡]
Wmax (W)	180.0 ± 21.1	180.0 ± 21.1	172.0 ± 19.3	172.0 ± 19.3	170.0 ± 17.0	170.0 ± 17.0	172.0 ± 21.5	172.0 ± 21.5
VO_2peak ($L.min^{-1}$)	2.93 ± 0.25	3.89 ± 0.68[b]	2.87 ± 0.28	4.15 ± 0.45[c]	2.48 ± 0.32	3.99 ± 0.52[c]	2.37 ± 0.30	4.05 ± 0.59[c¶§‡]
V_E ($L.min^{-1}$)	119.9 ± 18.1	116.1 ± 25.6	118.6 ± 19.0	117.3 ± 16.7	110.8 ± 24.5	109.5 ± 17.8	117.6 ± 17.5	113.6 ± 21.2
RR ($breaths.min^{-1}$)	53.5 ± 7.1	51.2 ± 5.7	53.2 ± 7.0	52.6 ± 6.0	49.6 ± 8.6	49.5 ± 5.6	52.7 ± 7.2	52.2 ± 7.7
HR ($beats.min^{-1}$)	182.2 ± 7.9	182.1 ± 8.7	182.7 ± 6.2	182.9 ± 6.2	178.6 ± 7.0	178.5 ± 6.5	180.9 ± 7.9	180.5 ± 7.9
$P_{ET}O_2$ (mmHg)	71.3 ± 2.6	96.4 ± 9.9[c]	64.4 ± 3.1	90.6 ± 13.4[c]	56.7 ± 3.4	91.4 ± 12.2[c]	51.8 ± 2.1	92.3 ± 11.5[c¶§‡]
$P_{ET}CO_2$ (mmHg)	29.0 ± 2.9	30.5 ± 3.0[a]	29.0 ± 2.9	30.1 ± 2.5[a]	28.7 ± 3.6	29.5 ± 3.5[a]	28.3 ± 2.4	30.2 ± 2.7[a]
RER	1.13 ± 0.08	0.92 ± 0.10[c]	1.12 ± 0.08	0.87 ± 0.12[c]	1.21 ± 0.11	0.84 ± 0.10[c]	1.35 ± 0.14	0.90 ± 0.15[c¶§‡]
VCO_2 ($L.min^{-1}$)	3.28 ± 0.28	3.29 ± 0.51	3.21 ± 0.34	3.25 ± 0.29	3.00 ± 0.47	3.02 ± 0.37	3.13 ± 0.40	3.16 ± 0.41[§]
RPM	61.7 ± 9.0	67.0 ± 12.5	63.8 ± 11.4	69.5 ± 10.2[b]	61.9 ± 11.3	68.1 ± 9.4[T]	58.3 ± 12.6	65.6 ± 13.9[T¶]
VM RMSraw (μV)	116.9 ± 45.3	122.7 ± 46.6	120.2 ± 42.5	119.8 ± 39.2	120.1 ± 49.4	125.3 ± 47.6	102.6 ± 47.0	108.4 ± 44.3
VL RMSraw (μV)	116.5 ± 38.1	123.6 ± 43.3	107.3 ± 52.5	110.8 ± 52.6	118.4 ± 50.2	122.7 ± 52.9	87.2 ± 36.1	94.5 ± 37.0[b¶]
Average RMSraw (μV)	116.7 ± 32.5	123.2 ± 35.9	113.8 ± 42.6	115.3 ± 40.3	119.3 ± 41.6	124.0 ± 43.1	94.9 ± 37.5	101.5 ± 36.3[a¶]
VM RMSNz (A.U.)	182.1 ± 53.9	191.7 ± 57.8	204.3 ± 70.8	205.8 ± 68.7	189.5 ± 57.3	197.9 ± 51.7	172.9 ± 70.7	184.7 ± 77.1[¶]
VL RMSNz (A.U.)	195.4 ± 52.6	206.8 ± 66.6	177.8 ± 41.3	183.4 ± 43.3	194.5 ± 70.0	199.4 ± 57.5	155.9 ± 55.7	167.3 ± 53.4[a¶]
Average RMSNz (A.U.)	188.7 ± 43.9	199.2 ± 52.7	191.1 ± 53.8	194.6 ± 50.8	192.0 ± 61.4	198.6 ± 51.6	164.4 ± 62.0	176.0 ± 63.9[¶]
VM TAINz (A.U.)	39.9 ± 15.7	43.6 ± 16.2[T]	42.8 ± 19.2	40.6 ± 11.2	42.1 ± 17.0	42.6 ± 14.5	36.1 ± 14.4	38.0 ± 16.4[¶]
VL TAINz (A.U.)	43.2 ± 19.3	42.4 ± 14.4	34.1 ± 9.0	35.3 ± 7.2	40.5 ± 15.2	40.9 ± 12.8	32.5 ± 13.8	34.1 ± 15.6
Average TAINz (A.U.)	41.5 ± 17.1	43.0 ± 15.1	38.4 ± 13.4	37.9 ± 8.4	41.3 ± 15.9	41.7 ± 13.5	34.3 ± 13.5	36.0 ± 15.5[¶]
VM MPF (Hz)	87.4 ± 20.1	84.9 ± 20.6	84.7 ± 20.2	86.0 ± 21.0	88.5 ± 14.6	87.0 ± 16.6	81.8 ± 15.2	81.7 ± 16.4
VL MPF (Hz)	71.4 ± 15.8	85.3 ± 21.9[c]	85.7 ± 19.4	85.6 ± 21.8	88.1 ± 15.0	86.3 ± 16.9	81.9 ± 15.5	82.1 ± 16.1[¶‡]
Average MPF (Hz)	79.4 ± 17.8	85.1 ± 21.2[b]	85.2 ± 19.8	85.8 ± 21.4	88.3 ± 14.8	86.6 ± 16.7	81.8 ± 15.3	81.9 ± 16.2[‡]
VM MdPF (Hz)	70.9 ± 16.2	69.9 ± 16.2	67.5 ± 13.6	68.7 ± 15.2	72.1 ± 11.8	70.3 ± 12.2	65.0 ± 10.6	66.1 ± 13.2
VL MdPF (Hz)	71.4 ± 15.8	68.8 ± 16.6[a]	67.9 ± 13.6	68.1 ± 16.2	71.4 ± 12.1	69.2 ± 12.7	65.5 ± 11.0	65.9 ± 12.5
Average MdPF (Hz)	71.1 ± 16.0	69.3 ± 16.4	67.7 ± 13.6	68.4 ± 15.6	71.8 ± 11.8	69.8 ± 12.3	65.3 ± 10.8	66.0 ± 12.8
VM Burst (ms)	375.6 ± 127.2	363.0 ± 130.0	377.9 ± 196.2	317.6 ± 83.8	372.8 ± 102.7	322.0 ± 73.8[a]	367.5 ± 85.1	319.2 ± 72.1[a¶]
VL Burst (ms)	381.7 ± 120.6	321.3 ± 83.7[a]	343.6 ± 109.4	309.1 ± 73.1[T]	366.7 ± 107.3	315.0 ± 72.4[T]	371.4 ± 97.1	309.3 ± 60.0[a¶]
Average Burst (ms)	378.6 ± 113.0	342.2 ± 92.2[T]	360.8 ± 150.4	313.3 ± 77.6	369.8 ± 104.6	318.5 ± 58.9[a]	369.5 ± 88.6	314.2 ± 63.9[a¶]
VM Timing (%)	49.1 ± 3.4	46.3 ± 7.7	48.2 ± 3.5	48.1 ± 4.4	48.6 ± 3.0	47.8 ± 3.6	49.4 ± 3.4	47.4 ± 4.3[a¶]
VL Timing (%)	49.5 ± 3.6	50.2 ± 2.2	49.4 ± 2.5	49.7 ± 2.1	50.4 ± 1.6	49.4 ± 2.4	50.5 ± 2.3	49.4 ± 2.8
Average Timing (%)	49.3 ± 3.0	48.3 ± 4.2	48.8 ± 2.7	48.9 ± 3.0	49.5 ± 2.1	48.6 ± 2.8[T]	50.0 ± 2.8	48.4 ± 3.4[a¶]

F_IO_2, inspiratory oxygen fraction; SpO_2, hemoglobin saturation in capillary blood measured by pulse oximetry; Wmax, power output at exhaustion; VO_2, oxygen consumption; V_E, pulmonary ventilation; RR, respiratory rate; HR, heart rate; $P_{ET}O_2$, end-tidal O_2 pressure; $P_{ET}CO_2$, end-tidal CO_2 pressure; RER, respiratory exchange ratio; VCO_2,CO_2 production; RPM, revolutions per minute; VL, vastus lateralis; VM, vastus medialis; RMSraw, raw root mean square; RMSNz, normalized root mean square; TAINz: normalized total activation index (arbitrary units, A.U.); MPF, mean power frequency; MdPF, median power frequency; Burst: contraction burst duration; Timing, start of activation expressed as percentage of total revolution duration. [a]$P < 0.05$; [b]$P < 0.01$; [c]$P < 0.001$; and [T]$P < 0.1$ (F_IO_2 = 73 mmHg vs. new gas mixture). [¶]$P < 0.05$ ANOVA breathing gas switch main effect; [§]$P < 0.05$ ANOVA oxygenation level main effect; [‡]$P < 0.05$ ANOVA breathing gas switch x oxygenation level interaction: n = 10.

that both transitions occurred at comparable exercise intensities. Moreover, our investigation has also demonstrated that an increase in MA after the increase of P_IO_2 at fatigue in hypoxia is not indispensable for the ergogenic effects elicited by the increase of P_IO_2. Collectively, our results suggest that severe hypoxia depresses the capacity of the central nervous system to activate the musculature during whole-body exercise to exhaustion, by a mechanism that can be swiftly reversed by increasing the P_IO_2.

Severe Hypoxia Reduces the Level of Muscle Activation Attainable during Incremental Exercise to Exhaustion

In support of a central predominance of task failure mechanisms is the rapid relief of fatigue with the increase of P_IO_2, e.g., when subjects at exhaustion are asked to continue the exercise once the hypoxic gas mixture they are breathing is swiftly switched to normoxic room air (Calbet et al., 2003a) or hyperoxic gas (Amann et al., 2007). This concurs with the demonstration of a

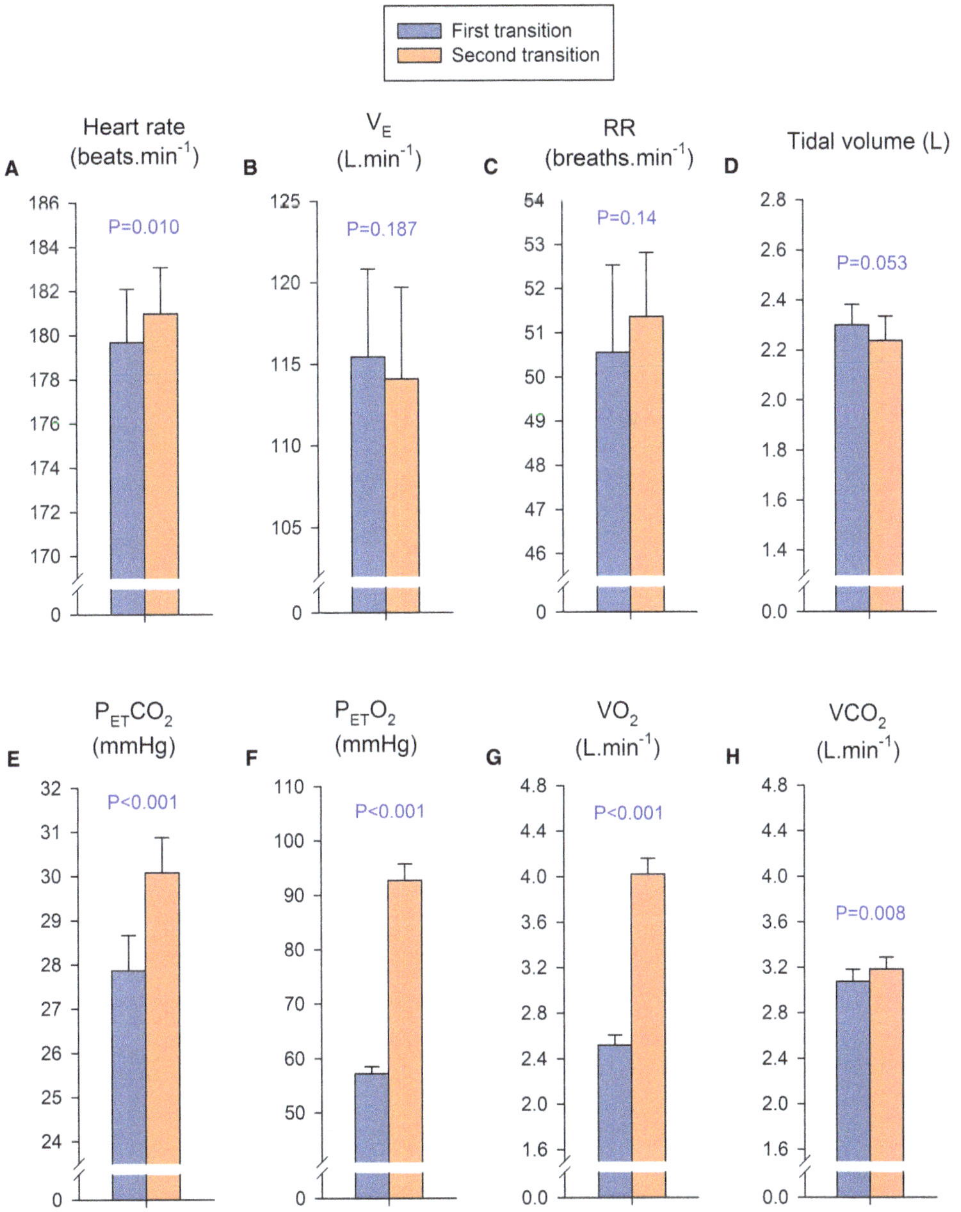

FIGURE 4 | Cardiorespiratory variables during the first and second transition. In the first transition, the P_IO_2 was increased from severe hypoxia ($P_IO_2 = 73$ mmHg) to less hypoxic levels, while during the second transition the P_IO_2 was increased from different levels of hypoxia to normoxia. We calculated a mean value for the four P_IO_2 conditions of the first transition (blue bars) and compared it with the mean value of the four conditions of the second transition (orange bars), including in the analysis only the breath-by-breath data collected during the first 10 s of each transition. The mean response of the first transition was compared with the mean response of the second transition with a Student's paired *t*- test. It is important to remark that in both transitions the absolute exercise intensity was similar (170–173 W), however there is a remarkable difference in VO_2 which is explained by the massive passage of O_2 from the alveoli to the lung capillaries, driven by the much higher $P_{ET}O_2$ during the second transition. This massive diffusion of O_2 is facilitated by the low SaO_2 of the hemoglobin arriving to the lung capillaries at maximal exercise in hypoxia (Calbet et al., 2016). **(A)** Heart rate; **(B)** B pulmonary ventilation (V_E); **(C)** respiratory rate (RR); **(D)** tidal volumen; **(E)** end-tidal CO_2 pressure ($P_{ET}CO_2$); **(F)** end-tidal O_2 pressure; ($P_{ET}O_2$), **(G)** Oxygen uptake (VO_2); **(H)** CO_2 production (VCO_2). Each bar corresponds to the mean of 10 subjects; error bars represent the standard error of the mean.

greater functional reserve at task failure in SAH than in normoxia (Amann et al., 2007; Calbet et al., 2015a; Morales-Alamo et al., 2015; Torres-Peralta et al., 2016). However, increased P_IO_2 does not relieve fatigue when administered at exhaustion during whole-body exercise in moderate hypoxia ($F_IO_2 = 0.15$, equivalent to 2700 m above sea level) (Amann et al., 2007) or during exercise recruiting a small muscle mass in severe hypoxia (Calbet and Lundby, 2009).

It has been reported that a greater level of supraspinal fatigue occurs at task failure during whole-body (Goodall et al., 2010)

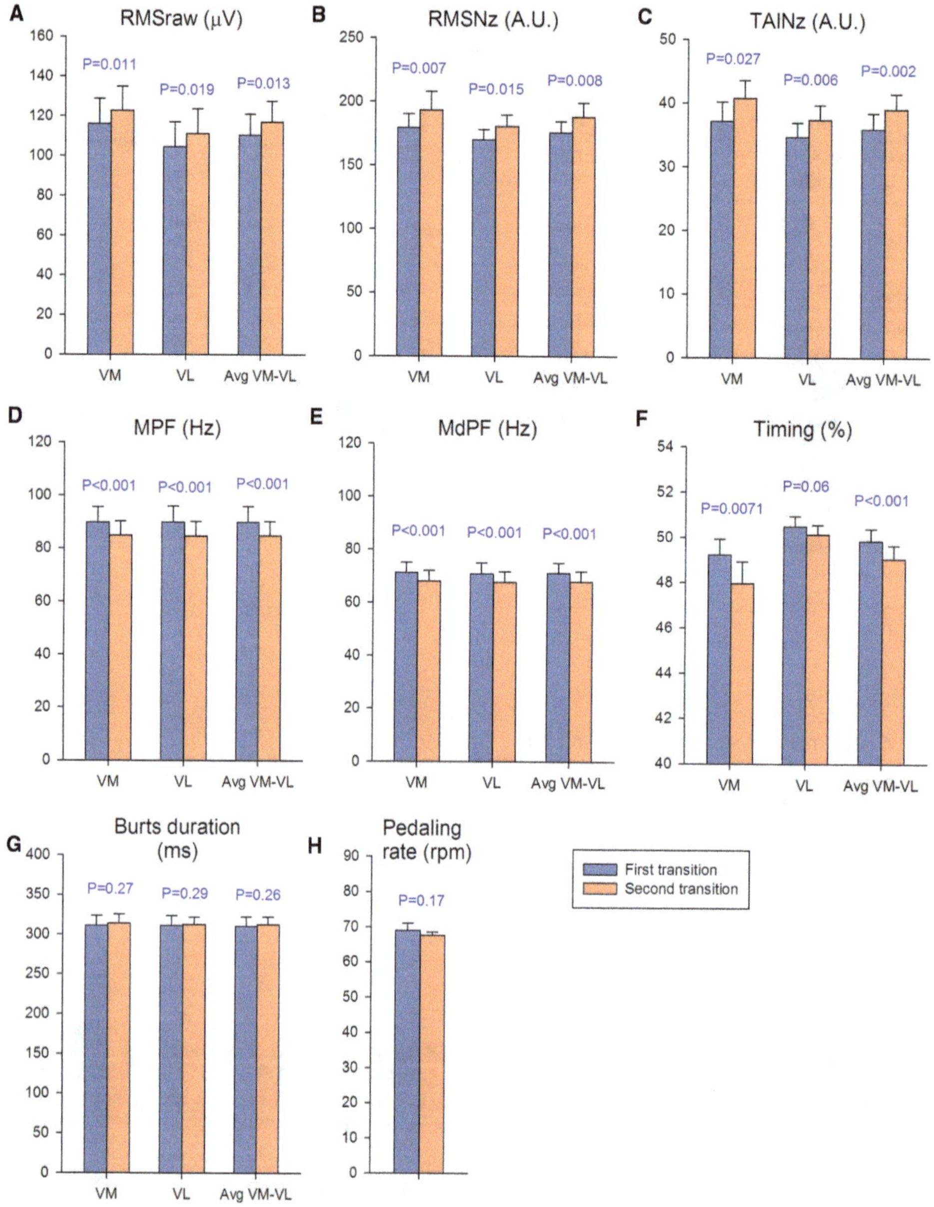

FIGURE 5 | Muscle activation and pedaling rate during the first and second transitions. We calculated a mean value for the four P_IO_2 conditions of the first transition (blue bars) and compared it with the mean value calculated using the four conditions of the second transition (orange bars). The mean response of the first transition was compared with the mean response of the second transition with a Student's paired *t*-test. VM, *vastus medialis*; VL, *vastus lateralis*; **(A)** RMSraw, raw root mean square; **(B)** RMSNz, normalized root mean square; **(C)** TAINz, normalized total activation index; **(D)** MPF, mean power frequency; **(E)** MdPF, median power frequency; **(F)** Timing, start of activation expressed as percentage of total revolution duration; **(G)** burts duration; **(H)** pedaling rate. Each bar corresponds to the mean of 10 subjects; error bars represent the standard error of the mean.

and knee-extension exercise (Goodall et al., 2010) in hypoxia than in normoxia. This effect is more accentuated with increased severity of hypoxia (Goodall et al., 2010). Nevertheless, in contrast to our observations, quadriceps MA (EMG_{RMS}) declined during repeated isometric muscle contractions (60% of the maximal voluntary contraction, 5 s/5 s contraction/recovery) to similar levels in severe hypoxia ($F_IO_2 = 0.10$) and in normoxia (Goodall et al., 2010). A crucial difference between whole-body and small muscle mass (knee extension) exercise in hypoxia is that for a given P_IO_2, pulmonary gas exchange is more perturbed during whole-body than small muscle mass exercise, as reflected by the larger alveolo-arterial O_2 difference (A-aDO_2) observed during whole-body compared to small muscle mass exercise (Calbet et al., 2009b). The larger A-aDO_2 combined with a greater right-shift of the ODC during whole-body exercise in severe hypoxia causes more desaturation for a given PaO_2

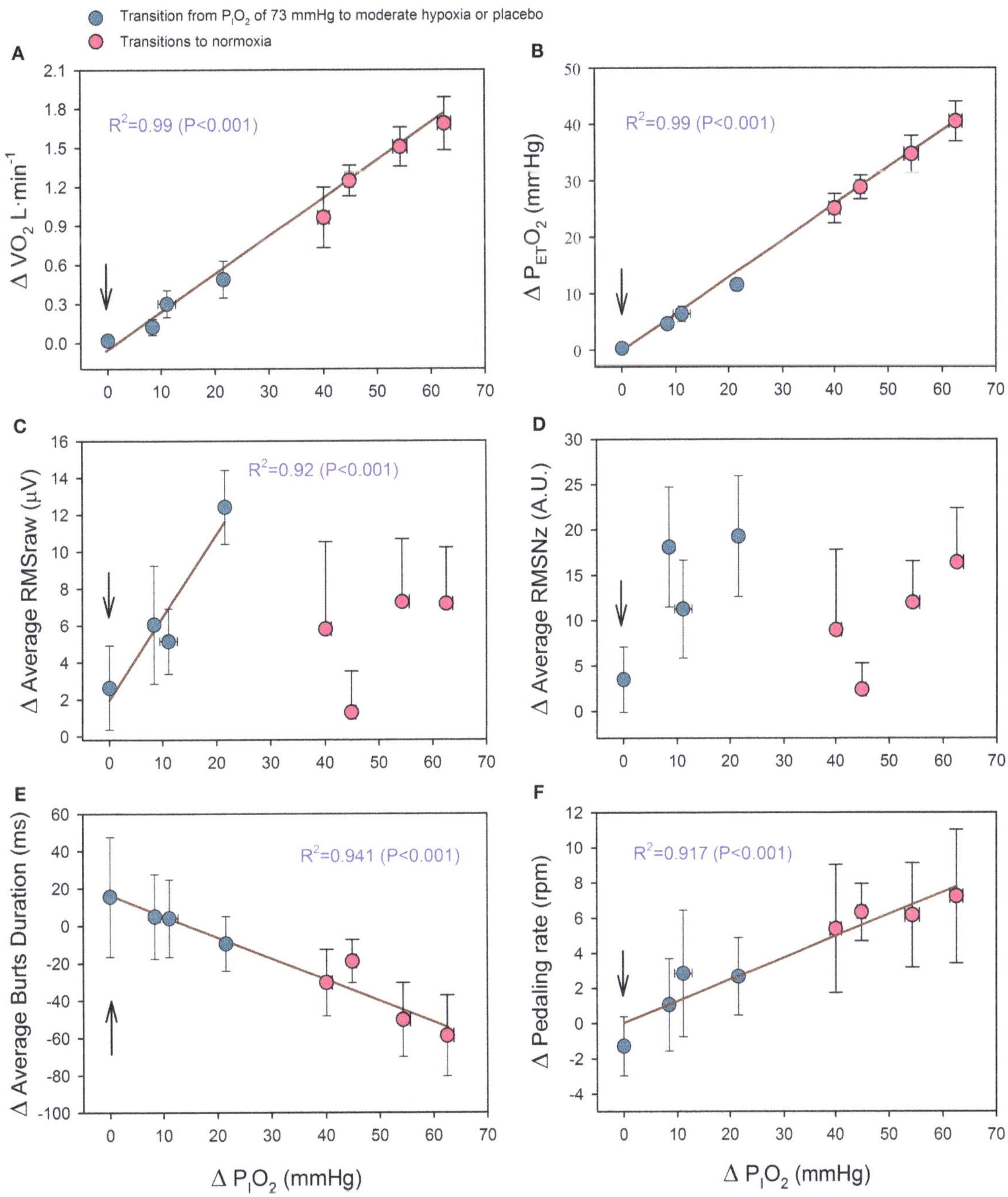

FIGURE 6 | Relationship between the magnitude of the P_IO_2 change (in mmHg) in transition from hypoxia to a higher P_IO_2 and the increases of: (A) oxygen uptake (VO_2), (B) end-tidal O_2 pressure ($P_{ET}O_2$), (C) average raw root mean square (RMSraw) of *vastus medialis* and *vastus lateralis*, (D) average normalized root mean square (RMSNz) of *vastus medialis* and *vastus lateralis*, (E) average burst duration of *vastus medialis* and *vastus lateralis*, and (E) pedaling rate. The vertical arrow indicates the placebo condition. Green circles: transitions from severe hypoxia (P_IO_2 = 73 mmHg) to placebo (vertical arrow) and moderate hypoxia; red circles: transitions from different levels of hypoxia (P_IO_2 of 73, 82, 92, and 99 mmHg) to normoxia. Each point corresponds to the mean of 10 subjects; error bars represent the standard error of the mean.

during whole-body than small muscle exercise in severe hypoxia (Calbet et al., 2009b). Consequently, with an F_IO_2 close to 0.10, SpO_2 at exhaustion was 78% during knee extension exercise in a study by Goodall et al. (2010) and 63% in the current investigation (Calbet et al., 2015a). In the present experiments, SpO_2 was 79% at exhaustion when the P_IO_2 was 99 mmHg, a level of hypoxemia for which acute oxygenation at exhaustion did not enhance muscle activation. Although no definitive conclusion on which variable, PaO_2 or SaO_2, plays a more important role in the reduction of MA during exercise in severe hypoxia, our data combined with those of Goodall et al. (2010) indicate that MA is lower at exhaustion in hypoxia than in normoxia when the levels of SaO_2 fall below ~70%, regardless of P_IO_2.

Mechanisms by Which Hypoxia Could Reduce Muscle Activation Close to Exhaustion

Hypothetically, hypoxia could attenuate MA through two main mechanisms. Severe hypoxia could trigger inhibitory feedback at spinal and supraspinal levels reducing the discharge rate of spinal motoneurons compared to normoxia. Alternatively, severe hypoxia could limit or reduce the recruitment of high-threshold motor units. Regarding the first mechanism, animal studies have shown that levels of PaO_2 similar to those observed in this investigation at exhaustion in SAH (Calbet et al., 2015a) increase the baseline discharge frequency of group III and especially of group IV muscle afferents in resting cats (Hill et al., 1992; Lagier-Tessonnier et al., 1993) and rabbits (Arbogast et al., 2000). Increased firing rates by group III/IV muscle afferents may cause reflex inhibition of the α-motoneuron pool (for review see Amann and Kayser, 2009) and, hence, reduced muscle activation. In the present investigation, MPF and MdPF were lower during the second that during the first transition (**Figures 6D** and **F**), coinciding with a greater attenuation of fatigue, likely due to the almost 5 times greater average ΔP_IO_2 during the second than the first transition. This finding does not necessarily indicates a change in motor activation, since MPF and MdPF are poor indices of motor unit recruitment patterns (Farina et al., 2014), and MPF and MdPF may be affected by peripheral factors, as recently demonstrated (Torres-Peralta et al., 2016). In agreement with our interpretation, increased metaboreflex activation during ischemic intermittent isometric muscle knee-extension contractions to exhaustion had no clear inhibitory effects on EMG_{RMS} values (Millet et al., 2009).

Regarding the second mechanism, hypoxia may reduce the oxygenation of the prefrontal, premotor, and motor cortex leading to a mismatch between energy demand and aerobic ATP re-synthesis, which could limit the corticospinal motor drive (Rasmussen et al., 2007; Verges et al., 2012). In agreement with this idea, our subjects developed a lower mean power output during the first 10 s of sprint exercise (30 s Wingate test) in severe hypoxia ($P_IO_2 = 73$ mmHg) than in normoxia, despite the fact that leg VO_2 measured by the direct Fick method, was similar regardless of F_IO_2 (Calbet et al., 2015a). Interestingly, the duration of the contraction bursts was reduced and the start of the contraction bursts slightly advanced in the pedaling cycle with the transition from exhaustion in severe hypoxia to exercise in normoxia (**Table 3**). Likewise, subjects increased their pedaling rate in response to an increase of P_IO_2 at exhaustion. Interestingly, this effect was linearly dependent on the increase in P_IO_2 (**Figure 6F**). The latter implies that enhanced oxygenation (P_aO_2 and/or S_aO_2) at exhaustion swiftly alters the pattern of muscle activation/recruitment, likely allowing for a greater recruitment of faster motor units (Holt et al., 2014). This also points toward a central regulatory mechanism. In contrast, there was no improvement in any variable during the placebo transition, indicating that the level of oxygenation (P_aO_2 and/or S_aO_2) and the central command barely changed. Had the placebo transition reduced the perception of effort, a change would have been expected in the cardiorespiratory response to exercise (Robertson, 1982; Calbet et al., 2015b; Cochrane et al., 2015). Since all subjects believed that they were receiving oxygen-enriched gas at all transitions, included the placebo transition, and no subject was able to guess whether a gas mixture other than normoxia was administered, we can rule out psychological factors as being responsible for the changes in MA elicited by increased P_IO_2. In turn, psychological factors likely explain the ~42 additional seconds that the subjects were able to exercise during the placebo transition.

Although iEMG increases with increasing angular velocity during concentric contractions (Westing et al., 1991; Amiridis et al., 1996), this factor alone cannot explain the increased MA elicited by increased P_IO_2 in our experiment. In fact, pedaling rate did not increase significantly in the transition from severe hypoxia to moderate hypoxia (i.e., P_IO_2 of 92, and 99 mmHg), while MA was increased.

Limitations

Although the amplitude of the surface EMG signal can provide a useful approximation of the amplitude component of the neural drive to muscle during some controlled conditions including dynamic exercise (Farina et al., 2014; Coelho et al., 2015), it has limitations. For example, the EMG signal is affected by the thickness of the subcutaneous adipose tissue, the spatial resolution is low overrepresenting superficial muscles fibers, may be altered by cross-talk from neighboring muscles, and is affected by the electrical properties of the sarcolemma, which may change during exercise (Farina et al., 2014). None of these factors is expected to change much within the first 10 s of increased P_IO_2 in our experimental conditions because exercise intensity was maintained at the same level during the first 2 min following the change in P_IO_2. The fact that the EMG amplitude of an interference signal is less than that obtained by summing the amplitudes of the individual motor unit action potentials, a phenomenon referred to as amplitude cancelation, also limits the interpretation of our results. Amplitude cancelation increases monotonically as the neural drive to muscle is elevated, affecting mostly the low-threshold motor units (Mottram et al., 2005; Farina et al., 2014). In our experimental conditions, reduced amplitude cancelation during the first 10 s of the transitions from task failure to increased P_IO_2, as a mechanism to explain the increase in EMG amplitude, is also unlikely since increasing P_IO_2 is expected to facilitate the neural drive to the muscles. To circumvent these limitations we have focused on assessing changes during the last 10 s of a given hypoxic condition and the first 10 s of the change to a higher P_IO_2. With such a short period, and given the stability of load at the start of the transition, the metabolic changes in the muscles should have been minuscule. This minimized the potential alteration of the EMG due to modification of the electrical properties of the muscle fibers and local metabolic factors during the first 10 s of the transition to a higher P_IO_2.

Another limitation of this study is due to the use of finger pulse oximetry rather than the direct assessment of SaO_2, which is less accurate at SaO_2 below 75–85% (Trivedi et al., 1997; Kolb et al., 2004). Another drawback of finger pulse oximetry is related to the slow response time of all pulse oximeters (Trivedi et al., 1997), with the delay being higher for finger than earlobe placements (Trivedi et al., 1997; Hamber et al., 1999). Consequently, the SpO_2 values recorded during the first 10 s of the transitions from hypoxia to higher P_IO_2 underestimated the actual SaO_2 values. Nevertheless, we should emphasize that the readings of our pulse oximeter were closely correlated to the SaO_2 values, when measured simultaneously under steady conditions in the same subjects included in this study ($SaO_2 = 1.005 \times SpO_2 - 0.76$, $n = 74$, SaO_2 range: 53.9–96.5%, $R^2 = 0.99$). Since during the transitions VO_2 increased linearly with the increase of P_IO_2 (**Figure 6A**), oxygen transport from the lungs to the muscles and the central nervous system must have also been enhanced.

In summary, this investigation demonstrates that close to task failure, MA is lower during IE test to exhaustion in SAH than in normoxia. We have shown that increasing P_IO_2 at exhaustion reduces fatigue and allows for the continuation of exercise in moderate and severe acute hypoxia, regardless of the effects of oxygenation on muscle activation. In hypoxia, MA at task failure is increased within 10 s of oxygenation when task failure occurred at levels of hypoxia equivalent to an altitude close to 5200 m above sea level ($P_IO_2 \sim 73$ mmHg), and when the P_IO_2 is increased to levels ≥ 92 mmHg and SaO_2 above 70%. Overall, these findings indicate that one of the central mechanisms by which severe hypoxia may cause central fatigue and task failure is by reducing the capacity for maximal muscle activation. The fact that exercise could be continued at exhaustion in severe hypoxia with the administration of a placebo-gas mixture demonstrates that this central mechanism has a cognitive component.

AUTHOR CONTRIBUTIONS

Conception and design of the experiments: JC; pre-testing, experimental preparation, data collection, and analysis: RT, DM, JL, IP, JP, and JC; EMG analysis: RT, MG, and MI. The first version of the manuscript was written by RT and JC. All co-authors read and approved the final version of the manuscript.

ACKNOWLEDGMENTS

This study was supported by a grant from the Ministerio de Educación y Ciencia of Spain (DEP2009-11638 and FEDER). Especial thanks are given to José Navarro de Tuero for his excellent technical assistance.

REFERENCES

Amann, M., and Calbet, J. A. (2008). Convective oxygen transport and fatigue. *J. Appl. Physiol.* 104, 861–870. doi: 10.1152/japplphysiol.01008.2007

Amann, M., and Kayser, B. (2009). Nervous system function during exercise in hypoxia. *High. Alt. Med. Biol.* 10, 149–164. doi: 10.1089/ham.2008.1105

Amann, M., Romer, L. M., Subudhi, A. W., Pegelow, D. F., and Dempsey, J. A. (2007). Severity of arterial hypoxaemia affects the relative contributions of peripheral muscle fatigue to exercise performance in healthy humans. *J. Physiol.* 581, 389–403. doi: 10.1113/jphysiol.2007.129700

Amiridis, I. G., Martin, A., Morlon, B., Martin, L., Cometti, G., Pousson, M., et al. (1996). Co-activation and tension-regulating phenomena during isokinetic knee extension in sedentary and highly skilled humans. *Eur. J. Appl. Physiol. Occup. Physiol.* 73, 149–156. doi: 10.1007/BF00262824

Arbogast, S., Vassilakopoulos, T., Darques, J. L., Duvauchelle, J. B., and Jammes, Y. (2000). Influence of oxygen supply on activation of group IV muscle afferents after low-frequency muscle stimulation. *Muscle Nerve* 23, 1187–1193.

Baum, B. S., and Li, L. (2003). Lower extremity muscle activities during cycling are influenced by load and frequency. *J. Electromyogr. Kinesiol.* 13, 181–190. doi: 10.1016/S1050-6411(02)00110-4

Calbet, J. A., Boushel, R., Radegran, G., Sondergaard, H., Wagner, P. D., and Saltin, B. (2003a). Determinants of maximal oxygen uptake in severe acute hypoxia. *Am. J. Physiol. Regul.* 284, R291–R303. doi: 10.1152/ajpregu.00155.2002

Calbet, J. A., Boushel, R., Radegran, G., Sondergaard, H., Wagner, P. D., and Saltin, B. (2003b). Why is VO_2max after altitude acclimatization still reduced despite normalization of arterial O_2 content? *Am. J. Physiol. Regul.* 284, R304–R316. doi: 10.1152/ajpregu.00156.2002

Calbet, J. A., Gonzalez-Alonso, J., Helge, J. W., Sondergaard, H., Munch-Andersen, T., Saltin, B., et al. (2015b). Central and peripheral hemodynamics in exercising humans: leg vs. arm exercise. *Scand. J. Med. Sci. Sports* 25(Suppl. 4), 144–157. doi: 10.1111/sms.12604

Calbet, J. A. L., Lundby, C., and Boushel, R. (2016). Integrative conductance of oxygen during exercise at altitude. *Adv. Exp. Med. Biol.* 903, 395–408. doi: 10.1007/978-1-4899-7678-9_26

Calbet, J. A., Losa-Reyna, J., Torres-Peralta, R., Rasmussen, P., Ponce-Gonzalez, J. G., Sheel, A. W., et al. (2015a). Limitations to oxygen transport and utilization during sprint exercise in humans: evidence for a functional reserve in muscle O_2 diffusing capacity. *J. Physiol.* 593, 4649–4664. doi: 10.1113/JP270408

Calbet, J. A., and Lundby, C. (2009). Air to muscle O_2 delivery during exercise at altitude. *High. Alt. Med. Biol.* 10, 123–134. doi: 10.1089/ham.2008.1099

Calbet, J. A., Radegran, G., Boushel, R., and Saltin, B. (2009b). On the mechanisms that limit oxygen uptake during exercise in acute and chronic hypoxia: role of muscle mass. *J. Physiol.* 587, 477–490. doi: 10.1113/jphysiol.2008.162271

Calbet, J. A., Robach, P., and Lundby, C. (2009a). The exercising heart at altitude. *Cell. Mol. Life Sci.* 66, 3601–3613. doi: 10.1007/s00018-009-0148-6

Cochrane, K. C., Housh, T. J., Bergstrom, H. C., Jenkins, N. D., Johnson, G., Schmidt, R. J., et al. (2015). Physiological responses during cycle ergometry at a constant perception of effort. *Int. J. Sports Med.* 36, 466–473. doi: 10.1055/s-0034-1396826

Coelho, A. C., Cannon, D. T., Cao, R., Porszasz, J., Casaburi, R., Knorst, M. M., et al. (2015). Instantaneous quantification of skeletal muscle activation, power production, and fatigue during cycle ergometry. *J. Appl. Physiol.* 118, 646–654. doi: 10.1152/japplphysiol.00948.2014

Farina, D., Merletti, R., and Enoka, R. M. (2014). The extraction of neural strategies from the surface EMG: an update. *J. Appl. Physiol.* 117, 1215–1230. doi: 10.1152/japplphysiol.00162.2014

Goodall, S., Gonzalez-Alonso, J., Ali, L., Ross, E. Z., and Romer, L. M. (2012). Supraspinal fatigue after normoxic and hypoxic exercise in humans. *J. Physiol.* 590, 2767–2782. doi: 10.1113/jphysiol.2012.228890

Goodall, S., Ross, E. Z., and Romer, L. M. (2010). Effect of graded hypoxia on supraspinal contributions to fatigue with unilateral knee-extensor contractions. *J. Appl. Physiol.* 109, 1842–1851. doi: 10.1152/japplphysiol.00458.2010

Goodall, S., Twomey, R., Amann, M., Ross, E. Z., Lovering, A. T., Romer, L. M., et al. (2014). AltitudeOmics: exercise-induced supraspinal fatigue is attenuated in healthy humans after acclimatization to high altitude. *Acta Physiol.* *210*, 875–888. doi: 10.1111/apha.12241

Hamber, E. A., Bailey, P. L., James, S. W., Wells, D. T., Lu, J. K., and Pace, N. L. (1999). Delays in the detection of hypoxemia due to site of pulse oximetry probe placement. *J. Clin. Anesth.* 11, 113–118. doi: 10.1016/S0952-8180(99)00010-0

Hill, J. M., Pickar, J. G., Parrish, M. D., and Kaufman, M. P. (1992). Effects of hypoxia on the discharge of group III and IV muscle afferents in cats. *J. Appl. Physiol.* 73, 2524–2529.

Holt, N. C., Wakeling, J. M., and Biewener, A. A. (2014). The effect of fast and slow motor unit activation on whole-muscle mechanical performance: the size principle may not pose a mechanical paradox. *Proc. Biol. Sci.* 281:20140002. doi: 10.1098/rspb.2014.0002

Hug, F., and Dorel, S. (2009). Electromyographic analysis of pedaling: a review. *J. Electromyogr. Kinesiol.* 19, 182–198. doi: 10.1016/j.jelekin.2007.10.010

Kayser, B., Narici, M., Binzoni, T., Grassi, B., and Cerretelli, P. (1994). Fatigue and exhaustion in chronic hypobaric hypoxia: influence of exercising muscle mass. *J. Appl. Physiol.* 76, 634–640.

Kolb, J. C., Farran, P., Norris, S. R., Smith, D., and Mester, J. (2004). Validation of pulse oximetry during progressive normobaric hypoxia utilizing a portable chamber. *Can. J. Appl. Physiol.* 29, 3–15. doi: 10.1139/h04-001

Lagier-Tessonnier, F., Balzamo, E., and Jammes, Y. (1993). Comparative effects of ischemia and acute hypoxemia on muscle afferents from tibialis anterior in cats. *Muscle Nerve* 16, 135–141. doi: 10.1002/mus.880160203

Merletti, R., and Hermens, H. (2000). Introduction to the special issue on the SENIAM European concerted action. *J. Electromyogr. Kinesiol.* 10, 283–286. doi: 10.1016/S1050-6411(00)00019-5

Millet, G. Y., Aubert, D., Favier, F. B., Busso, T., and Benoit, H. (2009). Effect of acute hypoxia on central fatigue during repeated isometric leg contractions. *Scand. J. Med. Sci. Sports* 19, 695–702. doi: 10.1111/j.1600-0838.2008.00823.x

Morales-Alamo, D., Losa-Reyna, J., Torres-Peralta, R., Martin-Rincon, M., Perez-Valera, M., Curtelin, D., et al. (2015). What limits performance during whole-body incremental exercise to exhaustion in humans? *J. Physiol.* 593, 4631–4648. doi: 10.1113/JP270487

Mottram, C. J., Jakobi, J. M., Semmler, J. G., and Enoka, R. M. (2005). Motor-unit activity differs with load type during a fatiguing contraction. *J. Neurophysiol.* 93, 1381–1392. doi: 10.1152/jn.00837.2004

Ozgunen, K. T., Celik, U., and Kurdak, S. S. (2010). Determination of an optimal threshold value for muscle activity detection in EMG analysis. *J. Sports Sci. Med.* 9, 620–628.

Rasmussen, P., Dawson, E. A., Nybo, L., van Lieshout, J. J., Secher, N. H., and Gjedde, A. (2007). Capillary-oxygenation-level-dependent near-infrared spectrometry in frontal lobe of humans. *J. Cereb. Blood Flow Metab.* 27, 1082–1093. doi: 10.1038/sj.jcbfm.9600416

Robertson, R. J. (1982). Central signals of perceived exertion during dynamic exercise. *Med. Sci.* 14, 390–396. doi: 10.1249/00005768-198205000-00014

Scharhag-Rosenberger, F., Carlsohn, A., Lundby, C., Schuler, S., Mayer, F., and Scharhag, J. (2014). Can more than one incremental cycling test be performed within one day? *Eur. J. Sport Sci.* 14, 459–467. doi: 10.1080/17461391.2013.853208

Solomonow, M., Baten, C., Smit, J., Baratta, R., Hermens, H., D'Ambrosia, R., et al. (1990). Electromyogram power spectra frequencies associated with motor unit recruitment strategies. *J. Appl. Physiol.* 68, 1177–1185.

Torres-Peralta, R., Losa-Reyna, J., Gonzalez-Izal, M., Perez-Suarez, I., Calle-Herrero, J., Izquierdo, M., et al. (2014). Muscle activation during exercise in severe acute hypoxia: role of absolute and relative intensity. *High. Alt. Med. Biol.* 15, 472–482. doi: 10.1089/ham.2014.1027

Torres-Peralta, R., Morales-Alamo, D., Gonzalez-Izal, M., Losa-Reyna, J., Perez-Suarez, I., Izquierdo, M., et al. (2016). Task failure during exercise to exhaustion in normoxia and hypoxia is due to reduced muscle activation caused by central mechanisms while muscle metaboreflex does not limit performance. *Front. Physiol.* 6:414. doi: 10.3389/fphys.2015.00414

Trivedi, N. S., Ghouri, A. F., Lai, E., Shah, N. K., and Barker, S. J. (1997). Pulse oximeter performance during desaturation and resaturation: a comparison of seven models. *J. Clin. Anesth.* 9, 184–188. doi: 10.1016/S0952-8180(97)00037-8

Verges, S., Rupp, T., Jubeau, M., Wuyam, B., Esteve, F., Levy, P., et al. (2012). Cerebral perturbations during exercise in hypoxia. *Am. J. Physiol. Regul.* 302, R903–R916. doi: 10.1152/ajpregu.00555.2011

Wang, W., Wang, Z., Faith, M. S., Kotler, D., Shih, R., and Heymsfield, S. B. (1999). Regional skeletal muscle measurement: evaluation of new dual-energy X-ray absorptiometry model. *J. Appl. Physiol.* 87, 1163–1171.

Westing, S. H., Cresswell, A. G., and Thorstensson, A. (1991). Muscle activation during maximal voluntary eccentric and concentric knee extension. *Eur. J. Appl. Physiol. Occup. Physiol.* 62, 104–108. doi: 10.1007/BF00626764

20

Changes in Muscle and Cerebral Deoxygenation and Perfusion during Repeated Sprints in Hypoxia to Exhaustion

*Sarah J. Willis, Laurent Alvarez, Grégoire P. Millet**† and Fabio Borrani*†*

Faculty of Biology and Medicine, Institute of Sport Sciences, University of Lausanne, Lausanne, Switzerland

***Correspondence:**
Grégoire P. Millet
gregoire.millet@unil.ch

† These authors have contributed equally to this work.

During supramaximal exercise, exacerbated at exhaustion and in hypoxia, the circulatory system is challenged to facilitate oxygen delivery to working tissues through cerebral autoregulation which influences fatigue development and muscle performance. The aim of the study was to evaluate the effects of different levels of normobaric hypoxia on the changes in peripheral and cerebral oxygenation and performance during repeated sprints to exhaustion. Eleven recreationally active participants (six men and five women; 26.7 ± 4.2 years, 68.0 ± 14.0 kg, 172 ± 12 cm, 14.1 ± 4.7% body fat) completed three randomized testing visits in conditions of simulated altitude near sea-level (~380 m, F_IO_2 20.9%), ~2000 m (F_IO_2 16.5 ± 0.4%), and ~3800 m (F_IO_2 13.3 ± 0.4%). Each session began with a 12-min warm-up followed by two 10-s sprints and the repeated cycling sprint (10-s sprint: 20-s recovery) test to exhaustion. Measurements included power output, vastus lateralis, and prefrontal deoxygenation [near-infrared spectroscopy, delta (Δ) corresponds to the difference between maximal and minimal values], oxygen uptake, femoral artery blood flow (Doppler ultrasound), hemodynamic variables (transthoracic impedance), blood lactate concentration, and rating of perceived exertion. Performance (total work, kJ; −27.1 ± 25.8% at 2000 m, $p < 0.01$ and −49.4 ± 19.3% at 3800 m, $p < 0.001$) and pulse oxygen saturation (−7.5 ± 6.0%, $p < 0.05$ and −18.4 ± 5.3%, $p < 0.001$, respectively) decreased with hypoxia, when compared to 400 m. Muscle Δ hemoglobin difference ([Hbdiff]) and Δ tissue saturation index (TSI) were lower ($p < 0.01$) at 3800 m than at 2000 and 400 m, and lower Δ deoxyhemoglobin resulted at 3800 m compared with 2000 m. There were reduced changes in peripheral [Δ[Hbdiff], ΔTSI, Δ total hemoglobin ([tHb])] and greater changes in cerebral (Δ[Hbdiff], Δ[tHb]) oxygenation throughout the test to exhaustion ($p < 0.05$). Changes in cerebral deoxygenation were greater at 3800 m than at 2000 and 400 m ($p < 0.01$). This study confirms that performance in hypoxia is limited by continually decreasing oxygen saturation, even though exercise can be sustained despite maximal peripheral deoxygenation. There may be a cerebral autoregulation of increased perfusion accounting for the decreased arterial oxygen content and allowing for task continuation, as shown by the continued cerebral deoxygenation.

Keywords: repeated sprint ability, altitude, oxygenation, NIRS, maximal exercise, convection, diffusion, blood flow

INTRODUCTION

During exercise, the circulatory system is challenged to improve oxygen delivery of the working tissues. Oxygen delivery is known to be regulated by physiological mechanisms of both convective (as decrease in arterial oxygen content in hypoxic conditions due to a lower inspired fraction of oxygen; di Prampero, 2003; Sweeting et al., 2017; Villar and Hughson, 2017) and diffusive (as blood flow is regulated via vascular vasodilation based on the metabolic demand of exercise and transports to the muscle for perfusion and to the mitochondria for energy metabolism; Calbet, 2000; di Prampero, 2003; Laughlin and Joyner, 2003; Walker et al., 2007) factors. It has been demonstrated that diminishing the oxygen availability has a detrimental effect on endurance performance as well as on the ability to repeat maximal and short sprints without adequate recovery (Balsom et al., 1994; Smith and Billaut, 2010, 2012; Girard et al., 2011; Billaut and Buchheit, 2013).

As exercise intensity increases, there is a progressive muscle deoxygenation to a minimal point or plateau close to maximal power output or exhaustion (Grassi et al., 1999; Neary et al., 2001; Subudhi et al., 2007). In hypoxic conditions, this plateau in deoxyhemoglobin concentration has been considered an indication of maximal skeletal muscle oxygen extraction as a product of reduced oxygen availability (Esaki et al., 2005; Legrand et al., 2005). The peripheral muscle tissue was shown to regulate this oxygen extraction in order to longer maintain the balance between oxygen delivery and consumption in hypoxic conditions (Subudhi et al., 2007; Smith and Billaut, 2010, 2012). Researchers have also reported that maintaining a high muscle oxygen extraction during low arterial oxygen pressure conditions facilitates the development of hypoxemia in trained individuals (Van Thienen and Hespel, 2016).

Systemic hypoxemia is considered to be a strong contributor to cerebral deoxygenation, (Nielsen et al., 2002; Amann and Calbet, 2008; Amann and Kayser, 2009) which has been shown to occur also during repeated sprint exercise (Billaut and Smith, 2010). Cerebral deoxygenation has been considered as an influential factor for decreasing exercise intensity or cessation of exercise (Smith and Billaut, 2010). Furthermore, low brain oxygenation due to insufficient oxygen delivery and/or lower pressure gradient of arterial oxygen has an influence on the diffusive delivery of oxygen to the sarcomere and mitochondria, which may induce a central fatigue (Amann and Calbet, 2008). The arterial blood pressure (i.e., cerebral perfusion pressure) increases during exercise, and with rapid or forceful muscle contractions may exceed the limits of cerebral autoregulation (maintenance of blood flow to the brain under conditions of changing blood pressure), thus exposing a potential risk of high blood pressure combined with increased blood flow in the brain (Bill and Linder, 1976; MacDougall et al., 1985; Calbet et al., 2015a; Curtelin et al., 2017). In addition, cerebral blood flow provides an important signal to the central nervous system (CNS) which may become a supplemental limiting factor for exercise at altitude in addition to cardiorespiratory capacity and muscle fatigue (Kayser, 2003; Imray et al., 2005). Moreover, the CNS is sensitive to the factors of partial pressure of arterial oxygen, arterial oxygen content, and arterial oxygen saturation, which together (along with many other factors) influence the cardiac output and thus have an impact on brain function (Calbet et al., 2003). Indeed, cerebral function during exercise (especially supramaximal intensity) may have a large influence on fatigue in addition to the decrease in peripheral muscle performance (Shibuya et al., 2004; Amann et al., 2007; Subudhi et al., 2007; Amann and Calbet, 2008; Smith and Billaut, 2010). However, there is still uncertainty regarding cerebral oxygenation and the effect on performance as well as cessation of exercise during repeated sprints in hypoxia.

Changes in oxygenation and the hemodynamics of these tissues can be non-invasively recorded using near-infrared spectroscopy (NIRS) for real-time measures (Van Beekvelt et al., 2001). Previous reports have examined peripheral and cerebral oxygenation with NIRS during repeated sprint exercise, however, none of these studies have been performed with repeated sprint exercise to exhaustion in hypoxic conditions [series of repeated sprints, (Racinais et al., 2007; Smith and Billaut, 2010, 2012; Billaut and Buchheit, 2013); or incremental ramp test to exhaustion, (Amann et al., 2007; Subudhi et al., 2007)]. In addition, recent research has eluded that there may be greater blood volume shifts in the muscle during repeated sprint exercise possibly due to greater arteriolar dilation together with increased capillary volume (De Smet et al., 2017). Therefore, there are factors contributing to the end of exercise within maximal repeated sprints to exhaustion which remain unknown.

Thus, the aim of the present study was to investigate changes in peripheral and cerebral oxygenation during maximal repeated sprints to exhaustion as well as the physiological effects of different levels of hypoxia. The hypothesis was that performance would be impaired in hypoxia due to decreased convective oxygen delivery. Additionally, the changes in peripheral and cerebral de/re-oxygenation during sprints/recoveries were hypothesized to be greater as hypoxia increased, and that cerebral oxygenation variables may challenge blood flow regulation at the end of exercise.

METHODS

Participants

Eleven healthy, recreationally active volunteers participated in this study (six men and five women; 26.7 ± 4.2 years, 68.0 ± 14.0 kg, 172 ± 12 cm, 14.1 ± 4.7% body fat). Participants were required to train at least 4 h per week and be accustomed to maximal intensity exercise. Exclusion criteria for participation included any skeletal or muscular injury in the last 3 months,

---

Abbreviations: F_IO_2, fraction of inspired oxygen; NIRS, near-infrared spectroscopy; Δ, delta change over time; RSAT, repeated sprint ability test; $\dot{V}O_2$, maximal oxygen uptake; $\dot{V}_E$, minute ventilation; $\dot{V}_E/\dot{V}O_2$, ventilatory equivalent for oxygen; $\dot{V}_E/\dot{V}CO_2$, ventilatory equivalent for carbon dioxide; RER, respiratory exchange ratio; BF, breathing frequency; SV, stroke volume; HR, heart rate; Q, cardiac output; SVR, systemic vascular resistance; EDV, end diastolic volume; EF, ejection fraction; RPE, rate of perceived exertion; O_2Hb, oxyhemoglobin; HHb, deoxyhemoglobin; tHb, total hemoglobin; Hbdiff, hemoglobin difference; TSI, tissue saturation index; $P_{a,CO2}$, partial pressure of arterial carbon dioxide; $P_{a,O2}$, partial pressure of arterial oxygen.

pain, or any other medical condition which could compromise the study. Participants gave written informed consent after being informed of the procedures and risks involved. The experimental protocol was approved by the Ethical Commission for Human Research CER-VD 138/15 and conducted according to the Declaration of Helsinki.

Study Design

In a randomized, single-blinded experimental protocol, participants reported to the laboratory for a total of four sessions (one familiarization and three testing visits). The testing visits were performed in simulated altitude of sea level (~380 m, F_IO_2 20.9%), ~2000 m (F_IO_2 16.5 ± 0.4%), and ~3800 m (F_IO_2 13.3 ± 0.4%). Each session was completed in a normobaric hypoxic chamber (ATS Altitude Training, Sydney, Australia) built in the laboratory. This chamber utilizes a system containing a compressor connected to air filters which enable the regulation of the level of oxygen (simulated altitude settings as noted above). Participants were asked to avoid strenuous activity as well as caffeine or alcohol consumption 24 h before each visit. All visits were scheduled at the same time of day and at least 48 h apart to limit fatigue.

Familiarization

During the familiarization visit, anthropometric data (body height, body mass, and skin fold measurement) were collected along with the completion of the informed consent and health questionnaires. Skin fold measurements were obtained by an experienced technician using the seven-site formula from the 2014 ACSM guidelines (ACSM, 2014). Afterwards, participants were seated on an electronically braked cycling ergometer (Lode Excalibur Sport Ergometer, Lode B.V., Netherlands) and dimensions were recorded for standardization during subsequent sessions. After a 5-min warm-up at 1.5 $W{\cdot}kg^{-1}$, participants performed two 10-s maximal sprints with 3 min of active recovery between. Following an additional 5-min passive recovery, participants were familiarized with the repeated sprint ability test (RSAT), as described in detail below.

Testing Visits

The protocol of the testing visit is illustrated in **Figure 1**. Each session began in the normobaric hypoxic chamber with a 12-min warm-up (6 min at 50 W, 6 min at 100 W) at a cadence of 85 rpm. Following which, the two maximal 10-s warm-up sprints were performed (similar to the familiarization visit) with 3 min of active recovery between sprints. After a 5-min passive recovery, the measurements for pre-RSAT were collected. These measurements (described in detail below) included resting Doppler blood flow and estimates of cardiovascular function synchronized at the same moment. Participants were then fitted with a mask to measure oxygen uptake. Participants then performed the RSAT to exhaustion. Upon completion of the test, measurements were taken in the following sequence: Doppler blood flow at 1-min from end of RSAT in synchronization with cardiovascular function, blood lactate concentration, and rating of perceived exertion (RPE) values.

Repeated Sprint Ability Test

After the normalization and warm-up period described above, participants performed the RSAT as previously described previously (Faiss et al., 2013). Participants began pedaling at 20 W with a cadence of 85 rpm for 1 min, followed immediately by the RSAT of 10-s all-out maximal sprint and 20-s active recovery (1:2 work-to-rest ratio) until volitional exhaustion or task failure (cadence <70 rpm) similar to Faiss et al. (2013). Immediately at the end of each 10-s sprint, the ergometer automatically switched to a resistance of 20 W for the 20-s recovery. Participants were given very strong verbal encouragement and were not given any indication of the number of sprints performed. All sprints were performed using the "Wingate mode" from the manufacturer with an individually fixed torque factor of 0.8 $Nm{\cdot}kg^{-1}$. Participants were instructed to perform each sprint as hard and fast as possible and perform as many sprints as possible while also maintaining a similar body position. In order to avoid any pacing strategy, the first two sprints were controlled to obtain at least 95% of the best sprint from the two warm-up sprints performed, which was the case for each test. Mean power (W), number of sprints performed, and total work (kJ) were obtained for further analysis, as well as the calculation of fatigue index or percent decrement ($S_{dec}(\%) = [1 - ((S_1 + S_2 + S_3 + \ldots + S_{final})/(S_{best} \times \text{number of sprints}))] \times 100$), where S_1 corresponds to sprint 1, etc., (Glaister et al., 2008). During RSAT, pulse oxygen saturation was measured at the earlobe with an oximeter (8000Q2 Sensor, Nonin Medical Inc., Amsterdam, The Netherlands) and recorded at 5 Hz, the minimum of which was used for further analysis. The RPE was evaluated using the Borg scale (6–20) as a perception of effort in both the legs and the breathing immediately after the test.

Metabolic Measurements

Breath-by-breath pulmonary gas-exchange data were collected continuously (Medgraphics CPX, Loma Linda, CA, USA). Oxygen consumption ($\dot{V}O_2$), ventilation ($\dot{V}_E$), ventilatory equivalent for oxygen ($\dot{V}_E/\dot{V}O_2$), and for carbon dioxide ($\dot{V}_E/\dot{V}CO_2$), respiratory exchange ratio (RER), and breath frequency (BF) were computed and stored for further analyses. The system was calibrated with a 3-L syringe (M9474, Medikro Oy, Finland) and known gas mixtures of O_2 and CO_2 prior to each measurement. Heart rate was monitored at 5 Hz with a telemetry based heart rate monitor (Polar RS400, Kempele, Finland) and the maximum recorded was used for further analysis. During the RSAT, the highest 30-s average of oxygen uptake was computed and used for further analysis. In addition, blood lactate concentration was assessed at the earlobe post-RSAT. After the skin was cleaned and dried, a lancet was used to take a small droplet (0.2 µl) into the strip for analysis (Lactate Scout, EKF Diagnostics, GmbH, Leipzig, Germany).

Cardiovascular Measurements

Estimates of cardiovascular variables were obtained throughout the entire protocol using Physioflow® (Manatec type PF05L1, Paris, France). The measuring device is based on a bioimpedance method which continuously calculates stroke volume (SV), heart rate (HR), cardiac output (Q), systemic vascular resistance (SVR),

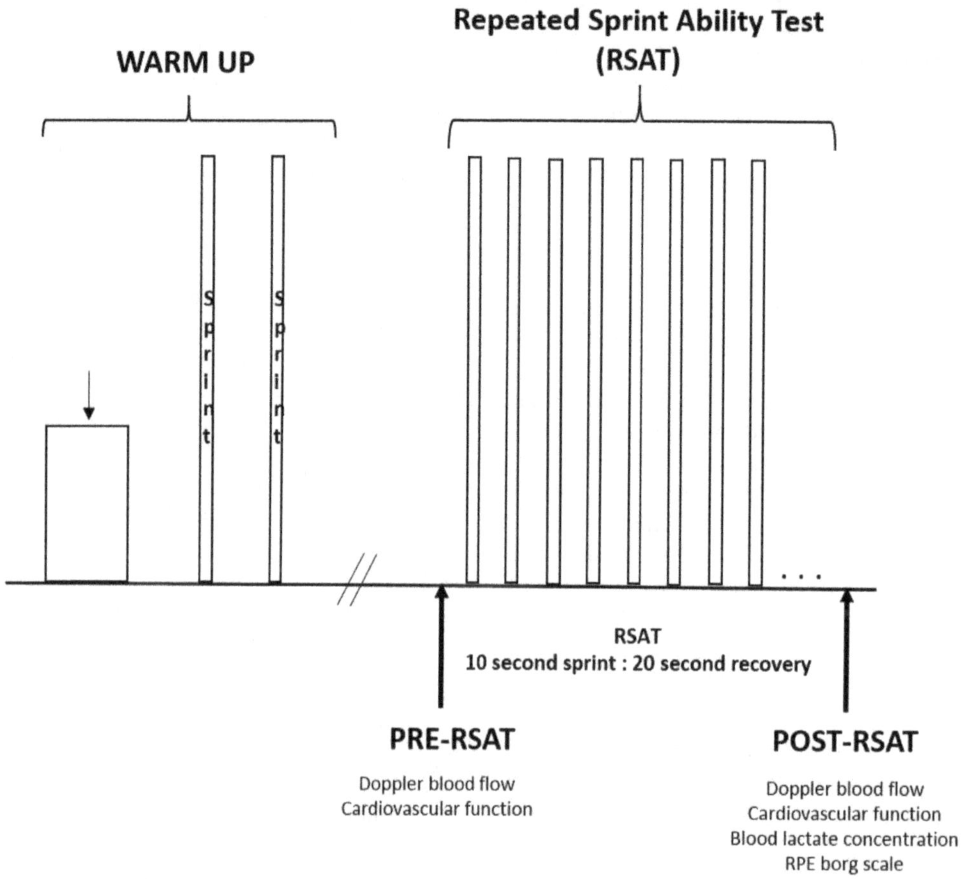

FIGURE 1 | General protocol of warm up and repeated sprint ability test to exhaustion.

end diastolic volume (EDV), and ejection fraction (EF) to detect changes in transthoracic impedance during cardiac ejection. These parameters were analyzed at the same moment (average of 30 s) as the pre- and post- Doppler blood flow measurements. While in the cycling position at rest, Doppler blood flow measurements were collected by an experienced technician on the left femoral artery with a linear probe (L12-5L60N) using EchoWave II 3.4.4 software (Telemed Medical Systems, Telemed Ltd. Lithuania, Milano, Italy) ~5 min pre-, as well as at 1-min post-RSAT. A video image was obtained for 30 s and subsequent analysis was performed to take an average of 10 frames, meaning a measurement every ~1.5 s. Measurements of the blood flow were calculated within the software via a measurement of the vessel diameter (mm) and the blood velocity ($cm \cdot s^{-1}$).

Near-Infrared Spectroscopy Measurements

Muscle oxygenation was evaluated using the near-infrared spectroscopy (NIRS) technique as described previously by Boushel and Piantadosi (2000). The PortaMon and PortaLite devices (Artinis, Zetten, The Netherlands) were used to measure muscle oxygenation of the vastus lateralis (PortaMon) and of the prefrontal cortex (PortaLite) at wavelengths between 760 and 850 nm. All devices were placed into a tight transparent plastic wrap to avoid humidity and create a waterproof barrier for proper function and signal quality. The PortaMon was placed on the lower third of the vastus lateralis and attached with double sided tape, then wrapped with tension against the leg to reduce movement during exercise. The position was marked with a permanent pen and images were taken to reproduce the placement in subsequent visits. The PortaLite was attached on the surface of the left prefrontal cortex with double sided tape, then the subject was fitted with a head wrap to create a dark environment and maintain a stable position of the probe. Measurements included a standard differential pathlength factor of 4.0 for the vastus lateralis as there is a lack of any clear standard value for the quadriceps during cycling sprints (Faiss et al., 2013) and 6.0 for the prefrontal cortex, similar to van der Zee et al. (1992) and Amann et al. (2007). All signals were recorded at the maximum frequency for each device (10 Hz for PortaMon and 50 Hz for PortaLite) and then exported at 10 Hz for further analysis (Oxysoft 3.0.53, Artinis, The Netherlands). For analysis, a 4th-order low-pass zero-phase Butterworth filter (cutoff frequency 0.2 Hz) was implemented to reduce artifacts and smooth perturbations in the signal from pedal strokes. Detection of maximum and minimum was performed automatically using deoxyhemoglobin as reference value for the start point of sprints. This allowed determination of successive sprint and recovery phases to be identified, and sprint phases to be further analyzed. The change (Δ) for each sprint was defined as the difference between maximum and minimum values for each sprint. Delta concentrations of oxyhemoglobin ($\Delta[O_2Hb]$), deoxyhemoglobin ($\Delta[HHb]$), hemoglobin difference ($\Delta[Hbdiff]$), total hemoglobin ($\Delta[tHb]$), and tissue saturation index (ΔTSI, %) were obtained. Finally, the analysis was normalized to the duration of the set to exhaustion; i.e., percentage of sprints performed (i.e., 20, 40, 60, 80, 100%), and a linear interpolation was calculated when there was a fractional number of sprints, since each participant performed a different number of sprints in each condition.

Statistical Analysis

Cardiovascular estimates and blood flow measurements were evaluated with a linear mixed effects analysis of the relationship between condition (400, 2000, 3800 m) and time (pre or post). Fixed effects included condition and time, while participant was set as a random effect. Measurements of oxygenation were also evaluated with a linear mixed model analysis with fixed effects of condition and set duration (20, 40, 60, 80, 100% of sprints performed) with participants as the random effect. The remaining variables including: performance, metabolic gas exchange, pulse oxygen saturation, blood lactate, and RPE were also analyzed with a linear mixed model setting condition as the fixed effect and participant as the random effect. Visual inspection of residual plots did not reveal obvious deviations from homoscedasticity or normality. All analyses were performed using R (R Core Team, 2017, Foundation for Statistical Computing, Vienna, Austria) and nlme4 (Pinheiro et al., 2017). *P*-values were set to 0.05 and were obtained by likelihood ratio tests of the full model with the effect in question against the model without the effect in question. Contrasts were obtained using least-squares means for mixed models [library lsmeans, (Lenth, 2016)] employing Tukey method. Values are represented in tables and figures as mean ± standard deviation.

TABLE 1 | Performance and respiratory values during repeated sprint test to exhaustion in simulated altitude of 400, 2000, and 3800 m.

	400 m	2000 m	3800 m
Number of sprints	29.8 ± 13.7 34 (13–47)	19.8 ± 10.2$^{\#}$ 38 (9–47)	15.4 ± 9.5$^{\#\#\#}$ 26 (7–33)
Mean power (W)	543 ± 135 403 (332–736)	557 ± 150 456 (344–801)	511 ± 139$^{\&}$ 480 (320–800)
Fatigue index (% decrement)	26.5 ± 7.2 22 (14–36)	23.6 ± 7.1 21 (13–34)	26.4 ± 8.0 28 (12–40)
Total work (kJ)	162 ± 81 256 (50–306)	107 ± 41$^{\#\#}$ 137 (31–168)	78 ± 48$^{\#\#\#}$ 25 (166–191)
Maximal heart rate (bpm)	185 ± 9 29 (174–203)	183 ± 11 34 (165–199)	178 ± 8$^{\#\#\#\&}$ 25 (166–191)
SpO_2 (%)	93.8 ± 4.5 14 (86–100)	86.7 + 6.4$^{\#}$ 18 (78–96)	76.5 ± 6.0$^{\#\#\#\&\&\&}$ 18 (70–88)
$\dot{V}O_2$ (ml·kg^{-1}·min^{-1})	40.1 ± 4.1 14.0 (34.5–8.5)	36.4 ± 4.3$^{\#\#\#}$ 11.5 (30.3–41.8)	32.0 ± 3.7$^{\#\#\#\&\&\&}$ 9.8 (27.0–36.8)
RER	1.11 ± 0.06 0.19 (1.01–1.20)	1.19 ± 0.08$^{\#\#}$ 0.22 (1.10–1.32)	1.22 ± 0.09$^{\#\#\#}$ 0.26 (1.06–1.32)
$\dot{V}_E$ (L·min^{-1})	137 ± 28 98.8 (93.6–192.4)	137 ± 30 108.2 (90.6–198.8)	135 ± 35$^{\#\&}$ 117.2 (80.8–198)
$\dot{V}_E/\dot{V}O_2$	50.7 ± 4.5 13.1 (43.1–56.2)	56.0 ± 4.8$^{\#\#\#}$ 14.4 (48.3–62.7)	60.0 ± 6.6$^{\#\#\#\&\&}$ 21.9 (48.4–70.3)
$\dot{V}_E/\dot{V}CO_2$	45.8 ± 4.4 12.4 (39.9–52.3)	47.0 ± 4.1 11.9 (40.4–52.3)	49.3 ± 3.2$^{\#}$ 8.8 (45.0–53.8)
BF (br·min^{-1})	66.9 ± 5.0 16 (59–75)	64.2 ± 3.7 13 (58–71)	63.9 ± 6.5 22 (54–76)
RPE legs (Borg 6-20)	17.7 ± 2.1 5 (15–20)	18.5 ± 1.3 4 (16–20)	17.8 ± 1.9 6 (14–20)
RPE breathing (Borg 6-20)	18.3 ± 1.4 4 (16–20)	19.2 ± 0.8 2 (18–20)	18.3 ± 2.3 8 (12–20)
Blood lactate (mmol·L^{-1})	9.5 ± 5.2 16.9 (4.6–21.5)	11.6 ± 4.8 14.9 (6.2–21.1)	10.7 ± 5.2 13.7 (4.6–18.3)

Mean ± SD. Range (minimum-maximum). $^{\#\#\#}p < 0.001$, $^{\#\#}p < 0.01$, $^{\#}p < 0.05$ *for difference with 400 m.* $^{\&\&\&}p < 0.001$, $^{\&\&}p < 0.01$, $^{\&}p < 0.05$ *for difference with 2000 m.* SpO_2*, pulse oxygen saturation;* $\dot{V}O_2$*, oxygen uptake; RER, respiratory exchange ratio;* $\dot{V}_E$*, minute ventilation; BF, breathing frequency; RPE, rating of perceived exertion.*

RESULTS

Performance

All performance data are presented in **Table 1**. The number of sprints performed to exhaustion decreased by 26.9 ± 29.5% at 2000 m ($p < 0.05$) and 44.9 ± 22.8% at 3800 m ($p < 0.001$) when compared to 400 m. Similarly, the total work was decreased by 27.1 ± 25.8% ($p < 0.01$) and 49.4 ± 19.3% ($p < 0.001$), respectively. As expected, the pulse oxygen saturation also decreased 7.5 ± 6.0% at 2000 m ($p < 0.05$) and 18.4 ± 5.3% at 3800 m ($p < 0.001$), when compared to 400 m.

Metabolic Responses

Metabolic data are also presented in **Table 1**. During the repeated sprint to exhaustion, the peak oxygen uptake was reduced by 9.3 ± 5.5% at 2000 m ($p < 0.001$) and 19.8 ± 5.7% at 3800 m ($p < 0.001$), when compared to 400 m. There was a higher respiratory exchange ratio (RER, $\dot{V}CO_2/\dot{V}O_2$) with increased altitude ($p < 0.01$). In addition, the ventilatory equivalent for oxygen ($\dot{V}_E/\dot{V}O_2$) increased by 10.6 ± 4.6% at 2000 m and 17.9 ± 5.0% at 3800 m, ($p < 0.001$), respectively.

Cardiovascular Responses

There was a main effect of time (pre-post) for stroke volume (SV, $p < 0.05$), heart rate (HR, $p < 0.001$), and cardiac output (Q, $p < 0.001$) which all increased, while the systemic vascular resistance (SVR) was decreased ($p < 0.001$). There were no main effects of condition and no interactions present. All cardiovascular results are shown in **Table 2**. The average increase in femoral artery blood flow from pre- to post- repeated sprint to exhaustion was 71% at 400 m, 34% at 2000 m, and 24% at 3800 m when compared with the resting measurement pre-RSAT.

Peripheral Oxygenation

As indicated in **Figure 2**, for the vastus lateralis, there was a main effect of condition which resulted in a lower $\Delta[Hbdiff]$ and ΔTSI with the highest deoxygenation at 3800 m when compared

TABLE 2 | Average cardiovascular values pre- and 1-min post- repeated sprint ability test (RSAT) representing a main effect difference post-RSAT in simulated altitude of 400, 2000, and 3800 m.

	400 m		2000 m		3800 m	
	Pre-	**Post-**	**Pre-**	**Post-**	**Pre-**	**Post-**
SV	89 ± 11	101 ± 22*	77 ± 16	92 ± 22*	94 ± 18	98 ± 21*
	29 (74–103)	63 (73–136)	52 (52–104)	61 (69–130)	62 (74–136)	63 (76–139)
HR (bpm)	94 ± 17	136 ± 16***	97 ± 16	130 ± 25***	95 ± 16	123 ± 15***
	49 (72–121)	62 (108–170)	55 (69–124)	71 (107–178)	58 (67–125)	44 (101–145)
Q ($L \cdot min^{-1}$)	8.4 ± 2.0	14.0 ± 4.2***	7.6 ± 2.7	12.4 ± 5.5***	8.8 ± 1.9	12.0 ± 2.4***
	6.8 (5.4–12.2)	14.4 (7.9–22.3)	8.1 (4.8–12.9)	14.8 (8.4–23.2)	6.4 (6.3–12.7)	6.6 (8.9–15.5)
SVR ($dyn.s \cdot cm^{-5}$)	817 ± 173	508 ± 140***	999 ± 302	621 ± 182***	843 ± 165	611 ± 101***
	466 (588–1,054)	403 (324–727)	928 (582–1,510)	541 (338–879)	577 (623–1,200)	260 (508–768)
EDV (ml)	114 ± 18	134 ± 31*	107 ± 11	122 ± 22*	124 ± 32	121 ± 25*
	51 (89–140)	90 (91–181)	30 (94–124)	62 (98–160)	99 (95–194)	77 (96–173)
EF (%)	78.7 ± 3.3	77.6 ± 14.2	71.6 ± 12.7	75.6 ± 2.9	76.9 ± 8.3	81.0 ± 3.7
	8.8 (73.6–82.4)	50.8 (40.8–91.6)	37.5 (46.4–83.9)	26.7 (58.9–85.6)	26.3 (64.7–91.0)	11.1 (74.1–85.2)
Blood Flow ($ml \cdot min^{-1}$)£	405 ± 276	694 ± 716	633 ± 555	847 ± 588	631 ± 699	782 ± 744
	771 (14–785)	1,990 (11–2,001)	1,836 (9–1,845)	1,626 (138–1,764)	2,013 (5–2,018)	1,913 (19–1,932)

*Mean ± SD Range (minimum-maximum). Measures were obtained at rest prior to RSAT (pre-), and at 1-min post-RSAT. £Blood flow for one subject was obtained from the popliteal artery, thus the range of values is high. ***p < 0.001, *p < 0.05 for difference with pre-. SV, stroke volume; HR, heart rate; Q, cardiac output; SVR, systemic vascular resistance; EDV, end diastolic volume; EF, ejection fraction.*

with 400 and 2000 m ($p < 0.05$). Additionally, the main effect of condition was indicated for Δ[HHb] and Δ[tHb] in which resulted in greater changes in the 2000 m condition ($p < 0.05$) compared with 400 and 3800 m. There was a main effect of set duration near the end of the sprint test to exhaustion ($p < 0.05$) with Δ[Hbdiff], ΔTSI, and Δ[tHb] decreasing toward end of the test. Absolute maximal TSI values are shown in **Figure 4**, with a main effect of hypoxic condition and a continual decrease as hypoxia severity increased ($p < 0.001$) as well as a main effect of set duration near exhaustion ($p < 0.05$). No interactions were present.

Cerebral Oxygenation

In the prefrontal cortex (**Figure 3**), there was a main effect of condition for Δ[HHb] with a smaller decrease (smaller change) at 3800 m when compared with 400 and 2000 m ($p < 0.01$). Additionally, a main effect of condition resulted with greater Δ[Hbdiff] at both 2000 and 3800 m, compared with 400 m ($p < 0.05$). Similarly, there was higher ΔTSI at both 2000 and 3800 m when compared with 400 m ($p < 0.01$). There was a main effect of set duration near the end of the sprint test to exhaustion ($p < 0.05$) with Δ[Hbdiff] and Δ[tHb] increasing in the last 20% of the sprint test. In addition, for Δ[Hbdiff], there was a significant interaction effect between condition and set duration ($F = 2.706, p < 0.01$).

DISCUSSION

The main findings of this study were:

1. There was a continual decrease in convective factors of oxygen delivery (e.g., decreases in pulse oxygen saturation and peak oxygen uptake) with increased hypoxia severity, which was linked with impairment in performance (number of sprints and total work) across conditions.
2. There were reduced changes in peripheral oxygenation values at 3800 m indicating a possible limitation of the oxygen transport system (i.e., circulatory) which was non-linear as hypoxia increased, likely indicating different responses as altitude increases. This may suggest a threshold between 2000 and 3800 m regarding the means of oxygen transport, which supports previous research stating 2000 m moderate and 3800 m is high altitude (Bartsch et al., 2008).
3. Cerebral deoxygenation demonstrated greater changes at 3800 m compared with 400 and 2000 m, as well as an increased change in blood volume in the final 20% of the set duration (at exhaustion). This may indicate that central autoregulation occurs in order to continue exercise despite limited peripheral and cerebral oxygen delivery, until a certain point of limited diffusion at which protective mechanisms cease exercise.

Decreased Convective Oxygen Delivery

With increased altitude, there was an expected and logical decrease in convective factors of oxygen transport. Specifically, there was a decreased pulse oxygen saturation (level of the capillary) and decreased peak oxygen uptake (pulmonary and systemic circulation) with conditions of decreased oxygen. Maximal heart rate was also decreased significantly at 3800 m. Interestingly, there was no increase with altitude in minute ventilation or breathing frequency. However, since the exercise was maximal and to exhaustion, any difference between altitude levels would have been minor. The ventilatory efficiency index

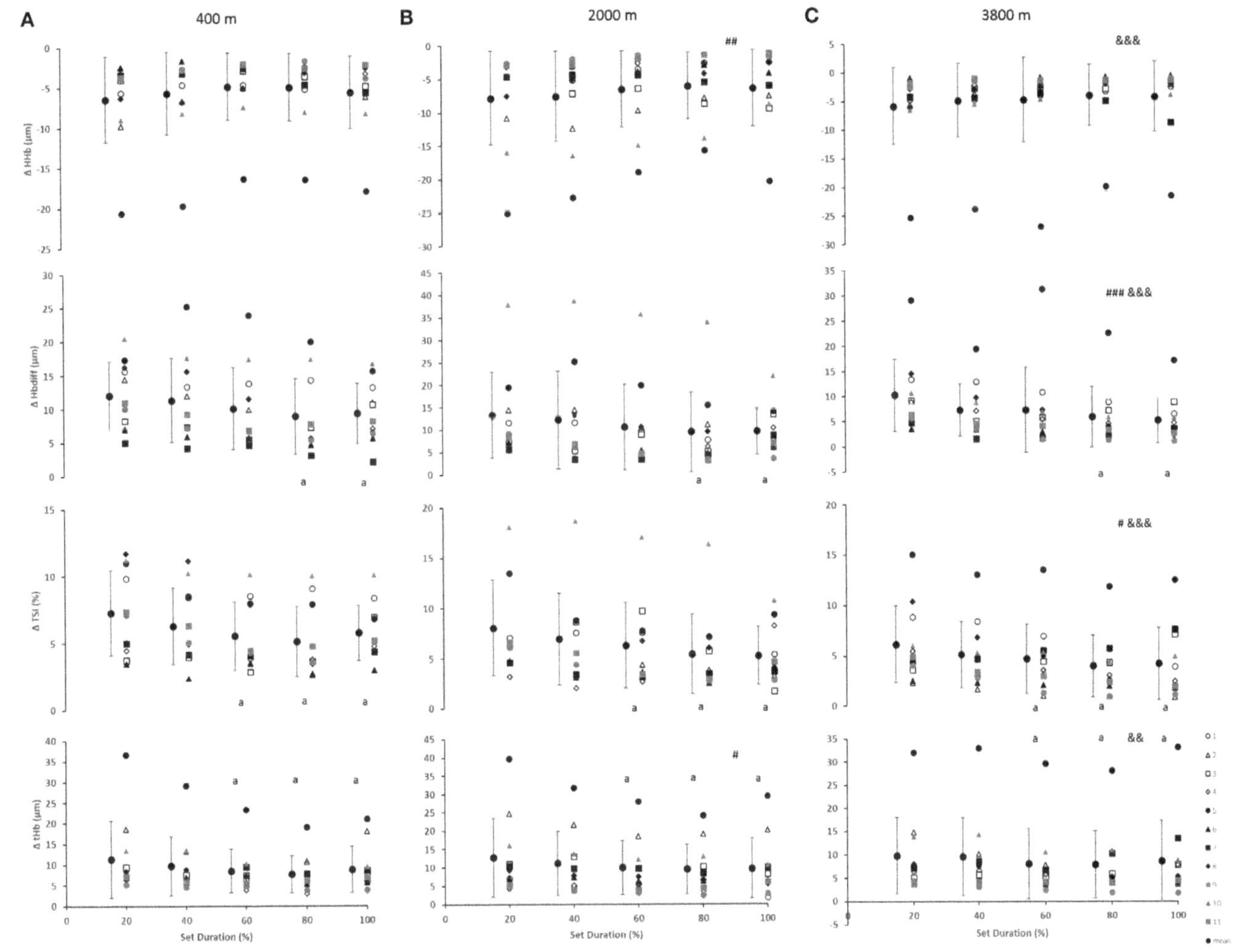

FIGURE 2 | Near-infrared spectroscopy (NIRS) results representing the average maximum-minimum delta (Δ) value during the percentage of sprints completed to exhaustion for the individual response of the vastus lateralis in simulated altitude of **(A)** 400 m, **(B)** 2000 m, and **(C)** 3800 m. Mean ± SD. $^{###}p < 0.001$, $^{##}p < 0.01$, $^{#}p < 0.05$ for difference with 400 m; $^{\&\&\&}p < 0.001$, $^{\&\&}p < 0.01$ for difference with 2000 m. Symbol: a for difference with 20%.

($\dot{V}_E/\dot{V}O_2$) was increased with altitude naturally due to a decrease in oxygen uptake (**Table 1**), similar as previously shown (Calbet et al., 2009). It has been suggested that the first limitation of performance in hypoxia is the delivery of oxygen primarily by factors of convection (which resulted in the present study) and subsequently by means of diffusion capacities at the muscle and mitochondrial (Calbet et al., 2009, 2015b) as well as pulmonary level (Sarkar et al., 2017). Additionally, there were no differences in the hemodynamic response with repeated sprints to exhaustion between altitude conditions (SV, Q, HR, SVR, EDV, EF) and also no acute peripheral vasodilation as noted by femoral arterial blood flow. Peak cardiac output has been shown to remain similar between different levels of hypoxia as a possible counteraction for the reduction in arterial content of oxygen (Calbet et al., 2009). Furthermore, this study demonstrated that the limitation of oxygen delivery resulted in an impairment in performance across conditions. There were no changes in the rating of perceived exertion of the leg or breathing or changes in blood lactate concentration between conditions, indicating that the maximal efforts of the tests were similar despite the differences in total work. These results suggest there are some factor(s) allowing performance to be at least partly maintained despite continued decreases in pulse oxygen saturation and oxygen uptake due to regulatory mechanisms facilitating the oxygen delivery as the severity of hypoxia increases. This can be partly explained by the oxygen-hemoglobin dissociation curve and the shift of the curve based on the affinity for oxygen. As demonstrated by Calbet and colleagues, the offloading of oxygen from hemoglobin does not require a right-shift in the oxygen-hemoglobin dissociation curve indicating less of a role of the Bohr effect (Calbet et al., 2015b).

Limitations of Peripheral Oxygenation

The change in vastus lateralis oxygenation values were less at 3800 m indicating less of a change from maximum to minimum during sprints, meaning there was a further limitation of the oxygen transport system (i.e., circulatory) in comparison to the other conditions of 400 and 2000 m (**Figure 2**). Indeed, the

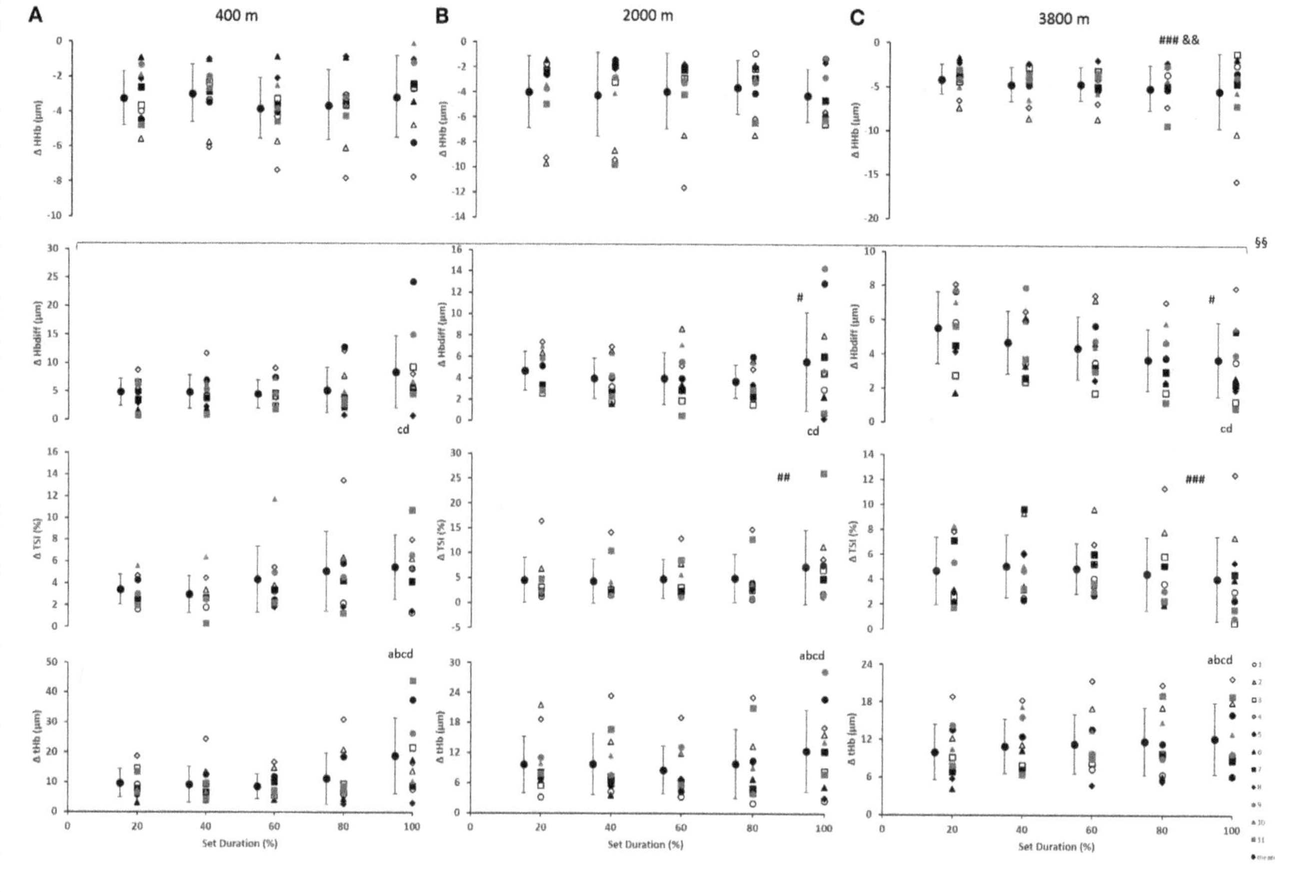

FIGURE 3 | Near-infrared spectroscopy (NIRS) results representing the average maximum-minimum delta (Δ) value during the percentage of sprints completed to exhaustion for the individual response of the prefrontal cortex in simulated altitude of **(A)** 400 m, **(B)** 2000 m, and **(C)** 3800 m. Mean ± SD. ###$p < 0.001$, #$p < 0.05$ for difference with 400 m; &&$p < 0.01$ for difference with 2000 m. Symbol: a for difference with 20%, b for difference with 40%, c for difference with 60%, and d for difference with 80%. §§Significant ($p < 0.01$) interaction (condition × set duration) was present.

absolute maximal values of TSI indicated a continual limitation of oxygen as hypoxia increased, which decreased toward the end of the test (**Figure 4**). In fact, an inconsistent decrease in Δ[HHb] was demonstrated as the severity of hypoxia increased, indicating a possible threshold between 2000 and 3800 m where peripheral oxygenation becomes limited. An increase in [HHb] in hypoxia has been shown to increase the metabolic demand of exercise (Costes et al., 1996) and is considered as a counteraction for the reduced oxygen availability (Legrand et al., 2005). This is likely due to increased local acidosis reducing hemoglobin's affinity for oxygen through the Bohr effect (Nielsen et al., 2002). Furthermore, previous research has demonstrated that the role of this acidosis is minimal regarding the mechanisms of oxygen offloading during exercise, which supports the result of the current study with no change in blood lactate concentration between conditions, as seen in **Table 1** (Calbet et al., 2015b).

All changes in peripheral oxygenation (Δ[HHb], Δ[tHb], and ΔTSI) were continually decreasing toward the end of the test (**Figure 1**). In the present study, there was a plateau in Δ[HHb], which has been previously suggested to be an indication of maximal skeletal muscle oxygen extraction (Esaki et al., 2005). However, it has also been shown that the peripheral muscle can continue to extract oxygen even in conditions of reduced oxygen availability (Smith and Billaut, 2010, 2012). This supports previous research that suggested the plateau in peripheral deoxygenation was not a reason for the exhaustion and the end of exercise, but rather an indication of an equilibrium between the oxygen delivery and extraction/consumption over higher work rates (Subudhi et al., 2007). This confirms the result of the current study that performance can continue despite limited convective oxygen transport (decreased oxygen uptake and pulse oxygen saturation) as well as despite maximal levels of peripheral deoxygenation. The decreased Δ[HHb] in the vastus lateralis at 3800 m in the present study suggests that a compensatory larger extraction may at least partly counterbalance the lower convective oxygen supply and therefore reduce the diffusion limitation, as previously suggested (Cerretelli, 1976; Wagner, 2000).

Moreover, Amann and colleagues have suggested that when substantial peripheral muscle fatigue has occurred in normoxia or moderate hypoxia, there is no capacity to reverse the magnitude and thus, exercise is terminated via reduction in the central motor output for prevention of further development of peripheral fatigue beyond a critical level (in accordance with

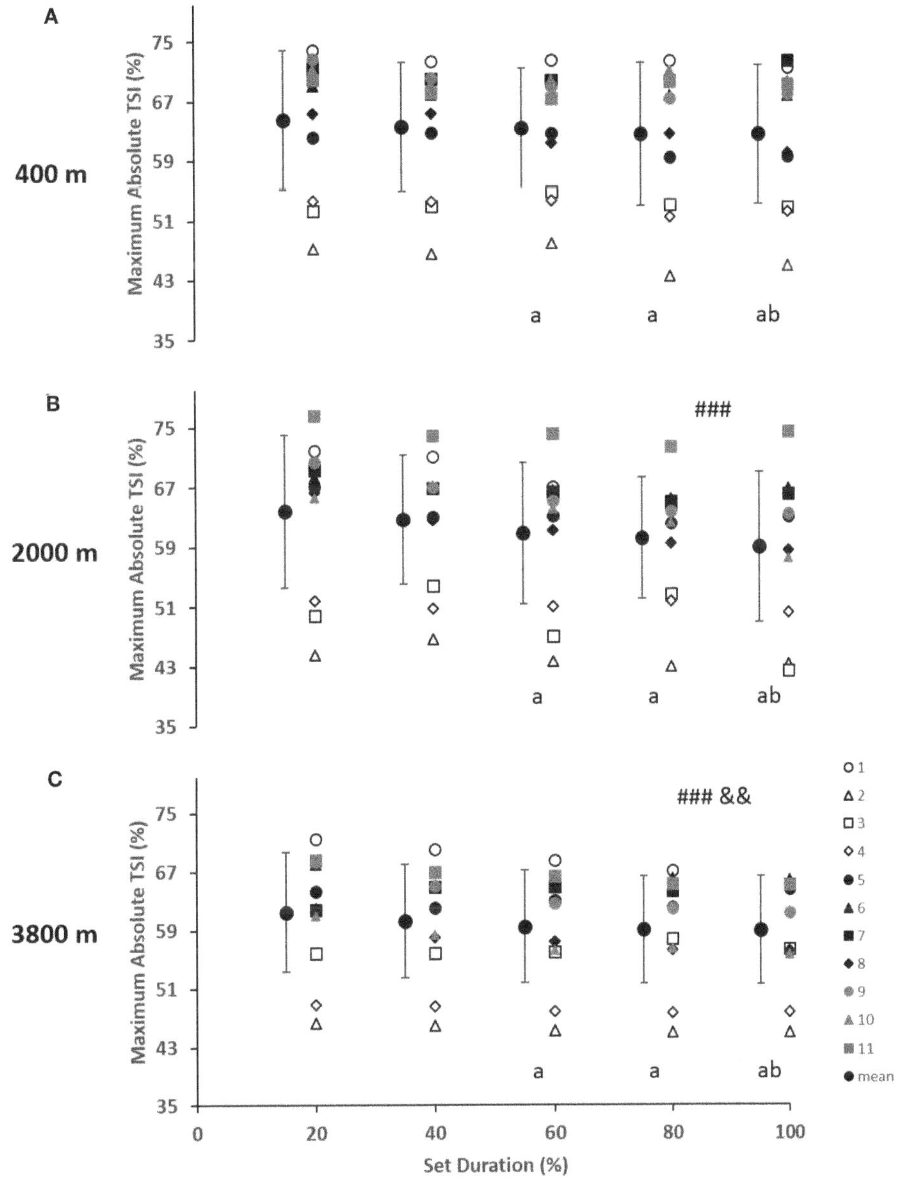

FIGURE 4 | Near-infrared spectroscopy (NIRS) results representing the average maximum value of tissue saturation index (%) during the percentage of sprints completed to exhaustion for the individual response of the vastus lateralis in simulated altitude of **(A)** 400 m, **(B)** 2000 m, and **(C)** 3800 m. Mean ± SD. ###$p < 0.001$ for difference with 400 m; &&$p < 0.01$ for difference with 2000 m. Symbol: a for difference with 20%, and b for difference with 40%.

their previous research; Amann et al., 2006, 2007; Romer et al., 2007). In addition, researchers have suggested an influence of the central nervous system over the active muscles in hypoxia (Amann et al., 2007), as there is decreased central command at low oxygen fraction (Millet et al., 2009). This mechanism could partially contribute to the greater performance detriments with lower oxygenation levels (range of 70–75% arterial oxygen saturation), which is likely regulated by differences in the partial pressure of arterial oxygen ($P_{a,O2}$) rather than changes in arterial content or hemoglobin concentration (Horstman et al., 1980; Calbet et al., 2002; Lundby and Damsgaard, 2006).

Limitations of Cerebral Oxygenation

Greater decreases in prefrontal cortex deoxygenation (Δ[HHb]) were demonstrated at 3800 m. Cerebral changes in oxygenation were limited (lower) at both 2000 and 3800 m, in comparison to the 400 m condition. Furthermore, greater changes in [tHb], a well-known indicator of regional blood volume and perfusion (Van Beekvelt et al., 2001; Faiss et al., 2013), and Δ[Hbdiff] were seen at the end of the test (i.e., exhaustion, last 20% of sprints) with increased changes at both 2000 and 3800 m for Δ[Hbdiff]. These data together illustrate the oxygen delivery regulation of the brain.

Previous research has indicated that in hypoxic conditions there is a greater diffusive limitation due to a lower gradient of the partial pressure of oxygen (Wagner, 1993). In hypoxia, the brain adjusts for a lower arterial oxygen content by increasing the extraction of oxygen (Gonzalez-Alonso et al., 2004; Rasmussen et al., 2007) and increasing cerebral blood flow at rest (Lassen, 1959; Willie et al., 2012). While during exercise, there are the additional factors of hypocapnia and increased arterial blood pressure which contribute to the impact of oxygenation and brain function in hypoxia (Curtelin et al., 2017). Curtelin et al. (2017) found that the priority is placed on maintaining cerebral oxygen delivery even though there is also a need to regulate cerebral blood flow to avoid an excessive increase in blood pressure. During sprint exercise in hypoxia, the combination of increased mean arterial pressure and cardiac output increases perfusion of the muscle tissue while simultaneously challenging the brain with the risk of hyperperfusion (Bill and Linder, 1976; Deegan et al., 2010). As demonstrated in the present study, there were greater changes in the perfusion (Δ[tHb]) in the end of the test, which was likely tolerated despite higher perfusion pressure and reduced partial pressure of arterial carbon dioxide ($P_{a,CO2}$) during sprint exercise in severe hypoxia in order to protect brain function in low oxygen conditions with the counter-risk of increased hemodynamic injury (Curtelin et al., 2017). This change was mostly present in the normoxic condition, however, there was a main effect difference at the end of exercise. Further, this finding may provide insight to the reason for exercise cessation. Moreover, the evidence of previous research showing a 66% decrease in cerebral $P_{a,O2}$ with acute hypoxia cannot be ignored (Calbet et al., 2009). In fact, it was found that the low $P_{a,O2}$ may be as low as 10 Torr in some areas of the brain (Calbet et al., 2003). This low $P_{a,O2}$ would suggest there is a low pressure gradient, however it remains unknown about the diffusion distance and the possible diffusive limitation of oxygen delivery to the brain at altitude (Hornbein et al., 1989; Dunn et al., 2016). There is likely a coupling between arterial blood pressure and perfusion pressure (gradient between arterial and venous blood pressure) related to pressure, flow, and resistance to determine the mechanisms of the diffusion limitation of cerebral oxygen delivery during exhaustive exercise in hypoxia.

The results of the present study confirm that exercise performance in hypoxia can continue despite limited peripheral convective oxygen delivery, with the continuation of performance due to a functional reserve in muscle oxygen diffusing capacity (Calbet et al., 2015b). Meanwhile, the brain increases blood flow to account for decreased arterial oxygen content and to maintain oxygen delivery to preserve the brain's function (central motor output) and thus task continuation despite the progression of central fatigue (Amann et al., 2007; Curtelin et al., 2017). Progressive changes continue until an underlying threshold is reached where the pressure of increased perfusion of the brain surpasses a critical threshold and likely leads to exercise cessation due to increased mean arterial pressure and hyperperfusion. However, these mechanisms are speculative and therefore further research is warranted.

Limitations of the Study

Researchers acknowledge that the current results are influenced by an elevation of skin blood flow during exercise, which is due to the nature of the device placed on the surface of the skin (Subudhi et al., 2007). Therefore, it is probable that the current results would underestimate tissue deoxygenation. Moreover, it is likely that the changes found would be greater in these variables and would not alter the conclusions made here. The difference between hemoglobin and myoglobin is not known with the use of the NIRS, it is therefore not possible to distinguish the differences between blood-muscle oxygen transport in the current study. Furthermore, the reliability of probe placement was minimized with permanent markings and picture identification, however, there is day-to-day variation in these parameters of about 8.0–9.4% (Kishi et al., 2003; Kolb et al., 2004). It is assumed that [O_2Hb] and [HHb] are in existing equilibrium where an increase in one simultaneously decreases the other. This assumption is based on maintaining [tHb] constant. As most of the body's arterial blood volume is oxygenated, [tHb] is closely related to [O_2Hb] if the consumption of oxygen remains constant, which can be reflected by HHb concentration (Van Beekvelt et al., 2001; Subudhi et al., 2007). During exercise, these variables are in constant flux and for that reason, the NIRS measurements should be considered with scrutiny. In addition, the test-retest reliability of the blood flow measurements from the femoral artery conducted pre- and post-RSAT have not been previously reported, thus it is important to consider in interpretation of these results. As this study involved non-invasive measurements as part of a larger protocol, there is a lack of data corresponding to changes in blood gases, blood pressure, and cerebral blood flow which would certainly improve the interpretation of these results.

CONCLUSION

In summary, this study confirms that performance in hypoxia is limited by continually decreasing convective oxygen delivery while exercise can continue despite maximal peripheral deoxygenation. The limitation of peripheral oxygenation was not linear across varying hypoxic conditions possibly indicating a threshold at which point oxygen delivery has a stronger effect on the periphery between 2000 and 3800 m. There may be a cerebral autoregulation that increases cerebral perfusion at exhaustion to account for decreased arterial oxygen content (as shown across all conditions) and allow for task continuation (greater cerebral deoxygenation at 3800 m in comparison to 400 and 2000 m).

AUTHOR CONTRIBUTIONS

All authors listed have made substantial, direct, and intellectual contributions to this work. In addition, all authors have approved this work for publication.

ACKNOWLEDGMENTS

Authors wish to thank all the participants for their time, effort, enthusiasm, and cooperation on this project.

REFERENCES

ACSM (2014). *ACSM's Guidelines for Exercise Testing and Prescription*. Baltimore, MD: Lippincott Williams and Wilkins.

Amann, M., and Calbet, J. A. (2008). Convective oxygen transport and fatigue. *J. Appl. Physiol.* 104, 861–870. doi: 10.1152/japplphysiol.01008.2007

Amann, M., Eldridge, M. W., Lovering, A. T., Stickland, M. K., Pegelow, D. F., and Dempsey, J. A. (2006). Arterial oxygenation influences central motor output and exercise performance via effects on peripheral locomotor muscle fatigue in humans. *J. Physiol.* 575(Pt 3), 937–952. doi: 10.1113/jphysiol.2006.113936

Amann, M., and Kayser, B. (2009). Nervous system function during exercise in hypoxia. *High Alt. Med. Biol.* 10, 149–164. doi: 10.1089/ham.2008.1105

Amann, M., Romer, L. M., Subudhi, A. W., Pegelow, D. F., and Dempsey, J. A. (2007). Severity of arterial hypoxaemia affects the relative contributions of peripheral muscle fatigue to exercise performance in healthy humans. *J. Physiol.* 581(Pt 1), 389–403. doi: 10.1113/jphysiol.2007.129700

Balsom, P. D., Gaitanos, G. C., Ekblom, B., and Sjodin, B. (1994). Reduced oxygen availability during high intensity intermittent exercise impairs performance. *Acta Physiol. Scand.* 152, 279–285. doi: 10.1111/j.1748-1716.1994.tb09807.x

Bartsch, P., Saltin, B., Dvorak, J., and Federation Internationale de Football, A. (2008). Consensus statement on playing football at different altitude. *Scand. J. Med. Sci. Sports* 18(Suppl. 1), 96–99. doi: 10.1111/j.1600-0838.2008.00837.x

Bill, A., and Linder, J. (1976). Sympathetic control of cerebral blood flow in acute arterial hypertension. *Acta Physiol. Scand.* 96, 114–121. doi: 10.1111/j.1748-1716.1976.tb10176.x

Billaut, F., and Buchheit, M. (2013). Repeated-sprint performance and vastus lateralis oxygenation: effect of limited O(2) availability. *Scand. J. Med. Sci. Sports* 23, e185–e193. doi: 10.1111/sms.12052

Billaut, F., and Smith, K. (2010). Prolonged repeated-sprint ability is related to arterial O2 desaturation in men. *Int. J. Sports Physiol. Perform.* 5, 197–209. doi: 10.1123/ijspp.5.2.197

Boushel, R., and Piantadosi, C. A. (2000). Near-infrared spectroscopy for monitoring muscle oxygenation. *Acta Physiol. Scand.* 168, 615–622. doi: 10.1046/j.1365-201x.2000.00713.x

Calbet, J. A. (2000). Oxygen tension and content in the regulation of limb blood flow. *Acta Physiol. Scand.* 168, 465–472. doi: 10.1046/j.1365-201x.2000.00698.x

Calbet, J. A., Boushel, R., Radegran, G., Sondergaard, H., Wagner, P. D., and Saltin, B. (2003). Determinants of maximal oxygen uptake in severe acute hypoxia. *Am. J. Physiol. Regul. Integr. Comp. Physiol.* 284, R291–R303. doi: 10.1152/ajpregu.00155.2002

Calbet, J. A., Gonzalez-Alonso, J., Helge, J. W., Sondergaard, H., Munch-Andersen, T., Saltin, B., et al. (2015a). Central and peripheral hemodynamics in exercising humans: leg vs arm exercise. *Scand. J. Med. Sci. Sports* 25(Suppl. 4), 144–157. doi: 10.1111/sms.12604

Calbet, J. A., Losa-Reyna, J., Torres-Peralta, R., Rasmussen, P., Ponce-Gonzalez, J. G., Sheel, A. W., et al. (2015b). Limitations to oxygen transport and utilization during sprint exercise in humans: evidence for a functional reserve in muscle O2 diffusing capacity. *J. Physiol.* 593, 4649–4664. doi: 10.1113/JP270408

Calbet, J. A., Radegran, G., Boushel, R., and Saltin, B. (2009). On the mechanisms that limit oxygen uptake during exercise in acute and chronic hypoxia: role of muscle mass. *J. Physiol.* 587, 477–490. doi: 10.1113/jphysiol.2008.162271

Calbet, J. A., Radegran, G., Boushel, R., Sondergaard, H., Saltin, B., and Wagner, P. D. (2002). Effect of blood haemoglobin concentration on V(O2,max) and cardiovascular function in lowlanders acclimatised to 5260 m. *J. Physiol.* 545(Pt 2), 715–728. doi: 10.1113/jphysiol.2002.029108

Cerretelli, P. (1976). Limiting factors to oxygen transport on Mount Everest. *J. Appl. Physiol.* 40, 658–667.

Costes, F., Barthelemy, J. C., Feasson, L., Busso, T., Geyssant, A., and Denis, C. (1996). Comparison of muscle near-infrared spectroscopy and femoral blood gases during steady-state exercise in humans. *J. Appl. Physiol.* 80, 1345–1350.

Curtelin, D., Morales-Alamo, D., Torres-Peralta, R., Rasmussen, P., Martin-Rincon, M., Perez-Valera, M., et al. (2017). Cerebral blood flow, frontal lobe oxygenation and intra-arterial blood pressure during sprint exercise in normoxia and severe acute hypoxia in humans. *J. Cereb. Blood Flow Metab.* doi: 10.1177/0271678X17691986. [Epub ahead of print].

Deegan, B. M., Devine, E. R., Geraghty, M. C., Jones, E., Olaighin, G., and Serrador, J. M. (2010). The relationship between cardiac output and dynamic cerebral autoregulation in humans. *J. Appl. Physiol.* 109, 1424–1431. doi: 10.1152/japplphysiol.01262.2009

di Prampero, P. E. (2003). Factors limiting maximal performance in humans. *Eur. J. Appl. Physiol.* 90, 420–429. doi: 10.1007/s00421-003-0926-z

De Smet, S., van Herpt, P., D'Hulst, G., Van Thienen, R., Van Leemputte, M., and Hespel, P. (2017). Physiological adaptations to hypoxic vs. normoxic training during intermittent living high. *Front. Physiol.* 8:347. doi: 10.3389/fphys.2017.00347

Dunn, J. O. C., Mythen, M. G., and Grocott, M. P. (2016). Physiology of oxygen transport. *BJA Educ.* 16, 341–348. doi: 10.1093/bjaed/mkw012

Esaki, K., Hamaoka, T., Radegran, G., Boushel, R., Hansen, J., Katsumura, T., et al. (2005). Association between regional quadriceps oxygenation and blood oxygen saturation during normoxic one-legged dynamic knee extension. *Eur. J. Appl. Physiol.* 95, 361–370. doi: 10.1007/s00421-005-0008-5

Faiss, R., Leger, B., Vesin, J. M., Fournier, P. E., Eggel, Y., Deriaz, O., et al. (2013). Significant molecular and systemic adaptations after repeated sprint training in hypoxia. *PLoS ONE* 8:e56522. doi: 10.1371/journal.pone.0056522

Girard, O., Mendez-Villanueva, A., and Bishop, D. (2011). Repeated-sprint ability - part I: factors contributing to fatigue. *Sports Med.* 41, 673–694. doi: 10.2165/11590550-000000000-00000

Glaister, M., Howatson, G., Pattison, J. R., and McInnes, G. (2008). The reliability and validity of fatigue measures during multiple-sprint work: an issue revisited. *J. Strength Cond. Res.* 22, 1597–1601. doi: 10.1519/JSC.0b013e318181ab80

Gonzalez-Alonso, J., Dalsgaard, M. K., Osada, T., Volianitis, S., Dawson, E. A., Yoshiga, C. C., et al. (2004). Brain and central haemodynamics and oxygenation during maximal exercise in humans. *J. Physiol.* 557(Pt 1), 331–342. doi: 10.1113/jphysiol.2004.060574

Grassi, B., Quaresima, V., Marconi, C., Ferrari, M., and Cerretelli, P. (1999). Blood lactate accumulation and muscle deoxygenation during incremental exercise. *J. Appl. Physiol.* 87, 348–355.

Hornbein, T. F., Townes, B. D., Schoene, R. B., Sutton, J. R., and Houston, C. S. (1989). The cost to the central nervous system of climbing to extremely high altitude. *N. Engl. J. Med.* 321, 1714–1719. doi: 10.1056/NEJM198912213212505

Horstman, D., Weiskopf, R., and Jackson, R. E. (1980). Work capacity during 3-wk sojourn at 4,300 m: effects of relative polycythemia. *J. Appl. Physiol. Respir. Environ. Exerc. Physiol.* 49, 311–318.

Imray, C. H., Myers, S. D., Pattinson, K. T., Bradwell, A. R., Chan, C. W., Harris, S., et al. (2005). Effect of exercise on cerebral perfusion in humans at high altitude. *J. Appl. Physiol.* 99, 699–706. doi: 10.1152/japplphysiol.00973.2004

Kayser, B. (2003). Exercise starts and ends in the brain. *Eur. J. Appl. Physiol.* 90, 411–419. doi: 10.1007/s00421-003-0902-7

Kishi, K., Kawaguchi, M., Yoshitani, K., Nagahata, T., and Furuya, H. (2003). Influence of patient variables and sensor location on regional cerebral oxygen saturation measured by INVOS 4100 near-infrared spectrophotometers. *J. Neurosurg. Anesthesiol.* 15, 302–306. doi: 10.1097/00008506-200310000-00002

Kolb, J. C., Ainslie, P. N., Ide, K., and Poulin, M. J. (2004). Protocol to measure acute cerebrovascular and ventilatory responses to isocapnic hypoxia in humans. *Respir. Physiol. Neurobiol.* 141, 191–199. doi: 10.1016/j.resp.2004.04.014

Lassen, N. A. (1959). Cerebral blood flow and oxygen consumption in man. *Physiol. Rev.* 39, 183–238.

Laughlin, M. H., and Joyner, M. (2003). Closer to the edge? Contractions, pressures, waterfalls and blood flow to contracting skeletal muscle. *J. Appl. Physiol.* 94, 3–5. doi: 10.1152/japplphysiol.00829.2002

Legrand, R., Ahmaidi, S., Moalla, W., Chocquet, D., Marles, A., Prieur, F., et al. (2005). O2 arterial desaturation in endurance athletes increases muscle deoxygenation. *Med. Sci. Sports Exerc.* 37, 782–788. doi: 10.1249/01.MSS.0000161806.47058.40

Lenth, R. V. (2016). Least-squares means: the R package lsmeans. *J. Stat. Softw.* 69:33. doi: 10.18637/jss.v069.i01

Lundby, C., and Damsgaard, R. (2006). Exercise performance in hypoxia after novel erythropoiesis stimulating protein treatment. *Scand. J. Med. Sci. Sports* 16, 35–40. doi: 10.1111/j.1600-0838.2004.00434.x

MacDougall, J. D., Tuxen, D., Sale, D. G., Moroz, J. R., and Sutton, J. R. (1985). Arterial blood pressure response to heavy resistance exercise. *J. Appl. Physiol.* 58, 785–790.

Millet, G. Y., Aubert, D., Favier, F. B., Busso, T., and Benoit, H. (2009). Effect of acute hypoxia on central fatigue during repeated isometric leg contractions. *Scand. J. Med. Sci. Sports* 19, 695–702. doi: 10.1111/j.1600-0838.2008.00823.x

Neary, J. P., Hall, K., and Bhambhani, Y. N. (2001). Vastus medialis muscle oxygenation trends during a simulated 20-km cycle time trial. *Eur. J. Appl. Physiol.* 85, 427–433. doi: 10.1007/s004210100481

Nielsen, H. B., Bredmose, P. P., Stromstad, M., Volianitis, S., Quistorff, B., and Secher, N. H. (2002). Bicarbonate attenuates arterial desaturation during maximal exercise in humans. *J. Appl. Physiol.* 93, 724–731. doi: 10.1152/japplphysiol.00398.2000

Pinheiro, J., Bates, D., DebRoy, S., Sarkar, D., and R Core Team. (2017). *nlme: Linear and Nonlinear Mixed Effects Models [Online]*. Available online at: https://CRAN.R-project.org/package=nlme (Accessed August 16, 2017).

R Core Team (2017). *R: A Language and Environment for Statistical Computing.* Vienna: R Foundation for Statistical Computing. Available online at: http://www.R-project.org/

Racinais, S., Bishop, D., Denis, R., Lattier, G., Mendez-Villaneuva, A., and Perrey, S. (2007). Muscle deoxygenation and neural drive to the muscle during repeated sprint cycling. *Med. Sci. Sports Exerc.* 39, 268–274. doi: 10.1249/01.mss.0000251775.46460.cb

Rasmussen, P., Dawson, E. A., Nybo, L., van Lieshout, J. J., Secher, N. H., and Gjedde, A. (2007). Capillary-oxygenation-level-dependent near-infrared spectrometry in frontal lobe of humans. *J. Cereb. Blood Flow Metab.* 27, 1082–1093. doi: 10.1038/sj.jcbfm.9600416

Romer, L. M., Haverkamp, H. C., Amann, M., Lovering, A. T., Pegelow, D. F., and Dempsey, J. A. (2007). Effect of acute severe hypoxia on peripheral fatigue and endurance capacity in healthy humans. *Am. J. Physiol. Regul. Integr. Comp. Physiol.* 292, R598–R606. doi: 10.1152/ajpregu.00269.2006

Sarkar, M., Niranjan, N., and Banyal, P. K. (2017). Mechanisms of hypoxemia. *Lung India* 34, 47–60. doi: 10.4103/0970-2113.197116

Shibuya, K., Tanaka, J., and Ogaki, T. (2004). Muscle oxygenation kinetics at the onset of exercise do not depend on exercise intensity. *Eur. J. Appl. Physiol.* 91, 712–715. doi: 10.1007/s00421-004-1045-1

Smith, K. J., and Billaut, F. (2010). Influence of cerebral and muscle oxygenation on repeated-sprint ability. *Eur. J. Appl. Physiol.* 109, 989–999. doi: 10.1007/s00421-010-1444-4

Smith, K. J., and Billaut, F. (2012). Tissue oxygenation in men and women during repeated-sprint exercise. *Int. J. Sports Physiol. Perform.* 7, 59–67. doi: 10.1123/ijspp.7.1.59

Subudhi, A. W., Dimmen, A. C., and Roach, R. C. (2007). Effects of acute hypoxia on cerebral and muscle oxygenation during incremental exercise. *J. Appl. Physiol.* 103, 177–183. doi: 10.1152/japplphysiol.01460.2006

Sweeting, A. J., Billaut, F., Varley, M. C., Rodriguez, R. F., Hopkins, W. G., and Aughey, R. J. (2017). Variations in hypoxia impairs muscle oxygenation and performance during simulated team-sport running. *Front. Physiol.* 8:80. doi: 10.3389/fphys.2017.00080

Van Beekvelt, M. C., Colier, W. N., Wevers, R. A., and Van Engelen, B. G. (2001). Performance of near-infrared spectroscopy in measuring local O(2) consumption and blood flow in skeletal muscle. *J. Appl. Physiol.* 90, 511–519.

van der Zee, P., Cope, M., Arridge, S. R., Essenpreis, M., Potter, L. A., Edwards, A. D., et al. (1992). Experimentally measured optical pathlengths for the adult head, calf and forearm and the head of the newborn infant as a function of inter optode spacing. *Adv. Exp. Med. Biol.* 316, 143–153. doi: 10.1007/978-1-4615-3404-4_17

Van Thienen, R., and Hespel, P. (2016). Enhanced muscular oxygen extraction in athletes exaggerates hypoxemia during exercise in hypoxia. *J. Appl. Physiol.* 120, 351–361. doi: 10.1152/japplphysiol.00210.2015

Villar, R., and Hughson, R. L. (2017). Vascular conductance and muscle blood flow during exercise are altered by inspired oxygen fraction and arterial perfusion pressure. *Physiol. Rep.* 5:e13144. doi: 10.14814/phy2.13144

Wagner, P. D. (1993). Algebraic analysis of the determinants of VO2,max. *Respir. Physiol.* 93, 221–237. doi: 10.1016/0034-5687(93)90007-W

Wagner, P. D. (2000). Diffusive resistance to O2 transport in muscle. *Acta Physiol. Scand.* 168, 609–614. doi: 10.1046/j.1365-201x.2000.00712.x

Walker, L., Eng, B., McFarlane, A., and Waye, J. S. (2007). High oxygen affinity hemoglobin variant in a Canadian family: Hb Bunbury [beta94(FG1)Asp->Asn, GAC->AAC]. *Hemoglobin* 31, 101–103. doi: 10.1080/03630260601059241

Willie, C. K., MacLeod, D. B., Shaw, A. D., Smith, K. J., Tzeng, Y. C., Eves, N. D., et al. (2012). Regional brain blood flow in man during acute changes in arterial blood gases. *J. Physiol.* 590, 3261–3275. doi: 10.1113/jphysiol.2012.228551

21

Similar Inflammatory Responses Following Sprint Interval Training Performed in Hypoxia and Normoxia

Alan J. Richardson[1]*, Rebecca L. Relf*[1]*, Arron Saunders*[1] *and Oliver R. Gibson*[2]*

[1] *Environmental Extremes Lab, Centre for Sport and Exercise Science and Medicine, University of Brighton, Eastbourne, UK,* [2] *Centre for Human Performance, Exercise, and Rehabilitation, Brunel University London, Uxbridge, UK*

***Correspondence:**
Oliver R. Gibson
oliver.gibson@brunel.ac.uk

Sprint interval training (SIT) is an efficient intervention capable of improving aerobic capacity and exercise performance. This experiment aimed to determine differences in training adaptations and the inflammatory responses following 2 weeks of SIT (30 s maximal work, 4 min recovery; 4–7 repetitions) performed in normoxia or hypoxia. Forty-two untrained participants [(mean ± *SD*), age 21 ±1 years, body mass 72.1 ±11.4 kg, and height 173 ±10 cm] were equally and randomly assigned to one of three groups; control (CONT; no training, $n = 14$), normoxic (NORM; SIT in FiO_2: 0.21, $n = 14$), and normobaric hypoxic (HYP; SIT in FiO_2: 0.15, $n = 14$). Participants completed a $\dot{V}O_{2peak}$ test, a time to exhaustion (TTE) trial (power = 80% $\dot{V}O_{2peak}$) and had hematological [hemoglobin (Hb), haematocrit (Hct)] and inflammatory markers [interleukin-6 (IL-6), tumor necrosis factor-α (TNFα)] measured in a resting state, pre and post SIT. $\dot{V}O_{2peak}$ ($mL.kg^{-1}.min^{-1}$) improved in HYP (+11.9%) and NORM (+9.8%), but not CON (+0.9%). Similarly TTE improved in HYP (+32.2%) and NORM (+33.0%), but not CON (+3.4%) whilst the power at the anaerobic threshold (AT; $W.kg^{-1}$) also improved in HYP (+13.3%) and NORM (+8.0%), but not CON (–0.3%). AT ($mL.kg^{-1}.min^{-1}$) improved in HYP (+9.5%), but not NORM (+5%) or CON (–0.3%). No between group change occurred in 30 s sprint performance or Hb and Hct. IL-6 increased in HYP (+17.4%) and NORM (+20.1%), but not CON (+1.2%), respectively. TNF-α increased in HYP (+10.8%) NORM (+12.9%) and CON (+3.4%). SIT in HYP and NORM increased $\dot{V}O_{2peak}$, power at AT and TTE performance in untrained individuals, improvements in AT occurred only when SIT was performed in HYP. Increases in IL-6 and TNFα reflect a training induced inflammatory response to SIT; hypoxic conditions do not exacerbate this.

Keywords: high intensity training, altitude, endurance, inflammation, cytokine

INTRODUCTION

With a training volume and energy expenditure significantly less than traditional aerobic endurance training, sprint interval training (SIT) is considered a time-efficient method of improving cardiometabolic health (Gillen et al., 2016), skeletal muscle oxidative capacity and exercise performance (Gibala et al., 2006; Burgomaster et al., 2008). SIT is characterized by repeated bouts of exercise at a supramaximal intensity, interspersed by recovery periods (Burgomaster et al., 2005). This training induces a cascade of physiological adaptations, predominantly occurring at the muscle (metabolic adaptations), which can occur in as little as 2 weeks (Burgomaster et al., 2005; Gibala et al., 2006). Identified mechanisms facilitating improved exercise capacity via enhanced VO_2 and O_2 transport capacity include increased oxidative (Gibala et al., 2006) and glycolytic enzyme activity (Talanian et al., 2007; Daussin et al., 2008), muscle buffering capacity, glycogen content (Burgomaster et al., 2005) and increased skeletal muscle capillariation (De Smet et al., 2016; Montero and Lundby, 2016). Augmentation of exercise performance as a result of mitochondrial (Little et al., 2010) and vascular (Rakobowchuk et al., 2008) adaptations alongside improving hormonal responses (Kon et al., 2015), and insulin sensitivity (Richards et al., 2010), have reinforced SIT as a powerful training stimulus in diseased (Whyte et al., 2010), healthy untrained (Burgomaster et al., 2006; Gibala et al., 2006), and trained (Macpherson and Weston, 2015) populations.

Hypoxia has been widely observed as a potent stimuli for improving functional outcomes allied to exercise capacity (Rusko et al., 2004), with ascents ~2500 m identified as optimal (Chapman et al., 2014) using a LHTL model for improving endurance training. A number of review articles have supported the various applications for hypoxia in trained individuals (Wilber, 2007; Millet et al., 2010, 2013). Conversely, recent discussion has proposed a limited potential for the additional benefits of adding a hypoxic stimulus to training in trained populations (Lundby et al., 2012; McLean et al., 2014). This notion may however be, too broad to suggest hypoxia is entirely ineffective. Rather the benefits of the additional hypoxic stimulus likely elicit specific adaptations allied to the protocol which has been implemented, e.g., improved repeated sprint ability after repeated sprint training in hypoxia (Faiss et al., 2013b). It has been proposed that the addition of hypoxic stress during interval training is a mechanism to further enhance performance (Faiss et al., 2013a). The application of an additional stimuli to training (i.e., hypoxia) is challenging given the necessity to maintain an optimal training stimulus, e.g., training intensity (Millet and Faiss, 2012) and optimal level of altitude (Goods et al., 2014) for beneficial adaptations. Preliminary research supports the notion that performing SIT in hypoxia may enhance the magnitude of adaptation when compared to equivalent training prescription in normoxia (Puype et al., 2013). Mechanistically, SIT in hypoxia vs. normoxia provides additive stress resulting from an increased metabolic demand to exercise and increased relative stress during recovery thus potentiating greater adaptations (Buchheit et al., 2012). Training in hypoxia still maintains the favorable time efficiencies compared to traditional continuous lower intensity training, which makes the intervention favorable for a number of applications across populations (Gibala et al., 2012). The 30 s exercise duration of each bout of SIT requires a ~55% contribution from aerobic metabolism (Billaut and Bishop, 2009), this typically elicits greater performance detriments when training in hypoxia vs. normoxia, however prolonged recovery facilitates near complete recovery with the intention of maintaining sprint training specific stimuli (Millet and Faiss, 2012). This important balance between work:rest ratios theoretically preserves specific training stimuli associated with SIT, e.g., upregulated oxygen signaling genes and fast twitch fiber recruitment (Millet and Faiss, 2012), whilst increasing the metabolic disturbances required for adaptations to glycolytic pathways (Puype et al., 2013). Recent literature has identified that SIT in hypoxia augments adaptation during a 6 week training periods (Puype et al., 2013), however SIT in hypoxia over a 2 week training intervention may offer little additional benefit when compared to equivalent training in normoxia (Richardson and Gibson, 2015). Additional benefits of hypoxia have however also been shown in other repeated sprint training interventions of 2 (Faiss et al., 2015) to 4 weeks (Faiss et al., 2013b; Galvin et al., 2013; Kasai et al., 2015). This training modality, dose-response relationship remains to be fully determined in hypoxia, though it is known that 2 weeks is a sufficient time period to elicit adaptations in normoxia (Burgomaster et al., 2005, 2008).

Combinations of SIT and hypoxia induce significant physiological stress (Puype et al., 2013), which may impact recovery and therefore subsequent training or competition performance may be impaired (Goods et al., 2015). Interleukin-6 (IL-6) and tumor necrosis factor (TNFα) are pro-inflammatory cytokines both of which increase following equivalent training performed in hypoxia and normoxia (Svendsen et al., 2016). Plasma IL-6 increases with high intensity interval training (HIIT; Croft et al., 2009) and with increasing severity of hypoxia (Schobersberger et al., 2000; Turner et al., 2016), while TNFα appears to remain unchanged in response to passive hypoxic exposures (Turner et al., 2016). IL-6 has an important anti-inflammatory and adaptation-signaling role during the post-exercise recovery phase, with a greater increase in IL-6 post-hypoxic exercise reflective of a greater training stress (Fischer, 2006; Scheller et al., 2011). Given the failure for 2 weeks of SIT in hypoxia to elicit greater adaptations than SIT in normoxia (Richardson and Gibson, 2015) identification of the pro-inflammatory response to both interventions would facilitate greater understanding of the magnitude of additional training stimuli induced by hypoxia. Additionally, should a greater inflammatory response be identified, in the absence of improved adaptive response than equivalent training in normoxia, the use of SIT in hypoxia may be counterproductive.

The aims of this study were to investigate differences in the magnitude of training adaptations (VO_{2max}, time to exhaustion, Anaerobic Threshold) and inflammatory responses (IL-6 and TNFα), to 2 weeks of SIT performed in normoxia and hypoxia. It was hypothesized that due to the short 2-week (Richardson and Gibson, 2015), vs. longer 6 week (Puype et al., 2013), duration of the SIT, no differences in the magnitude of training adaptations would be observed. Additionally it was hypothesized that SIT performed in hypoxia will elicit greater inflammatory responses than SIT performed in normoxia due to an increased physiological stress caused by an inhibited aerobic contribution during recovery.

METHODS

Subjects

Forty-two untrained, but recreationally active individuals (27 males, 15 females) age 21 ± 1 years, body mass 72.1 ± 11.4 kg, and height 173 ± 10 cm volunteered to take part in this experiment (**Table 1**). No differences in anthropometric or fitness measures were found between groups ($p > 0.05$). Participants were informed of the procedures to be employed in the study and associated risks, which had the approval of the University of Brighton Research Ethics Committee (ESREGC/06/14). All participants provided written, informed consent. The participants were non-smokers and had not spent time above 2000 m in the 2 months prior to the study. Participants were advised to refrain from alcohol and caffeine for 24 h prior to testing and to maintain their normal unstructured training habits (<2 hr.wk) throughout the study.

Experimental Design

The 42 participants were randomly assigned and equally split for number ($n = 14$) and sex (9 males, 5 females), to one of the three intervention groups; a normoxic (NORM) (FiO_2: 0.2093) environment, a moderate normobaric hypoxic (HYP) (FiO_2: 0.15, range 0.148–0.152; $FiCO_2$: 0.0008, range 0.0003–0.0028) environment and a control (CONT) normoxic non-training group (**Table 1**). All testing was performed in a nitrogen enriched normobaric hypoxic chamber with temperature (19°C) and humidity (40%) regulated by air conditioning (Altitude Centre, London, UK).

Familiarization of the Wingate anaerobic test (WAnT) and time to exhaustion (TTE) was performed prior to any of the experimental testing. Preliminary testing involved participants completing in sequence, a peak oxygen consumption ($\dot{V}O_{2peak}$) incremental test, a time to exhaustion cycle test (TTE) and a Wingate anaerobic test (WAnT), with 24 h separating each test. Prior to each $\dot{V}O_{2peak}$ test, venous blood was taken to measure haematocrit (Hct), hemoglobin (Hb), Interleukin- 6 (IL-6), and TNFα, see **Figure 1**. The SIT consisted of six WAnT sessions over a 2-week period with 24–48 h between each session (**Figure 1**). Each training session followed that an established SIT protocol (Burgomaster et al., 2005), consisting of an increasing number of WAnTs [four to seven 30 s "all out" efforts on a cycle ergometer interspersed with 4 min warm up/recovery (60 W)]. Throughout training heart rate [HR, bts.min^{-1} (Polar FT1, Polar Electro, Kempele, Finland)], peripheral arterial oxygen saturation [SpO_2, % (PalmSat 2500, Nonin Medical Inc., Minnesota, USA)], and rating of perceived exertion [RPE; Borg Scale 6–20 (Borg, 1982)] were measured immediately after each WAnT and every minute thereafter during recovery. Those in the CONT group maintained usual physical activity regimes for the 2 week period. Forty-eight hours after the final SIT session all participants repeated the $\dot{V}O_{2peak}$, TTE and WAnT protocols, each separated by 24 h.

TABLE 1 | Participant baseline values for anthropometric and aerobic capacity measures.

	CONT	NORM	HYP
Body Mass (Kg)	70.3 ± 13	73.3 ± 11	72.5 ± 10
Height (cm)	172 ± 10	174 ± 11	174 ± 8
Age (years)	20 ± 1	20 ± 1	20 ± 1
Hb (g.dL^{-1})	14.5 ± 1.4	14.2 ± 1.5	14.6 ± 1.8
Hct (%)	44 ± 2	45 ± 2	44 ± 2
TTE (s)	606 ± 280	589 ± 372	633 ± 330
$\dot{V}O_{2peak}$ (mL.kg^{-1}.min^{-1})	42.1 ± 9.7	42.2 ± 8.6	43.6 ± 7.9

Hb, B-Hemoglobin; Hct, Hematocrit; TTE - Time to Exhaustion.

Preliminary and Post Testing

Participants performed an incremental test to volitional exhaustion on an electromagnetically-braked cycle (Schoberer Rad Messtechnik equipped with 8 strain gauges, SRM, Germany), with the zero offset calibration procedure performed on the SRM PowerMeter prior to each test, to determine $\dot{V}O_{2peak}$. Starting at 100 W, there was a stepwise increase in power of 20 W.min^{-1}. Expired gases were obtained using a breath by breath gas analyser (Metamax 3X, Cortex, Germany). HR and RPE were taken at the end of every stage. Anaerobic threshold was computer-determined with additional visual inspection to determine the first breakpoint in ventilatory parameters.

Twenty-four hours later, participants performed a TTE at an intensity corresponding to 80% peak power output (PPO) attained during the pre-SIT assessment of $\dot{V}O_{2peak}$, on a cycle ergometer at a target cadence of 80 revs.min^{-1} (Monark, model 864, Sweden). The test was terminated at volitional exhaustion when the participants' cadence fell below 40 revs·min^{-1}; exercise duration (seconds) was then determined. Capillary blood was collected from the fingertip pre and 2 min post TTE for analysis of blood lactate (2300 Stat Plus, YSI Life Sciences, USA).

Prior to each $\dot{V}O_{2peak}$ test 10 mL of blood was collected from the ante-cubital fossa. Whole blood (~50 μL) was divided into two heparinised capillary tubes (Hawksley & Sons Ltd., England) then centrifuged (Hematospin 1300, Hawksley & Sons Ltd., England) at 1000 rpm for 1.5 min to calculate the haematocrit using a micro haematocrit reader (Hawksley & Sons Ltd., England); the average of duplicate samples was recorded. Hemoglobin concentration (B-Hemoglobin Photometer, Hemocue, Sweden) was determined via the average of triplicate samples (B-Hemoglobin Microvettes, Hemocue, Sweden). The remaining blood was transferred into two 5 mL EDTA tubes and centrifuged at 5000 rpm for 10 min. Plasma was then extracted into microvettes and stored at –86°C. IL-6 and TNFα concentrations were analyzed using Enzyme-linked immunosorbent assays in accordance with manufacturer instructions (DuoSet ELISA Development System; R&D Systems Inc., Abingdon, UK) with corrections made for the change in plasma volume (Dill and Costill, 1974). The technical error of measurement (TEM) between duplicate samples for IL-6 was 7.1%, with a unit error value of 2.76 pg.mL^{-1} and for TNFα it was 4.1%, with a unit error value of 518.7 pg.mL^{-1}.

WAnT

Each WAnT, performed 24 h following the TTE, consisted of 30 s of "all out" maximal cycling on a friction-loaded cycle ergometer (Monark Ergomedic Peak Bike 894e, Monark Exercise AB, Sweden). The load was calculated as 7.5% body mass [0.075 kg/kg.bm^{-1}, (Bar-Or, 1987)]. The onset of each sprint was marked with a "3-2-1. GO!" countdown, and participants were instructed to cycle for ~2 s against the ergometers inertial

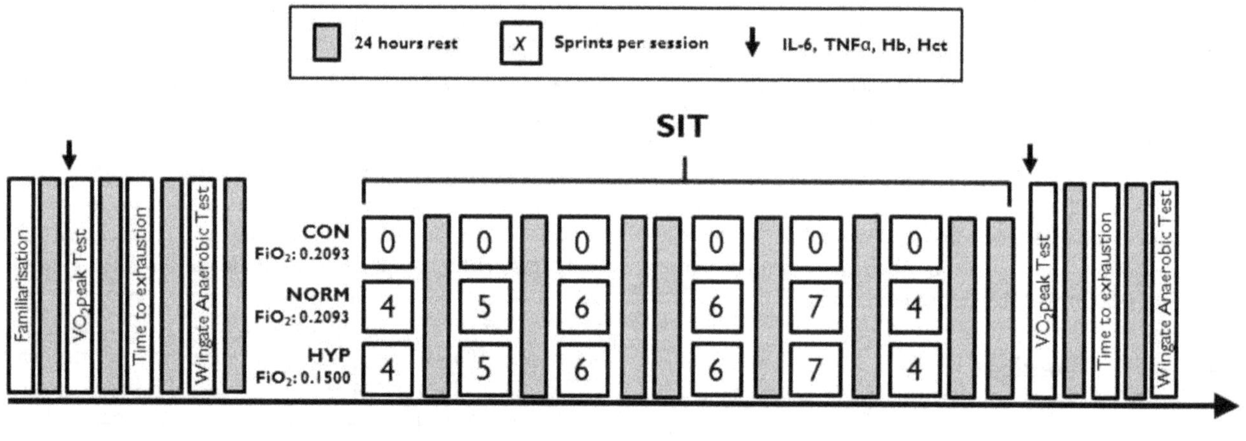

FIGURE 1 | Schematic of the testing and sprint interval training protocol for each training group.

resistance before the full load was released at 70 rpm. Participants were required to stay seated on the saddle and were verbally encouraged throughout the test. Each sprint was followed by a 4 min recovery period—participants were required actively recover (unloaded cycling at 60 revs.min^{-1}). Peak power output, average 30-s power output (total work), and fatigue index [also known as rate of power decline; ((Peak Power Output−Min Power Output)/Peak Power Output) × 100) (%)] were recorded by Monark Anaerobic Test software (ver. 3.2.7.0, Monark Exercise AB, Sweden).

Sprint Interval Training

All SIT was performed on a cycle ergometer (Monark, model 864, Sweden) against a resistance of 0.075 kg.kg^{-1} body mass, from a rolling start of 70 revs·min^{-1}. Participants were verbally encouraged throughout. The sprints were interspersed with a 4 min active recovery period of cycling at 60 W. Power measures were recorded using Monark Anaerobic Test software (Monark, Sweden) continuously throughout the sprints. The number of sprints increased from four to seven over the 2 weeks (total six sessions). Training days were interspersed with one rest day (**Figure 1**). SpO_2 and HR were monitored using a finger pulse oximeter (Nonin 2500, Nonin Medical Inc., USA) 1 min after every sprint.

Statistical Analysis

Data were tested for normality, skewness and kurtosis. Data were normally distributed unless otherwise stated. A Two Way Mixed Design ANOVA was performed separately on each of the independent variables; $\dot{V}O_{2peak}$, TTE, Peak Power, Mean Power, Fatigue index (from WAnT test), IL-6, TNFα, Hb, and Hct, to determine whether there was a significant change between the three conditions (HYP, NORM, and CON) over two time-points (pre and post). The mean sessional recovery HR and SpO_2 observed following each SIT were analyzed using a mixed 2-way ANOVA using the Greenhouse-Geisser correction to determine whether there was a significant change between the two training conditions (HYP and NORM) over the six SIT sessions. Adjusted Bonferroni comparisons were used as *post-hoc* analyses for all ANOVA. Partial eta squared was used to calculate effect sizes (np^2; small = 0.01, medium = 0.06, large = 0.13) were calculated to analyse the magnitude and trends with data. All data were reported as Mean ± *SD*. All statistical tests followed a significance level of $p < 0.05$. The statistical package used was SPSS (SPSS Inc., Chicago, USA, version 20.0).

RESULTS

Endurance Capacity

$\dot{V}O_{2peak}$ was significantly different from pre to post-training ($p = 0.001$, $np^2 = 0.44$), and between different training groups ($p = 0.002$, $np^2 = 0.28$, **Figure 2**). *Post-hoc* analysis observed increases in HYP ($p = 0.001$; +0.39 ± 0.29 L.min^{-1}; 43.6 ± 8.0 to 48.8 ± 9.2 mL.kg^{-1}.min^{-1}) and NORM ($p = 0.002$; +0.32 ± 0.38 L.min^{-1}; 42.2 ± 8.6 to 46.0 ± 7.5 mL.kg^{-1}.min^{-1}), but not for CONT ($p = 0.906$; 42.1 ± 9.7 to 42.2 ± 9.7 mL.kg^{-1}.min^{-1}). Relative power at $\dot{V}O_{2peak}$ (W.kg^{-1}) was greater pre to post ($p = 0.001$, $np^2 = 0.42$) overall and for the pre-post∗group interaction ($p = 0.004$, $np^2 = 0.25$). *Post-hoc* analysis observed increases in HYP ($p = 0.001$; 3.90 ± 0.72 to 4.20 ± 0.80 W.kg^{-1}) and NORM ($p = 0.001$; 3.54 ± 0.73 to 3.86 ± 0.86 W.kg^{-1}), but not for CONT ($p = 0.872$; 3.75 ± 0.56 to 3.76 ± 0.70 W.kg^{-1}).

The anaerobic threshold (AT) increased pre to post SIT ($p = 0.001$, $np^2 = 0.30$) overall and for the pre-post∗group interaction ($p = 0.001$, $np^2 = 0.29$). *Post-hoc* analysis only observed increases in HYP ($p = 0.001$; 22.6 ± 4.1 to 24.6 ± 4.2 mL.kg^{-1}.min^{-1}) and not NORM ($p = 0.050$; 22.9 ± 4.7 to 24.0 ± 4.8 mL.kg^{-1}.min^{-1}) or CONT ($p = 0.417$; 22.7 ± 5.6 to 22.4 ± 4.9 mL.kg^{-1}.min^{-1}). Relative power at AT was greater pre to post-training ($p = 0.001$, $np^2 = 0.313$) overall and for the pre-post∗group interaction ($p = 0.006$, $np^2 = 0.23$). *Post-hoc* analysis observed increases in both HYP ($p = 0.001$; 2.00 ± 0.36 to 2.26 ± 0.45 W.kg^{-1}) and NORM ($p = 0.017$; 1.88 ± 0.40 to 2.04 ± 0.49 W.kg^{-1}) but no change in CONT ($p = 0.925$; 1.98 ± 0.35 to 1.97 ± 0.37 W.kg^{-1}).

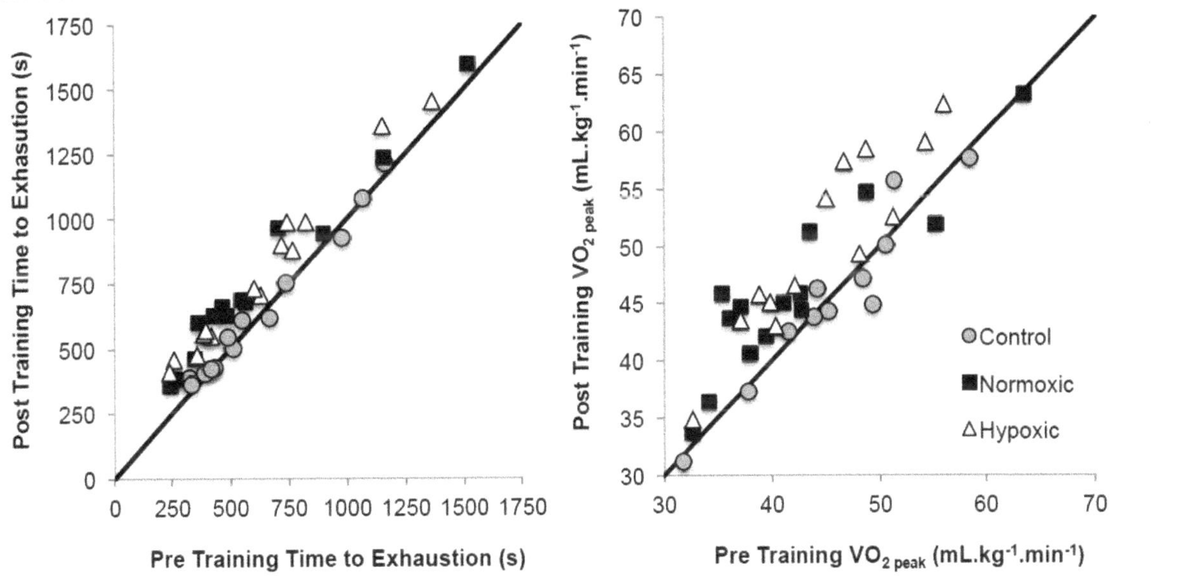

FIGURE 2 | Pre training to post training time to exhaustion and $\dot{V}O_{2peak}$ changes for the three training groups. Solid black lines demonstrates the line of equality.

TTE was significantly different from pre to post test ($p = 0.001$, $np^2 = 0.82$) overall, and for the pre-post∗group interaction ($p = 0.001$, $np^2 = 0.64$, **Figure 2**). *Post-hoc* analysis observed increases in HYP ($p = 0.001$; 633 ± 330 to 787 ± 326 s) and NORM ($p = 0.001$; 589 ± 373 to 729 ± 351 s), but not for CONT ($p = 0.212$; 607 ± 280 to 620 ± 274 s).

Power Capacity during WAnT

Peak power was not different during the WAnT from pre to post-training ($p = 0.530$, $np^2 = 0.010$) or between different training groups (CONT; 11.2 ± 3.0 to 10.9 ± 2.2 $W.kg^{-1}$, NORM; 11.0 ± 1.3 to 11.4 ± 1.4 $W.kg^{-1}$, HYP; 11.7 ± 2.4 to 11.9 ± 2.4 $W.kg^{-1}$) ($p = 0.052$, $np^2 = 0.141$).

Similarly, mean power was not different from pre to post-training ($p = 0.653$, $np^2 = 0.005$), or between training groups (CONT; 3.8 ± 0.8 to 3.7 ± 0.8 $W.kg^{-1}$, NORM; 4.0 ± 1.1 to 4.1 ± 0.9 $W.kg^{-1}$, HYP; 3.6 ± 1.3 to 3.8 ± 1.2 $W.kg^{-1}$) ($p = 0.319$, $np^2 = 0.057$).

Fatigue Index was found to be significantly reduced from pre to post-training ($p = 0.001$, $np^2 = 0.968$), although there was no significant difference between training groups CONT; 62.7 ± 10.7 to 62.9 ± 12.3%, NORM; 63.5 ± 9.2 to 61.8 ± 9.4%, HYP; 65.1 ± 12.6 to 62.3 ± 10.1%) ($p = 0.851$, $np^2 = 0.008$).

Hematological and Inflammatory Markers

Hb was significantly different from pre to post-training ($p = 0.036$, $np^2 = 0.11$). However, this increase was not different between training groups ($p = 0.082$, $np^2 = 0.12$) for CONT (14.6 ± 1.5 to 14.6 ± 1.5 $g.dL^{-1}$), NORM (14.3 ± 1.5 to 14.3 ± 1.3 $g.dL^{-1}$), and HYP (14.7 ± 1.8 to 15.0 ± 1.7 $g.dL^{-1}$).

Hct was not different from pre to post-training ($p = 0.701$, $np^2 = 0.00$) or between groups ($p = 0.215$, $np^2 = 0.08$) for CONT (44.0 ± 2.8 to 43.7 ± 2.4%), NORM (44.9 ± 2.1 to 45.0 ± 2.7%), and HYP (45.7 ± 2.8 to 46.0 ± 3.1%).

Blood lactate increased in all TTE tests ($p = 0.001$, $np^2 = 0.29$). Post TTE blood lactate values increased significantly with NORM ($p = 0.01$ 5.07 ± 0.77 to 5.62 ± 1.01 $mmol.L^{-1}$), and HYP training ($p = 0.010$; 5.24 ± 0.9 to 5.76 ± 0.82 $mmol.L^{-1}$), but not in CONT ($p = 0.101$; 6.42 ± 0.8 to 6.52 ± 0.95 $mmol.L^{-1}$).

IL-6 was significantly different from pre to post test ($p = 0.001$, $np^2 = 0.39$) and this increase was different between training groups ($p = 0.007$, $np^2 = 0.23$). *Post-hoc* analysis observed increases for HYP ($p = 0.001$; 1.7 ± 0.2 to 2.0 ± 0.2 $pg.mL^{-1}$) and NORM ($p = 0.003$; 1.7 ± 0.2 to 2.0 ± 0.3 $pg.mL^{-1}$), but not for CONT ($p = 0.836$; 1.7 ± 0.2 to 1.7 ± 0.2 $pg.mL^{-1}$).

TNFα was significantly different from pre to post test ($p = 0.006$, $np^2 = 0.175$), however, was not significantly different between training groups ($p = 0.151$, $np^2 = 0.09$) (NORM; 3.0 ± 0.6 to 3.4 ± 0.9 $pg.mL^{-1}$; HYP; 3.1 ± 0.8 to 3.3 ± 0.6 $pg.mL^{-1}$; CONT; 2.7 ± 0.7 to 2.8 ± 0.6 $pg.mL^{-1}$).

Training Markers

Recovery HR was not different between sessions ($p = 0.250$; $np^2 = 0.11$) or for the different training groups ($p = 0.420$; $np^2 = 0.04$, **Figure 3**). SpO_2 was different between sessions ($p = 0.001$; $np^2 = 0.30$) and significantly less with HYP training ($p = 0.001$; $np^2 = 0.20$). *Post-hoc* analysis of SpO_2 is presented in **Figure 3** for clarity.

DISCUSSION

The aim of this experiment was to quantify the improvements in aerobic capacity and aerobic performance following 2 weeks of SIT in normoxia, and hypoxia in comparison to a non-trained control group. In support of previous work in the field, we have

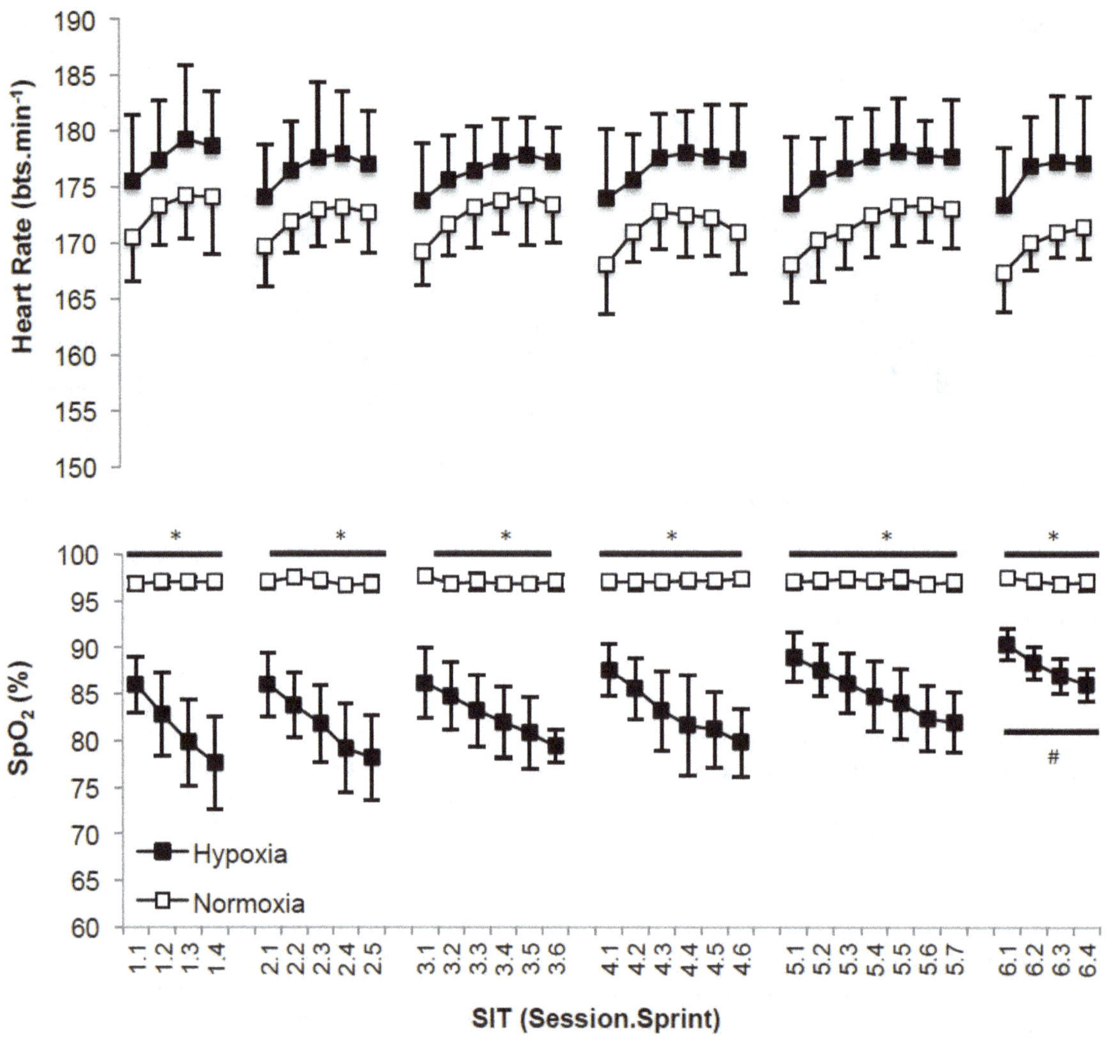

FIGURE 3 | (Mean ± *SD*) SpO_2 and heart rate values after each sprint for all training sessions. *Denotes significant difference ($p < 0.05$) between conditions within session. #Denotes significant difference ($p < 0.05$) from first, second, third, fourth and fifth sessions.

demonstrated that SIT improved $\dot{V}O_{2peak}$, power at AT and TTE to comparable magnitude associated with interval training in normoxia (Burgomaster et al., 2005; Gibala et al., 2006; Hazell et al., 2010), and hypoxia (Galvin et al., 2013; Puype et al., 2013; Gatterer et al., 2014; Brocherie et al., 2015; Richardson and Gibson, 2015; De Smet et al., 2016). In contrast to our hypothesis, an additive effect of performing SIT in hypoxia vs. normoxia was observed with regards to the AT, with no changes observed in NORM and CONT. Equality of increases in IL-6 48 h following normoxic and hypoxic SIT, also opposed our initial hypothesis. This change in concentration reflecting a training induced inflammatory response absent in controls, but with no greater, undesirable inflammatory response observed in hypoxia.

Adaptations to Aerobic Capacity and Exercise Performance

In the present study $\dot{V}O_{2peak}$, TTE, and power at the AT increased following SIT in HYP and NORM suggesting improved oxidative phosphorylation had occurred (Burgomaster et al., 2005, 2006). Interestingly, when considering AT expressed at $mL.kg^{-1}.min^{-1}$ this adaptation only occurred in HYP (+9.5%), not NORM (+5.0%). Puype et al. (2013) acknowledged that their 6-week intervention improved the power corresponding to the AT (quantified from a 4 $mmol.L^{-1}$ lactate concentration) by ~7% (in normoxia) and 9% (in hypoxia) only following hypoxic, and not normoxic training. This adaptation was associated with an increase in muscle phosphofructokinase (PFK; hypoxia = +59%, normoxia = +17%). It was reported that VO_{2max} increased (hypoxia = +7.4%; normoxia = +5.8%) and TTE improved (hypoxia = +5.0%; normoxia = +2.9%) compared to controls, but with no difference when performing the training in hypoxia vs. normoxia (Puype et al., 2013). These observations are in line with our experiment. Our data is also supportive of an increased AT following SIT (Puype et al., 2013), and therefore increased glycolytic capacity via elevated PFK. Methodological differences in identifying the threshold, and the three-fold protocol duration of Puype et al. (2013) provide a rationale for the contrast between significant changes in the power at the AT following training in hypoxia (Puype et al., 2013) and the absence of a further improvement in power at the AT in comparison to normoxia as observed by ourselves. The improved AT ($mL.kg^{-1}.min^{-1}$) following SIT in hypoxia in comparison to SIT in normoxia in our study may have also been acknowledged by Puype et al. (2013), unfortunately this was not quantified. SIT, or similar training, elicits known metabolic adaptations, e.g., increased oxidative (Gibala et al., 2006) and glycolytic enzyme activity (Talanian et al., 2007; Daussin et al., 2008), improved muscle buffering capacity, elevated intramuscular glycogen content (Burgomaster et al., 2005) and increased skeletal muscle capillarisation (Puype et al., 2013). These are likely induced from the performance of the sprints within the protocol, with hypoxia potentiating greater metabolic disturbances in vs. normoxia (Faiss et al., 2013b; Galvin et al., 2013; Puype et al., 2013). Even greater improvements in glycolytic function may have been identified by increased mean power and improved fatigue index during the WaNT (Puype et al., 2013), however this was not case suggesting the mode of training was not structured effectively to facilitate this. Increased lactate in response to improved TTE suggests a greater tolerance to metabolic acidosis via group III/IV afferents (Amann et al., 2015) with SIT not demonstrating improved lactate clearance as supported by evidence elsewhere (Juel et al., 2004). The absence of a difference in peak and mean power, and fatigue index during the WAnT demonstrate that SIT in normoxia and hypoxia was effective at improving aerobic metabolic pathways. Mechanisms supporting the physiological ($\dot{V}O_{2peak}$) and performance (TTE) responses in our normobaric hypoxic environment do not appear hematological given the lack of intragroup difference in Hb and Hct (**Table 2**), this is in agreement with the proposal of others (Richalet and Gore, 2008), reinforcing the metabolic adaptive pathway. The measurement of Hb and Hct would however be improved by assessing total Hb mass thus accounting for changes otherwise lost when measuring the concentration (Burge and Skinner, 1995; Schmidt and Prommer, 2005). Based upon the expected lack of hematological adaptations between groups, aforementioned modulators of oxygen utilization at the muscle are most likely improved by SIT irrespective of the FiO_2 in which it is performed. Interestingly, improvements in SpO_2 were observed within the HYP group by the 6th session (**Figure 3**). This suggests some level of acclimation to hypoxia had occurred. SIT may therefore be effective at mitigating desaturation known to occur during repeated/intermittent sprint performance in hypoxia (Bowtell et al., 2014; Turner et al., 2014). Accordingly, future work investigating training adaptations to SIT could consider the benefits of hypoxic SIT to prepare athletes, rather than untrained individuals as in the present experiment, for competition in hypoxia (Girard et al., 2013; Millet et al., 2013). Concurrent mechanistic work may also wish to consider whether our equal pre to post-intervention measures of Hb and Hct data confirms a lack of hematological adaptation i.e., HB_{mass}, in favor of improved metabolic pathways (Faiss et al., 2013b). Additionally exploration of the mechanisms by which preservation of SpO_2 occurs in response to SIT in hypoxia may also be considered. With no clear additional benefit of performing 2 weeks of SIT in hypoxia rather than normoxia (on $\dot{V}O_{2peak}$, and TTE performance lasting ~10 min, **Table 2**), implementing this training appears largely unreasoned from a performance perspective at the present time, particularly given the challenge of facilitating training in this environment.

TABLE 2 | Change (%) in aerobic capacity, time to exhaustion (TTE), bloods and inflammatory measures in each group.

	CONT	NORM	HYP
$\dot{V}O_{2peak}$	0.9 ± 11.4	9.8 ± 9.4*	11.9 ± 6.7*
Power at $\dot{V}O_{2peak}$	−0.1 ± 5.9	8.8 ± 7.8*	7.7 ± 6.0*
AT	−0.4 ± 4.4	5.0 ± 8.2	9.5 ± 7.1*
Power at AT	−0.3 ± 12.4	8.0 ± 10.2*	13.3 ± 8.5*
TTE	3.4 ± 7.3	32.3 ± 19.0*	32.2 ± 20.7*
WAnT Peak Power	−1.7 ± 7.0	3.6 ± 3.7	1.8 ± 5.9
WAnT Mean Power	−2.4 ± 5.4	3.1 ± 9.3	4.2 ± 10.6
WAnT Fatigue Index	0.5 ± 11.4	−2.6 ± 4.7	−3.4 ± 9.5
IL-6	1.2 ± 11.8	20.1 ± 22.1*	17.4 ± 15.3*
TNFα	3.5 ± 17.5	12.9 ± 16.9*	10.8 ± 16.3*
Hb	0.1 ± 1.6	0.7 ± 4.3	2.7 ± 3.0
Hct	−0.7 ± 2.0	0.4 ± 2.7	0.7 ± 1.9

AT, Anaerobic Threshold; TTE, Time to Exhaustion; WAnT, Wingate Anaerobic Test; IL-6, Interleukin 6; TNFα, Tumor Necrosis Factor; Hb, Hemoglobin; Hct, Hematocrit.
**Denotes significant change with training.*

Inflammatory Responses to SIT in Normoxia and Hypoxia

The increase in basal IL-6 following both normoxic and hypoxic SIT (**Table 2**) reflects the intensity and duration of the activity as widely observed elsewhere (Fischer, 2006). The functional significance of an increased IL-6 is complex (Gleeson and Bishop, 2000), with increased exercise requirements (Croft et al., 2009) and increasing metabolic stress, e.g., via hypoxia in isolation, or hypoxia related increases in the relative exercise intensity (Schobersberger et al., 2000) typically eliciting larger responses. IL-6 has an important anti-inflammatory and adaptation signaling role during the post-exercise recovery phase (Svendsen et al., 2016), with a greater increase in IL-6 post-hypoxic exercise reflective of a greater training stress (Fischer, 2006; Scheller et al., 2011). A reduction of IL-6 is a known training adaptation (Fischer, 2006); the elevation of the cytokine 48 h following the final training session however indicates that recovery/adaptation was incomplete. Irrespective of the consequential effects of increased basal IL-6, the current data appeases concerns that training in hypoxia as having an impairment upon individuals when compared to equivalent normoxic training. The increase in TNF-α alongside IL-6 is similar to other data demonstrating relationships between these inflammatory biomarkers and exercise (Gleeson and Bishop, 2000). Interestingly, a similar magnitude of inflammatory response to SIT was observed for TNFα as IL-6, however this was not statistically different to controls despite the ~12% difference between NORM and HYP, and CON. This disparity between IL-6 and TNFα may be due to the greater within group variability observed with this inflammatory marker (~25%) or the lack of hypoxia specific TNFα induction during passive (Turner et al., 2016) or active (Svendsen et al., 2016) exposures. Nonetheless performing SIT in hypoxia did not exacerbate the inflammatory response in comparison to normoxia, and is therefore unlikely to be detrimental to subsequent training or performance. A more precise quantification of training load within each group, and subsequently ensuring equality of load between groups, would give further confidence in the equality of inflammatory responses to SIT performed in either normoxia or hypoxia. Should absolute or relative internal/external training load be different between SIT performed in normoxia or hypoxia, then this may influence the interpretation of the inflammatory markers and suggest that hypoxia reduces or exacerbates the responses.

Similar basal inflammatory markers IL-6 and TNFα 24 h post the final SIT suggests that the increased stress of training in hypoxia is equal to that of normoxia and would not be detrimental to the individual. This equality of cytokine response is in agreement with the comparable magnitude of increases in IL-6 (hypoxia = +57%, normoxia = +56%) and lack of change in TNFα 2 h after a 75 min submaximal cycle in either condition (Svendsen et al., 2016). Accordingly the benefits of hypoxic SIT to prepare athletes for competition in hypoxia (Millet et al., 2013) can be determined at least equal to that of equivalent training in normoxia, without further compromising subsequent activities. Given the abundance of cellular and molecular pathways associated with SIT and HIIT, and hypoxia, this experiment presents a constrained overview of the responses. To optimize the application of SIT in hypoxia, future work should consider measurement of a wider spectrum of blood and muscle markers of training adaptations associated with SIT, and hypoxia both in isolation, and in combination. Additionally, further analysis of the impact of SIT in hypoxia on stress markers should be considered at a basal level (as determined within the present experiment) but also regarding the kinetics of a within session increase and the subsequent time-course to return to baseline prior to, and beyond our 48 h measurement point.

CONCLUSION

Two weeks of SIT in hypoxia improves peak oxygen uptake, time to exhaustion and power at the anaerobic threshold, to a similar magnitude as equivalent training in normoxia. Improvements in the anaerobic threshold itself were only elicited in response to SIT in hypoxia, and not normoxia, highlighting the additional benefit of training in this environment. Equality of increases in basal IL-6 and TNFα following SIT in hypoxia and normoxia suggests that hypoxia does not exacerbate inflammatory processes.

AUTHOR CONTRIBUTIONS

AR, RR, AS, and OG conceived and design the experiment. RR and AS performed the data collection. AR, RR, AS, and OG performed the statistical analysis and interpretation of data. AR, RR, AS, and OG participated in drafting the article or revising it critically for important intellectual content. AR, RR, AS, and OG approved the final manuscript.

REFERENCES

Amann, M., Sidhu, S. K., Weavil, J. C., Mangum, T. S., and Venturelli, M. (2015). Autonomic responses to exercise: group III/IV muscle afferents and fatigue. *Auton. Neurosci.* 188, 19–23. doi: 10.1016/j.autneu.2014.10.018

Bar-Or, O. (1987). The wingate anaerobic test. *Sport Med.* 4, 381–394. doi: 10.2165/00007256-198704060-00001

Billaut, F., and Bishop, D. (2009). Muscle fatigue in males and females during multiple-sprint exercise. *Sports Med.* 39, 257–278. doi: 10.2165/00007256-200939040-00001

Borg, G. A. (1982). Psychophysical bases of perceived exertion. *Med. Sci. Sports Exerc.* 14, 377–381. doi: 10.1249/00005768-198205000-00012

Bowtell, J. L., Cooke, K., Turner, R., Mileva, K. N., and Sumners, D. P. (2014). Acute physiological and performance responses to repeated sprints in varying degrees of hypoxia. *J. Sci. Med. Sport* 17, 399–403. doi: 10.1016/j.jsams.2013.05.016

Brocherie, F., Millet, G. P., Hauser, A., Steiner, T., Rysman, J., Wehrlin, J. P., et al. (2015). "Live high-train low and high" hypoxic training improves team-sport performance. *Med. Sci. Sports Exerc.* 47, 2140–2149. doi: 10.1249/MSS.0000000000000630

Buchheit, M., Kuitunen, S., Voss, S. C., Williams, B. K., Mendez-Villanueva, A., and Bourdon, P. C. (2012). Physiological strain associated with high-intensity hypoxic intervals in highly trained young runners. *J. Strength Cond. Res.* 26, 94–105. doi: 10.1519/JSC.0b013e3182184fcb

Burge, C. M., and Skinner, S. L. (1995). Determination of hemoglobin mass and blood volume with CO: evaluation and application of a method. *J. Appl. Physiol.* 79, 623–631.

Burgomaster, K. A., Heigenhauser, G. J. F., and Gibala, M. J. (2006). Effect of short-term sprint interval training on human skeletal muscle carbohydrate metabolism during exercise and time-trial performance. *J. Appl. Physiol.* 100, 2041–2047. doi: 10.1152/japplphysiol.01220.2005

Burgomaster, K. A., Howarth, K. R., Phillips, S. M., Rakobowchuk, M., Macdonald, M. J., McGee, S. L., et al. (2008). Similar metabolic adaptations during exercise after low volume sprint interval and traditional endurance training in humans. *J. Physiol.* 586, 151–160. doi: 10.1113/jphysiol.2007.142109

Burgomaster, K. A., Hughes, S. C., Heigenhauser, G. J. F., Bradwell, S. N., Gibala, M. J., Kirsten, A., et al. (2005). Six sessions of sprint interval training increases muscle oxidative potential and cycle endurance capacity in humans. *J. Appl. Physiol.* 1, 1985–1990. doi: 10.1152/japplphysiol.01095.2004

Chapman, R. F., Karlsen, T., Resaland, G. K., Ge, R.-L., Harber, M. P., Witkowski, S., et al. (2014). Defining the "dose" of altitude training: how high to live for optimal sea level performance enhancement. *J. Appl. Physiol.* 116, 595–603. doi: 10.1152/japplphysiol.00634.2013

Croft, L., Bartlett, J. D., MacLaren, D. P. M., Reilly, T., Evans, L., Mattey, D. L., et al. (2009). High-intensity interval training attenuates the exercise-induced increase in plasma IL-6 in response to acute exercise. *Appl. Physiol. Nutr. Metab.* 34, 1098–1107. doi: 10.1139/H09-117

Daussin, F. N., Zoll, J., Dufour, S. P., Ponsot, E., Lonsdorfer-Wolf, E., Doutreleau, S., et al. (2008). Effect of interval versus continuous training on cardiorespiratory and mitochondrial functions: relationship to aerobic performance improvements in sedentary subjects. *Am. J. Physiol. Regul. Integr. Comp. Physiol.* 295, R264–R272. doi: 10.1152/ajpregu.00875.2007

De Smet, S., Van Thienen, R., Deldicque, L., James, R., Sale, C., Bishop, D. J., et al. (2016). Nitrate intake promotes shift in muscle fiber type composition during sprint interval training in hypoxia. *Front. Physiol.* 7:233. doi: 10.3389/fphys.2016.00233

Dill, D. B., and Costill, D. L. (1974). Calculation of percentage changes in volumes of blood, plasma, and red cells in dehydration. *J. Appl. Physiol.* 37, 247–248.

Faiss, R., Girard, O., and Millet, G. (2013a). Advancing hypoxic training in team sports: from intermittent hypoxic training to repeated sprint training in hypoxia. *Br. J. Sports Med.* 47(Suppl. 1), i45–i50. doi: 10.1136/bjsports-2013-092741

Faiss, R., Léger, B., Vesin, J.-M., Fournier, P.-E., Eggel, Y., Dériaz, O., et al. (2013b). Significant molecular and systemic adaptations after repeated sprint training in hypoxia. *PLoS ONE* 8:e56522. doi: 10.1371/journal.pone.0056522

Faiss, R., Willis, S., Born, D.-P., Sperlich, B., Vesin, J.-M., Holmberg, H.-C., et al. (2015). Repeated double-poling sprint training in hypoxia by competitive cross-country skiers. *Med. Sci. Sports Exerc.* 47, 809–817. doi: 10.1249/MSS.0000000000000464

Fischer, C. P. (2006). Interleukin-6 in acute exercise and training: what is the biological relevance? *Exerc. Immunol. Rev.* 12, 6–33. Available online at: http://www.medizin.uni-tuebingen.de/transfusionsmedizin/institut/eir/content/2006/6/article.pdf

Galvin, H. M., Cooke, K., Sumners, D. P., Mileva, K. N., and Bowtell, J. L. (2013). Repeated sprint training in normobaric hypoxia. *Br. J. Sports Med.* 47, i74–i79. doi: 10.1136/bjsports-2013-092826

Gatterer, H., Philippe, M., Menz, V., Mosbach, F., Faulhaber, M., and Burtscher, M. (2014). Shuttle-run sprint training in hypoxia for youth elite soccer players: a pilot study. *J. Sports Sci. Med.* 13, 731–735. Available online at: http://www.jssm.org/gecjssm-13-731.xml.xml

Gibala, M. J., Little, J. P., Macdonald, M. J., and Hawley, J. A. (2012). Physiological adaptations to low-volume, high-intensity interval training in health and disease. *J. Physiol.* 590, 1077–1084. doi: 10.1113/jphysiol.2011.224725

Gibala, M. J., Little, J. P., van Essen, M., Wilkin, G. P., Burgomaster, K., Safdar, A., et al. (2006). Short-term sprint interval versus traditional endurance training: similar initial adaptations in human skeletal muscle and exercise performance. *J. Physiol.* 575, 901–911. doi: 10.1113/jphysiol.2006.112094

Gillen, J. B., Martin, B. J., MacInnis, M. J., Skelly, L. E., Tarnopolsky, M. A., and Gibala, M. J. (2016). Twelve weeks of sprint interval training improves indices of cardiometabolic health similar to traditional endurance training despite a five-fold lower exercise volume and time commitment. *PLoS ONE* 11:e0154075. doi: 10.1371/journal.pone.0154075

Girard, O., Amann, M., Aughey, R., Billaut, F., Bishop, D. J., Bourdon, P., et al. (2013). Position statement–altitude training for improving team-sport players' performance: current knowledge and unresolved issues. *Br. J. Sports Med.* 47, i8–i16. doi: 10.1136/bjsports-2013-093109

Gleeson, M., and Bishop, N. C. (2000). Special feature for the Olympics: effects of exercise on the immune system: modification of immune responses to exercise by carbohydrate, glutamine and anti-oxidant supplements. *Immunol. Cell Biol.* 78, 554–561. doi: 10.1111/j.1440-1711.2000.t01-6-.x

Goods, P. S. R., Dawson, B., Landers, G. J., Gore, C. J., Croft, K., and Peeling, P. (2015). Effect of repeat-sprint training in hypoxia on post-exercise interleukin-6 and F_2-isoprostanes. *Eur. J. Sport Sci.* doi: 10.1080/17461391.2015.1123776. [Epub ahead of print].

Goods, P. S. R., Dawson, B. T., Landers, G. J., Gore, C. J., and Peeling, P. (2014). Effect of different simulated altitudes on repeat-sprint performance in team-sport athletes. *Int. J. Sports Physiol. Perform.* 9, 857–862. doi: 10.1123/ijspp.2013-0423

Hazell, T. J., Macpherson, R. E. K., Gravelle, B. M. R., and Lemon, P. W. R. (2010). 10 or 30-s sprint interval training bouts enhance both aerobic and anaerobic performance. *Eur. J. Appl. Physiol.* 110, 153–160. doi: 10.1007/s00421-010-1474-y

Juel, C., Klarskov, C., Nielsen, J. J., Krustrup, P., Mohr, M., and Bangsbo, J. (2004). Effect of high-intensity intermittent training on lactate and H+ release from human skeletal muscle. *Am. J. Physiol. Endocrinol. Metab.* 286, E245–E251. doi: 10.1152/ajpendo.00303.2003

Kasai, N., Mizuno, S., Ishimoto, S., Sakamoto, E., Maruta, M., Goto, K., et al. (2015). Effect of training in hypoxia on repeated sprint performance in female athletes. *Springerplus* 4, 310. doi: 10.1186/s40064-015-1041-4

Kon, M., Nakagaki, K., Ebi, Y., Nishiyama, T., and Russell, A. P. (2015). Hormonal and metabolic responses to repeated cycling sprints under different hypoxic conditions. *Growth Horm. IGF Res.* 25, 121–126. doi: 10.1016/j.ghir.2015.03.002

Little, J. P., Safdar, A., Wilkin, G. P., Tarnopolsky, M. A., and Gibala, M. J. (2010). A practical model of low-volume high-intensity interval training induces mitochondrial biogenesis in human skeletal muscle: potential mechanisms. *J. Physiol.* 588, 1011–1022. doi: 10.1113/jphysiol.2009.181743

Lundby, C., Millet, G. P., Calbet, J. A., Bärtsch, P., and Subudhi, A. W. (2012). Does "altitude training" increase exercise performance in elite athletes? *Br. J. Sports Med.* 46, 792–795. doi: 10.1136/bjsports-2012-091231

Macpherson, T. W., and Weston, M. (2015). The effect of low-volume sprint interval training on the development and subsequent maintenance of aerobic fitness in soccer players. *Int. J. Sports Physiol. Perform.* 10, 332–338. doi: 10.1123/ijspp.2014-0075

McLean, B. D., Gore, C. J., and Kemp, J. (2014). Application of "live low-train high" for enhancing normoxic exercise performance in team sport athletes. *Sports Med.* 44, 1275–1287. doi: 10.1007/s40279-014-0204-8

Millet, G., Faiss, R., Brocherie, F., and Girard, O. (2013). Hypoxic training and team sports: a challenge to traditional methods? *Br. J. Sports Med.* 47, i6–i7. doi: 10.1136/bjsports-2013-092793

Millet, G. P., and Faiss, R. (2012). Hypoxic conditions and exercise-to-rest ratio are likely paramount. *Sports Med.* 42, 1081–1083. doi: 10.2165/11640210-000000000-00000

Millet, G., Roels, B., Schmitt, L., Woorons, X., and Richalet, J. P. (2010). Combining hypoxic methods for peak performance. *Sports Med.* 40, 1–25. doi: 10.2165/11317920-000000000-00000

Montero, D., and Lundby, C. (2016). Effects of exercise training in hypoxia versus normoxia on vascular health. *Sports Med.* doi: 10.1007/s40279-016-0570-5. [Epub ahead of print].

Puype, J., Van Proeyen, K., Raymackers, J.-M., Deldicque, L., and Hespel, P. (2013). Sprint interval training in hypoxia stimulates glycolytic enzyme activity. *Med. Sci. Sports Exerc.* 45, 2166–2174. doi: 10.1249/MSS.0b013e31829734ae

Rakobowchuk, M., Tanguay, S., Burgomaster, K. A., Howarth, K. R., Gibala, M. J., and MacDonald, M. J. (2008). Sprint interval and traditional endurance training induce similar improvements in peripheral arterial stiffness and flow-mediated dilation in healthy humans. *Am. J. Physiol. Regul. Integr. Comp. Physiol.* 295, R236–R242. doi: 10.1152/ajpregu.00069.2008

Richalet, J.-P., and Gore, C. J. (2008). Live and/or sleep high:train low, using normobaric hypoxia. *Scand. J. Med. Sci. Sports* 18, 29–37. doi: 10.1111/j.1600-0838.2008.00830.x

Richards, J. C., Johnson, T. K., Kuzma, J. N., Lonac, M. C., Schweder, M. M., Voyles, W. F., et al. (2010). Short-term sprint interval training increases insulin sensitivity in healthy adults but does not affect the thermogenic response to beta-adrenergic stimulation. *J. Physiol.* 588, 2961–2972. doi: 10.1113/jphysiol.2010.189886

Richardson, A. J., and Gibson, O. R. (2015). Simulated hypoxia does not further improve aerobic capacity during sprint interval training. *J. Sports Med. Phys. Fitness* 55, 1099–1106. Available online at: http://www.minervamedica.it/en/journals/sports-med-physical-fitness/article.php?cod=R40Y2015N10A1099

Rusko, H. K., Tikkanen, H. O., and Peltonen, J. E. (2004). Altitude and endurance training. *J. Sports Sci.* 22, 928–944. discussion: 945. doi: 10.1080/02640410400005933

Scheller, J., Chalaris, A., Schmidt-Arras, D., and Rose-John, S. (2011). The pro- and anti-inflammatory properties of the cytokine interleukin-6. *Biochim. Biophys. Acta* 1813, 878–888. doi: 10.1016/j.bbamcr.2011.01.034

Schmidt, W., and Prommer, N. (2005). The optimised CO-rebreathing method: a new tool to determine total haemoglobin mass routinely. *Eur. J. Appl. Physiol.* 95, 486–495. doi: 10.1007/s00421-005-0050-3

Schobersberger, W., Hobisch-Hagen, P., Fries, D., Wiedermann, F., Rieder-Scharinger, J., Villiger, B., et al. (2000). Increase in immune activation, vascular endothelial growth factor and erythropoietin after an ultramarathon run at moderate altitude. *Immunobiology* 201, 611–620. doi: 10.1016/S0171-2985(00)80078-9

Svendsen, I. S., Hem, E., and Gleeson, M. (2016). Effect of acute exercise and hypoxia on markers of systemic and mucosal immunity. *Eur. J. Appl. Physiol.* 116, 1219–1229. doi: 10.1007/s00421-016-3380-4

Talanian, J. L., Galloway, S. D. R., Heigenhauser, G. J. F., Bonen, A., and Spriet, L. L. (2007). Two weeks of high-intensity aerobic interval training increases the capacity for fat oxidation during exercise in women. *J. Appl. Physiol.* 102, 1439–1447. doi: 10.1152/japplphysiol.01098.2006

Turner, G., Gibson, O. R., and Maxwell, N. S. (2014). Simulated moderate hypoxia reduces intermittent sprint performance in games players. *J. Sports Med. Phys. Fitness* 54, 566–574. Available online at: http://www.minervamedica.it/en/journals/sports-med-physical-fitness/article.php?cod=R40Y2014N05A0566

Turner, G., Gibson, O. R., Watt, P. W., Pringle, J. S. M., Richardson, A. J., and Maxwell, N. S. (2016). The time course of endogenous erythropoietin, IL-6, and TNFα in response to acute hypoxic exposures. *Scand. J. Med. Sci. Sports.* doi: 10.1111/sms.12700. [Epub ahead of print].

Whyte, L. J., Gill, J. M. R., and Cathcart, A. J. (2010). Effect of 2 weeks of sprint interval training on health-related outcomes in sedentary overweight/obese men. *Metab. Clin. Exp.* 59, 1421–1428. doi: 10.1016/j.metabol.2010.01.002

Wilber, R. (2007). Application of altitude/hypoxic training by elite athletes. *Med. Sci. Sports Exerc.* 39, 1610–1624. doi: 10.1249/mss.0b013e3180de49e6

22

Walking in Hypoxia: An Efficient Treatment to Lessen Mechanical Constraints and Improve Health in Obese Individuals?

Olivier Girard[1, 2], Davide Malatesta[2] and Grégoire P. Millet[2]*

[1] *Athlete Health and Performance Research Center, Aspetar Orthopaedic and Sports Medicine Hospital, Doha, Qatar,* [2] *Faculty of Biology and Medicine, Institute of Sport Sciences, University of Lausanne, Lausanne, Switzerland*

Keywords: obesity, altitude training, hypoxic exercise, walking, mechanical loading

***Correspondence:**
Olivier Girard
oliv.girard@gmail.com

Obesity is defined as a body mass index >30 kg/m^2 and is a major health burden in many parts of the world (Finucane et al., 2011). The incidence of worldwide obesity is escalating at an increasing rate and has more than doubled since 1980. To tackle body fat accumulation and its clinical complications (e.g., diabetes, hypertension, heart disease), aggressive prevention strategies that are mainly based on dieting and lifestyle change have been implemented (Bray et al., 2016). Regular physical exercise such as walking is also generally recommended to increase energy expenditure (Donnelly et al., 2009). Despite an increasing and on-going body of research on cardio-metabolic disorders associated with the obese phenotype (Atkinson, 2014), many questions remain unanswered. Adherence to prescribed or spontaneous exercise remains low in obese patients (Dalle Grave et al., 2011), which raises specific questions on the effectiveness (Malhotra et al., 2015), as well as the objective (Browning and Kram, 2007) and subjective (Annesi, 2000) difficulties of exercising in these patients.

Due to discomfort, it remains unclear how excessive adipose tissue contributes to lower levels of physical activity as well as lower mobility and functional performance. Furthermore, obesity may increase joint stresses during simple locomotion tasks such as walking, which can lead to aberrant mechanics, reduced range of motion in the joints and eventually musculoskeletal pathologies (e.g., lower-extremity osteoarthritis, rheumatoid arthritis and/or low back pain) (Wearing et al., 2006; Browning, 2012; Sheehan and Gormley, 2012). For many obese patients, the reality of musculoskeletal disorders such as knee osteoarthritis may outweigh the eventual benefits of physical activity and weight loss. Altogether, non-compliance by obese patients to current exercise prescriptions and recommendations (Donnelly et al., 2009) suggests that existing exercise regimes do not necessarily meet the needs of this population. Alternative strategies are therefore required and their effectiveness must be clinically validated.

Hypoxic exposure results in any inspired pressure of oxygen under a normoxic value of 150 mmHg (Conkin and Wessel, 2008), while exercising is considered a new therapeutic strategy (Kayser and Verges, 2013; Millet et al., 2016). Until now, the combination of hypoxia and exercise stressors had mainly been investigated in normal weight patients (body mass index <25 kg/m^2) or lean individuals. The focus of the very few existing studies that included obese patients was on metabolic and body composition changes and not on walking or biomechanical improvement (Netzer et al., 2008; Haufe et al., 2010; Wiesner et al., 2010; Gatterer et al., 2015). Therefore, while cardio-metabolic adaptation was the main target of available studies on obesity (Atkinson, 2014; Verges et al., 2015), biomechanical investigations where hypoxia would be manipulated are also necessary. This is potentially useful to advance basic science as well as to develop effective physical activity recommendations to achieve energy expenditure goals while reducing the risk of musculoskeletal injury in obese patients (**Figure 1**).

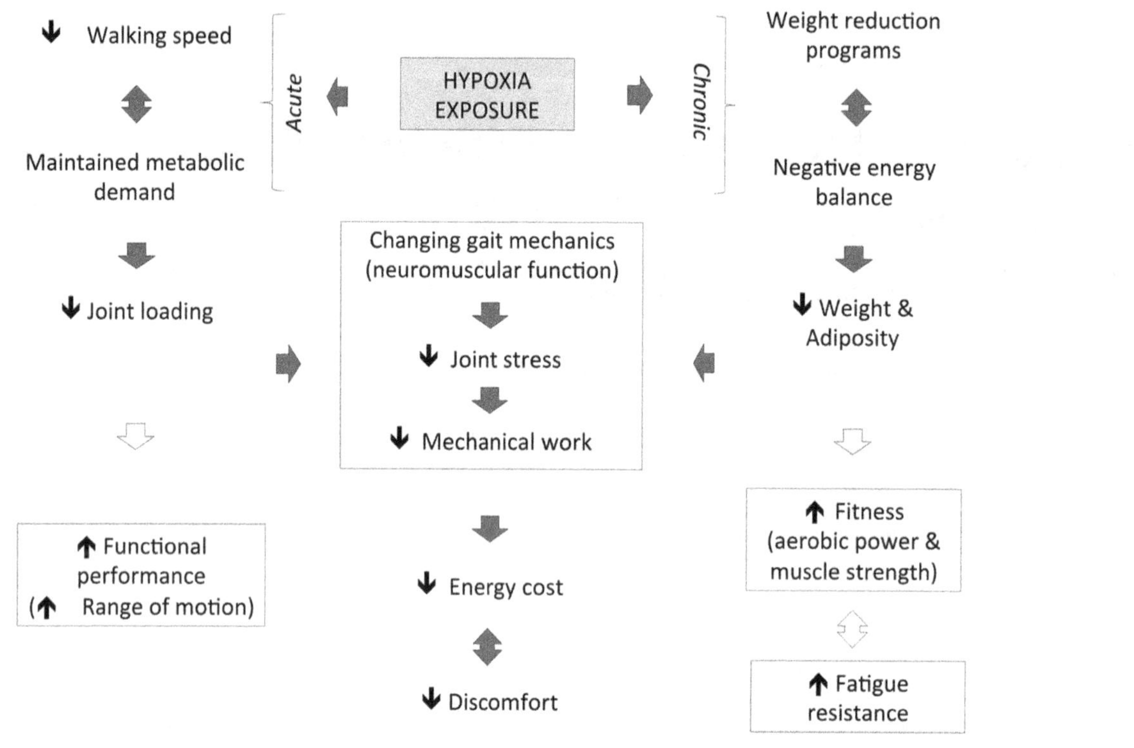

FIGURE 1 | Illustration of the hypothetical effects of hypoxia exposure on neuro-mechanical constraints associated with walking in obese patients

LOCOMOTION MECHANICS IN OBESE PATIENTS

Compared to lean individuals, preferred walking speeds have been consistently reported to be slower (i.e., typically 10–15%) in obese patients, with walking speeds that also appear inversely related to body mass index (Browning and Kram, 2005; Malatesta et al., 2009). This is presumably because of disproportionately heavier limbs, reduced relative muscle strength and a greater need to maintain balance during ambulation (Sheehan and Gormley, 2012). Obese patients tend to walk with a longer period of double support (i.e., both feet on the ground) and they swing their legs more rapidly (e.g., shorter swing time) with more lateral circumduction (e.g., wider step width) as well as abnormal (e.g., altered distribution) lower-extremity joint loads, absolute ground reaction forces (e.g., excessive peak forces and higher loading rates) and forefoot pressures when compared with non-obese individuals walking at identical speeds (Devita and Hortobágyi, 2003; Wearing et al., 2006; Browning, 2012). To date, there is no clear consensus on the precise nature of mechanical "mal-adaptations" associated with obesity (Sheehan and Gormley, 2012). Hence, whether a more erect sagittal plane posture and greater knee adduction, hip abduction and foot eversion are seen in obese vs. lean individuals remains controversial. As obese patients typically display a large variability in their mechanical stride parameters, it is difficult to identify common characteristics of walking patterns in this population (Wearing et al., 2006). Despite their greater body mass, absolute joint torques at the hip and knee are relatively similar to those of non-obese individuals, while ankle joint torques are approximately twice as large (Wearing et al., 2006). These biomechanical differences require that physical therapists and clinicians should make specific recommendations when prescribing physical exercise to obese patients.

WEIGHT-PERTURBATION INTERVENTIONS

Increasing the level of physical activity is likely a crucial intervention for an efficient prevention and treatment of obesity (Donnelly et al., 2009). The importance of reducing fat-mass accumulation in obese patients is indisputable; but surprisingly, only a few studies addressing the positive effects of weight loss on changes in walking biomechanics exist. Notwithstanding, massive weight loss produces dramatic reductions in knee forces during walking but when patients walk faster, these favorable reductions become substantially attenuated (Devita et al., 2016).

Because of various interventions (e.g., exercise training, Peyrot et al., 2010) or bariatric surgery (Hortobágyi et al., 2011), mechanical alterations (e.g., lower knee joint loads) and reductions in musculoskeletal pain may minimize the net energy cost. The combination of slower walking speeds and moderate inclines (0.75 m/s, 6°) is another intervention that is metabolically similar to a "normal" level of walking (1.50 m/s, 0°), yet it is associated with reduced net-muscle moments and loading rates (Ehlen et al., 2011). Furthermore, a faster stride frequency when walking speed is held constant (an example of "gait retraining") likely increases (~5%) energy expenditure without negatively affecting walking mechanics (Russell et al., 2010). Finally, a 10% weight loss through dietary intervention reduced knee compression by 200 N and reduced pain and disability in obese adults with knee osteoarthritis (Messier et al., 2013). Reducing potentially harmful forces in the knee during walking would improve locomotion in obese individuals.

In clinical rehabilitation settings, reducing musculoskeletal loading using lower body-pressure treadmills has an unprecedented popularity. For example, a 2016 meta-analysis indicated that peak and active vertical ground-reaction forces were consistently reduced in artificially weight-reduced healthy individuals; unweighting also provided some horizontal assistance and altered regional loading within the foot toward a forefoot strike (Farina et al., 2017). A potential drawback is that decreased speed with body-weight support will also reduce energy expenditure (e.g., oxygen uptake and heart rate readings) and muscle activation (i.e., with different responses between both stabilizer and propulsive muscles), likely minimizing any stimulus training effect. Use of a lower-body positive-pressure treadmill requires wearing tight neoprene shorts that are then attached to the treadmill and probably limits the range of motion of certain lower extremity joints and balance. One also cannot rule out that an improper arm swing leads to modified gait mechanics.

HYPOXIC EXPOSURE

Browning and Kram (2007) calculated that obese patients would need to walk at approximately 1.1 m/s (i.e., close to their preferred walking speed) to have a biomechanically equivalent joint load as lean individuals walking at 1.4 m/s. Consequently, obese patients would have to walk faster than their preferred walking speed to increase exercise intensity and to match the current physical activity guidelines (Donnelly et al., 2009). However, lower-extremity joint loads and the associated risk of musculoskeletal disorders likely increase with walking speed (Browning and Kram, 2007). In this context, acute hypoxia exposure may become advantageous as the mechanical load during physical exercise under hypoxic vs. normoxic conditions would be significantly reduced to achieve the same metabolic effect. In short, hypoxia enabled obese patients to achieve a higher metabolic demand, while a lower walking speed was also likely more protective of the muscles/joints in obese patients with orthopedic comorbidities (Wiesner et al., 2010).

To limit the negative effect of increased level walking speed on mechanical constraints, it is important to determine if walking in an O_2-deprived environment at a slower speed represents an effective strategy to reduce the load across the lower extremity joints, while providing adequate (i.e., similar to faster walking speeds near sea level) physiological stimulus for weight management. In healthy older community dwellers, changes of time-based gait parameters (e.g., slower cadence, longer stride time, and larger temporal gait variability) from the beginning to the end of a 40-min treadmill walk occurred, but these fatigue-related effects were similar to a 2,600-m simulated altitude or those near sea-level (Drum et al., 2016). Conversely and while exposed to hypoxia, obese subjects may re-organize their neuromuscular function to produce gait patterns that result in different knee joint loading. Based on the findings of studies conducted in healthy populations with lower-body positive-pressure treadmills, we postulated that most muscles that are involved in body-support would demonstrate a reduction in muscle activity as mechanical constraints would decrease with acute hypoxia exposure. Changes in muscle activity are not directly proportional to the changes in "unweighting" for all muscles, and vary widely across muscles [i.e., activation is not decreased in certain muscles (e.g., tibialis anterior, rectus femoris) until considerable unweighting occurs, Sainton et al., 2015, while others (e.g., hip adductor; Hunter et al., 2014) will barely change] and include the severity of hypoxic stress. This type of exercise intervention may be particularly useful to develop familiarity and compliance with regular physical exercise, especially when ambulation becomes less painful (Hootman et al., 2002; Ekkekakis and Lind, 2006).

Hypoxic conditioning consisting of chronic hypoxic exposure or sessions of intermittent exposure to moderate hypoxia repeated over several weeks may induce hematological, vascular, metabolic and neurological effects (Verges et al., 2015). This is presently considered as a promising therapeutic modality for several pathological states (e.g., heart failure, stroke, spinal cord injury patients) including obesity (Urdampilleta et al., 2012; Kayser and Verges, 2013; Millet et al., 2016). Continuous hypoxic training (low intensity endurance exercise for 90 min at 60% of the heart rate at maximum aerobic capacity, three times per week for 8 weeks; inspired fraction of $O_2 = 15\%$) in overweight subjects (body mass index >27 kg/m^2) leads to larger (+1.14 vs. 0.03 kg) weight loss than similar training in normoxic environments (Netzer et al., 2008). The effectiveness of such a low-intensity intervention remains questionable over a longer period of 8 months since Gatterer et al. (2015) did not report higher reductions in body weight between hypoxic and normoxic interventions. However, the biomechanical consequences of chronic hypoxic interventions on the walking pattern of obese patients are simply unknown.

To date, epidemiological reports associate the moderate altitude of residence to lower obesity prevalence without clear underlying mechanisms (Voss et al., 2014; Woolcott et al., 2016). Recently, it was reported that O_2 variations in organic systems may lead to considerable (3%) weight loss (yet of undefined composition) and improve metabolic and cardiorespiratory health (Netzer et al., 2008; Kayser and Verges, 2013; Kong et al., 2014). This leads to the suggestion that sustained hypoxia may be of benefit to weight management programs in obese patients (Millet et al., 2016). For prolonged exposure, the so-called "altitude anorexia" mechanisms that lead to a reduced appetite in altitude cannot be ruled out (Tschop and Morrison, 2001). The explanation for this phenomenon remains unclear but has been related to a modification in appetite regulation hormones (Shukla et al., 2005).

PERSPECTIVES

Acute Hypoxia

- On a lower-body positive-pressure treadmill, faster speeds are required to reach similar exercise intensities than on a normal treadmill (Farina et al., 2017). Reportedly, faster walking and running speeds (6–16 km/h) rather than increases in percent body weight (50–100%) cause a greater maximum plantar force on a lower-body positive-pressure treadmill (Thomson et al., 2017). These observations are limited in scope to healthy male runners. When combined, acute hypoxia exposure (normobaric hypoxia) to artificially increase the metabolic load and exercise on body positive-pressure or aquatic treadmills to decrease the mechanical strain might be clinically relevant. Deeper investigations of obese patients walking at slower speeds (e.g., ranging 0.5–3.5 km/h) with and without hypoxic exposure are required and are likely to alter the relationship between speed and muscle unweighting on mechanical strain as reported in similar studies (Thomson et al., 2017). While exercising at simulated altitudes ranging from 2,500 to 3,500 m is commonly implemented (Haufe et al., 2010; Kong et al., 2014; Gatterer et al., 2015), the optimal degree of hypoxic severity (i.e., maximize physiological adaptations with limited negative consequences) is unknown (e.g., Urdampilleta et al., 2012 for intermittent hypoxic exercise recommendations), and requires further study. However, it is likely that due to the maladaptive side effects associated with hypoxia (i.e., sleep apnea, intermittent hypoxemia), obese patients would not tolerate a high-altitude (Dempsey and Morgan, 2015). For safety reasons, we speculate that hypoxic training could be performed at a simulated altitude lower than 3,500 m.
- Thus far, the available obesity-related studies investigated gait mechanics prior to any signs of fatigue. Perturbations in muscle force generation could reduce the ability of fatigued muscle groups to attenuate to ground reaction impact forces, thereby exaggerating gait abnormalities, and likely increasing the fall risks during locomotor tasks (Himes and Reynolds, 2012). To date, there is a dearth of information pertaining to the changes in gait and balance control over time as obese patients start to fatigue. It is also unknown whether there is a cumulative effect of hypoxic exposure and exercise-induced fatigue on locomotion mechanics that may increase fall risks in obese individuals who are exercising for a prolonged time at moderate altitude.
- Walking includes an inherent fall risk based only on the mere exposure to gradients and surface variations (e.g., stair climbing, rocky paths) that would influence the load applied to the weight-bearing joints of obese individuals. Surface electromyography (EMG) recording during various locomotive tasks would elucidate muscle activation strategies used by obese patients to cope with these situations, including whether hypoxia exposure modifies neuromuscular responses. While the surface EMG may be feasible in severely obese individuals (Minetto et al., 2013), decomposition of surface EMG signals into time-frequency components, wavelet components and degrees-of-freedom force functions may provide further insight into the contributions from the neuromuscular system (Hamid Nawab et al., 2010).

Chronic Hypoxia

- Weight loss is an important method for the treatment of obesity and its associated comorbidities. It is possible to measure the net energy cost of level-walking in obese patients by investigating the effect of decreased body mass on gait pattern and external mechanical work (i.e., simple inverted pendulum modeling to approximate the energy required to raise and accelerate the center of mass; Malatesta et al., 2013). To date, moderate-intensity continuous training is the type of physical activity most frequently recommended to obese patients (Donnelly et al., 2009). That said, growing evidence suggests that high-intensity interval training is a time-efficient approach in this population (Kong et al., 2016). However, this training was rated as less pleasant and less enjoyable than an isocaloric session of moderate-intensity continuous exercise (Decker and Ekkekakis, 2017). Future studies are warranted that compare the effects of various exercise modalities/intensities in addition to hypoxia exposure on the changes in gait pattern.
- Hypoxic training embraces different methods as "live high–train high," "live high–train low," or "live high–train low" interspersed with hypoxic training for additional sessions ("live high–train low and high") that can be conducted in normobaric or hypobaric (natural) conditions with the use of artificial devices or by ascending to elevated terrestrial environments (Millet et al., 2013). To our knowledge, there are no studies that compared the influence of these different altitude-training methods on the weight loss and gait mechanics in obese patients. Consequently, how different physiological adaptations and different degrees of body mass loss associated with various hypoxic training methods would specifically affect gait pattern in obese patients remains undetermined.
- Walking and hiking for hours at low-to-moderate intensity in mountainous areas is a popular and safe outdoor activity, even for obese patients (Neumayr et al., 2014), and should therefore be recommended to increase physical activity in this population. The potential identification of a significant difference between simulated (i.e., normobaric hypoxia) and terrestrial (i.e., hypobaric hypoxia) altitudes is also clinically relevant. Interestingly, Degache et al. (2012) reported that real altitude superiorly decreased postural stability. Investigations that compare normobaric to hypobaric hypoxia in obese patients are currently lacking.

CONCLUSION

Obese patients should be enthusiastically encouraged to engage in regular physical activity for the improvement of cardio-metabolic health, with exercises selected that minimize the joint load and pain as much as possible. Walking at slower speeds under hypoxic conditions would reduce joint loading (and the risk of musculoskeletal injury/pathology), while ensuring an adequate exercise stimulus for weight management. Alternatively, hypoxic conditioning may be an appropriate form of exercise training for obese patients as it can lead to effective weight loss due to a negative energy balance. These acute and chronic hypoxic-related interventions would contribute to the support of an appropriate and individualized prescription for obese patients to reduce the biomechanical load involved in walking and eventually improve training adherence (**Figure 1**).

AUTHOR CONTRIBUTIONS

All authors listed, have made substantial, direct and intellectual contribution to the work, and approved it for publication.

REFERENCES

Annesi, J. J. (2000). Effects of minimal exercise and cognitive behavior modification on adherence, emotion change, self-image, and physical change in obese women. *Percept. Mot. Skills* 91, 322–336. doi: 10.2466/pms.2000.91.1.322

Atkinson, R. L. (2014). Current status of the field of obesity. *Trends Endocrinol. Metab.* 25, 283–284. doi: 10.1016/j.tem.2014.03.003

Bray, G. A., Fruhbeck, G., Ryan, D. H., and Wilding, J. P. (2016). Management of obesity. *Lancet* 387, 1947–1956. doi: 10.1016/S0140-6736(16)00271-3

Browning, R. C. (2012). Locomotion mechanics in obese adults and children. *Curr. Obes. Rep.* 1, 152–159. doi: 10.1007/s13679-012-0021-z

Browning, R. C., and Kram, R. (2005). Energetic cost and preferred speed of walking in obese vs. normal weight women. *Obes. Res.* 13, 891–899. doi: 10.1038/oby.2005.103

Browning, R. C., and Kram, R. (2007). Effects of obesity on the biomechanics of walking at different speeds. *Med. Sci. Sports Exerc.* 39, 1632–1641. doi: 10.1249/mss.0b013e318076b54b

Conkin, J., and Wessel, J. H. (2008). Critique of the equivalent air altitude model. *Aviat. Space Environ. Med.* 79, 975–982. doi: 10.3357/ASEM.2331.2008

Dalle Grave, R., Calugi, S., Centis, E., El Ghoch, M., and Marchesini, G. (2011). Cognitive-behavioral strategies to increase the adherence to exercise in the management of obesity. *J. Obes.* 2011:348293. doi: 10.1155/2011/348293

Decker, E. S., and Ekkekakis, P. (2017). More efficient, perhaps, but at what price? Pleasure and enjoyment responses to high-intensity interval exercise in low-active women with obesity. *Psychol. Sport Exerc.* 28, 1–10. doi: 10.1016/j.psychsport.2016.09.005

Degache, F., Larghi, G., Faiss, R., Deriaz, O., and Millet, G. P. (2012). Hypobaric versus normobaric hypoxia: same effects on postural stability? *High Alt. Med. Biol.* 13, 40–45. doi: 10.1089/ham.2011.1042

Dempsey, J. A., and Morgan, B. J. (2015). Humans in hypoxia: a conspiracy of maladaptation?! *Physiology (Bethesda)* 30, 304–316. doi: 10.1152/physiol.00007.2015

Devita, P., and Hortobágyi, T. (2003). Obesity is not associated with increased knee joint torque and power during level walking. *J. Biomech.* 36, 1355–1362. doi: 10.1016/S0021-9290(03)00119-2

Devita, P., Rider, P., and Hortobágyi, T. (2016). Reductions in knee joint forces with weight loss are attenuated by gait adaptations in class III obesity. *Gait Posture* 45, 25–30. doi: 10.1016/j.gaitpost.2015.12.040

Donnelly, J. E., Blair, S. N., Jakicic, J. M., Manore, M. M., Rankin, J. W., and Smith, B. K. (2009). Appropriate physical activity intervention strategies for weight loss and prevention of weight regain for adults. *Med. Sci. Sports Exerc.* 41, 459–471. doi: 10.1249/MSS.0b013e3181949333

Drum, S. N., Faude, O., de Fay du Lavallaz, E., Allemann, R., Nève, G., and Donath, L. (2016). Acute effects of walking at moderate normobaric hypoxia on gait and balance performance in healthy community-dwelling seniors: a randomized controlled crossover study. *Arch. Gerontol. Geriatr.* 67, 74–79. doi: 10.1016/j.archger.2016.06.022

Ehlen, K. A., Reiser, R. F., and Browning, R. C. (2011). Energetics and biomechanics of inclined treadmill walking in obese adults. *Med. Sci. Sports Exerc.* 43, 1251–1259. doi: 10.1249/MSS.0b013e3182098a6c

Ekkekakis, P., and Lind, E. (2006). Exercise does not feel the same when you are overweight: the impact of self-selected and imposed intensity on affect and exertion. *Int. J. Obes.* 30, 652–660. doi: 10.1038/sj.ijo.0803052

Farina, K. A., Wright, A. A., Ford, K. R., Wirfel, L. A., and Smoliga, J. M. (2017). Physiological and biomechanical responses to running on lower body positive pressure treadmills in healthy populations. *Sports Med.* 47, 261–275. doi: 10.1007/s40279-016-0581-2

Finucane, M. M., Stevens, G. A., Cowan, M. J., Danaei, G., Lin, J. K., Paciorek, C. J., et al. (2011). National, regional, and global trends in body-mass index since 1980: systematic analysis of health examination surveys and epidemiological studies with 960 country-years and 9·1 million participants. *Lancet* 377, 557–567. doi: 10.1016/S0140-6736(10)62037-5

Gatterer, H., Haacke, S., Burtscher, M., Faulhaber, M., Melmer, A., Ebenbichler, C., et al. (2015). Normobaric intermittent hypoxia over 8 months does not reduce body weight and metabolic risk factors - a randomized, single blind, placebo-controlled study in normobaric hypoxia and normobaric sham hypoxia. *Obes. Facts* 8, 200–209. doi: 10.1159/000431157

Haufe, S., Wiesner, S., Engeli, S., Luft, F. C., and Jordan, J. (2010). Influences of normobaric hypoxia training on metabolic risk markers in human subjects. *Med. Sci. Sports Exerc.* 40, 1939–1944. doi: 10.1249/MSS.0b013e31817f1988

Himes, C. L., and Reynolds, S. L. (2012). Effect of obesity on falls, injury, and disability. *J. Am. Geriatr. Soc.* 60, 124–129. doi: 10.1111/j.1532-5415.2011.03767.x

Hootman, J. M., Macera, C. A., Ainsworth, B. E., Addy, C. L., Martin, M., and Blair, S. N. (2002). Epidemiology of musculoskeletal injuries among sedentary and physically active adults. *Med. Sci. Sports Exerc.* 34, 838–844. doi: 10.1097/00005768-200205000-00017

Hortobágyi, T., Herring, C., Pories, W. J., Rider, P., and Devita, P. (2011). Massive weight loss-induced mechanical plasticity in obese gait. *J. Appl. Physiol.* 111, 1391–1399. doi: 10.1152/japplphysiol.00291.2011

Hunter, I., Seeley, M. K., Hopkins, J. T., Carr, C., and Franson, J. J. (2014). EMG activity during positive-pressure treadmill running. *J. Electromyogr. Kinesiol.* 24, 348–352. doi: 10.1016/j.jelekin.2014.01.009

Kayser, B., and Verges, S. (2013). Hypoxia, energy balance and obesity: from pathophysiological mechanisms to new treatment strategies. *Obes. Rev.* 14, 579–592. doi: 10.1111/obr.12034

Kong, Z., Fan, X., Sun, S., Song, L., Shi, Q., and Nie, J. (2016). Comparison of high-intensity interval training and moderate-to-vigorous continuous training for cardiometabolic health and exercise enjoyment in obese young women: a randomized controlled trial. *PLoS ONE* 11:e0158589. doi: 10.1371/journal.pone.015858

Kong, Z., Zang, Y., and Hu, Y. (2014). Normobaric hypoxia training causes more weight loss than normoxia training after a 4-week residential camp for obese young adults. *Sleep Breath.* 18, 591–597. doi: 10.1007/s11325-013-0922-4

Malatesta, D., Vismara, L., Menegoni, F., Galli, M., Romei, M., and Capodaglio, P. (2009). Mechanical external work and recovery at preferred walking speed in obese subjects. *Med. Sci. Sports Exerc.* 41, 426–434. doi: 10.1249/MSS.0b013e31818606e7

Malatesta, D., Vismara, L., Menegoni, F., Grugni, G., and Capodaglio, P. (2013). Effect of obesity onset on pendular energy transduction at spontaneous walking speed: Prader-Willi versus nonsyndromal obese individuals. *Obesity (Silver Spring)* 21, E586–591. doi: 10.1002/oby.20455

Malhotra, A., Noakes, T., and Phinney, S. (2015). It is time to bust the myth of physical inactivity and obesity: you cannot outrun a bad diet. *Br. J. Sports Med.* 49, 967–968. doi: 10.1136/bjsports-2015-094911

Messier, S. P., Mihalko, S. L., Legault, C., Miller, G. D., Nicklas, B. J., DeVita, P., et al. (2013). Effects of intensive diet and exercise on knee joint loads, inflammation, and clinical outcomes among overweight and obese adults with knee osteoarthritis: the IDEA randomized clinical trial. *J. Am. Med. Assoc.* 310, 1263–1273. doi: 10.1001/jama.2013.277669

Millet, G. P., Brocherie, F., Faiss, R., and Girard, O. (2013). Hypoxic training and team sports: a challenge to traditional methods? *Br. J. Sports Med.* 47, 6–7. doi: 10.1136/bjsports-2013-092793

Millet, G. P., Debevec, T., Brocherie, F., Malatesta, D., and Girard, O. (2016). Therapeutic use of exercising in hypoxia: promises and limitations. *Front. Physiol.* 7:224. doi: 10.3389/fphys.2016.00224

Minetto, M. A., Botter, A., Šprager, S., Agosti, F., Patrizi, A., Lanfranco, F., et al. (2013). Feasibility study of detecting surface electromyograms in severely obese patients. *J. Electromyogr. Kinesiol.* 23, 285–295. doi: 10.1016/j.jelekin.2012.09.008

Nawab, S. H., Chang, S. S., and De Luca, C. J. (2010). High-yield decomposition of surface EMG signals. *Clin. Neurophysiol.* 121, 1602–1615. doi: 10.1016/j.clinph.2009.11.092

Netzer, N. C., Chytra, R., and Küpper, T. (2008). Low intense physical exercise in normobaric hypoxia leads to more weight loss in obese people than low intense physical exercise in normobaric sham hypoxia. *Sleep Breath* 12, 129–134. doi: 10.1007/s11325-007-0149-3

Neumayr, G., Fries, D., Mittermayer, M., Humpeler, E., Klingler, A., Schobersberger, W., et al. (2014). Effects of hiking at moderate and low altitude on cardiovascular parameters in male patients with metabolic syndrome: Austrian Moderate Altitude Study. *Wilderness Environ. Med.* 25, 329–334. doi: 10.1016/j.wem.2014.01.003

Peyrot, N., Morin, J.-B., Thivel, D., Isacco, L., Taillardat, M., Belli, A., et al. (2010). Mechanical work and metabolic cost of walking after weight loss in obese adolescents. *Med. Sci. Sports Exerc.* 42, 1914–1922. doi: 10.1249/MSS.0b013e3181da8d1e

Russell, E. M., Braun, B., and Hamill, J. (2010). Does stride length influence metabolic cost and biomechanical risk factors for knee osteoarthritis in obese women? *Clin. Biomech.* 25, 438–443. doi: 10.1016/j.clinbiomech.2010.01.016

Sainton, P., Nicol, C., Cabri, J., Barthelemy-Montfort, J., Berton, E., and Chavet, P. (2015). Influence of short-term unweighing and reloading on running kinetics and muscle activity. *Eur. J. Appl. Physiol.* 115, 1135–1145. doi: 10.1007/s00421-014-3095-3

Sheehan, K., and Gormley, J. (2012). Gait and increased body weight (potential implications for musculoskeletal disease). *Phys. Ther. Rev.* 17, 91–98. doi: 10.1179/1743288X11Y.0000000057

Shukla, V., Singh, S. N., Vats, P., Singh, V. K., Singh, S. B., and Banerjee, P. K. (2005). Ghrelin and leptin levels of sojourners and acclimatized lowlanders at high altitude. *Nutr. Neurosci.* 8, 161–165. doi: 10.1080/10284150500132823

Thomson, A., Einarsson, E., Witvrouw, E., and Whiteley, R. (2017). Running speed increases plantar load more than per cent body weight on an AlterG® treadmill. *J. Sports Sci.* 35, 277–282. doi: 10.1080/02640414.2016.1163401

Tschop, M., and Morrison, K. M. (2001). Weight loss at high altitude. *Adv. Exp. Med. Biol.* 502, 237–247. doi: 10.1007/978-1-4757-3401-0_16

Urdampilleta, A., Gonzalez-Muniesa, P., Portillo, M. P., and Martinez, J. A. (2012). Usefulness of combining intermittent hypoxia and physical exercise in the treatment of obesity. *J. Physiol. Biochem.* 68, 289–304. doi: 10.1007/s13105-011-0115-1

Verges, S., Chacaroun, S., Godin-Ribuot, D., and Baillieul, S. (2015). Hypoxic conditioning as a new therapeutic modality. *Front. Pediatr.* 3:58. doi: 10.3389/fped.2015.00058

Voss, J. D., Allison, D. B., Webber, B. J., Otto, J. L., and Clark, L. L. (2014). Lower obesity rate during residence at high altitude among a military population with frequent migration: a quasi experimental model for investigating spatial causation. *PLoS ONE* 9:e93493. doi: 10.1371/journal.pone.0093493

Wearing, S. C., Hennig, E. M., Byrne, N. M., Steele, J. R., and Hills, A. P. (2006). The biomechanics of restricted movement in adult obesity. *Obes. Rev* 7, 13–24. doi: 10.1111/j.1467-789X.2006.00215.x

Wiesner, S., Haufe, S., Engeli, S., Mutschler, H., Haas, U., Luft, F. C., et al. (2010). Influences of normobaric hypoxia training on physical fitness and metabolic risk markers in overweight to obese subjects. *Obesity (Silver Spring)* 18, 116–120. doi: 10.1038/oby.2009.193

Woolcott, O. O., Gutierrez, C., Castillo, O. A., Elashoff, R. M., Stefanovski, D., and Bergman, R. N. (2016). Inverse association between altitude and obesity: a prevalence study among andean and low-altitude adult individuals of Peru. *Obesity (Silver Spring)* 24, 929–937. doi: 10.1002/oby.21401

Permissions

All chapters in this book were first published by Frontiers; hereby published with permission under the Creative Commons Attribution License or equivalent. Every chapter published in this book has been scrutinized by our experts. Their significance has been extensively debated. The topics covered herein carry significant findings which will fuel the growth of the discipline. They may even be implemented as practical applications or may be referred to as a beginning point for another development.

The contributors of this book come from diverse backgrounds, making this book a truly international effort. This book will bring forth new frontiers with its revolutionizing research information and detailed analysis of the nascent developments around the world.

We would like to thank all the contributing authors for lending their expertise to make the book truly unique. They have played a crucial role in the development of this book. Without their invaluable contributions this book wouldn't have been possible. They have made vital efforts to compile up to date information on the varied aspects of this subject to make this book a valuable addition to the collection of many professionals and students.

This book was conceptualized with the vision of imparting up-to-date information and advanced data in this field. To ensure the same, a matchless editorial board was set up. Every individual on the board went through rigorous rounds of assessment to prove their worth. After which they invested a large part of their time researching and compiling the most relevant data for our readers.

The editorial board has been involved in producing this book since its inception. They have spent rigorous hours researching and exploring the diverse topics which have resulted in the successful publishing of this book. They have passed on their knowledge of decades through this book. To expedite this challenging task, the publisher supported the team at every step. A small team of assistant editors was also appointed to further simplify the editing procedure and attain best results for the readers.

Apart from the editorial board, the designing team has also invested a significant amount of their time in understanding the subject and creating the most relevant covers. They scrutinized every image to scout for the most suitable representation of the subject and create an appropriate cover for the book.

The publishing team has been an ardent support to the editorial, designing and production team. Their endless efforts to recruit the best for this project, has resulted in the accomplishment of this book. They are a veteran in the field of academics and their pool of knowledge is as vast as their experience in printing. Their expertise and guidance has proved useful at every step. Their uncompromising quality standards have made this book an exceptional effort. Their encouragement from time to time has been an inspiration for everyone.

The publisher and the editorial board hope that this book will prove to be a valuable piece of knowledge for researchers, students, practitioners and scholars across the globe.

List of Contributors

Jin-zhuo Ning, Fan Cheng, Wei-min Yu, Ting Rao, Yuan Ruan, Run Yuan, Xiao-bin Zhang, Yang Du and Cheng-cheng Xiao
Department of Urology, Renmin Hospital of Wuhan University, Wuhan, China

Wei Li
Department of Anesthesiology, Renmin Hospital of Wuhan University, Wuhan, China

Dong Zhuo
Department of Urology, Wannan Medical College, Wuhu, China

Chang Liu, Lu Liu, Er-Long Zhang, Bind-da Sun, Gang Xu, Jian Chen and Yu-qi Gao
Institute of Medicine and Hygienic Equipment for High Altitude Region, College of High Altitude Military Medicine, Army Medical University, Third Military Medical University, Chongqing, China
Key Laboratory of High Altitude Environmental Medicine, Army Medical University, Third Military Medical University, Ministry of Education, Chongqing, China
Key Laboratory of High Altitude Medicine, People's Liberation Army, Chongqing, China

Bao Liu
Institute of Medicine and Hygienic Equipment for High Altitude Region, College of High Altitude Military Medicine, Army Medical University, Third Military Medical University, Chongqing, China
Key Laboratory of High Altitude Environmental Medicine, Army Medical University, Third Military Medical University, Ministry of Education, Chongqing, China
Key Laboratory of High Altitude Medicine, People's Liberation Army, Chongqing, China
The 12th Hospital of Chinese People's Liberation Army, Kashi, China

David Morales-Alamo, Borja Guerra, Marcos Martin-Rincon, Miriam Gelabert-Rebato, Cecilia Dorado and José A. L. Calbet
Department of Physical Education, University of Las Palmas de Gran Canaria, Las Palmas de Gran Canaria, Spain
Research Institute of Biomedical and Health Sciences, Las Palmas de Gran Canaria, Spain

Alfredo Santana
Research Institute of Biomedical and Health Sciences, Las Palmas de Gran Canaria, Spain
Clinical Genetics Unit, Complejo Hospitalario Universitario Insular-Materno Infantil de Las Palmas de Gran Canaria, Las Palmas de Gran Canaria, Spain

Fernando A. Moraga
Laboratorio de Fisiología, Hipoxia y Función Vascular, Departamento de Ciencias Biomédicas, Facultad de Medicina, Universidad Católica del Norte, Coquimbo, Chile

Iván López and Daniel Soza
Safety Group, Atacama Large Millimeter Submillimeter Array, Calama, Chile

Alicia Morales and Jessica Noack
Departamento de Ciencias de la Salud, Escuela de Enfermería, Universidad Santo Tomás, Santiago, Chile

Andrew P. Holmes, Clare J. Ray, Andrew M. Coney and Prem Kumar
Institute of Clinical Sciences, College of Medical and Dental Sciences, University of Birmingham, Birmingham, United Kingdom

Sandy MacMillan and A. Mark Evans
Centre for Discovery Brain Sciences and Centre for Cardiovascular Science, College of Medicine and Veterinary Medicine, University of Edinburgh, Edinburgh, United Kingdom

Kiumars Shamloo, Juan Chen, Jasmine Sardar, Rinzhin T. Sherpa, Rajasekharreddy Pala and Kimberly F. Atkinson
Department of Biomedical and Pharmaceutical Sciences, Chapman University, Irvine, CA, United States

William J. Pearce and Lubo Zhang
Departments of Basic Sciences, Physiology and Pharmacology, Lawrence D. Longo MD Center for Perinatal Biology, Loma Linda University School of Medicine, Loma Linda, CA, United States

Surya M. Nauli
Department of Biomedical and Pharmaceutical Sciences, Chapman University, Irvine, CA, United States
Division of Nephrology and Hypertension, Department of Medicine, University of California, Irvine, Irvine, CA, United States

Lara Muralt, Michael Furian, Mona Lichtblau, Sayaka S. Aeschbacher, Maya Bisang, Stefanie Ulrich, Tsogyal D. Latshang and Silvia Ulrich
Department of Respiratory Medicine, University Hospital Zurich, Zurich, Switzerland
Kyrgyz-Swiss High Altitude Clinic and Medical Research Center, Tuja-Ashu, Kyrgyzstan

Ross A. Clark
School of Health and Sports Science, University of the Sunshine Coast, Sunshine Coast, QLD, Australia

Bermet Estebesova, Ulan Sheraliev, Nuriddin Marazhapov, Batyr Osmonov and Talant M. Sooronbaev
Kyrgyz-Swiss High Altitude Clinic and Medical Research Center, Tuja-Ashu, Kyrgyzstan
Department of Respiratory Medicine, National Center for Cardiology and Internal Medicine, Bishkek, Kyrgyzstan

Konrad E. Bloch
Department of Respiratory Medicine, University Hospital Zurich, Zurich, Switzerland
Kyrgyz-Swiss High Altitude Clinic and Medical Research Center, Tuja-Ashu, Kyrgyzstan
Department of Respiratory Medicine, National Center for Cardiology and Internal Medicine, Bishkek, Kyrgyzstan

Ginés Viscor, Joan R. Torrella and Teresa Pages
Physiology Section, Department of Cell Biology, Physiology and Immunology, Faculty of Biology, Universitat de Barcelona, Barcelona, Spain

Luisa Corral, Antoni Ricart, Casimiro Javierre and Josep L. Ventura
Exercise Physiology Unit, Department of Physiological Sciences, Faculty of Medicine and Health Sciences, Universitat de Barcelona, L'Hospitalet de Llobregat, Barcelona, Spain

Bernardo J. Krause
Division of Pediatrics, Faculty of Medicine, Pontificia Universidad Católica de Chile, Santiago, Chile

Paola Casanello
Division of Pediatrics, Faculty of Medicine, Pontificia Universidad Católica de Chile, Santiago, Chile
Division of Obstetrics & Gynecology, Faculty of Medicine, Pontificia Universidad Católica de Chile, Santiago, Chile

Ana C. Dias, Paulina Arias, Victoria Velarde, German A. Arenas and Rodrigo Iturriaga
Laboratorio de Neurobiología, Facultad de Ciencias Biológicas, Pontificia Universidad Católica de Chile, Santiago, Chile

Marcelo D. Preite
Departamento de Química Orgánica, Facultad de Química, Pontificia Universidad Católica de Chile, Santiago, Chile

Raúl Pulgar-Sepúlveda and Fernando C. Ortiz
Instituto de Ciencias Biomédicas, Facultad de Ciencias de la Salud, Universidad Autónoma de Chile, Santiago, Chile

Rodrigo Varas
Instituto de Ciencias Biomédicas, Facultad de Ciencias de la Salud, Universidad Autónoma de Chile, Santiago, Chile
Facultad de Ciencias de la Salud, Universidad Autónoma de Chile, Talca, Chile

Rodrigo Iturriaga
Laboratorio de Neurobiología, Facultad de Ciencias Biológicas, Pontificia Universidad Católica de Chile, Santiago, Chile

Rodrigo Del Rio
Laboratory of Cardiorespiratory Control, Department of Physiology, Pontificia Universidad Católica de Chile, Santiago, Chile
Centro de Envejecimiento y Regeneración, Pontificia Universidad Católica de Chile, Santiago, Chile
Centro de Excelencia en Biomedicina de Magallanes, Universidad de Magallanes, Punta Arenas, Chile

Thâmila Kamila de Souza Medeiros, Daniela Monteiro Baptista da Silva, Ovidiu Constantin Baltatu and Luciana Aparecida Campos
Center of Innovation, Technology and Education at Anhembi Morumbi University - Laureate International Universities, São José dos Campos, Brazil
School of Health Sciences at Anhembi Morumbi University - Laureate International Universities, São José dos Campos, Brazil

Mirela Dobre
Division of Nephrology and Hypertension, University Hospitals, Cleveland, OH, United States

Andrei Brateanu
Medicine Institute, Cleveland Clinic, Cleveland, OH, United States

Olivier Girard
ISSUL, Institute of Sport Sciences, Faculty of Biology and Medicine, University of Lausanne, Lausanne, Switzerland
Athlete Health and Performance Research Centre, Orthopaedic and Sports Medicine Hospital, Aspetar, Doha, Qatar

Franck Brocherie and Grégoire P. Millet
ISSUL, Institute of Sport Sciences, Faculty of Biology and Medicine, University of Lausanne, Lausanne, Switzerland

Yanchun Wang
Department of Health Care and Geriatrics, Lanzhou General Hospital of Lanzhou Military Region, Lanzhou, China

Xiao-Han Ding
Department of Health Care and Geriatrics, Lanzhou General Hospital of Lanzhou Military Region, Lanzhou, China
Department of Geriatric Cardiology, Chinese PLA General Hospital, Beijing, China

Bin Cui, Jun Qin, Ji-Hang Zhang, Shi-Yong Yu, Xiao-Hui Zhao and Lan Huang
Department of Cardiology, Xinqiao Hospital, Army Medical University (Third Military Medical University), Chongqing, China

Rong-Sheng Rao
Department of Ultrasonography, Xinqiao Hospital, Army Medical University (Third Military Medical University), Chongqing, China

Aaron C. Petersen, Alice J. Sweeting and Robert J. Aughey
Institute of Sport, Exercise and Active Living, Victoria University, Melbourne, VIC, Australia

Mathew W. H. Inness
Institute of Sport, Exercise and Active Living, Victoria University, Melbourne, VIC, Australia
Western Bulldogs Football Club, Melbourne, VIC, Australia

François Billaut
Institute of Sport, Exercise and Active Living, Victoria University, Melbourne, VIC, Australia
Département de Kinesiologie, Université Laval, Quebec City, QC, Canada

Emily J. Walker
Institute of Sport, Exercise and Active Living, Victoria University, Melbourne, VIC, Australia
Collingwood Football Club, Melbourne, VIC, Australia

Ruud Van Thienen, Evi Masschelein, Gommaar D'Hulst and Peter Hespel
Exercise Physiology Research Group, Department of Kinesiology, KU Leuven, Leuven, Belgium

Oliver R. Gibson
Centre for Human Performance, Exercise, and Rehabilitation, Brunel University London, Uxbridge, UK

Martine Thomis
Physical Activity, Sports and Health Research Group, Department of Kinesiology, KU Leuven, Leuven, Belgium

Alexandra Jochmans-Lemoine, Susana Revollo, Jorge Soliz and Vincent Joseph
Centre de Recherche de l'Institut Universitaire de Cardiologie et de Pneumologie de Québec, Université Laval, Quebec City, QC, Canada

Gabriella Villalpando, Ibana Valverde and Marcelino Gonzales
Instituto Boliviano de Biologia de Altura, Universidad Mayor de San Andrés, La Paz, Bolivia

Sofien Laouafa
Centre de Recherche de l'Institut Universitaire de Cardiologie et de Pneumologie de Québec, Université Laval, Quebec City, QC, Canada
Centre National de la Recherche Scientifique, UMR 5023, Université Claude Bernard Lyon 1, Villeurbanne, France

Matthew I. Black
School of Sport, Exercise and Health Sciences, Loughborough University, Loughborough, UK

Christopher R. Potter, Cain C. T. Clark and Stephen B. Draper
HE Sport, University Centre, Hartpury College, Gloucestershire, UK

Jo Corbett
Department of Sport and Exercise Science, University of Portsmouth, Portsmouth, UK

Jesús G. Ponce-González
Department of Physical Education, University of Las Palmas de Gran Canaria, Las Palmas, Spain

Rafael Torres-Peralta, José Losa-Reyna, David Morales-Alamo, Ismael Pérez-Suárez and José A. L. Calbet
Department of Physical Education, University of Las Palmas de Gran Canaria, Las Palmas, Spain
Research Institute of Biomedical and Health Sciences, Instituto Universitario de Investigaciones Biomédicas y Sanitarias, Las Palmas, Spain

Miriam González-Izal and Mikel Izquierdo
Department of Health Sciences, Public University of Navarra, Tudela, Spain

Alan J. Richardson, Rebecca L. Relf and Arron Saunders
Environmental Extremes Lab, Centre for Sport and Exercise Science and Medicine, University of Brighton, Eastbourne, UK

Olivier Girard
Athlete Health and Performance Research Center, Aspetar Orthopaedic and Sports Medicine Hospital, Doha, Qatar
Faculty of Biology and Medicine, Institute of Sport Sciences, University of Lausanne, Lausanne, Switzerland

Sarah J. Willis, Laurent Alvarez, Fabio Borrani, Davide Malatesta and Grégoire P. Millet
Faculty of Biology and Medicine, Institute of Sport Sciences, University of Lausanne, Lausanne, Switzerland

Index

www.ingramcontent.com/pod-product-compliance
Lightning Source LLC
LaVergne TN
LVHW082149200926
848484LV00008B/2128